Basic Clinical Radiobiology

FOURTH EDITION

Edited by

Michael Joiner
Professor of Radiobiology
Wayne State University
USA

Albert van der Kogel
Professor of Radiobiology
Radboud University Nijmegen Medical Centre
The Netherlands

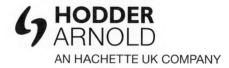
HODDER
ARNOLD
AN HACHETTE UK COMPANY

First published in Great Britain in 1993 by Edward Arnold.
Second edition published in Great Britain in 1997 by Arnold.
Third edition published in Great Britain in 2002 by Hodder Arnold.
This fourth edition published in Great Britain in 2009 by Hodder Arnold,
an imprint of Hodder Education, an Hachette UK Company, 338 Euston Road, London NW1 3BH.

http://www.hoddereducation.com

Whilst the advice and information in this book are believed to be true and accurate at the date of
going to press, neither the author[s] nor the publisher can accept any legal responsibility or liability
for any errors or omissions that may be made. In particular (but without limiting the generality of
the preceding disclaimer) every effort has been made to check drug dosages; however it is still
possible that errors have been missed. Furthermore, dosage schedules are constantly being revised
and new side-effects recognized. For these reasons the reader is strongly urged to consult the drug
companies' printed instructions before administering any of the drugs recommended in this book.

British Library Cataloguing in Publication Data
A catalogue record for this book is available from the British Library

Library of Congress Cataloging-in-Publication Data
A catalog record for this book is available from the Library of Congress

ISBN   978 0 340 929 667

3 4 5 6 7 8 9 10

Commissioning Editor: Gavin Jamieson
Project Editor: Francesca Naish
Production Controller: Joanna Walker
Cover Designer: Helen Townson
Indexer: Laurence Erington

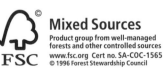

Typeset in 10/12 pt Minion by Macmillan Publishing Solutions
Printed and bound in the UK by MPG Books

What do you think about this book? Or any other Hodder Arnold title?
Please visit our website: www.hoddereducation.com

Contents

Contributors

M Baumann
Department of Radiation Oncology and OncoRay Center
for Radiation Research in Oncology
Medical Faculty and University Hospital Carl Gustav
Carus
Technical University Dresden
Dresden
Germany

AC Begg
Division of Experimental Therapy
Netherlands Cancer Institute
Amsterdam
The Netherlands

SM Bentzen
Departments of Human Oncology, Medical Physics,
Biostatistics and Medical Informatics
University of Wisconsin School of Medicine and Public
Health
Madison, Wisconsin
USA

W Dörr
Department of Radiation Oncology
Medical Faculty and University Hospital Carl Gustav
Carus
Technical University Dresden
Dresden
Germany

V Grégoire
Department of Radiation Oncology and Centre for
Molecular Imaging and Experimental Radiotherapy
Université Catholique de Louvain, St. Luc University
Hospital
Brussels
Belgium

K Haustermans
Department of Radiation Oncology, Leuven Cancer
Institute
University Hospital Gasthuisberg
Leuven
Belgium

MR Horsman
Department of Experimental Clinical
Oncology
Aarhus University Hospital
Aarhus
Denmark

MC Joiner
Department of Radiation Oncology and Karmanos
Cancer Institute
Wayne State University School of
Medicine
Detroit, Michigan
USA

M Koritzinsky
Department of Radiation Oncology, University of
Toronto
Princess Margaret Hospital/Ontario Cancer Institute,
University Health Network
Toronto, Ontario
Canada

J Lee
Centre for Molecular Imaging and Experimental
Radiotherapy
Université Catholique de Louvain, St. Luc University
Hospital
Brussels
Belgium

J Overgaard
Department of Experimental Clinical Oncology
Aarhus University Hospital
Aarhus
Denmark

GG Steel
Institute of Cancer Research
Royal Marsden Hospital
Sutton, Surrey
UK

FA Stewart
Division of Experimental Therapy
Netherlands Cancer Institute
Amsterdam
The Netherlands

KR Trott
Department of Oncology
University College
London
UK

AJ van der Kogel
Department of Radiation Oncology
Radboud University Nijmegen Medical
Centre
Nijmegen
The Netherlands

BG Wouters
Departments of Radiation Oncology and Medical
Biophysics, University of Toronto
Princess Margaret Hospital/Ontario Cancer Institute,
University Health Network
Toronto, Ontario
Canada

D Zips
Department of Radiation Oncology
Medical Faculty and University Hospital Carl Gustav
Carus
Technical University Dresden
Dresden
Germany

Preface

This is the fourth edition of *Basic Clinical Radiobiology*, which was first published in 1993. It is a teaching book which is directed at an international audience but has arisen and evolved largely from courses organized by the European Society for Therapeutic Radiology and Oncology (ESTRO) for students of radiotherapy, radiation physics and radiobiology. In this new edition, as previously, we have included as contributors many of the radiation oncologists and biologists from both Europe and North America who currently teach this material for those ESTRO courses that continue to take place now typically twice a year and attract students from all over the world.

The first three editions of this book were under the editorship of Gordon Steel, but in this new edition Gordon has passed the editing pen to his two senior co-teachers, who have both been involved in these international courses since their inception in 1990. We acknowledge and thank Gordon for his tremendous effort and expert stewardship over the first three editions, and we hope very much that, in this new edition, we have managed to maintain the high standard of content, presentation and accessibility that has always been an integral part of this project.

This new edition is the most extensive revision to *Basic Clinical Radiobiology* yet. New chapters have been added which review image-guided radiotherapy, biological response modifiers, the tumour microenvironment, and radiation-induced second cancers. Substantial additions have been made to the description of the pathogenesis of normal tissue side-effects, the molecular description of the DNA damage response, cell death, and molecular targeting and individualization. With clinical trials demonstrating that tumour-targeted molecules can improve the therapeutic ratio, these topics have become important in teaching radiation biology and questions on these subject areas are appearing in board examinations for radiation oncology and medical physics.

At the same time, we continue to provide in-depth coverage of the more established subjects of dose responses and fractionation including the linear-quadratic framework, time factors and dose-rate effects, volume effects and retreatment tolerance, tumour radiobiology, combined radiotherapy and chemotherapy, and the oxygen effect. Also well-covered are high-linear energy transfer (LET) effects, but now with additional presentation of the status of clinical usage of light ions and protons, which centres are starting to adopt in their radiotherapy practices.

Thus, with including the essential core material while adequately covering the rapidly expanding field of molecular radiobiology, both necessary for a full understanding of clinical radiotherapy, this new edition of the book is larger than the previous editions. Yet, we believe we have achieved the same high level of accessibility and ease of reading that have always been the hallmarks of this book and which we hope will once again make *Basic Clinical Radiobiology* a valuable companion to all people involved in radiation oncology, whatever their contribution and level of expertise.

Michael Joiner
Albert van der Kogel

Introduction: the significance of radiobiology and radiotherapy for cancer treatment

MICHAEL C. JOINER, ALBERT J. VAN DER KOGEL AND G. GORDON STEEL

1.1 THE ROLE OF RADIOTHERAPY IN THE MANAGEMENT OF CANCER

Radiotherapy has consistently remained one of the two most effective treatments for cancer, with more than half of all patients estimated to receive radiotherapy at some point during their management (Tobias, 1996; Delancy *et al.*, 2005). Surgery, which has the longer history, is also the primary form of treatment in many tumour types and leads to good therapeutic results in a range of early non-metastatic tumours. Radiotherapy is a good alternative to surgery for the long-term control of many tumours of the head and neck, lung, cervix, bladder, prostate and skin, in which it often achieves a reasonable probability of tumour control with good cosmetic results. In addition to these examples of the curative role of radiation therapy, many patients gain valuable palliation by radiation. Chemotherapy is the third most important treatment modality at the present time. Following the early use of nitrogen mustard during the 1920s it has emerged to the point where a large choice of drugs is available for the management of cancer, although no more than 10–20 agents are in common use. Many patients receive chemotherapy at some point in their management and useful symptom relief and disease arrest are often obtained. Last, targeted agents (also called small or smart molecules) are being introduced into clinical practice, and some [e.g. epithelial growth factor receptor (EGFR) inhibitors] have been associated with radiotherapy and shown promising clinical results.

Table 1.1, adapted from Delaney *et al.* (2005), illustrates the proportions of patients who should optimally receive radiotherapy for cancers in different sites, derived from evidence-based guidelines. The following is a brief outline exampling the role of radiotherapy in different disease sites:

- *Breast* – early breast cancers, not known to have metastasized, are usually treated by surgery (e.g. lumpectomy or tumourectomy) and this has a tumour control rate in the region of 50–70 per cent. Postoperative radiotherapy given to the breast and regional lymph nodes increases control by up to 20 per cent and improves long-term survival. Hormonal therapy and chemotherapy also have significant impact on patient survival. In patients who have evidence

Table 1.1 Optimal radiotherapy utilization rate by cancer type*

Tumour type	Proportion of all cancers (%)	Proportion of patients receiving radiotherapy (%)	Patients receiving radiotherapy (% of all cancers)
Breast	13	83	10.8
Lung	10	76	7.6
Melanoma	11	23	2.5
Prostate	12	60	7.2
Gynaecological	5	35	1.8
Colon	9	14	1.3
Rectum	5	61	3.1
Head and neck	4	78	3.1
Gall bladder	1	13	0.1
Liver	1	0	0.0
Oesophageal	1	80	0.8
Stomach	2	68	1.4
Pancreas	2	57	1.1
Lymphoma	4	65	2.6
Leukaemia	3	4	0.1
Myeloma	1	38	0.4
Central nervous system	2	92	1.8
Renal	3	27	0.8
Bladder	3	58	1.7
Testis	1	49	0.5
Thyroid	1	10	0.1
Unknown primary	4	61	2.4
Other	2	50	1.0
Total	100	–	52.3

*From Delaney *et al.* (2005), with permission.

of metastatic spread at the time of diagnosis the outlook is poor.

- *Lung* – most locally advanced lung tumours are inoperable and, in these, the 5-year survival rate for radiotherapy combined with chemotherapy is in the region of 5 per cent. However, studies have shown high local tumour control after high-dose radiotherapy for early disease in patients not suitable for surgery.
- *Prostate* – surgery and radiotherapy have a similar level of effectiveness, with excellent long-term outcome. Early-stage disease is often treated with radiotherapy alone, either by external beam or by brachytherapy, with 5-year disease-specific control rates more than 95 per cent. Locally, more advanced tumours may require an association between anti-hormonal

treatment and external radiotherapy. Chemotherapy makes a limited contribution to local tumour control.

- *Cervix* – disease that has developed beyond the *in situ* stage is often treated by a combination of intracavitary and external-beam radiotherapy; in more advanced stages radiotherapy is frequently combined with chemotherapy. The control rate varies widely with the stage of the disease, from around 70 per cent in stage I to perhaps 7 per cent in stage IV.
- *Head and neck* – early-stage disease can be cured with either surgery or radiotherapy (external-beam and/or brachytherapy). For more advanced disease, radiotherapy is typically delivered with alternative fractionation (e.g. accelerated treatment or hyperfractionation), or with concomitant

chemoradiotherapy. More recently concomitant association of EGFR inhibitors (e.g. cetuximab) and radiotherapy has also been validated. Post-operative radiotherapy or concomitant chemo-radiotherapy is also often used after primary surgery for locally advanced diseases.

- *Lymphoma* – in early-disease Hodgkin's lymphoma, radiotherapy alone achieves a control rate of around 80–90 per cent, but now is more often associated with chemotherapy allowing for smaller irradiated volumes and lower doses of radiation.
- *Bladder* – the success of surgery or radiotherapy varies widely with stage of the disease; both approaches give 5-year survival rates in excess of 50 per cent. For early-stage bladder cancer, organ-preserving (partial) bladder irradiation is a good alternative to surgery with comparable local control rates.
- *Other tumour sites* – radiotherapy alone or combined with chemotherapy is also frequently used as a postoperative modality in brain tumours, pancreatic tumours or sarcomas, or as a preoperative modality in oesophageal, rectal or gastric tumours.

Substantial numbers of patients with common cancers achieve long-term tumour control largely by the use of radiation therapy. Informed debate on the funding of national cancer programmes requires data on the relative roles of the main treatment modalities. Broad estimates by DeVita *et al.* (1979) and Souhami and Tobias (1986) suggested that local treatment, which includes surgery and/or radiotherapy, could be expected to be successful in approximately 40 per cent of these cases; in perhaps 15 per cent of all cancers radiotherapy would be the principal form of treatment. In contrast, many patients do receive chemotherapy but their contribution to the overall cure rate of cancer may be only around 2 per cent, with some prolongation of life in perhaps another 10 per cent. This is because the diseases in which chemotherapy alone does well are rare. If these figures are correct, it may be that around seven times as many patients currently are cured by radiotherapy as by chemotherapy. This is not to undervalue the important benefits of chemotherapy in a number of chemosensitive diseases and as an adjuvant treatment, but to stress the greater role of radiotherapy as a curative agent (Tubiana, 1992).

Considerable efforts are being devoted at the present time to the improvement of radiotherapy and chemotherapy. Wide publicity is given to the newer areas of drug development such as lymphokines, growth factors, anti-oncogenes and gene therapy. But if we were to imagine aiming to increase the cure rate of cancer by, say, 2 per cent, it would seem on a realistic estimation that this would be more likely to be achieved by increasing the results of radiotherapy from say 15 per cent to 17 per cent than by doubling the results achieved by chemotherapy.

There are four main ways in which such an improvement in radiotherapy might be obtained:

1. by raising the standards of radiation dose prescription and delivery to those currently in use in the best radiotherapy centres;
2. by improving radiation dose distributions beyond those that have been conventionally achieved, either using techniques of conformal radiotherapy and intensity modulation with photons or by the use of proton or carbon-ion beams;
3. by integrating image-guidance into daily treatment delivery;
4. by exploiting radiobiological initiatives.

The proportion of radiotherapists world-wide who work in academic centres is probably less than 5 per cent. They are the clinicians who may have access to new treatment technology, for example ion beam therapy and image guidance, or to new radiosensitizers or to new agents for targeted therapy. Chapters of this book allude to these exciting developments which may well have a significant impact on treatment success in the future. However, it should not be thought that the improvement of radiation therapy lies exclusively with clinical research in the specialist academic centres. It has widely been recognized that by far the most effective way of improving cure rates on a national or international scale is by quality assurance in the prescription and delivery of radiation treatment. Chapters 8–10 of this book deal with the principles on which fractionation schedules should be optimized, including how to respond to unavoidable gaps in treatment. For many radiotherapists this will be the most important part of this book, for even in the smallest department it is possible, even without access to greatly increased funding, to move closer to optimum fractionation practices.

1.2 THE ROLE OF RADIATION BIOLOGY

Experimental and theoretical studies in radiation biology contribute to the development of radiotherapy at three different levels, moving in turn from the most general to the more specific:

- *Ideas* – providing a conceptual basis for radiotherapy, identifying mechanisms and processes that underlie the response of tumours and normal tissues to irradiation and which help to explain observed phenomena. Examples are knowledge about hypoxia, reoxygenation, tumour cell repopulation or mechanisms of repair of DNA damage.
- *Treatment strategy* – development of specific new approaches in radiotherapy. Examples are hypoxic cell sensitizers, targeted agents, high-linear energy transfer (LET) radiotherapy, accelerated radiotherapy and hyperfractionation.
- *Protocols* – advice on the choice of schedules for clinical radiotherapy. For example, conversion formulae for changes in fractionation or dose rate, or advice on whether to use chemotherapy concurrently or sequentially with radiation. We may also include under this heading methods for predicting the best treatment for the individual patient (individualized radiotherapy).

There is no doubt that radiobiology has been very fruitful in the generation of new ideas and in the identification of potentially exploitable mechanisms. A variety of new treatment strategies have been produced but, unfortunately, few of these have so far led to demonstrable clinical gains. In regard to the third of the levels listed above, the newer conversion formulae based on the linear-quadratic (LQ) equation seem to be successful. However, beyond this, the ability of laboratory science to guide the radiotherapist in the choice of specific protocols is limited by the inadequacy of the theoretical and experimental models: it will always be necessary to rely on clinical trials for the final choice of a protocol.

1.3 THE TIME-SCALE OF EFFECTS IN RADIATION BIOLOGY

Irradiation of any biological system generates a succession of processes that differ enormously in time-scale. This is illustrated in Fig. 1.1 in which these processes are divided into three phases (Boag, 1975), described below.

Physical phase

The physical phase consists of interactions between charged particles and the atoms of which the tissue is composed. A high-speed electron takes about 10^{-18}s to traverse the DNA molecule and about 10^{-14}s to pass across a mammalian cell. As it does so it interacts mainly with orbital electrons, ejecting

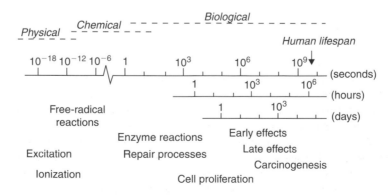

Figure 1.1 Time-scale of the effects of radiation exposure on biological systems.

some of them from atoms (ionization) and raising others to higher energy levels within an atom or molecule (excitation). If sufficiently energetic, these secondary electrons may excite or ionize other atoms near which they pass, giving rise to a cascade of ionization events. For 1 Gy of absorbed radiation dose, there are in excess of 10^5 ionizations within the volume of every cell of diameter 10 μm.

Chemical phase

The chemical phase describes the period in which these damaged atoms and molecules react with other cellular components in rapid chemical reactions. Ionization and excitation lead to the breakage of chemical bonds and the formation of broken molecules known as 'free radicals'. These are highly reactive and they engage in a succession of reactions that lead eventually to the restoration of electronic charge equilibrium. Free-radical reactions are complete within approximately 1 ms of radiation exposure. An important characteristic of the chemical phase is the competition between scavenging reactions, for example with sulphydryl compounds that inactivate the free radicals, and fixation reactions that lead to stable chemical changes in biologically important molecules.

Biological phase

The biological phase includes all subsequent processes. These begin with enzymatic reactions that act on the residual chemical damage. The vast majority of lesions, for example in DNA, are successfully repaired. Some rare lesions fail to repair and it is these that lead eventually to cell death. Cells take time to die; indeed after small doses of radiation they may undergo a number of mitotic divisions before dying. It is the killing of stem cells and the subsequent loss of the cells that they would have given rise to that causes the early manifestations of normal-tissue damage during the first weeks and months after radiation exposure. Examples are breakdown of the skin or mucosa, denudation of the intestine and haemopoietic damage (see Chapter 13, Section 13.2). A secondary effect of cell killing is compensatory cell proliferation, which occurs both in normal tissues and in tumours. At later times after

the irradiation of normal tissues the so-called 'late reactions' appear. These include fibrosis and telangiectasia of the skin, spinal cord damage and blood vessel damage. An even later manifestation of radiation damage is the appearance of second tumours (i.e. radiation carcinogenesis). The time-scale of the observable effects of ionizing radiation may thus extend up to many years after exposure.

1.4 RESPONSE OF NORMAL AND MALIGNANT TISSUES TO RADIATION EXPOSURE

Much of the text of this book will focus on the effects of radiation exposure that become apparent to the clinician or the patient during the weeks, months and years after radiotherapy. These effects are seen both in the tumour and in the normal tissues that are unavoidably included within the treatment plan and exposed to radiation. The primary tasks of radiation biology, as applied to radiotherapy, are to explain observed phenomena, and to suggest improvements to existing therapies (as outlined in Section 1.2).

The response of a tumour is seen by *regression*, often followed by *regrowth* (or recurrence), but perhaps with failure to regrow during the normal lifespan of the patient (which we term cure or, more correctly, *local control*). These italicized terms describe the tumour responses that we seek to understand. The cellular basis of tumour response, including tumour control, is dealt with in Chapter 7.

The responses of normal tissues to therapeutic radiation exposure range from those that cause mild discomfort to others that are life-threatening. The speed at which a response develops varies widely from one tissue to another and often depends on the dose of radiation that the tissue receives. Generally speaking, the haemopoietic and epithelial tissues manifest radiation damage within weeks of radiation exposure, while damage to connective tissues becomes important at later times. A major development in the radiobiology of normal tissues during the 1980s was the realization that early and late normal-tissue responses are differently modified by a change in dose fractionation and this gave rise to the current interest in hyperfractionation (see Chapter 10, Section 10.3).

The first task of a radiobiologist is to measure a tissue response accurately and reliably. The term assay is used to describe such a system of measurement. Assays for tumour response are described in Chapter 7, Section 7.2. For normal tissues, the following three general types of assay are available:

- *Scoring of gross tissue effects* – it is possible to grade the severity of damage to a tissue using an arbitrary scale as is done, for example, in Figs 13.7 and 13.9. In superficial tissues this approach has been remarkably successful in allowing isoeffect relationships to be determined.
- *Assays of tissue function* – for certain tissues, functional assays are available that allow radiation effects to be documented. Examples are the use of breathing rate as a measure of lung function in mice, ethylenediaminetetraacetic acid (EDTA) clearance as a measure of kidney damage (Fig. 8.4), or blood counts as an indicator of bone marrow function.
- *Clonogenic assays* – in some tumours and some normal tissues it has been possible to develop methods by which the colony of cells that derive

from a single irradiated cell can be observed. In tumours this is particularly important because of the fact that regrowth of a tumour after sub-curative treatment is caused by the proliferation of a small number of tumour cells that retain colony-forming ability. This important area of radiation biology is introduced in Chapter 4.

1.5 RESPONSE CURVES, DOSE–RESPONSE CURVES AND ISOEFFECT RELATIONSHIPS

The damage that is observed in an irradiated tissue increases, reaches a peak, and then may decline (Fig. 1.2a). How should we quantify the magnitude of this response? We could use the measured response at some chosen time after irradiation, such as the time of maximum response, but the timing of the peak may change with radiation dose and this would lead to some uncertainty in the interpretation of the results. A common method is to calculate the cumulative response by integrating this curve from left to right (Fig. 1.2b). Some normal tissue

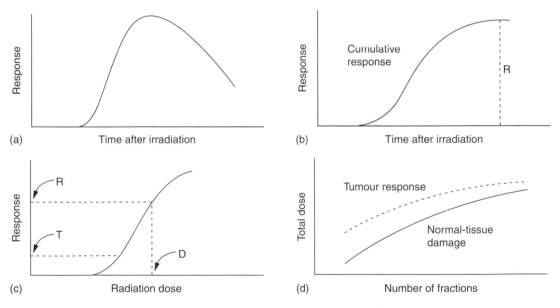

Figure 1.2 Four types of chart leading to the construction of an isoeffect plot. (a) Time-course of development of radiation damage in a normal tissue. (b) The cumulative response. (c) A dose–response relationship, constructed by measuring the response (*R*) for various radiation doses (*D*); acceptable clinical tolerance (*T*) of most tissues is towards the low end of the dose–response relationship. (d) Isoeffect plot for a fixed level of normal-tissue damage (also a similar plot for tumour response).

responses give a cumulative curve that rises to a plateau, and the height of the plateau is a good measure of the total effect of that dose of radiation on the tissue. Other normal-tissue responses, in particular the late responses seen in connective and vascular tissues, are progressive and the cumulative response curve will continue to rise (Figs 13.7 and 13.8). The quantification of clinical normal-tissue reactions is dealt with in Chapter 13, Section 13.4.

The next stage in a study of the radiation response of a tissue will be to vary the radiation dose and thus to investigate the dose–response relationship (Fig. 1.2c). Many examples of such curves are given throughout this book, for example Figs 5.6, 14.3 and 19.8. Cell survival curves (see Chapter 4, Section 4.3) are further examples of dose–response curves that are widely used in radiobiology. The position of the curve on the dose scale indicates the sensitivity of the tissue to radiation; its steepness also gives a direct indication of the change in response that will accompany an increase or decrease in radiation dose. These aspects of dose–response curves are dealt with in detail in Chapter 5.

The foregoing paragraphs have, for simplicity, referred to 'dose' as though we are concerned only with single radiation exposures. It is a well-established fact in radiation oncology that multiple radiation doses given over a period of a few weeks give a better curative response than can be achieved with a single dose. Diagrams similar to Fig. 1.2a–c can also be constructed for fractionated radiation treatment, although the results are easiest to interpret when the fractions are given over a time that is short compared with the time-scale of development of the response. If we change the schedule of dose fractionation, for example by giving a different number of fractions, changing the fraction size or changing radiation dose rate, we can then investigate the therapeutic effect in terms of an isoeffect plot (Fig. 1.2d). Experimentally this is done by performing multiple studies at different doses for each chosen schedule and calculating a dose–response curve. We then select some particular level of effect (R in Fig. 1.2c) and read off the total radiation dose that gives this effect. For effects on normal tissues the isoeffect will often be some upper limit of tolerance of the tissue, perhaps expressed as a probability of tissue failure (see Chapter 5, Section 5.1, and Chapter 14, Section 14.2) and perhaps choosing a

lower level of effect (T in Fig. 1.2c) will be more appropriate. The isoeffect plot shows how the total radiation dose for the chosen level of effect varies with dose schedule: examples are given in Figs 8.2 and 10.3, and recommendations for tolerance calculations are set out in Chapters 8 and 9. The dashed line in Fig. 1.2d illustrates how therapeutic conclusions may be drawn from isoeffect curves. If the curve for tumour response is flatter than for normal-tissue tolerance, then there is a therapeutic advantage in using a large number of fractions: a tolerance dose given using a small number of fractions will be far short of the tumour-effective dose, whereas for large fraction numbers it may be closer to an effective dose.

1.6 THE CONCEPT OF THERAPEUTIC INDEX

Any discussion of the possible benefit of a change in treatment strategy must always consider simultaneously the effects on tumour response and on normal-tissue damage. A wide range of factors enter into this assessment. In the clinic, in addition to quantifiable aspects of tumour response and toxicity, there may be a range of poorly quantifiable factors such as new forms of toxicity or risks to the patient, or practicality and convenience to hospital staff; there are also cost implications. These must all be balanced in the clinical setting. The role of radiation biology is to address the quantifiable biological aspects of a change in treatment.

In the research setting, this can be done by considering dose–response curves. As radiation dose is increased, there will be a tendency for tumour response to increase, and the same is also true of damage to normal tissues. If, for example, we measure tumour response by determining the proportion of tumours that are controlled, then we expect a sigmoid relationship to dose (for fractionated radiation treatment we could consider the total dose or any other measure of treatment intensity). This is illustrated in the upper part of Fig. 1.3. If we quantify damage to normal tissues in some way for the same treatment schedule, there will also be a rising curve of toxicity (lower panel). The shape of this curve is unlikely to be the same as that for tumour response and we probably will not wish to determine more

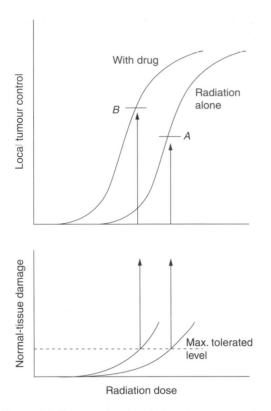

Figure 1.3 The procedure by which an improvement in therapeutic index might be identified, as a result of adding chemotherapy to radiotherapy (see text, Section 1.6).

than the initial part of this curve since a high frequency of severe damage is unacceptable. By analogy with what must be done in the clinic, we can then fix a notional upper limit of tolerance (see Chapter 14, Section 14.2). This fixes, for that treatment schedule, the upper limit of radiation dose that can be tolerated, for which the tumour response is indicated by the point in Fig. 1.3 labelled *A*.

Consider now the effect of adding treatment with a cytotoxic drug. We plan that this will increase the tumour response for any radiation dose and this will be seen as a movement to the left of the curve for tumour control (Fig. 1.3). However, there will probably also be an increase in damage to normal tissues which again will consist of a leftward movement of the toxicity curve. The relative displacement of the curves for the tumour and normal tissues will usually be different and this fact makes the amount of benefit from the chemotherapy very difficult to assess. How do we know whether there has been a real therapeutic

gain? For studies on laboratory animals there is a straightforward way of asking whether the combined treatment is better than radiation alone: for the same tolerance level of normal-tissue damage (the broken line) the maximum radiation dose (with drug) will be lower and the corresponding level of tumour control is indicated by point *B* in Fig. 1.3. If *B* is higher than *A* then the combination is better than radiation alone and represents a therapeutic gain, because it gives a greater level of tumour control for the same level of morbidity.

This example illustrates the radiobiological concept of therapeutic index: it is the tumour response for a fixed level of normal-tissue damage (see Chapter 5, Section 5.6). The term therapeutic window describes the (possible) difference between the tumour control dose and the tolerance dose. The concept can, in principle, be applied to any therapeutic situation or to any appropriate measures of tumour response or toxicity. Its application in the clinic is, however, not a straightforward matter, as indicated in Chapter 18, Section 18.1. Therapeutic index also carries the notion of 'cost–benefit' analysis. It is impossible to reliably discuss the potential benefit of a new treatment without reference to its effect on therapeutic index.

1.7 THE IMPORTANCE OF RADIATION BIOLOGY FOR THE FUTURE DEVELOPMENT OF RADIOTHERAPY

Radiation oncology, more than any of the other modalities for cancer treatment, is, to a large extent, a technical discipline. Improvements in the treatment of cancer with radiotherapy over recent decades have resulted mainly from improvements in technology, combining new methods of precision in dose delivery with new imaging tools. A major recent development has been the introduction of intensity modulation in combination with various functional imaging modalities such as functional magnetic resonance imaging (fMRI) and positron emission tomography(PET)/computed tomography (CT). This has led to new concepts such as 'biological target volume', 'dose painting' and 'theragnostic imaging' (see Chapter 20). These developments will undoubtedly lead to further improvements in tumour control rates and reductions in morbidity.

In parallel with these technological advances, new developments have taken place in radiobiology, encompassing the understanding of cancer biology in general, and the radiation response in particular. These fundamental and preclinical research efforts in biology hold great promise, just as the technical innovations, for improving the radiotherapy of cancer. It is even likely that the expected improvements from technical innovations will reach a limit, and the next breakthroughs will come from biological innovations, such as the application of molecularly targeted drugs (see Chapters 21 and 22) in combination with high-precision methods to deliver radiation.

It is interesting to note that the recent rapid progress in knowledge of the biology of cancer is itself also partly due to technological innovations, especially in high-throughput methods to study the genetics of the whole cell. There are now several methods to look at the genes (DNA) and expression of those genes (RNA and protein) in high numbers (tens of thousands) all at once. The trend here is away from the study of single genes or parameters towards genome-wide studies. The many different potential causes of failure, or of severe normal-tissue reactions, necessitates such multiparameter/multigene studies. Methods to selectively manipulate gene expression represent another revolution in biology, allowing one to quickly assess the importance of any given gene by reducing or eliminating its expression (RNA interference and microRNA methods). Radiation biologists are now exploiting these techniques to better understand the molecular pathways that determine how cells respond to damage. This should lead to identification not only of new targets, but of targets that are specifically deregulated in tumours, providing the all-important tumour specificity of therapy. This should also lead to the development of more robust and accurate predictors of which tumours or normal tissues will respond well to standard radiotherapy and which will not, which could significantly improve individualized radiotherapy (see Chapter 23).

Over the last decade we have seen a change from 'classic radiobiology', which has often focused on fractionation, the LQ model, and the phenomenology of repair in terms of 'sublethal' and 'potentially lethal' damage. However, fractionation remains an important core subject for the application of radiation therapy, and the development of the LQ model, together with elucidation of the importance of repopulation, has been central in understanding fractionation, leading to new and better clinical fractionation schemes and the ability to predict the response of normal tissue and tumours to non-standard schedules (see Chapters 8–12). It is of great interest to see a change developing in the established concept of high α/β values for tumours and acutely responding tissues, and low α/β values for late-responding tissues. This 'dogma' has now evolved into a more differentiated view, indicating that some tumours may have a lower α/β ratio than surrounding normal tissues, requiring a very different approach to the design of treatment schedules. This new knowledge is now being applied to the design of hypofractionated schedules, such as for the treatment of prostate tumours, which is a dramatic deviation from clinical practice in the last decades.

In a similar manner, simple descriptions of repair and recovery have been supplemented by increasing knowledge and understanding of the molecular pathways involved in various types of repair, including those for base damage, single-strand DNA breaks and double-strand breaks. This is leading to new ways to target deregulated repair pathways, with the promise of improving radiotherapy (see Chapter 23). In recent years, a link has been established between the EGFR pathway and DNA double-strand break repair. This is highly relevant to radiotherapy as blocking the EGFR has been shown to improve the effect of radiotherapy in head and neck cancer (see Chapter 21).

Hypoxia has always been a focus in radiation research, given its large influence on radiosensitivity (see Chapter 15). However, here again, phenomenology has now been replaced by a huge plethora of molecular studies illuminating how cells respond to hypoxia of different degrees and fluctuating over time (see Chapter 16). Hypoxia is also an important issue for other disciplines apart from cancer, and so an enormous amount of fundamental information has been contributed by these different areas, which radiation biologists can also exploit. This has led to several novel ways to either attack or exploit tumour hypoxia clinically (see Chapter 17).

Indirectly related to hypoxia is the tumour vasculature and blood supply, and this component of the tumour microenvironment has been a target for therapy for many years now. One approach is to block one of the most important growth factors involved in new vessel formation and the maintenance of blood vessels, vascular endothelial growth factor (VEGF). Another approach is to modify the function of mature blood vessels. Since radiation therapy is a balancing act between damage to tumours and normal tissues, sparing the latter has always attracted the attention of radiation scientists. The trends in radiation studies of normal tissues, as above, are to elucidate the molecular pathways determining response, and by an increased understanding to both predict and ameliorate severe side-effects (see Chapter 22).

Radiation oncology has always been at the interface of physics, biology and medicine, and, with new developments in the technology of high-precision beam delivery with functional and molecular imaging, these are exciting times. Clearly, today's radiation oncologists and clinical physicists need to obtain a solid understanding of both radiation biology and the new developments in molecular radiation oncology: that is the purpose of this book.

Key points

1. Radiotherapy is a very important curative and palliative modality in the treatment of cancer, with more than half of all patients estimated to receive radiotherapy at some point during their management.
2. The effects of radiation on mammalian tissues should be viewed as a succession of processes extending from microseconds to months and years after exposure. In choosing one endpoint of effect, it is important not to overlook the rest of this process.
3. Therapeutic index is always 'the name of the game' in curative cancer therapy.
4. Significant gains are still to be made by the optimization of biological and physical factors, particularly in the domain of 'biologically based treatment planning' and image-guided therapy.
5. Further gains will also accrue from the increasing knowledge of the molecular mechanisms underlying radiation responses, enabling tumour-specific targeting of radiosensitization.

■ BIBLIOGRAPHY

Boag JW (1975). The time scale in radiobiology. 12th Failla memorial lecture. In: Nygaard OF, Adler HI, Sinclair WK (eds) *Radiation research. Proceedings of the 5th International Congress of Radiation Research.* New York: Academic Press, 9–29.

Delaney G, Jacob S, Featherstone C, Barton M (2005). The role of radiotherapy in cancer treatment: estimating optimal utilization from a review of evidence-based clinical guidelines. *Cancer* **104:** 1129–37.

DeVita VT, Oliverio VT, Muggia FM *et al.* (1979). The drug development and clinical trials programs of the division of cancer treatment, National Cancer Institute. *Cancer Clin Trials* **2:** 195–216.

Souhami RL, Tobias JS (1986). *Cancer and its management.* Oxford: Blackwell Scientific.

Tobias JS (1996). The role of radiotherapy in the management of cancer – an overview. *Ann Acad Med Singapore* **25:** 371–9.

Tubiana M (1992). The role of local treatment in the cure of cancer. *Eur J Cancer* **28A:** 2061–9.

■ FURTHER READING

Bentzen SM, Thames HD (1995). A 100-year Nordic perspective on the dose-time problem in radiobiology. *Acta Oncol* **34:** 1031–40.

Feinendegen L, Hahnfeldt P, Schadt EE, Stumpf M, Voit EO (2008). Systems biology and its potential role in radiobiology. *Radiat Environ Biophys* **47:** 5–23.

Salminen E, Izewska J, Andreo P (2005). IAEA's role in the global management of cancer – focus on upgrading radiotherapy services. *Acta Oncol* **44:** 816–24.

Willers H, Beck-Bornholdt HP (1996). Origins of radiotherapy and radiobiology: separation of the influence of dose per fraction and overall treatment time on normal tissue damage by Reisner and Miescher in the 1930s. *Radiother Oncol* **38:** 171–3.

Irradiation-induced damage and the DNA damage response

BRADLY G. WOUTERS AND ADRIAN C. BEGG

2.1 DNA DAMAGE BY IONIZING RADIATION (AND OTHER SOURCES)

Ionizing radiation (IR) consisting of electromagnetic radiation, or photons, is the type of radiation most commonly used for the treatment of patients with radiotherapy. Typical energies of the photons produced by 4–25 MV linear accelerators found in radiotherapy departments range from less than 100 keV to several MeV (the maximum energy of the machine being used). From its name, the principal damaging effects of this type of radiation arise from its ability to ionize, or eject electrons, from molecules within cells. Almost all the photons produced by linear accelerators have sufficient energy to cause such ionizations. Most biological damage, however, is done by the ejected electrons themselves, which go on to cause further ionizations in molecules they collide with, progressively slowing down as they go. At the end of electron tracks, interactions with other molecules become more frequent, giving rise to clusters of ionizations (Goodhead, 2006). The pattern and density of ionizations and their relationship with the size of the DNA double helix is shown in Fig. 2.1. The clusters are such that many ionizations can occur within a few base pairs of the DNA. These clusters are a unique characteristic of IR, in contrast to other forms of radiation such as UV or DNA-damaging drugs such as topoisomerase inhibitors. Only a few per cent of the damage is clustered, but when these clusters occur in DNA, the cell has particular difficulty coping with the damage.

Ionized molecules are highly reactive and undergo a rapid cascade of chemical changes, which can lead to the breaking of chemical bonds. This can disrupt the structure of macromolecules such as DNA, leading to severe consequences if not repaired adequately or in time. Ionizing radiation deposits its energy randomly, thus causing damage to all molecules in the cell. However, there are multiple copies of most molecules (e.g. water, mRNA, proteins and others) and most undergo a continuous rapid turnover, limiting the consequences of damaging just a few molecules of one type. In contrast, DNA is present in only two copies, has very limited turnover, is the largest molecule thus providing the biggest target, and is central to all cellular functions. The consequence of permanent damage to DNA can therefore be serious and often lethal for the cell.

There is also compelling experimental evidence that the DNA is the principal target for radiation-induced cell killing. Elegant experiments have been carried out irradiating individual cells with small polonium needles producing short-range α-particles (Warters and Hofer, 1977). High doses could be given to plasma membranes and cytoplasm without causing cell death. However, as soon as the needle was placed so that the nucleus received even one or two α-particles, cell death resulted. Other experiments used radioactively labelled compounds to irradiate principally the plasma membrane (^{125}I-concanavalin), or principally the DNA (^{3}H-labelled thymidine), and compared this with homogeneous cell irradiation with X-rays. Cell death closely correlated only with dose to the nucleus, and not with either the plasma membrane or the cytoplasm (Table 2.1).

Because of the importance of DNA, cells and organisms have developed a complex series of processes and pathways for ensuring that the DNA remains intact and unaltered in the face of continuous attack from within (e.g. oxidation and alkylation owing to metabolism) and from the outside (e.g. ingested chemicals, UV and ionizing radiation) (Harper and Elledge, 2007). These include different forms of DNA repair to cope with the different forms of DNA damage induced by different agents.

Specialized repair systems have therefore evolved for detecting and repairing damage to bases [base excision repair (BER)], single-strand breaks [single-strand break repair (SSBR), closely related to BER], and double-strand breaks [homologous recombination (HR) and non-homologous end-joining (NHEJ)]. All these lesions are produced by ionizing radiation, and each of these repair pathways is described in more detail in Sections 2.7 and 2.8. There are also other DNA repair pathways, such as those for correcting mismatches of bases in DNA which can occur during replication, such as mismatch repair (MMR), and for repairing bulky lesions or DNA adducts such as those formed by UV light and some drugs such as cisplatin [nucleotide excision repair (NER)]. However, neither MMR nor NER appears to be important for ionizing radiation, since cells with mutations or deletions in genes on

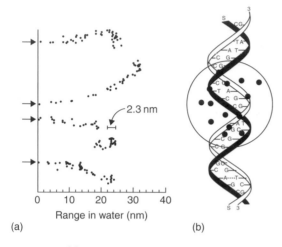

Figure 2.1 (a) Computer-simulated tracks of 1 keV electrons. Note the scale in relation to the 2.3 nm diameter of the DNA double helix (adapted from Chapman and Gillespie, 1981). (b) Illustrating the concept of a local multiply-damaged site produced by a cluster of ionizations impinging on DNA.

Table 2.1 Toxicity of radioisotopes depends upon their subcellular distribution

Radiation source/type	Radiation dose to part of the cell* (Gy)		
	Nucleus	Cytoplasm	Membranes
X-rays	3.3	3.3	3.3
^{3}H-Thymidine	3.8	0.27	0.01
^{125}I-Concanavalin	4.1	24.7	516.7

*For each of these three treatments a dose has been chosen that gives 50 per cent cell killing in Chinese hamster ovary (CHO) cells. The absorbed radiation doses to the nucleus, cytoplasm or membranes have then been calculated. ^{3}H-Thymidine is bound to DNA and ^{125}I-concanavalin to cell membranes. It is the nuclear dose that is constant and thus correlates with cell killing, not the cytoplasmic or membrane doses. From Warters et al. (1977) with permission.

these pathways are not more sensitive to IR. In contrast, mutations or deletions in BER, SSBR, HR or NHEJ genes can all, under certain circumstances, lead to increased radiosensitivity.

To give an idea of the scale of damage, 1 Gy of irradiation will cause in each cell approximately 10^5 ionizations, > 1000 damages to DNA bases, around 1000 single-strand DNA breaks (SSBs) and around 20–40 double-strand DNA breaks (DSBs). To put this into further perspective, 1 Gy will kill only about 30 per cent of cells for a typical mammalian cell line, including human. This relatively limited cytotoxicity, despite large numbers of induced lesions per cell, is the consequence of efficient DNA repair.

Cellular DNA comprises two opposing strands linked by hydrogen bonds and forming a double helical structure. Each strand is a linear chain of the four bases – adenine (A), cytosine (C), guanine (G) and thymine (T) – connected by sugar molecules and a phosphate group, the so-called sugar–phosphate backbone (Fig. 2.2). The order

of the bases is the code determining not only which protein is made but whether a gene is active (transcribed) or not. In turn, this double helix is wound at regular intervals around a complex of a specific class of proteins (histones), forming nucleosomes, resembling beads on a string. Many other proteins are also associated with the DNA; these control DNA metabolism, including transcription, replication and repair. The DNA plus its associated proteins is called chromatin. There are further levels of folding and looping, finally making up the compact structure of the chromosomes.

This structure poses various challenges to the cell for repairing DNA damage. First, specialized proteins have to be sufficiently abundant and mobile to detect damage within seconds or minutes of it occurring. Second, the chromatin usually needs to be remodelled (e.g. the structure opened up) to allow access of repair proteins (van Attikum and Gasser, 2005). This may entail removal of nucleosomes close to the break, among other changes. The correct repair, accessory and signalling proteins

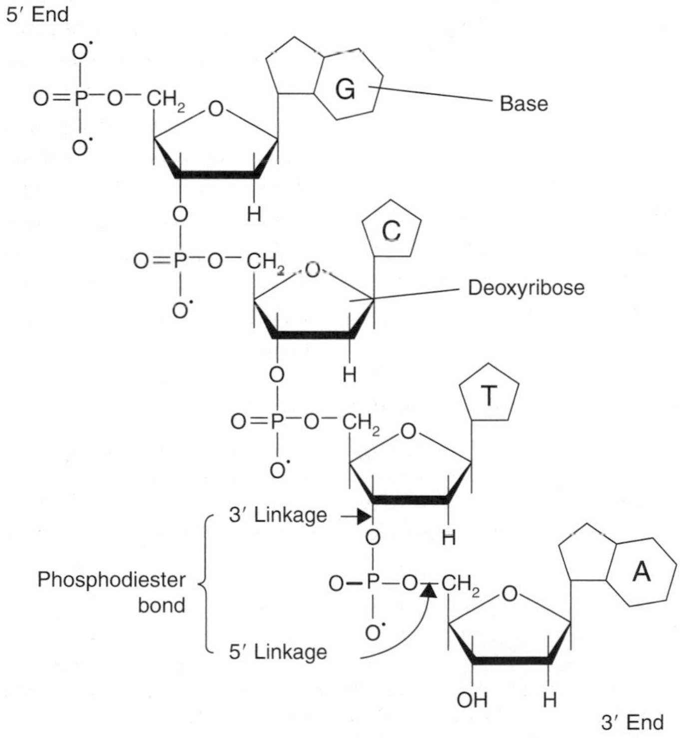

Figure 2.2 The structure of DNA, in which the four bases (G, C, T and A) are linked through sugar groups to the sugar–phosphate backbone.

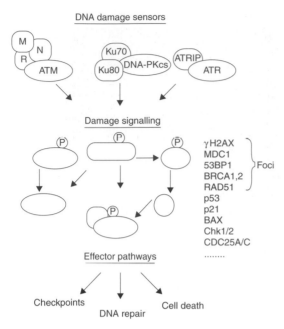

DNA damage sensors

Damage signalling

γH2AX
MDC1
53BP1 } Foci
BRCA1,2
RAD51
p53
p21
BAX
Chk1/2
CDC25A/C
....

Effector pathways

Checkpoints   Cell death
         DNA repair

Figure 2.3 The DNA damage response can be divided into sensors and effectors. The sensors consist of protein complexes which recognize DNA damage and include MRN–ATM, Ku–DNA-PKcs, and ATRIP–ATR (see text). These proteins signal to many other proteins which activate three important effector pathways: checkpoints, DNA repair and cell death. Examples of some of the proteins which signal from the sensors to the effector pathways are listed.

then need to be recruited, often mediated by histone modifications, and tightly coordinated. This includes stopping various processes such as transcription and cell-cycle progression to concentrate on repair. Repair progress needs to be continually monitored so that the chromatin will be reset to its original state after completion of repair, and then normal cellular processes resumed.

2.2 THE DNA DAMAGE RESPONSE

The DNA damage response (DDR) is a highly complex and coordinated system that determines the cellular outcome of DNA damage caused by radiation. The DDR is not a single pathway, but rather a group of highly interrelated signalling pathways, each of which controls different effects on the cell. This system can be divided into two parts, the sensors of DNA damage and the effectors of damage

response (Fig. 2.3). The sensors consist of a group of proteins that actively survey the genome for the presence of damage. These proteins then signal this damage to three main effector pathways that together determine the outcome for the cell. These effector pathways include (1) programmed cell death pathways that kill damaged cells, (2) DNA repair pathways that physically repair DNA breaks and (3) pathways that cause temporary (or permanent) blocks in the progress of cells through the cell cycle – the damage checkpoints.

2.3 SENSORS OF DAMAGE

Foci formation

The initial cellular response to DSBs is characterized by the physical recruitment of a large number of different proteins to the sites of DNA damage. This clustering or recruitment of various proteins can be visualized microscopically as small regions or speckles in the nucleus after DNA damage following staining with antibodies to these proteins (Fig. 2.4). These subnuclear regions are commonly referred to as ionizing radiation induced 'foci' (IRIF). A large number of the proteins involved in the DDR have been shown to form IRIF at or very near to the actual sites of DSBs. Consequently, it is thought that each focus represents a platform from which DNA repair and signalling to the other effectors of the DDR occurs.

One of the earliest events known to occur in the DDR is the phosphorylation of a protein called histone H2AX (Stucki and Jackson, 2006). This is a variant of histone H2A, a component of the core nucleosome structure around which DNA is packaged. H2AX is distributed throughout the entire nucleus and makes up about 10–15 per cent of total cellular histone H2A. Starting within a few minutes of DSB formation, H2AX becomes phosphorylated in a region that extends over an extensive region around the site of the unrepaired DSBs. This phosphorylated form, known as γH2AX, is necessary for the recruitment of many of the other proteins involved in the DDR and the resulting formation of IRIF. Cells that have been engineered to lack H2AX show substantial defects in IRIF formation and are radiosensitive. In recent years,

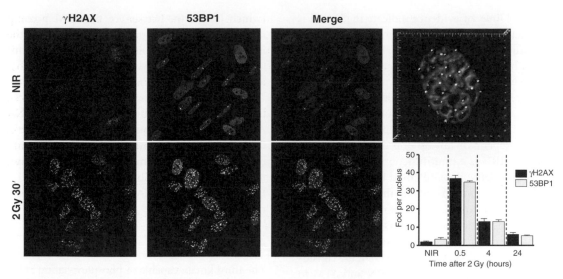

Figure 2.4 Examples of ionizing radiation-induced nuclear foci. Unirradiated and irradiated (2 Gy) cells have been fixed and stained with antibodies that recognize γH2AX and 53BP1, two proteins that interact at sites of DNA damage to form foci after induction of DNA double-strand breaks. These foci form rapidly and then resolve, consistent with the kinetics of DNA double-strand break rejoining. Photographs courtesy of Farid Jallai and Rob Bristow, Princess Margaret Hospital. See colour plate section for full colour images.

the presence of γH2AX foci, which can be detected using microscopy, has become a highly sensitive method for detecting the presence and/or repair of individual DSBs in irradiated cells.

The sensors of DSBs

Phosphorylation of H2AX at and around the sites of DSBs is one of the earliest events in the DDR, occurring within 5–30 min after DSB induction. This indicates that one or more kinases, enzymes which phosphorylate other proteins, are activated at the sites of DSBs. Three related kinases have been shown to be able to phosphorylate H2AX at sites of DSBs (Falck *et al.*, 2005).

ATM–MRN

The phosphorylation of H2AX at sites of DSBs produced by radiation occurs primarily by the ataxia telangiectasia mutated (ATM) protein. The gene that encodes this protein is mutated in the autosomal recessive syndrome ataxia telangiectasia (AT), which presents clinically as oculocutaneous telangiectasia and progressive cerebellar ataxia (O'Driscoll and Jeggo, 2006). These patients are frequently found to be highly radiosensitive and have an increased risk of developing cancer. Cells from AT patients or normal cells in which the ATM protein is inhibited are extremely radiosensitive, and are defective in H2AX phosphorylation, IRIF formation and many other aspects of the DDR.

Although there is still some debate about the exact sequence of events that occurs immediately after a DSB is created, it is now recognized that ATM requires at least one additional protein complex in order to 'find' the DSB and become activated. Recruitment of ATM to the DSB requires a protein complex known as MRN. This complex contains three proteins, MRE11, RAD50 and NBS1. The NBS1 protein is the product of the gene that is mutated in Nijmegen breakage syndrome (NBS). This syndrome is highly similar to AT and patients are also radiosensitive. Cells that lack NBS1 show similar defects in H2AX phosphorylation, IRIF formation and other aspects of the DDR. One of the key functions of NBS1 is to directly bind to ATM, and bring it to the sites of damage. Thus, when NBS1 is defective, ATM is unable to relocate to DSBs and is therefore unable to phosphorylate H2AX and initiate the DDR. This provides a molecular basis for the similarities between NBS and AT clinical syndromes.

Several lines of evidence indicate that MRN is the functional sensor of DSBs induced by radiation (Stucki and Jackson, 2006). First, the RAD50 protein has been shown to directly bind to DNA; second, NBS1 is required for recruitment of ATM to the break; third, MRN assembles at sites of DSBs faster than any other known protein; and fourth, MRN is the only known DNA repair complex that does not depend on any other protein to form foci at DSBs. MRN is a multifunctional complex. Not only does it sense the DSB, bind DNA and recruit ATM, it is also important for the 'processing' of the DSB. For example, it has exonuclease activity and can digest the ends of the DNA break which may not be compatible for ligation.

Thus, the earliest events in the DDR are considered to be the recruitment of MRN and ATM to DSBs. ATM is normally present in the cell, but in an inactive form. Activation of ATM occurs once it becomes associated with a DSB resulting in phosphorylation of H2AX at the site of the DSB. H2AX phosphorylation then spreads over relatively large chromatin regions (megabases) in both directions, an event that is regulated by an additional protein called MDC1. This protein acts as an adaptor/mediator by directly binding to both ATM and phosphorylated H2AX, and in this way is able to spread ATM phosphorylation of H2AX in both directions of the break. The spreading of this signal significantly alters the chromatin structure around the DSB and is thought to be important for assisting access of other DNA repair proteins to the break. The spreading also acts to 'amplify' the DSB signal. The presence of large areas of H2AX phosphorylation around a single DSB explains the relatively large foci that are observed microscopically.

DNA-PKcs-KU

In cells that completely lack the ATM protein, phosphorylation of H2AX and IRIF formation can still occur through an alternative mechanism but with somewhat delayed kinetics. In these cells, H2AX phosphorylation is mediated by the catalytic subunit of the DNA-dependent protein kinase (DNA-PKcs). DNA-PKcs is a kinase that is structurally related to ATM and which is very important in the non-homologous end joining pathway of DNA repair (see Section 2.7, NHEJ). In normal cells or in cells treated with an ATM inhibitor (which blocks the activity of the ATM protein), DNA-PKcs is unable to phosphorylate H2AX. Thus, in addition to its early role in activating components of the DDR, the ATM protein also appears to actively exclude DNA-PKcs at sites of DSBs.

The mechanism through which DNA-PKcs finds DSBs is very similar to that of ATM. Like ATM, DNA-PKcs is unable to act as a sensor of damage itself. This sensor function is carried out by the Ku70–Ku80 complex, which directly binds to the ends of DSBs. Binding of Ku70–Ku80 to DSBs then recruits DNA-PKcs allowing phosphorylation of H2AX.

ATR–ATRIP

The third kinase capable of phosphorylating H2AX is ATR, which stands for AT-related kinase. This enzyme does not appear to play any substantial role in the initial recognition of DSBs produced by radiation. Instead, it phosphorylates H2AX in response to other types of DNA damage and abnormalities such as single-stranded DNA and stalled or broken replication forks. It is thus very important for the types of damage that occur during normal DNA replication. The recruitment of ATR to sites of DNA damage requires another protein called ATRIP (ATR interacting protein). Thus, just like ATM and DNA-PKcs, ATR is recruited to sites of damage by a different protein that acts as the sensor of DNA damage.

Although ATR is not important in the initial detection of DSBs, it does play a role in this pathway after ATM is activated. As discussed above, the ATM–MRN complex leads to processing of the DNA at sites of DSBs. This processing can create stretches of single-stranded DNA, which will then activate ATR. Thus, ATR can be activated 'downstream' of ATM activation. Although highly related to ATM, ATR phosphorylates a distinct set of proteins that participate in the DDR. Consequently, components of the DDR effector pathways (DNA repair, checkpoints and cell death) are also dependent on ATR after radiation treatment.

2.4 SIGNALLING TO EFFECTOR PATHWAYS

Activation of ATM, DNA-PKcs and ATR leads to the phosphorylation not only of H2AX, but also of many other cellular proteins. Amazingly, recent studies have shown that as many as 700 proteins are substrates for the ATM and ATR kinases in response to DNA damage (Matsuoka *et al.*, 2007). Phosphorylation of these other proteins act as the 'signals' to activate the various different downstream effectors of the DDR (apoptosis, cell-cycle checkpoints and DNA repair). The ATM protein plays perhaps the most important role in transmitting these signals in response to radiation-induced DSBs and is thus considered to be a master regulator of the DDR.

2.5 PROGRAMMED CELL DEATH – APOPTOSIS

Two of the important proteins which are phosphorylated following activation of ATM are p53 and MDM2. p53 is one of the most commonly mutated tumour suppressors whose function is to regulate genes that control both cell-cycle checkpoints (see below) and programmed cell death through a programme known as apoptosis (see Chapter 3 for details). Consequently, activation of p53 after irradiation can lead either to a block in proliferation or directly to cell death (Fig. 2.5).

The p53 gene is regulated at the protein level by binding to its partner MDM2. This association leads to rapid ubiquitination and destruction of p53 through the proteasome pathway. Thus, in unstressed normal cells, p53 is made continuously but is degraded and is thus non-functional. Following DNA damage, ATM phosphorylates both p53 and MDM2. These events destabilize the p53–MDM2 interaction, and as a result the p53 protein is no longer degraded. In addition to this stabilization, direct phosphorylation of p53 by ATM leads to its activation as a transcription factor and thus the upregulation of its many target genes. These target genes include the pro-apoptotic genes BAX and PUMA, which in certain cells can be sufficient to induce cell death. Thus, in some cells, activation of the DDR itself can lead to rapid induction of cell death through apoptosis. The purpose of this DDR effector is likely to be similar to the function of p53 itself, namely tumour suppression. Because DNA damage can lead to dangerous mutations, it may be more beneficial to the organism to eliminate the cell rather than trying to repair the damage. This would be predicted to be especially important in rapidly proliferating tissues, and

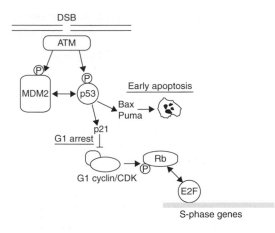

Figure 2.5 Cells irradiated in the G1 phase are influenced by the action of p53. Ataxia telangiectasia mutated (ATM) protein is activated by double-strand DNA breaks (DSBs) and phosphorylates both MDM2 and p53. This leads to stabilization and activation of p53, which then induces genes that can promote apoptosis (Bax, Puma) and induce checkpoints. Induction of p21 inhibits the action of cyclin–cyclin-dependent kinase (CDK) complexes that are necessary for the entry into S phase. Consequently cells are blocked at the G1/S border. In many cancer cells, p53 or other components of this checkpoint are mutated and so it is non-functional.

indeed these tissues tend to display radiation-induced apoptosis (see Chapter 3 for more details).

2.6 CHECKPOINT ACTIVATION

The second major effector pathway of the DDR is the activation of cell-cycle checkpoints. Treatment of cells with ionizing radiation causes delays in the movement of cells through the G1, S and G2 phases of the cell cycle (Table 2.2) (Kastan and Bartek, 2004). This occurs through the activation of DNA damage checkpoints, which are specific points in the cell cycle at which progression of the cell into the next phase can be blocked or slowed. The DDR activates four distinct checkpoints in response to irradiation that take place at different points within the cell cycle. Initially, these checkpoints were described as delays that would allow cells more time to repair DNA damage. This description is likely true to some extent, especially in terms of the importance of checkpoints in preventing mutations that might otherwise arise

Table 2.2 Radiation-induced cell-cycle checkpoints and their characteristics

Position	Primary signalling proteins	Applies to cells irradiated in	Features
G1	ATM, p53, p21	G1	Prevents entry into S
S	ATM, Chk1/Chk12, CDC25A/ CDC25C, BRCA1, BRCA2	S	Slows progression through S
G2-early	ATM, Chk1/Chk12, CDC25A/ CDC25C, BRCA1, BRCA2	G2	Prevents entry into mitosis
G2-late	ATR, Chk1, CDC25A/CDC25C	All phases	Accumulation of cells in G2

because of misrepair. However, there is little evidence to support a general role for checkpoints in influencing the overall radiosensitivity (cell survival) following single doses of radiation.

All movement through the cell cycle, be it in the G1, S, G2 or M phases, is driven by cyclin-dependent kinases (CDKs). The CDKs phosphorylate other proteins to initiate the processes required for progression thorough the cell cycle. A CDK is active only when associated with a cyclin partner (hence their name) and different cyclin–CDK complexes are active at different points within the cell cycle. For example, cyclinD–CDK4 is active in G1 and cyclinB–CDK1 is active in mitosis. Checkpoint activation requires inhibition of the cyclin–CDK complexes and for radiation this occurs through two main mechanisms. The first is by activation of other proteins that directly inhibit the cyclin–CDK complex; these are the cyclin-dependent kinase inhibitors (CDKIs). The second is by affecting phosphorylation and activity of the CDK enzyme itself. The activity of any given CDK is frequently affected by its phosphorylation status, and may be active in either the phosphorylated or dephosphorylated state depending on the specific CDK in question.

G1 arrest

Cells contain a checkpoint at the transition between the G1 and S phases that plays an important normal role in the decision of the cell to initiate cell division. This checkpoint is thus sensitive to growth factors, nutrients and other conditions that favour proliferation. The transition from G1 to S phase is controlled by the activation of the E2F transcription factor. This factor is important for regulating many

of the genes necessary to initiate DNA replication in S phase and in G1 is kept inactive by binding to the retinoblastoma protein (Rb). As cells normally move from G1 into S, the Rb protein becomes phosphorylated by G1 cyclin–CDKs including cyclinD–CDK4 and cyclinE–CDK2. This phosphorylation causes release of Rb from E2F, allowing E2F to function as a transcription factor and initiate S phase.

As discussed above, irradiation leads to an ATM-dependent stabilization and activation of p53. One of the genes that is upregulated by p53 is the CDKI p21 (CDKN1A). p21 inhibits the G1 cyclin–CDK complexes thereby preventing phosphorylation of Rb and entry into S phase. As a result, cells that are irradiated while in the G1 phase will exhibit a delay prior to entry into S phase that is dependent on both p53 and p21.

S-phase checkpoint

The remaining radiation-induced checkpoints are controlled by two highly related proteins known as Chk1 and Chk2 (Fig. 2.6) (Bartek et al., 2004). Chk1 and Chk2 are activated by phosphorylation and are direct targets of ATR and ATM respectively. Cells that are in S phase at the time of irradiation demonstrate a dose-dependent reduction in the rate of DNA synthesis and, as a result, the overall length of time that cells need to replicate their DNA substantially increases. The target for preventing S-phase progression is the CDK2 kinase, which must be in a dephosphorylated form to be active. The dephosphorylation of CDK2 is maintained by the phosphatases CDC25A and CDC25C. When Chk1 and Chk2 are activated, they phosphorylate CDC25A

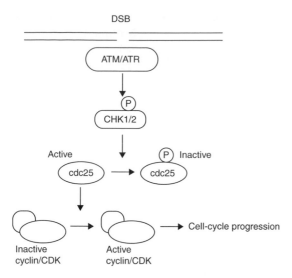

Figure 2.6 The S, early G2 and late G2 checkpoints are all activated by a similar mechanism. Ataxia telangiectasia mutated protein (ATM) and/or AT-related kinase (ATR) are activated by double-strand DNA breaks (DSBs) and phosphorylate the Chk1/2 kinases (see text). These kinases then phosphorylate and inactivate CDC25A/CDC25C. CDC25A/CDC25C are required for progression through S phase and into mitosis because they activate the required cyclin–cyclin-dependent kinase (CDK) complexes in both parts of the cell cycle. Thus when Chk1/2 are phosphorylated by ATM, cell-cycle checkpoints in both S and G2 are activated.

and CDC25CC leading to their destruction or inactivation. As a result, Chk1 and Chk2 activation by ATR and ATM results in an increase in the amount of phosphorylated CDK2 and thus slowed progression through S phase.

Although, ATM–Chk2 and ATR–Chk1 activation and inhibition of CDC25A/C is the main mechanism for initiation of the S-phase checkpoint, several other proteins in the DDR can also influence this response. This includes the BRCA1 and BRCA2 proteins, whose main function is in the homologous recombination branch of DNA repair (see Section 2.7). This suggests a complex relationship between checkpoint activation and DNA repair.

G2 early checkpoint

There are two additional checkpoints in G2, both of which operate along similar lines to that in S phase. The early G2 checkpoint is also ATM–Chk2–Cdc25A/C dependent and applies to cells that are irradiated while in G2. The checkpoint is activated by relatively low doses of radiation (1 Gy is enough) and results in a block of cell-cycle progression at the end of G2. The target of ATM–Chk2–Cdc25A/C signalling in this case is the mitotic cyclinB–CDK1 complex which, like CDK2 in S phase, must be dephosphorylated on specific sites to become active. It is called the early G2 checkpoint because it applies to cells that are irradiated while in G2 phase and rapidly blocks their movement into mitosis. As a result, there is a drop in the number cells within mitosis at short times after irradiation.

G2 late checkpoint

The late G2 checkpoint describes a long G2 delay that is observed after irradiation and is applicable to cells that have been previously irradiated while in the G1 or S phases. These cells may experience transient G1- and S-phase checkpoints, but when they arrive in the G2 phase many hours later they experience a second delay before entry into mitosis. Unlike the early G2 checkpoint, this delay is strongly dose-dependent, and can last many hours after high doses of radiation. In addition, unlike all the other damage checkpoints this late G2 checkpoint is independent of ATM. Instead, the principal signalling axis occurs from ATR to Chk1 to CDC25A/CDC25C. The late G2 checkpoint is thus mechanistically similar to the S and early G2 checkpoints, but likely arises from a fundamentally different type of DNA damage. Instead of being activated directly by DSBs, this checkpoint likely reflects a type of damage that persists after other DNA repair processes have occurred and which is sufficient to activate ATR.

Checkpoints, cancer and radiosensitivity

In a large proportion of tumour cells, one or more of the G1/S, S phase and early G2 checkpoints are disabled because of genetic changes that occur during tumourigenesis. In recent years, these checkpoint responses have been linked to a tumour suppressor function that must be disrupted to allow oncogene-induced proliferation. This is thought to occur following activation of growth-promoting oncogenes which induce 'inappropriate replication' and DNA damage from replication stress. When functional, the checkpoints block further proliferation of these cells and can thus actively suppress cancer development. This idea is supported by the finding that many early cancer lesions show widespread activation of checkpoint activity.

Mutations in genes such as p53, BRCA1 or other components of the DDR that influence checkpoint activation will result in the failure to delay cell-cycle progression in response to irradiation. This may have an important consequence for genetic instability after irradiation and tumour progression, but there is little evidence to suggest that lack of these checkpoints influences overall cellular radiosensitivity. Thus, although the G1/S, S and early G2 checkpoints are often described as providing extended time for repair, this extra time seems to be more important for the quality of repair rather than the amount of repair that takes place.

The late G2 checkpoint, which unlike all others is ATR rather than ATM dependent, is the only exception since evidence exists to support it as having a role in determining radiosensitivity. For example, inhibitors of ATR that prevent this checkpoint cause radiosensitization. Thus, for reasons that are still unclear, premature entry into mitosis of cells that are in the late G2 checkpoint results in increased cell death.

Although the G1/S, S and early G2 checkpoints may not affect the radiosensitivity of cells to single doses of radiation, they may affect the response to multiple (fractionated) doses. The presence of the checkpoints in normal cells, and absence in many tumour cells, will affect the redistribution of cells at time-points after irradiation and therefore indirectly the sensitivity of cells to subsequent doses of radiation. For example, consider two populations of cells that are identical with exception of the ability to block at the G1 checkpoint. Twenty-four hours after irradiation cells that lack this checkpoint may show reduced numbers of cells in G1 phase and more cells in S phase compared with cells that have an intact checkpoint. Since radiosensitivity is different in G1 and S phase, the two populations of cells may respond differently to subsequent irradiation at that time. Consequently, all checkpoints can potentially affect responses to radiotherapy given in multiple fractions.

2.7 DNA DSB REPAIR

As discussed above, DSBs are detected by specialized proteins which signal to the cell that damage has occurred, thereby initiating the DNA damage response. This response effectively focuses the cell's attention on the damage, stopping other processes such as transcription and cell-cycle progression, and, importantly, initiating repair. For DSBs, there are two main repair pathways, HR and NHEJ. These are quite different in the genes involved, the position in the cell cycle where they primarily act and in the speed and accuracy of repair. These processes are described in more detail below. Both affect the radiosensitivity of a cell.

HR

As the name implies, HR uses homologous undamaged DNA (that with an identical sequence) as the template to repair the DNA with the DSBs in it (West, 2003). By using DNA with the same sequence as a basis for repair, the process is error free. The general scheme is illustrated in Fig. 2.7. Briefly, single-strand regions are created around each side of the break, followed by their coating with specialized proteins. These single-stranded nucleoprotein filaments then invade undamaged double-stranded DNA on the neighbouring sister chromatid, forming a crossover, or bubble, structure. These bubbles are then expanded with specialized enzymes called helicases. The object of this process is to provide an undamaged DNA template of the same base sequence around the break site, so that DNA polymerases can then synthesize across the missing regions, thereby accurately repairing the break. The crossover structure then has to be reversed to reset the chromatin to its original configuration. This is done with specialized nucleases which cut, or resolve, the junctions, followed finally by connecting up, or ligating, adjacent ends with a ligase. The whole process takes several hours (up to

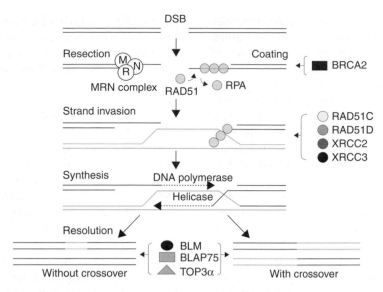

Figure 2.7 Schematic of double-strand DNA break (DSB) repair by homologous recombination (HR). The principal genes known to be involved are shown, although there are others not shown which are also involved in HR. Chromatin remodelling genes are not shown. The main feature is the use of an undamaged sister chromatid sequence (light coloured lines) as template for repair. The groups of genes (right and bottom centre) are involved with the processes indicated by the horizontal arrows.

6 hours or more) to complete. Some details of the genes involved in the process are given below.

The first step is to cut back one strand on each side of the break with an exonuclease, making a 3′ overhang, in order to create single-stranded regions which are necessary for subsequent strand invasion. The proteins involved in end resection include the MRN complex (described above under sensors of damage), MRE11 being the active component. The single-stranded DNA is immediately coated with RPA (replication protein A), a single-strand binding protein, which is a universal response of the cell to any single-stranded regions of DNA. This RPA is then displaced by a central protein in HR, namely RAD51. This results in the formation of a nucleo-protein filament of DNA coated with RAD51, which then undergoes the search for homologous DNA and strand invasion. Several RAD51 paralogues (genes arising from duplication of the parent gene but with modified sequence and function) help with these processes, including RAD51B, RAD51C, RAD51D, XRCC2 and XRCC3. Deletion or mutation of any of these genes can severely impair HR.

Helicases, including BLM and other members of the RecQ family, possibly with the help of RAD54,

then enlarge the subsequent 'bubble' structure (branch migration). The necessary DNA synthesis is carried out with DNA polymerases, the identity of which is still uncertain. One of the replicative polymerases is the likely candidate, however, since HR is mostly an error-free process, like replication, although some of the less accurate translesion synthesis polymerases have also been implicated in this process. The bubble structure then needs to be resolved by cutting the DNA at the crossover points, carried out by enzymes called resolvases. In bacteria and yeast, the identity of resolvases is known, but not in mammalian cells despite intense research. It is known that BLM exists in a complex with TopIIIa (a topoisomerase capable of untangling DNA) and a helper protein called BLAP75. There is now evidence that BLM pushes the two sides of the bubble towards each other via its helicase activity, leaving only a small crossover region, and that TopIIIa then untangles the DNA at this point, via its cutting and re-ligation activity that is common to topoisomerases, resulting in two separated sister chromatids. Finally, DNA ends are ligated probably with ligase 1, since eliminating the LIG1 gene reduces repair by HR.

In addition to those mentioned above, two other gene families are involved, well known for causing human repair deficiency syndromes, namely BRCA genes 1 and 2 and the Fanconi anaemia family (Zhang and Powell, 2005). Mutations or deletions in one or more of these genes compromises HR. BRCA2 has perhaps the most clearly defined function in regulating the binding of RAD51 to RPA-coated single-stranded DNA, a key step in HR. The Fanconi (*FANC*) genes also play a significant role in HR, although knocking out these genes has a milder effect than, for example, knocking out *BRCA2* or *RAD51* which can lead to cell and embryonic lethality. Cells with *FANC* gene mutations all show increased sensitivity to DNA crosslinking agents, repair of which depends on HR. However, mild or little increased sensitivity to ionizing radiation has been found in *FANC* mutant cells, although increased radiosensitivity under hypoxia has been reported, which may be a consequence of the increased crosslinks formed under hypoxic irradiation, again requiring HR repair. The 13 Fanconi genes can be divided into three groups: eight in a core complex (A, B, C, E, F, G, L and M), two substrates which are ubiquitinylated by the core complex (D2 and I) and three downstream targets (D1, J and N). DNA damage leads to ubiquitinylation of the D2–I complex, which binds and regulates BRCA2 (also known as FANCD1).

The role of BRCA1 is broader, although it clearly plays a role in HR. Together with its partner BARD1 it can ubiquitinylate other proteins (it is an E3 ubiquitin ligase), thus modifying their protein interacting properties, and thus their function. BRCA1–BARD1 appear in several complexes with other proteins, each playing a different role, including with BACH1 and TOPBP1 and others in replication inhibition (part of the intra-S checkpoint), with the MRN complex in NHEJ, with RAD52–BRCA2 in homologous recombination and with RNA polymerase II in transcription. Its ubiquitinylating function is necessary for each role.

NHEJ

As its name implies, NHEJ joins two DNA DSB ends together without requiring homologous DNA sequences (Lieber, 2008). This is a more

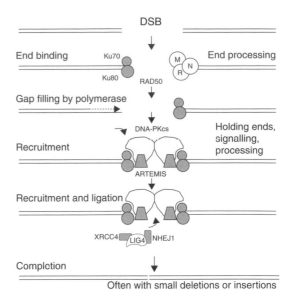

Figure 2.8 Schematic of double-strand DNA break (DSB) repair by non-homologous end-joining (NHEJ). The principal genes known to be involved are shown, although there are others not shown which are also involved in NHEJ. Chromatin remodelling genes are not shown. For clarity, processes such as end-binding have been shown on one side of the break only.

rapid process than HR but less accurate, with small deletions or insertions often resulting at the repaired break site. Although this can lead to mutations, it allows the cell to survive. An unrepaired DSB is often lethal through loss of a piece of chromosome at the next mitosis, with the potential loss of tens or hundreds of genes. In addition, only a minor fraction (a few per cent) of genomic DNA comprises gene coding or regulatory regions, so the chance of a break occurring in such regions is low, and these may also be silent (not expressed) and/or non-essential. Although NHEJ is 'quick and dirty', it is a good repair pathway for the cell to maximize its chance of survival.

The general scheme of NHEJ is shown in Fig. 2.8. The main steps in NHEJ, after sensing the DSB, involve nucleases to remove damaged DNA, polymerases to help repair and ligases to restore the continuity of the DNA chain. The first event in the sequence is binding of a Ku heterodimer (two different but related proteins: Ku70 and Ku80) to the DNA ends. This occurs within seconds of the break being formed because of high abundance of the Ku dimer and its high affinity for ends. The binding serves both to protect ends from degradation by exonucleases and to recruit the DNA-dependent protein kinase catalytic subunit (DNA-PKcs; officially called PRKDC), the second step in NHEJ.

Activation of PRKDC as a kinase occurs only when it is bound to the Ku complex at break sites. It has several substrates and several functions. It is a large protein and forms a physical bridge between the two ends, helping to keep them in close proximity for subsequent repair events. In addition, it phosphorylates a number of target proteins involved in checkpoints and repair. One of its targets is itself (autophosphorylation). There are a number of sites on the PRKDC protein which can be phosphorylated, some of which are autophosphorylated, while others are phosphorylated by ATM. Phosphorylation has been shown to be necessary for efficient repair by NHEJ since mutations at these sites make cells considerably more radiosensitive. Phosphorylation stimulates dissociation of the protein from DNA, or a change in conformation, allowing other repair factors access to the site, so that phosphorylation-mutant proteins remain at the site, blocking it for further repair.

PRKDC also exists in a complex with Artemis, which is recruited to DNA ends together with PRKDC. Artemis has endonuclease activity and its function is to clean up, or process, the DNA ends so they are suitable for ligation (Jeggo and Lobrich, 2005). The activation of PRKDC on end-binding leads not only to autophosphorylation but also to phosphorylation of Artemis, stimulating its nuclease activity. Break sites often show small deletions as a result. Artemis is apparently necessary for the repair of a minor fraction of DSBs. Another protein involved in end-processing in the NHEJ pathway is polynucleotide kinase (PNK), which is capable of trimming 'dirty' ends (e.g. those with the remnants of a sugar group instead of a 'clean' base with a 3′ phosphate). This action renders the ends ligatable with a ligase (see below).

Radiation often produces an overhang, or non-blunt, end, either directly or after end-processing. Such gaps can be filled by a polymerase to produce blunt-ended DNA ready for ligation. The translesion synthesis polymerases λ and μ have been shown to be capable of this and have been implicated in NHEJ. Polμ and another polymerase called terminal deoxynucleotidyl transferase (TdT) can also add a few nucleotides to a blunt end. DNA sequencing of breaks repaired by NHEJ therefore often shows small insertions. Whether replicative polymerases are also involved in these synthesis activities is not clear. The final step in repair is ligation of adjoining ends, which is carried out by ligase IV, aided by two other proteins, XRRC4 and XLF.

Making the choice between HR and NHEJ

Several factors determine which pathway is used to repair a damage-induced DSB. DNA damage detection proteins such as MRN and the Ku complex will compete for DNA ends and partially determine which pathway is subsequently used (Brugmans *et al.*, 2007). This is called passive competition, and there is evidence supporting such a model. However, there are other factors, one of the most obvious being template availability. Homologous recombination requires the availability of an homologous stretch of DNA, which the sister chromatid provides in S and G2. Although there is no sister chromatid in G1, there is an homologous chromosome, but this is often far away in molecular terms, making it a very difficult task for the HR machinery to find and use. Therefore HR is rare or absent in G1. A further illustration of the importance and use of HR is that cells often show increased radioresistance as they progress through S phase, being most resistant in late S, a time at which almost all DNA has a paired chromatid available for HR. Knocking out or reducing HR genes eliminates this late-S resistance (Tamulevicius *et al.*, 2007).

There are also active regulators of HR. As described above, end-resection at the break site, producing single-stranded DNA, is necessary for HR. End resection does not occur in G1, probably since it depends on specific CDKs, which are not active until late in G1. This further favours the NHEJ pathway in this phase. There are also anti-recombination genes in yeast with homologues in mammalian cells, with the job of preventing unwanted recombination, which can lead to genetic instability.

Finally, a comment on clinical relevance. Since HR is a pathway specific to S- and G2-phase cells, it occurs only in dividing cells. Conversely, NHEJ occurs in all phases of the cell cycle, and is thus neither phase specific nor cycle specific. The relevance for radiotherapy is that NHEJ is used by all cells and tissues, including those that are slowly dividing or non-dividing. This includes the dose-limiting late-reacting tissues such as spinal cord and stromal tissue, which give rise to fibrosis and telangiectasia. In attempting to find DNA-repair-inhibiting drugs to improve radiotherapy, targeting NHEJ is therefore likely to be a more risky strategy than inhibiting HR.

The link between SSBs and DSBs

Single-strand breaks can lead to the formation of DSBs in two main ways. First, ionizing radiation damage often occurs in clusters, such that some SSBs will also have damage to DNA bases in their near vicinity. During repair of the base damage by BER, SSBs are formed temporarily (see Section 2.8). It has been shown that, if base damage occurs on the opposite strand to a radiation-induced SSB, the temporary nick formed during BER can combine with the radiation break on the opposite strand causing a DSB. Second, if a SSB encounters a replication fork during S phase, this leads to collapse of the fork and a single-ended DSB. The cell attempts to repair these S-phase DSBs by HR. In this case NHEJ is not an option, since there is only one double-stranded end and not two, and so there is no adjacent end for the end-joining process. Thus HR provides a backup repair pathway for unrepaired SSBs.

The latter mechanism has clinical relevance, since it has been shown that drugs which inhibit poly-(ADP-ribose) polymerase (PARP), a SSB detector protein, are particularly effective in tumours with HR deficiencies, such as breast tumours with BCRA1 or BRCA2 deficiencies. The mechanism is probably that the PARP inhibitors suppress SSB repair, resulting in greater numbers of unrepaired SSBs, which therefore have a greater chance of hitting a replication fork. Under normal circumstances the resulting DSB would be repaired by HR, so the absence or reduction of

this backup pathway leads to a substantial increase in DSBs and thus cellular lethality.

2.8 OTHER DNA REPAIR PATHWAYS

Base excision repair and single-strand break repair (SSBR)

As mentioned in Section 2.1, DSBs, although the most lethal lesion induced by ionizing radiation, are not the most common. Base damage and SSBs far outweigh DSBs in number, being up to 50 times more frequent. Base damage and SSBs also occur without irradiation as a consequence of normal metabolism. It has been estimated that 100 000 such damages occur each day in every cell in the body. The repair pathways – BER and SSBR – have therefore evolved to repair such damage efficiently and maintain genome integrity (Fortini and Dogliotti, 2007).

An outline of the related BER and SSBR pathways is shown in Fig. 2.9. Briefly, in BER, most of the damaged bases in the DNA will be detected and removed by specialized proteins called glycosylases. There are several such enzymes, each specific for a particular type of base damage. They cut out the damaged base without cutting the DNA backbone, resulting in an abasic site. This will be recognized by another class of enzyme, AP endonuclease, which will cut the DNA backbone leaving a nick, or SSB. Subsequent repair follows one of two pathways: short patch or long patch. As their names imply, short patch repair involves replacing the damaged base only, while in long patch repair up to 10 nucleotides are cut out and replaced. Each requires DNA synthesis to replace the missing bases, carried out by DNA polymerase β for short patch repair and mainly DNA polymerases δ and ε (replicative enzymes) for long patch repair. As always, ligases complete the job: ligase 3 for short patch and ligase 1 for long patch. Repair of SSB is similar, although radiation itself causes the break rather than being a repair intermediate. Since these breaks are often 'dirty', with ends not recognized by ligases, there is an extra end-processing step, mainly by the enzyme PNK. Once a clean nick is produced, short or long patch repair can then follow, as for BER. This short summary does not include all proteins involved in the

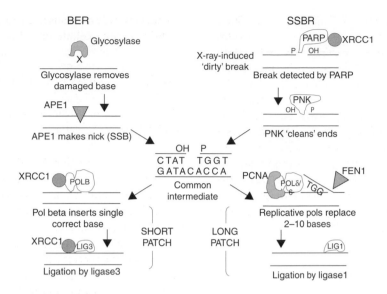

Figure 2.9 Schematic of the related pathways of base excision repair (BER) and single-strand break repair (SSBR). The X (top left) represents a damaged base. Different base damages are recognized and removed by different glycosylases as the first step in BER. Both pathways result in a common nicked intermediate, which is processed by one of two subpathways (short or long patch repair). APE1 apurinic/apyrimidinic endonuclease-1; PARP, poly (ADP-ribose) polymerase; PNK, polynucleotide kinase; POL, polymerase.

pathway. Two mentioned here briefly because of their importance are PARP-1, which efficiently and rapidly detects SSBs, and XRCC1, which is a helper protein for both PNK (damage processing) and ligase 3. Mutation, deletion or inhibition of either of these can lead to reduced repair and radiosensitization. Inhibition of PARP is particularly effective in HR-deficient tumours (see above), illustrating the relevance of the BER/SSBR pathways for possible clinical exploitation.

MMR and NER

The mismatch repair pathway corrects mispaired nucleotides (e.g. C with T). As with all repair pathways it comprises a recognition step, an excision and resynthesis step and ligation. Most studies with knockout cells for one or more mismatch repair genes have not found any increase in radiosensitivity. The details of the pathway will therefore not be described in detail here. However, this pathway clearly has relevance for cancer treatment, since MMR-deficient cells have altered sensitivity to some chemotherapy agents (e.g. cisplatin). In addition,

radiosensitization by thymidine analogues such as IUdR is enhanced in MMR-deficient cells because of inability to remove the modified base. The MMR status of cells is therefore of importance for outcome, not for radiotherapy alone, but for combinations of radiotherapy with some chemotherapy or radiosensitizing agents.

Nucleotide excision repair copes with bulky lesions, such as those caused by UV light (thymine dimers), and DNA adducts induced by cisplatin. However, as with MMR, knocking out NER genes has, in general, little effect on sensitivity to ionizing radiation, and so no detailed discussion of NER will be included here. There is one situation, however, where NER genes can affect the radiation response. Irradiation under hypoxia produces a greater number of DNA crosslinks than under oxic conditions. Such crosslinks require, among other factors, the excision activity of two NER genes, *ERCC1* and *XPF*. Defects in either of these genes can lead to modest increases in radiosensitivity of hypoxic cells. The status of the NER pathway is therefore relevant to radiotherapy in combination with certain chemotherapy agents, and possibly to hypoxic tumours treated with radiotherapy alone.

Key points

1. DNA is the critical target for radiation-induced cell killing.
2. Cells activate a DNA-damage response that consists of sensors and effectors.
3. Effector pathways include apoptosis, cell-cycle checkpoints and DNA repair.
4. DNA DSBs are the most important and difficult lesion to repair.
5. DSBs are repaired by both HR and NHEJ.

■ BIBLIOGRAPHY

Bartek J, Lukas C, Lukas J (2004). Checking on DNA damage in S phase. *Nat Rev Mol Cell Biol* **5**: 792–804.

Brugmans L, Kanaar R, Essers J (2007). Analysis of DNA double-strand break repair pathways in mice. *Mutat Res* **614**: 95–108.

Chapman JD, Gillespie CJ (1981). Radiation-induced events and their time-scale in mammalian cells. *Adv Radiat Biol* **9**: 143–98.

Falck J, Coates J, Jackson SP (2005). Conserved modes of recruitment of ATM, ATR and DNA-PKcs to sites of DNA damage. *Nature* **434**: 605–11.

Fortini P, Dogliotti E (2007). Base damage and single-strand break repair: mechanisms and functional significance of short- and long-patch repair subpathways. *DNA Repair (Amst)* **6**: 398–409.

Goodhead DT (2006). Energy deposition stochastics and track structure: what about the target? *Radiat Prot Dosimetry* **122**: 3–15.

Harper JW, Elledge SJ (2007). The DNA damage response: ten years after. *Mol Cell* **28**: 739–45.

Jeggo PA, Lobrich M (2005). Artemis links ATM to double strand break rejoining. *Cell Cycle* **4**: 359–62.

Kastan MB, Bartek J (2004). Cell-cycle checkpoints and cancer. *Nature* **432**: 316–23.

Lieber MR (2008). The mechanism of human nonhomologous DNA end joining. *J Biol Chem* **283**: 1–5.

Matsuoka S, Ballif BA, Smogorzewska A *et al.* (2007). ATM and ATR substrate analysis reveals extensive protein networks responsive to DNA damage. *Science* **316**: 1160–6.

O'Driscoll M, Jeggo PA (2006). The role of double-strand break repair – insights from human genetics. *Nat Rev Genet* **7**: 45–54.

Stucki M, Jackson SP (2006). gammaH2AX and MDC1: anchoring the DNA-damage-response machinery to broken chromosomes. *DNA Repair (Amst)* **5**: 534–43.

Tamulevicius P, Wang M, Iliakis G (2007). Homology-directed repair is required for the development of radioresistance during S phase: interplay between double-strand break repair and checkpoint response. *Radiat Res* **167**: 1–11.

van Attikum H, Gasser SM (2005). The histone code at DNA breaks: a guide to repair? *Nat Rev Mol Cell Biol* **6**: 757–65.

Warters RL, Hofer KG (1977). Radionuclide toxicity in cultured mammalian cells. Elucidation of the primary site for radiation-induced division delay. *Radiat Res* **69**: 348–58.

Warters RL, Hofer KG, Harris CR, Smith JM (1997). Radionuclide toxicity in cultured mammalian cells: elucidation of the primary site of radiation damage. *Curr Top Radiat Res* **12**: 389–407.

West SC (2003). Molecular views of recombination proteins and their control. *Nat Rev Mol Cell Biol* **4**: 435–45.

Zhang J, Powell SN (2005). The role of the BRCA1 tumor suppressor in DNA double-strand break repair. *Mol Cancer Res* **3**: 531–9.

■ FURTHER READING

Caldecott KW (2007). Mammalian single-strand break repair: mechanisms and links with chromatin. *DNA Repair (Amst)* **6**: 443–53.

Löbrich M, Jeggo PA (2007). The impact of a negligent G2/M checkpoint on genomic instability and cancer induction. *Nat Rev Cancer* **7**: 861–9.

Cell death after irradiation: how, when and why cells die

BRADLY G. WOUTERS

3.1 DEFINITIONS OF CELL DEATH

The successful use of radiation to treat cancer results primarily from its ability to cause the death of individual tumour cells. As discussed in Chapter 2, the biological consequences of irradiation, including cell death, are highly influenced by pathways within the DNA damage response (DDR) system. The DDR determines not only the sensitivity of cells to die following irradiation, but also the type of cell death that occurs, and the timing of cell death. Because the DDR differs among different types of normal and tumour cells (and perhaps even within different populations of tumour cells), the manifestation of cell death can also differ widely among different cell types.

It is important to define what is meant by cell death in the context of radiobiology and cancer therapy. For many years, little attention was paid towards differences in the mechanisms or types of cell death after irradiation or other cancer treatments. This was in part because many of the pathways that influence cell death were unknown and because cell death is typically very hard to assess. Quantification is complicated by the fact that cells die at various times after irradiation, often after

one or two trips around the cell cycle, and among surviving cells that continue to proliferate. Instead, researchers have focused on assessing clonogenic survival, which is defined as the ability of a cell to proliferate indefinitely after irradiation. This is a much more robust and relevant parameter to assess radiation effect since any cell that retains proliferative capacity can cause failure to locally control the tumour (discussed in more detail in Chapters 4 and 5). Consequently, cell death in the context of radiobiology is generally equated with any process that leads to the permanent loss of clonogenic capacity. This is a rather wide inclusion criterion for cell death, and obviously does not have meaning when applied to terminally differentiated cell types that do not proliferate, such as nerve and muscle cells. For these types of cells, it makes more sense to consider the specific types of cell death that lead to destruction of the cell, or to evaluate how radiation alters the function of these cells. Nonetheless, loss of reproductive capacity is a widely applicable definition for cell death in radiobiology and is highly relevant for the proliferating cells, including those in tumours and in many of the normal tissues of relevance for radiotherapy.

3.2 HOW CELLS DIE: PROGRAMMED CELL DEATH AND MITOTIC CATASTROPHE

It is now clear that cells can die by many different mechanisms following irradiation. Increased attention to the mechanisms of cell death occurred following the discovery of a genetically 'programmed' form of cell death known as apoptosis. This form of cell death results in rapid and normally complete destruction and removal of the cell, and is considered as a 'choice' made by the cell itself often as a consequence of damage, stress or as a barrier against tumourigenesis. Furthermore, this pathway can be activated directly by the DDR, and is thus a strong determinant of radiation-induced cell death for certain cell types. Since the discovery of apoptosis, several other pathways under genetic control have been identified that can contribute to loss of reproductive capacity after irradiation, including autophagy, senescence, and even necrosis (Okada and Mak, 2004). Each of these pathways can be distinguished at the molecular and morphological level (see Table 3.1) and each can potentially contribute to radiosensitivity in certain cell types and contexts. Importantly, the pathways that control these programmed forms of cell death are differentially activated in different tissue types, and are frequently altered in cancer. Consequently, differential activation of cell death pathways constitutes a main contributor to variation in radiation response among different cells, tumours, and tissues.

In addition to these genetically controlled programmes, a long-recognized contributor to cell death after irradiation is mitotic catastrophe in which cells fail to complete mitosis correctly. Applying our definitions above, mitotic catastrophe can be considered a form of cell death of its own, the so-called mitotic death, when it is severe enough to prevent mitosis completely or alter cell function sufficiently to prevent further proliferation. Mitotic catastrophe may also result in further chromosomal and DNA damage sufficient to activate the other forms of cell death.

Apoptosis

Apoptosis is a highly regulated form of cell death that can be initiated either as a result of conditions occurring within the cell itself (such as those after DNA damage) or from signals generated externally such as those from a surrounding tissue or immune cell (Taylor *et al.*, 2008). Apoptosis is an essential and normal part of many physiological processes including embryonic development, the immune system, and maintenance of tissue homeostasis. Consequently, alterations in the control of apoptosis contribute to several human diseases, including cancer.

Apoptosis is both morphologically and molecularly distinct from other forms of cell death (see Table 3.1). Morphologically, it is characterized by membrane blebbing, condensation, and digestion of the DNA into small fragments. During this process, cellular contents are also fragmented into many membrane-enclosed apoptotic bodies, which, *in vivo*, are taken up by phagocytes. This prevents leakage of potentially damaging cellular proteins and destruction of tissue architecture that is a familiar feature of necrosis.

The molecular participants in the apoptotic pathway can be divided into two groups: the sensors and effectors. The sensor molecules are involved in making the decision to initiate apoptosis whereas the effectors are responsible for carrying out that decision. Apoptotic cell death is characterized by the sequential activation of several different enzymes known as caspases. These proteins are initially expressed in an inactive form (procaspase) and are also kept in check by a family of inhibitors of apoptosis (IAP) proteins. Apoptosis begins following the activation of a 'sensor' caspase such as caspase 8 or 9, which generates the initial signal to induce apoptosis. These caspases subsequently activate a common set of other 'effector' caspases (e.g. caspase 3), which then cleave a large set of cellular proteins leading to the ultimate destruction of the cell.

Apoptosis that initiates from caspase 8 activation is termed the 'extrinsic' pathway because it is normally activated upon the binding of an extracellular ligand and subsequent activation of a death receptor present in the cellular membrane. Examples of these death-inducing ligands include tumuor necrosis factor (TNF), TNF-related apoptosis-inducing ligand (TRAIL), and FAS ligand, which bind to the TNF receptor, TRAIL receptor and FAS receptor respectively. This extrinsic pathway of apoptosis is

Table 3.1 The characteristics of different types of cell death*

Type of cell death	Morphological changes			Biochemical features	Common detection methods
	Nucleus	Cell membrane	Cytoplasm		
Apoptosis	Chromatin condensation; nuclear fragmentation; DNA laddering	Blebbing	Fragmentation (formation of apoptotic bodies)	Caspase-dependent	Electron microscopy; TUNEL staining; annexin staining; caspase-activity assays; DNA-fragmentation assays; detection of increased number of cells in sub-G1/G0; detection of changes in mitochondrial membrane potential
Autophagy	Partial chromatin condensation; no DNA laddering	Blebbing	Increased number of autophagic vesicles	Caspase-independent; increased lysosomal activity	Electron microscopy; protein-degradation assays; assays for marker–protein translocation to autophagic membranes
Necrosis	Clumping and random degradation of nuclear DNA	Swelling; rupture	Increased vacuolation; organelle degeneration; mitochondrial swelling	–	Electron microscopy; nuclear staining (usually negative); detection of inflammation and damage in surrounding tissues
Senescence	Distinct heterochromatic structure (senescence-associated heterochromatic foci)	–	Flattening and increased granularity	SA-β-gal activity	Electron microscopy; SA-β-gal staining; growth-arrest assays
Mitotic catastrophe	Multiple micronuclei; nuclear fragmentation; dicentric chromosomes	–	–	Caspase-independent (at early stage) abnormal CDK1/cyclin B activation	Electron microscopy; assays for mitotic markers (MPM2); TUNEL staining

CDK1, cyclin-dependent kinase 1; SA-β-gal, senescence-associated galactose; TUNEL, terminal deoxynucleotidyl transferase dUTP nick end labelling.

*Adapted from Okada and Mak (2004). Adapted by permission from Macmillan Publishers Ltd.

not induced by radiation to any significant degree, but is a candidate target for combining novel drugs with radiation (see Chapters 21 and 23).

Apoptosis that initiates from caspase 9 is termed the 'intrinsic' pathway because it is activated within the cell in response to various forms of cell damage. The activation of caspase 9 is controlled in large part by the balance of pro- and anti-apoptotic proteins that reside in or near the mitochondria. Under normal conditions this balance is in favour of the anti-apoptotic factors (such as BCL2), and activation of caspase 9 is prevented. Conditions that alter this balance lead to release of cytochrome c and other molecules from the mitochondria into the cytoplasm resulting in formation of a structure known as the apoptosome, and subsequently activation of caspase 9. After irradiation, this balance can be tipped in favour of apoptosis owing, in part, to p53 activation and induction of pro-apoptotic proteins such as BAX and PUMA.

Activation of apoptosis is highly dependent on the balance of the pro and anti-apoptotic proteins and this balance varies widely among different cell types and tumours. This explains why irradiation causes apoptosis only in certain normal tissues, despite the fact that p53 is activated in response to DNA damage in nearly all normal cells. For example, fibroblast cells almost never undergo apoptosis despite demonstrating p53 and BAX induction. In these cells, induction of BAX is not sufficient to initiate release of cytochrome c and thus activation of caspase 9. These cells may have a larger proportion of anti-apoptotic molecules like those from the BCL2 family, or they may have higher levels of the IAP proteins, which block caspase activation. Consequently, apoptosis plays little or no role in the radiosensitivity of these cell types. In contrast other normal cells, such as lymphocytes and thymocytes, readily undergo apoptosis following irradiation. In these cells, p53 induction of BAX is sufficient to cause cytochrome c release from the mitochondria and induction of apoptosis. Thus, the importance of apoptosis and the genes controlling it such as p53 is highly context dependent.

In tumours, an additional mechanism for variation in apoptosis sensitivity arises from the fact that many of the genes that regulate apoptosis are frequently altered in cancer. For example, many tumours show loss of p53 function, and are thus unable to initiate apoptosis through this pathway. Apoptosis is an important cellular defence against cancer development and loss of apoptotic sensitivity is recognized as an essential hallmark of cancer. Consequently, apoptotic sensitivity is often reduced in cancer compared with normal tissues although it can vary significantly among different tumours. Since radiation and other anticancer agents are capable of activating apoptosis, it has been widely suggested that apoptotic sensitivity is also an important contributor to radiosensitivity. However, this may or may not be correct, depending upon the relative importance of other forms of cell death.

Autophagy

Autophagy is a term that literally means 'self-eating' and describes a process in which cells digest parts of their own cytoplasm in order to generate small macromolecules and energy. The molecular basis of autophagy and its relationship to cell survival mechanisms is an active area of current research. Autophagy is controlled by more than 20 known gene products (Atg proteins) which initiate the formation of a double-membrane bound structure that grows and engulfs cytoplasmic components forming cytoplasm-filled vacuoles called autophagasomes (Klionsky, 2007). These fuse with lysosomes to initiate the degradation of the enclosed material into primary components and energy that can be used to fuel metabolism.

Autophagy is activated in response to several different situations, the best characterized of which occurs in response to growth factor or nutrient removal (starvation). This process is regulated by the mammalian target of rapamycin (mTOR) kinase, which is a general sensor of nutrient status integrating upstream signalling pathways that sense energy levels, oxygen and growth factor signalling. In this situation, autophagy is thought to sustain overall survival during times of low nutrient environment by causing the limited digestion of cytoplasmic elements to sustain metabolic processes. As such, one would expect that autophagy promotes cell survival, rather than cell death.

However, in contrast to this pro-survival role, activation of autophagy can also lead to a distinct form of programmed cell death, sometimes referred to as type II death (type I being apoptosis). Some aspects of this form of death are morphologically similar to apoptosis, although no caspase activation or DNA cleavage occurs. Autophagy also appears to function as a tumour suppressor, in much the same way that apoptosis does. The Beclin 1 gene is part of a complex required to initiate autophagy, and its loss leads to enhanced cancer development in mice. This gene is also altered in some human cancers, as are several tumour suppressors recently linked to autophagy including p53 and PTEN. These data suggest that autophagy acts in some way as a barrier to cancer formation, likely in part through its ability to promote cell death in transformed cells.

Autophagy has also been observed following treatment with many anti-cancer agents including radiation, suggesting that it may be an important mechanism of cell killing by these agents (Rubinsztein *et al.*, 2007). However, it is not yet clear whether the observed autophagy represents an attempt by the cell for survival or is an induced form of cell death. There also appears to be some relationship between autophagy and apoptosis, because autophagy is more readily observed in cells with defects in apoptosis. Consequently, similar to what has been discussed for apoptosis, the contribution of autophagy to cell death is also expected to be highly cell specific.

Necrosis

It has been said that if apoptosis represents 'death by suicide', then necrosis is 'death by injury'. Necrosis has historically been considered to be an inappropriate or accidental death that occurs under conditions that are extremely unfavourable, such as those incompatible with a critical normal physiological process. Examples of conditions that can activate necrosis include extreme changes in pH, energy loss and ion imbalance. Consequently, necrosis is generally thought of as an uncontrollable, irreversible and chaotic form of cell death. It is characterized by cellular swelling, membrane deformation, organelle breakdown and the release of lysosomal enzymes which attack the cell. These conditions can occur following infection, inflammation or ischaemia. Necrosis is also frequently

observed in human tumours and can be induced following treatment with certain DNA-damaging agents, including radiation.

More recently, a number of studies have suggested that necrosis is also a regulated process that can be modulated. For example, induction of necrosis seems to be dependent on cellular energy stores, such as NAD, and ATP. Furthermore, cell stress and cell signalling including oxidative stress, calcium levels and p53 activation have been shown to influence lysosomal membrane permeability. Permeabilization leads to intracellular acidification and release of various enzymes that can promote necrosis. Although it is not clear how the cell controls necrosis following irradiation, the frequency with which this is observed does vary among different cell types. This suggests that, just as for all the other forms of cell death, cellular pathways control the sensitivity of its activation.

Senescence

Cellular senescence is the term given to the observation that over time normal cells permanently lose their ability to divide. These cells remain present, metabolically intact and may or may not display functional changes. Senescence was first described by Leonard Hayflick in cultured primary cells that exhibit an initial period of exponential growth, followed by a permanent arrest termed replicative senescence or the Hayflick limit (Hayflick, 1965). Replicative senescence is associated with the aging process and correlates with the gradual shortening of telomeres at the ends of chromosomes during the exponential growth period.

In addition to this replicative form of senescence, 'premature' senescence can also be elicited by various cellular stresses such as those caused by oncogene activation or by radiation-induced DNA damage (Campisi and d'Adda di Fagagna, 2007). In both situations, the cells enter a permanent cell-cycle arrest characterized morphologically by a flattened cytoplasm and increased granularity or biochemically by an increase in senescence-associated β-galactosidase expression. Senescence-inducing stresses typically do not induce shortening of the telomeres, but instead are controlled by a number of molecular pathways that are only partially understood. As is the case for replicative senescence, cells that undergo senescence after irradiation are not metabolically 'dead', but because they have permanently ceased proliferation they are unable to contribute to tissue or tumour recovery.

The best understood part of accelerated senescence induction involves the activation of cell-cycle inhibitor proteins such as those activated by the DDR system after radiation. In some cell types, a transient G1 checkpoint activation owing to p53 induction of the p21 cyclin-dependent kinase inhibitor (CDKI) can lead to a secondary permanent arrest in G0 that is mediated by the CDKI p16 and the retinoblastoma tumour suppressor protein RB. This arrest may also be associated with chromatin changes and widespread gene silencing giving rise to senescent cells characterized by having increased areas of heterochromatin.

In much the same way as apoptosis, the propensity of different cell types and different tumours to undergo senescence is highly variable. Premature senescence occurs frequently in fibroblast cells after irradiation (which do not undergo apoptosis) and likely contributes in part to radiation-induced skin fibrosis. Both premature and replicative senescence also act as potential barriers to cancer development and consequently the pathways that control this process are frequently altered in cancer. However, it would appear that the pathways that control replicative and premature senescence are at least partly distinct since some tumour cells can be induced to undergo radiation-induced senescence although they have clearly acquired mechanisms to prevent replicative senescence. Nonetheless, the two pathways share some common features that may be altered during carcinogenesis. Consequently, there is a wide variation in the ability of cancer cells to initiate senescence after irradiation, depending upon the genetic changes within that individual cancer.

Mitotic catastrophe

Mitotic catastrophe is a term that has evolved over recent years to encompass the type of cell death that results from, or follows, aberrant mitosis. This is morphologically associated with the accumulation of multinucleated, giant cells containing uncondensed chromosomes and with the presence of chromosome aberrations and micronuclei. This process is thought to occur when cells proceed through mitosis in an inappropriate manner owing to entry of cells into mitosis with unrepaired or misrepaired DNA damage. This is frequently the case in cells following irradiation, which often display a host of different types of chromosome aberrations when they enter mitosis. Death, as defined here by the loss of replicative potential, can occur simply from a physical inability to replicate and separate the genetic material correctly, or to the loss of genetic material associated with this process. This is determined in large part by the types of chromosome aberrations that may be present in irradiated cells.

In addition to acting as a mechanism of cell death, mitotic catastrophe can also serve as a trigger for other cell death pathways, independently of the initial damage cause by irradiation. Thus, mitotic catastrophe which results in cell fusion, polyploidy, or failure to perform cytokinesis may subsequently lead to cell death by apoptosis, senescence, autophagy or necrosis. In this case, the attempt to undergo mitosis leads to the activation of the cell death programme, and not the initial DNA damage that was present prior to mitosis (Chu et al., 2004). The important distinction is that cell death is caused by the mitotic catastrophe, rather than as a direct cellular response to the initial DNA damage itself.

Several checkpoints in G2 and throughout mitosis exist to prevent mitotic catastrophe. These include two genetically distinct G2 checkpoints that are activated by the DDR following radiation-induced DNA damage (discussed in Chapter 2). Cells that show defects in checkpoint activation enter into mitosis prematurely and die through mitotic catastrophe. The failure to prevent entry into mitosis is thought to account for much of the enhanced radiosensitivity observed in ATM-deficient cells. Bypass of these checkpoints permits premature entry into mitosis even if the DNA has not been fully replicated or repaired, leading to an enhancement of mitotic catastrophe. Additional mitotic checkpoints ensure proper spindle assembly and attachment prior to cytokinesis. The spindle checkpoint is regulated by a number of different kinases, including the aurora kinases (A, B and C), polo kinases (PLK1, 2 and 3) as well as the

BUB1 and BUBR1 spindle checkpoint kinases. Deregulation of these kinases has been shown to lead to enhanced mitotic catastrophe. Many of the genes involved in the DDR and mitotic checkpoints are altered during cancer and, consequently, the propensity to undergo mitotic catastrophe can also vary significantly among different tumours.

3.3 WHEN AND WHY CELLS DIE AFTER IRRADIATION

The relative importance of the different forms of cell death after irradiation is often debated and is of importance when considering approaches to predicting radiation response (see Chapter 23) or when combining radiation with molecularly targeted agents (see Chapter 21). As outlined above, radiation has been demonstrated, in different cell types and circumstances, to induce all of the different known forms of cell death. Unfortunately, it is not possible to infer the importance of any particular cell death pathway simply by monitoring how a particular cell dies after being irradiated. Multiple cell death pathways may be activated within the same cell, but because a cell can die just once, the type of cell death that is observed will be that which occurs most rapidly and not necessarily that which is most sensitive to activation. For example, just because a cell dies by apoptosis after some given dose of radiation does

not imply that it would not have died by some other pathway if apoptosis had been disabled. In this regard, it is perhaps less important to consider how cells die after irradiation, but rather why cells die after irradiation. For this consideration it is possible to broadly classify cell death mechanisms into two classes: those that occur relatively soon after irradiation and before cell division, and those that occur comparatively late or after division (Fig. 3.1).

Early cell death: pre-mitotic

In a small minority of cell types, cell death occurs rapidly, within several hours after irradiation (Fig. 3.2) (Endlich *et al.*, 2000). This type of death, sometimes referred to as interphase death, is limited primarily to thymocytes, lymphocytes, spermatogonia, and other cells in rapidly proliferating tissues such as those in hair follicles, the small intestine, and in developing embryos. Early cell death is also observed in some types of cancers that arise from these cell types, including lymphomas, and may explain the unexpected effectiveness of radiotherapy protocols used in the treatment of this disease (e.g. two fractions of 2 Gy). In solid tumours, this type of cell death is rarely observed.

Early cell death results primarily from activation of pathways in response to the initial cellular damage caused by irradiation. The best example of this

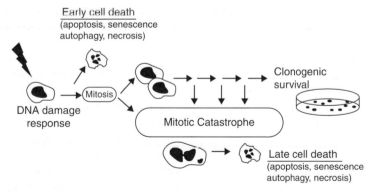

Figure 3.1 Schematic of cell death following irradiation. DNA damage induced by irradiation elicits activation of the DNA damage response (DDR – see Chapter 2), which leads to induction of cell-cycle checkpoints and DNA repair. In certain rare cells this response also induces apoptosis or other forms of cell death. However, in most cases cells die only after attempting mitosis. Remaining or improperly repaired DNA damage causes mitotic catastrophe, which subsequently leads to cell death. Mitotic catastrophe and cell death can take place after the first attempt at cell division, or after several rounds of proliferation. Consequently, this form of cell death is considered late cell death.

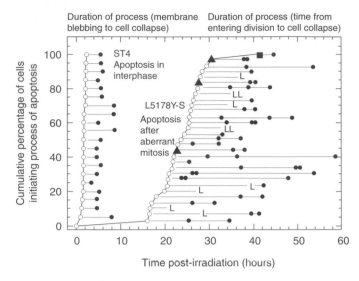

Figure 3.2 Data from Endlich *et al.* (2000) demonstrating early and late forms of cell death. The ST4 lymphoid cells die rapidly by apoptosis before mitosis. L5178Y–S cells also die by apoptosis following irradiation, but only after attempting to complete mitosis. In this case the initial DNA damage response is not sufficient to induce cell death and the cells die because of problems that occur during mitosis.

is the induction of apoptosis that is initiated as part of the DDR. The DDR is activated within minutes of irradiation, and this leads to p53 activation and to the upregulation of pro-apoptotic proteins. Of course, the DDR also induces pro-survival pathways at the same time, including DNA repair pathways and cell-cycle checkpoints. However, in this case these pro-survival pathways are largely irrelevant because apoptosis is initiated regardless of whether repair takes place or not. In this case, activation of apoptosis is a direct result of the initial levels of damage put into the cell. Consequently, for this early form of apoptosis, the genes that regulate this process can significantly influence radiosensitivity. Loss of p53, for example, leads to a defect in apoptosis, loss of the early form of cell death, and an increase in radioresistance.

Early activation of cell death pathways can also occur in certain cell types as a result of damage caused to cellular structures other than the DNA. In endothelial cells that make up blood vessels, relatively high radiation doses (above 15 Gy) have been reported to induce apoptosis as a result of damage to the cellular membrane and the activation of an enzyme known as ceramide synthase (Garcia-Barros *et al.*, 2003). Endothelial cells

contain very high amounts of this enzyme, and as a result after irradiation can produce large amounts of ceramide. As is the case for apoptosis induced by the DDR, ceramide-induced apoptosis results from pathways activated in response to initial damage caused by irradiation and is not sensitive to DNA repair and checkpoint pathways. Thus, for this form of cell death, the gene products that participate in the activation of apoptosis are important determinants of cellular radiosensitivity.

Late cell death: post-mitotic

The vast majority of proliferating normal and tumour cells die at a relatively long time after irradiation, usually after attempting mitosis one or more times (Fig. 3.2). Time-lapse video microscopy has clearly demonstrated that following a transient delay (owing to activation of checkpoints) most cells resume proliferation and progress through the cell cycle one, two or more times before eventually permanently ceasing proliferation (Forrester *et al.*, 1999). This has been known for more than 30 years and gave rise to the initial characterization of radiation-induced cell

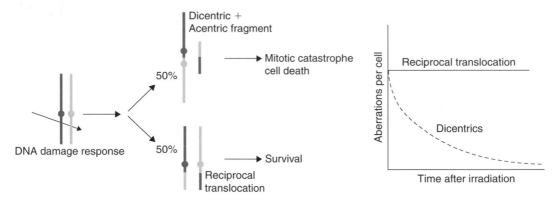

Figure 3.3 This figure, adapted from Brown and Attardi (2005), demonstrates the stochastic nature of cell death after irradiation. The DNA repair processes frequently lead to events in which chromosomes are not repaired correctly. It has been shown that irradiated cells produce approximately equal amounts of reciprocal translocations and dicentrics. The broken chromosomes in these cases are ligated to each other in a random or stochastic manner. Formation of a dicentric chromosome prevents proper mitosis and leads to cell death, whereas a reciprocal translocation that does not involve an important region of the genome is stable (sometimes for many decades). Thus, a population of irradiated cells will have approximately equal numbers of both types of aberrations and over time the cells with dicentrics will be lost owing to mitotic catastrophe-induced death. The initial amount of DNA damage and activation of the DNA damage response is the same in both types of cells but the outcome is very different. The outcome in this case is determined by the ability of the cells to avoid mitotic catastrophe. Adapted by permission from Macmillan Publishers Ltd.

death as reproductive or mitotic cell death. In this case, cell death does not occur until after the cell attempts to divide.

In cells that die at long irradiation times, the DDR activates both cell-cycle checkpoints and DNA repair systems that aid in the survival of the irradiated cells. In these cell types, the DDR is unable to induce apoptosis despite the fact that p53 or other pro-death pathways may be induced. Instead, DNA repair is allowed to take place and can have a large influence on the outcome and radiosensitivity of the cell. Consequently, most proliferating cells from animal models and patients with defects in DNA DSB repair show uniformly large increases in sensitivity to radiation-induced cell death.

Although DNA repair and checkpoint pathways play important roles in determining cell survival, cell death takes place at long times after irradiation takes place at times when the checkpoints are no longer active and when DNA repair processes have largely completed. The halftime for repair is approximately 2–4 hours for end-joining and perhaps somewhat longer from homologous recombination. Thus, only a very small fraction of

the initial DNA damage can be detected at times where cell death occurs. The signal for cell death in this case does not arise from the radiation-induced damage itself, but rather from the consequences of failure to properly complete mitosis. Mitotic catastrophe is therefore considered to be responsible for the majority of cell death in irradiated proliferating cells.

Why does irradiation cause proliferating cells to undergo mitotic catastrophe and cell death? This appears to result from the fact that, although DDR pathways remove much of the initial damage caused by irradiation, they are unable to prevent some cells with DNA breaks or DNA rearrangements from entering mitosis. The consequences of incomplete or improper DNA repair become readily visible as chromosomes condense in metaphase as a series of different types of chromosome aberrations. The fate of cells harbouring chromosome aberrations is largely determined by the nature of the chromosome aberration itself (Fig. 3.3) (Brown and Attardi, 2005). Studies have demonstrated approximately equal numbers of reciprocal translocations and non-reciprocal

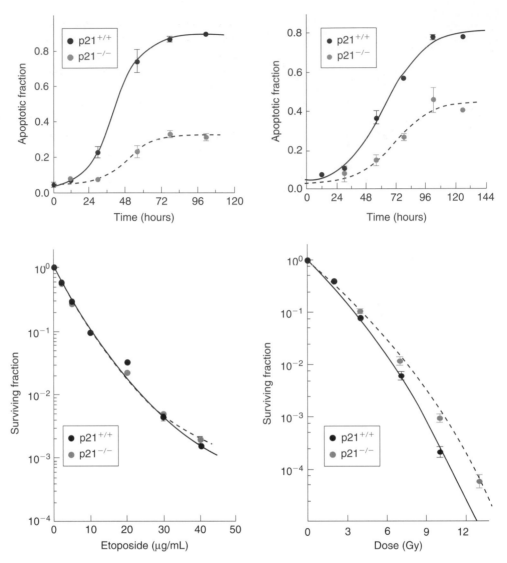

Figure 3.4 This figure, adapted from Wouters *et al.* (1997), demonstrates the discordance between assays of cell death and cell survival. The two cell lines differ only in the expression of the p21 cyclin-dependent kinase gene (*CDKN1A*). The p21 knockout cells show increased apoptosis after etoposide or irradiation (top panels) compared with the p21 wild-type cells. However, when assessed by clonogenic survival the p21 knockouts show a similar sensitivity to etoposide and a slight resistance to irradiation compared with the p21 wild-type cells. Here, apoptosis takes place after mitotic catastrophe and is just one mode of cell death that contributes to the loss of clonogenicity. Adapted with permission of American Association for Cancer Research.

translocations (a dicentric chromosome + acentric fragment) are formed after irradiation. Both of these types of aberrations result from misrepair in which chromosome ends are incorrectly ligated together in a largely stochastic process. However, whereas cells with dicentric and acentric fragments all die, those with reciprocal translocations often survive. The presence of two centromeres in dicentric chromosomes prevents their separation at metaphase, and consequently leads to mitotic catastrophe and eventually cell death. Some cells with dicentric chromosomes may manage to complete mitosis; however, loss of genetic material present in the acentric fragment (which forms a so-called

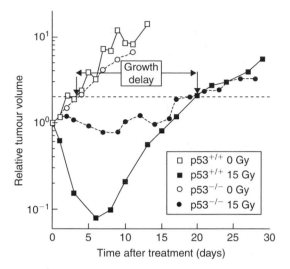

Figure 3.5 Although the mode of cell death may not affect the overall number of cells that die, it can dramatically affect the timing of their death. In this tumour regrowth experiment (from Brown and Wouters, 1999), tumours composed of p53 wild-type and knockout cells are irradiated and followed as a function of time. The unirradiated tumours grow at a similar rate. However, the p53 wild-type tumours undergo rapid apoptosis after irradiation and the tumours thus also shrink rapidly in size. The p53 knockout tumours do not undergo apoptosis and thus are considerably larger after irradiation during this first week. However, the total regrowth delay (measured when tumours reach twice their starting size) is identical for the two tumour types. This indicates that the total number of cells killed by irradiation is the same in both tumour types. In this case apoptosis alters the speed at which the cells die, but does not affect the total number of initially irradiated cells that will eventually die. Adapted with permission of American Association for Cancer Research.

micronuclei) in subsequent mitosis may lead to subsequent death later. This explains the good correlation that has been observed between the formation of dicentric chromosomes or micronuclei formation and cell survival. Reciprocal translocations do not cause problems at metaphase, and thus do not cause mitotic catastrophe or cell death. In fact, these types of aberrations can be found in cells from people exposed to irradiation many years later.

As mentioned previously, cells that experience mitotic catastrophe may ultimately undergo a secondary form of programmed cell death such as apoptosis, autophagy, necrosis or senescence. In this case this secondary form of death is not the cause, but simply the method through which cells die. This has led to a great deal of confusion about the importance of various forms of cell death, such as apoptosis, as determinants of radiosensitivity. Whereas activation of apoptosis and other programmed cell death programmes are responsible for why cells die at early times after irradiation, they are not similarly responsible for why cells die at long times after irradiation. As a result, alteration of a particular gene may dramatically alter the levels of radiation-induced apoptosis, without altering the overall ability of the cell to survive (Wouters *et al.*, 1997). In this case, cells are dying as the result of undergoing mitotic catastrophe and will die regardless of whether apoptosis is subsequently induced (Fig. 3.4).

Although apoptosis or other programmed cell death pathways may not affect overall survival after irradiation, they can dramatically influence the rate at which cells die and thus the early response of tumours to treatment (Brown and Wouters, 1999). Because apoptosis leads to rapid and complete destruction of the cell, tumours containing cells capable of undergoing apoptosis after mitotic catastrophe may shrink much faster than a similar tumour consisting of cells with the same overall radiosensitivity that do not similarly undergo apoptosis. For this reason, it is dangerous to draw any conclusions about tumour radiosensitivity from initial changes in tumour size after treatment (Fig. 3.5).

Time-lapse microscopy studies have demonstrated that, in cells which experience mitotic catastrophe, both the timing and nature of cell death is highly variable (Fig. 3.6) (Endlich *et al.*, 2000). As discussed earlier, a surviving cell is considered as one that can proliferate indefinitely. In tissue culture this is quantified by the ability to form a colony of a certain size after irradiation (usually 50 cells). Conversely, cell death in this context means that eventually all progeny of an irradiated cell will die. An irradiated cell that is destined to die (not produce a colony) may, however, still proceed through mitosis many times. The resulting daughter cells can die at very different times after irradiation. For example, following the first mitosis, one of the cells may die and the other may proceed through DNA

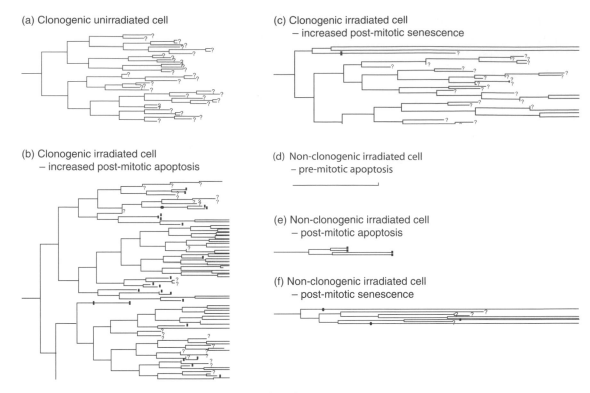

(a) Clonogenic unirradiated cell

(c) Clonogenic irradiated cell
– increased post-mitotic senescence

(b) Clonogenic irradiated cell
– increased post-mitotic apoptosis

(d) Non-clonogenic irradiated cell
– pre-mitotic apoptosis

(e) Non-clonogenic irradiated cell
– post-mitotic apoptosis

(f) Non-clonogenic irradiated cell
– post-mitotic senescence

Figure 3.6 This figure, adapted from Forrester *et al.* (1999), tracks the fate of several irradiated cells as a function of time (left to right) following exposure to radiation. (a) An unirradiated cell is shown as an example. Each cell division is indicated by a split of one line into two. After six or seven divisions enough cell progeny have been created to produce a colony that can be scored as a survivor. The initial cell is thus said to be clonogenic. Two cells that survive irradiation and eventually form colonies are shown in (b) and (c). In (b), the first division produces two daughter cells that both progress to mitosis and divide producing four cells. One of these four cells dies by apoptosis. Another one undergoes several more divisions but produces progeny that all eventually die. The other two cells both produce many surviving progeny that contribute to the long-term clonogenic potential of the initially irradiated cell. Note, that many of the progeny die in this case even though the initial cell has 'survived'. In (c) the irradiated cell is also clonogenic. In this case, one of the first two daughter cells produces cells which all eventually undergo senescence. Irradiated cells that are non-clonogenic are shown in (d), (e) and (f). In (d), a cell dies by apoptosis before mitosis. In (e) cells die by apoptosis after completing two divisions and in (e) cells undergo senescence after undergoing one or more mitoses. Adapted with permission of American Association for Cancer Research.

replication and mitosis to produce two more cells. Eventually, these cells will also die, although they may or may not attempt mitosis many times. Furthermore, the type of cell death that each daughter cell undergoes can be different. Consequently, a single irradiated cell can actually die through multiple modes of cell death! A similar situation also exists for irradiated cells that are destined to survive. These cells may also produce daughter cells with different survival potential. One daughter may die, while the other continues to proliferate and thus confers the status of 'survived' on the initially irradiated cell. Consequently, irradiated cells that die following cell division produce a pedigree of cells with different types that can only be tracked by time-lapse microscopy (Forrester *et al.*, 1999). Examples of cells destined for survival or death are shown in Fig. 3.6. This figure highlights the many problems associated with trying to quantify or ascribe a particular form of cell death after irradiation and the importance of the clonogenic survival assay for determining the ultimate response of individually irradiated cells.

'Bystander' death

A much less understood type of cell death that has been described in response to irradiation is known as bystander-induced death (Mothersill and Seymour, 2004). A number of experiments have challenged the widely held view that radiation kills cells exclusively by direct damage. The bystander effect describes a phenomenon in which cell death can occur in cells owing to irradiation of neighbouring cells. Evidence for this effect has come from studies using high linear energy transfer (LET) α-particles in which a larger fraction of cells die than are estimated to have been traversed. Supportive data have also been generated using microbeam irradiation, in which select cells or nuclei can be irradiated with particles (both α-particles and protons have been used) or soft X-rays. In these experiments, irradiation of a select group of cells leads to increased cell death in the unirradiated cells. In addition to cell death, bystander effects have also been observed for other known biological effects of irradiation, including DNA damage, chromosomal aberrations, mutation, transformation and gene expression.

The precise mechanism or importance of bystander effects has not yet been determined. Some studies have shown that transfer of media from irradiated cells to unirradiated cells can also cause the bystander effect. This would suggest that irradiated cells secrete factors that can be damaging to unirradiated cells. Other experiments have shown that bystander effects are more easily observed when cells are physically connected to irradiated cells by gap-junctions. This allows communication (transfer or molecules) directly between the cells. For example, irradiation may result in increased levels of long-lived reactive oxygen species that could be shared among irradiated and unirradiated cells. The bystander effect is probably most important at low doses of radiation which cause damage to only a small number of cells, and may thus be of most relevance to risk estimation.

> ## Key points
>
> 1. Most cell death is controlled or programmed in some way.
> 2. Major death pathways include apoptosis, senescence, autophagy and necrosis.
> 3. Measuring one form of cell death (e.g. apoptosis) will not necessarily correlate with how many cells die.
> 4. The form of cell death may influence the rate at which cells die and thus tumour regression.
> 5. Most cell death after radiation occurs late in response to mitotic catastrophe and not from the initial response to damage.

■ BIBLIOGRAPHY

Brown JM, Attardi LD (2005). The role of apoptosis in cancer development and treatment response. *Nat Rev Cancer* **5**: 231–7.

Brown JM, Wouters BG (1999). Apoptosis, p53, and tumor cell sensitivity to anticancer agents. *Cancer Res* **59**: 1391–9.

Campisi J, d'Adda di Fagagna F (2007). Cellular senescence: when bad things happen to good cells. *Nat Rev Mol Cell Biol* **8**: 729–40.

Chu K, Teele N, Dewey MW, Albright N, Dewey WC (2004). Computerized video time lapse study of cell cycle delay and arrest, mitotic catastrophe, apoptosis and clonogenic survival in irradiated 14-3-3sigma and CDKN1A (p21) knockout cell lines. *Radiat Res* **162**: 270–86.

Endlich B, Radford IR, Forrester HB, Dewey WC (2000). Computerized video time-lapse microscopy studies of ionizing radiation-induced rapid-interphase and mitosis-related apoptosis in lymphoid cells. *Radiat Res* **153**: 36–48.

Forrester HB, Vidair CA, Albright N, Ling CC, Dewey WC (1999). Using computerized video time lapse for quantifying cell death of X-irradiated rat embryo cells transfected with c-myc or c-Ha-ras. *Cancer Res* **59**: 931–9.

Garcia-Barros M, Paris F, Cordon-Cardo C *et al.* (2003). Tumor response to radiotherapy regulated by endothelial cell apoptosis. *Science* **300**: 1155–9.

Hayflick L (1965). The limited *in vitro* lifetime of human diploid cell strains. *Exp Cell Res* **37**: 614–36.

Klionsky DJ (2007). Autophagy: from phenomenology to molecular understanding in less than a decade. *Nat Rev Mol Cell Biol* **8**: 931–7.

Mothersill C, Seymour CB (2004). Radiation-induced bystander effects – implications for cancer. *Nat Rev Cancer* **4**: 158–64.

Okada H, Mak TW (2004). Pathways of apoptotic and non-apoptotic death in tumour cells. *Nat Rev Cancer* **4**: 592–603.

Rubinsztein DC, Gestwicki JE, Murphy LO, Klionsky DJ (2007). Potential therapeutic applications of autophagy. *Nat Rev Drug Discov* **6**: 304–12.

Taylor RC, Cullen SP, Martin SJ (2008). Apoptosis: controlled demolition at the cellular level. *Nat Rev Mol Cell Biol* **9**: 231–41.

Wouters BG, Giaccia AJ, Denko NC, Brown JM (1997). Loss of p21Waf1/Cip1 sensitizes tumors to radiation by an apoptosis-independent mechanism. *Cancer Res* **57**: 4703–6.

■ FURTHER READING

Steel GG (2001). The case against apoptosis. *Acta Oncol* **40**: 968–75.

Quantifying cell kill and cell survival

MICHAEL C. JOINER

4.1 CONCEPT OF CLONOGENIC CELLS

As explained in Chapter 13, Section 13.2, the maintenance of tissue size and therefore of tissue function in the normal renewal tissues of the body depends upon the existence of a small number of primitive 'stem cells' – cells that have the capacity to maintain their numbers while at the same time producing cells that can differentiate and proliferate to replace the rest of the functional cell population. Stem cells are at the base of the hierarchy of cells that make up the epithelial and haemopoietic tissues.

Carcinomas are derived from such hierarchical tissues, and our ability to recognize this in histological sections derives from the fact that these tumours often maintain many of the features of differentiation of the tissue within which they arose. Well-differentiated tumours do this to a greater extent than anaplastic tumours. It follows that not all the cells in a tumour are neoplastic stem cells: some have embarked on an irreversible process of differentiation. In addition, carcinomas contain many cells that make up the stroma (fibroblasts, endothelial cells, macrophages, etc.). Stem cells thus may constitute only a small proportion of the cells within a tumour.

When a tumour regrows after non-curative treatment, it does so because some neoplastic stem cells were not killed. Radiobiologists have therefore recognized that the key to understanding tumour response is to ask: How many stem cells are left? (if we can eradicate the last neoplastic stem cell then the tumour cannot regrow). It is almost impossible to recognize tumour stem cells *in situ*, and therefore assays have been developed that allow them to be detected after removal from the tumour. These assays generally detect stem cells by their ability to form a colony within some growth environment. We therefore call these 'clonogenic' or 'colony-forming' cells – cells that form colonies exceeding about 50 cells within a defined growth environment. The number 50 represents five or six generations of proliferation. It is chosen in order to exclude cells that have a limited growth potential as a result of having embarked on differentiation, or having been sublethally damaged by therapeutic treatment.

After exposure to radiation, damaged cells do not die immediately and they may produce a modest family of descendants. This is illustrated in Fig. 4.1. The growth of single mouse L-cells was observed under the microscope and one selected colony was irradiated with 200 röntgens of X-rays at the four-cell stage (Trott, 1972). The röntgen is an old radiation unit, roughly equivalent to 1 cGy. Subsequent growth was carefully recorded and in the figure each vertical line indicates the lifetime of a cell from birth at mitosis to its subsequent division. The two irradiated cells on the left and the right of this figure produced continuously expanding colonies, although some daughter cells had long intermitotic times. The other two irradiated cells fared badly: they underwent a number of irregular divisions, including a tripolar mitosis. But note that at the end of the experiment cells are present from each of the original four cells: the difference is that two produced expanding colonies and the other two did not. The first two were 'surviving clonogenic cells' and the other two are usually described as 'killed' by radiation, since their regrowth is probably unimportant for clinical outcome. It would be more precise to say that two of the cells lost their proliferative ability as a result of irradiation.

Some cells fail to undergo even one division after irradiation. Interphase cell death occurs in many cell types at very high radiation doses, and at conventional therapeutic dose levels it is characteristic of lymphoid cells and some cells in the intestinal crypts. Although interphase cell death and apoptosis are related concepts (see Chapter 3, Section 3.3) they are not synonymous for the same process. But the conventional radiobiological view is that it is loss of reproductive integrity that is the critical response to irradiation (either in tumour or normal-tissue cells): this occurs within a few hours of irradiation through damage to the genome, and the subsequent metabolic and death processes are 'downstream' of this event.

4.2 CLONOGENIC ASSAYS

Clonogenic assays have formed the basis of cellular response studies in tumours, and in some normal tissues. The basic idea is to remove cells from the tumour, place them in a defined growth environment and test for their ability to produce a sizeable colony of descendants. Many types of assay have been described; we illustrate the principle by a simple assay in tissue culture that is analogous to a microbiological assay.

A single-cell suspension of tumour cells is prepared and divided into two parts. One part is irradiated, the other kept as an unirradiated control. The two suspensions are then plated out in tissue culture under identical conditions, except that since we anticipate that radiation has killed some cells we will have to plate a larger number of the irradiated cells. We here envisage plating 100 control cells and 400 irradiated cells. After a suitable period of incubation the colonies are scored (Fig. 4.2). There are 20 control colonies, and we therefore say that the plating efficiency was $20/100 = 0.2$. The plating efficiency of the treated cells is lower: $8/400 = 0.02$. We calculate a surviving fraction as the ratio of these plating efficiencies:

$$\text{Surviving fraction} = \frac{\text{PE}_{\text{treated}}}{\text{PE}_{\text{control}}} = \frac{0.02}{0.2} = 0.1$$

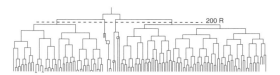

Figure 4.1 Pedigree of a clone of mouse L-cells irradiated with a dose of 200 R (i.e. röntgens) at the four-cell stage, illustrating the concept of surviving and non-surviving clonogenic cells. From Trott (1972), with permission.

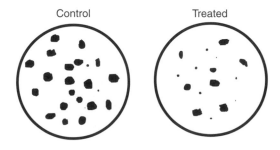

Figure 4.2 Illustrating the principle of measuring a cell surviving fraction.

thus correcting for the efficiency with which undamaged clonogenic cells are detected and for the different numbers of cells plated. Surviving fraction is often given as a percentage (10 per cent in this case).

The above description started with a suspension of tumour cells. In order to measure *in vivo* cell survival we take two groups of experimental tumours (often subcutaneously implanted tumours in mice), irradiate one and keep the other as a control; then, some time after irradiation, we make cell suspensions from both groups and plate them out under identical conditions as before. The difference here is that the cells are irradiated under *in vivo* conditions.

Although colony assays have formed a central place in tumour radiobiology they are not without artefacts. Bearing in mind that the numbers of cells plated will often differ between control and treated cultures, a key question is whether colony counts increase linearly with the number of cells plated. If they do not, then this will lead to errors in cell survival. The colonies in Fig. 4.2 have been drawn to illustrate a feature of colony assays that was mentioned in the previous section. Irradiation

not only reduces the colony numbers, it also increases the number of small colonies. Some of these small colonies may represent clones that eventually die out; others may arise from cells that have suffered non-lethal injury that reduces colony growth rate. Unless they reach the accepted cut-off of 50 cells they will not be counted, although their implications for the evaluation of radiation effects on tumours may be worthy of greater attention (Seymour and Mothersill, 1989).

4.3 CELL SURVIVAL CURVES

A cell survival curve is a plot of surviving fraction against dose (of radiation, cytotoxic drug or other cell-killing agent). Figure 4.3a shows that when plotted on linear scales the survival curve for cells irradiated in tissue culture is often sigmoid: there is a shoulder followed by a curve that asymptotically approaches zero survival. To indicate the sensitivity of the cells to radiation we could just read off the dose that kills say 50 per cent of the cells. This is sometimes called the ED_{50} (i.e. effect dose 50 per cent). Sometimes ED_{90} is used. In doing

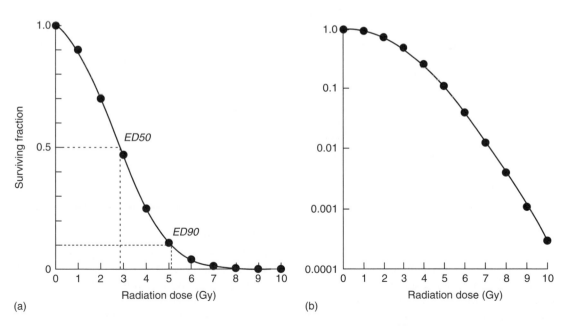

(a)

(b)

Figure 4.3 A typical cell survival curve for cells irradiated in tissue culture, plotted (a) on a linear survival scale. (b) The same data plotted on a logarithmic scale.

this we need make no assumptions about the shape of the curve.

There are two reasons why cell survival curves are more usually plotted on a logarithmic scale of survival:

1. If cell killing is random then survival will be an exponential function of dose, and this will be a straight line on a semi-log plot. Section 4.8 explains this in detail.
2. A logarithmic scale more easily allows us to see and compare the very low cell survivals required to obtain a significant reduction in tumour size, or local tumour control.

Such a plot is illustrated in Fig. 4.3b. The shapes of radiation survival curves and ways of describing their steepness are dealt with later in this chapter.

Note that, for the data shown in Fig. 4.3, radiation doses above 5 Gy reduce the survival of clonogenic cells to below 10 per cent. Measurement of radiosensitivity in terms of the parameter D_0 (see Section 4.8) is made on the exponential part of the survival curve, which in this case is above 5 Gy. These measurements are therefore made in a dose range where the surviving fraction is very low. Such D_0 values are relevant to the problem of exterminating the last few clonogenic cells, but if the cell population contains cells of differing radiosensitivity these values may not be typical of the radiosensitivity of the bulk of the tumour cell population.

4.4 ASSAYS FOR THE SURVIVAL OF CLONOGENIC CELLS

Many techniques have been described for detecting colony formation by tumour cells and thus for measuring cell survival. They almost all require first the production of single-cell suspensions. This is usually not straightforward, because tumour tissues differ widely in the ease with which they can be disaggregated. Enzymes such as trypsin, collagenase and pronase are often used and some tissues can be disaggregated mechanically.

Such techniques can also be used for the assay of colony-forming cells in normal tissues, especially the haemopoietic tissues that can easily be sampled and made into cell suspensions. In addition, a variety of *in situ* assays for normal-tissue

stem cells have been described (Potten, 1983). The following are some of the principal assays that have been used for tumour cells.

In vitro colony assays

Some tumour cells grow well attached to plastic tissue culture dishes or flasks. Others can be encouraged to do so by first laying down a feeder layer of lethally irradiated connective-tissue or tumour cells. For cells that have been established as an *in vitro* cell line this often works well but for studies on tumour samples taken directly from patients or animals it is commonly observed that normal-tissue fibroblasts grow better than the tumour cells and overgrow the cultures.

An alternative is to thicken the growth medium with agar or methylcellulose. This inhibits the growth of anchorage-requiring cell types, but many epithelial cells will still grow. A widely used assay of this type is that of Courtenay and Mills (1978) for human tumour cells. Agar cultures are grown in 15-mL plastic tubes overlaid with liquid medium that can regularly be replenished. The addition of rat red blood cells to the agar was found to promote the growth of a number of human tumour cell types. An important feature of the Courtenay–Mills assay was the use of a low oxygen tension (a gas phase of 90 per cent nitrogen, 5 per cent oxygen and 5 per cent carbon dioxide), which enhanced the plating efficiency of human tumour cells.

Spleen colony assay

Till and McCulloch (1961) showed that, when mouse bone marrow cells were injected intravenously into syngeneic recipients that had received sufficient whole-body irradiation to suppress endogenous haemopoiesis, colonies were produced in the spleen which derived from the stem cells in the graft. The colonies varied in morphology (erythroid, granulocyte or mixed) and these stem cells are therefore termed pluripotent. Their precise identity was not known and they are therefore often called colony-forming units (CFUs). Using this assay, Till and McCulloch obtained the first survival curve for bone marrow cells and found it to be very steep. The spleen colony assay has also been used for some types of mouse lymphoma cells.

Lung colony assay

This is analogous to the spleen colony assay and is applicable to any transplanted mouse tumour that readily forms colonies in the lung following intra-venous injection of a single-cell suspension. The cloning efficiency can often be increased by mixing the test cells with an excess (c. 10^6 per injection) of lethally irradiated tumour cells or plastic micro-spheres, which perhaps act by increasing the trap-ping of injected tumour cells in the lung. Not all the tumour cells grow: a few colonies per thousand tumour cells injected would be regarded as satis-factory. Although colonies are formed throughout the lung, they are usually scored only on the lung surface. The method was developed by Hill and Stanley (1975) on two experimental tumours and they give further experimental details.

Limiting-dilution assay

This is a non-cloning assay that was used in early radiation cell survival studies and which for some experimental tumours has the advantage of high sensitivity. The principle of the method is to pre-pare a suspension of tumour cells and to make a large number of subcutaneous implants into syn-geneic animals, covering a range of inoculum sizes and if possible spanning the level of 50 per cent tumour takes. The animals, usually mice, are then observed for a long enough period to record nearly every tumour that can grow from a single-cell implant. Take-rate is plotted against inoculum size and the point of 50 per cent takes is interpo-lated; this is usually called the 'TD$_{50}$' cell number. The experiment is performed simultaneously on treated cells and control cells and the surviving fraction is given by the ratio of the TD$_{50}$ values. The addition of an excess of lethally irradiated cells improves the take-rate; using this manoeuvre Steel and Adams (1975) found a TD$_{50}$ of 1–3 cells for the Lewis lung tumour and were thus able to

measure cell survival down to 10^{-6}. The method only works well in the absence of an immune response against the tumour grafts, which is a rel-atively uncommon situation especially with chem-ically and virally induced tumours.

Short-term *in vitro* assays

The need to develop *in vitro* assays that yield a quicker result than a true clonogenic assay arises from the interest in prediction of tumour response to treatment (see Chapter 23). A variety of assays have been proposed but their reliability and reproducibility have often been a limit to their clinical usefulness. Three common pitfalls are:

1. Biopsy samples of human tumours contain both tumour cells and normal connective tis-sue cells; both may grow under the assay condi-tions and it may be difficult to distinguish colony formation by tumour cells.
2. If the method requires the production of sin-gle-cell suspensions, great care must be taken to exclude cell clumps, as these may preferen-tially give rise to scorable colonies.
3. Radiation-killed cells take time to die (e.g. Fig. 4.1) and in a short-term assay they may be con-fused with genuine surviving tumour cells; therefore, the method may not easily distin-guish between radiosensitive cells and cells that die rapidly after irradiation.

Many basic principles underlying the predic-tion of tumour response are dealt with in the book edited by Chapman *et al.* (1989). Non-clonogenic assays for tumour cells include the following.

THE MICRONUCLEUS TEST

Tumour cells are cultured in the presence of cytochalasin-B, which blocks cytokinesis, creates binucleate cells, and thus allows nuclei that have undergone one post-treatment division to be identified. Micronuclei can be scored as small extranuclear bodies. Their frequency increases with radiation dose and gives a measure of radia-tion sensitivity (Streffer *et al.*, 1986). The reliabil-ity of the method is limited by the fact that diploid, polyploid and aneuploid cells may differ in their tolerance of genetic loss and therefore of micronucleus formation.

CELL GROWTH ASSAYS

A variety of methods have been used to measure the growth of cultures derived from treated and control tumour specimens, and thus to derive a measure of radiosensitivity or chemosensitivity. Incorporation of radioisotopes such as ^{3}H-thymidine has been widely used. A tetrazolium salt, 3-(4,5 dimethylthiazol-2-yl)-2,5-diphenyl tetrazolium bromide (MTT), is used to stain cell cultures and thus by a colorimetric assay to estimate the extent of growth (Carmichael et al., 1987; Wasserman and Twentyman, 1988). It can be used to evaluate growth in microtitre plates and with careful attention to technical factors it can yield a measure of radiosensitivity. The reagent 3-(4,5-dimethylthiazol-2-yl)-5-(3-carboxymethoxyphenyl)-2-(4-sulfophenyl)-2H-tetrazolium (MTS) is a development of MTT and forms soluble formazans upon bioreduction by the cells. This has the advantage that it eliminates the error-prone solubilization step which is required for the microculture tetrazolium assays which employ MTT (Goodwin et al., 1995). Such methods are vulnerable to the variable growth of fibroblasts, and for studies on leukaemic cells it may be preferable to stain the cells differentially and analyse the cultures microscopically (Bosanquet, 1991).

DNA DAMAGE ASSAYS

It is possible to measure DNA damage directly by antibody detection of foci of phosphorylated histone H2AX (γH2AX) in the cell nucleus, using image cytometry or flow cytometry. It has been found that the rate of γH2AX loss (a measure of DNA repair) correlates with cellular radiosensitivity measured with a clonogenic assay, although the relationship is by no means perfect (MacPhail et al., 2003). Moreover, the percentage of tumour cells that retain γH2AX foci 24 hours after single or fractionated doses of radiation appears to be an indicator of cellular radiosensitivity that might be useful in the clinic (Klokov et al., 2006).

Methods using precise cell counting

The methods described so far involve the plating of an aliquot of a cell suspension that on average will contain a known number of cells. The actual number of cells will vary according to Poisson statistics. For studies of the effects of low radiation doses (where the effects are small) greater statistical precision can be achieved by knowing exactly how many cells have been plated. This has been done using two main methods (see Section 4.14). A fluorescence-activated cell sorter (FACS) allows counted numbers of cells to be plated into culture dishes (Durand, 1986). An alternative is to use a microscopic live cell recognition system (Marples and Joiner, 1993), which allows the spatial coordinates of plated cells to be recorded; subsequently the colony formation by each individual cell can be examined. Both of these methods give high precision in the initial region of a cell survival curve and their use led to the identification of low-dose hyper-radiosensitivity (HRS) (see Section 4.14).

4.5 COMPARISON OF ASSAYS

Intercomparison of the results of assays of cell survival can provide an important check on their validity. This information can be valuable at both a practical and a fundamental level. At the practical level, it is logical to check a rapid short-term assay against the results of a more laborious but more reliable clonogenic assay. The more general question is whether assay of cell survival in two different growth environments does actually identify the same population of surviving tumour cells. It is usually cell survival in situ in the patient or in the experimental animal that we seek to determine, and to subject tumour cells to extraction procedures and to artificial growth environments might well produce artefacts. It is therefore reassuring that some careful comparisons between clonogenic assays in vitro, in the mouse lung and by subcutaneous transplantation have demonstrated good agreement for mouse tumours (Steel and Stephens, 1983).

4.6 DESCRIBING RELATIONSHIPS BETWEEN CELL SURVIVAL AND RADIATION DOSE

Research in experimental radiobiology covers studies at the cellular, animal and human levels. It deals at the fundamental level with the molecular, biochemical and biophysical nature of radiation damage. Descriptive models are a necessary part of radiobiology research: they provide a framework in which to analyse and compare data and ultimately to assist in building up consistent theories of radiation action both *in vitro* and *in vivo*. Models and mathematics are also sometimes necessary to relate experimental studies to clinical cancer treatment with the aim of improving therapy. In the following sections, we explain the most important models that are used to describe and analyse the relationship between cell survival and radiation dose.

4.7 A NOTE ON RADIATION RESPONSE AT THE MOLECULAR LEVEL

Radiation kills cells by producing secondary charged particles and free radicals in the nucleus which in turn produce a variety of types of damage in DNA. Evidence that damage to DNA is the primary cause of cell killing and mutation by radiation is set out in Chapter 2, Section 2.1. Each 1 Gy dose of low-linear energy transfer (LET) radiation produces over 1000 base damages, about 1000 initial single-strand breaks and approximately 20–40 initial double-strand breaks (DSBs). Some lesions are more important than others and radiation lethality correlates most significantly with the number of residual, unrepaired DSBs several hours after irradiation. If cell kill is modified by changing LET, oxygen level, thiol concentration or temperature, then for a fixed radiation dose only the number of DSBs reliably correlates with the change in cell kill. Single-strand breaks, base damage and DNA–protein crosslinks do not reflect the change in cell kill for all of these modifiers. The DNA DSB is therefore thought to be the most important type of cellular damage. Just one residual DSB (or 'hit') in a vital section of DNA may be sufficient to produce a significant chromosome aberration and thus to sterilize the cell.

4.8 TARGET THEORY

A simple way of picturing how radiation might kill cells is the idea that there may be specific regions of the DNA that are important to maintain the reproductive ability of cells. These sensitive regions could be thought of as specific targets for radiation damage so that the survival of a cell after radiation exposure would be related to the number of targets inactivated. There are two versions of this idea that have commonly been used. The first version of the theory proposed that just one hit by radiation on a single sensitive target would lead to death of the cell. This is called single-target single-hit inactivation, and it leads to the form of survival curve shown in Fig. 4.4a. The survival curve is exponential (i.e. a straight line in a semi-logarithmic plot of cell survival against dose). To derive an equation for this survival curve, Poisson statistics can be applied. The presumption is that during irradiation there are a very large number of hits on different cells taking place, but the probability (p) of the next hit occurring in a given cell is very small. Thus for each cell,

$$p(\text{survival}) = p(0 \text{ hits}) = \exp(-D/D_0)$$

where D_0 is defined as the dose that gives an average of one hit per target. A dose of D_0 Gy reduces survival from 1 to 0.37 (i.e. to e^{-1}), or from 0.1 to 0.037, etc. D/D_0 is the average number of hits per target (and in this case per cell). This is the reason why (as in Fig. 4.7, later) a scale of cell survival is sometimes labelled $-\ln(S)$: this is a scale of the natural logarithm of surviving fraction and it is also the equivalent number of 'lethal lesions' per cell.

In this example (Fig. 4.4a) $D_0 = 1.6$ Gy. Straight survival curves of this sort are usually found for the inactivation of viruses and bacteria. They may also be appropriate in describing the radiation response of some very sensitive human cells (normal and malignant) and also the radiation response at very low dose rates (see Chapter 12, Section 12.3) and response to high LET radiations (see Chapter 6, Section 6.3). This type of

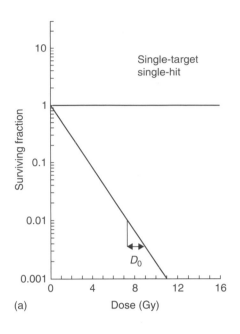

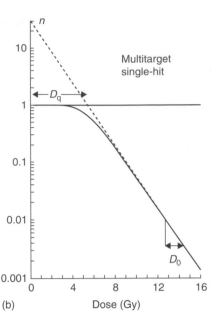

(a)

(b)

Figure 4.4 The two most common types of target theory. (a) Single-target inactivation; (b) multitarget inactivation.

'single-target single-hit' survival curve model is therefore actually valid outside of the 'target theory' framework. It describes the simple situation where if an individual cell receives an amount of radiation greater than D_0 then it will die, otherwise it will survive.

For mammalian cells in general, their response to radiation is usually described by 'shouldered' survival curves. In an attempt to model this type of response, a more general version of target theory was proposed called multitarget single-hit inactivation. In this extended target idea, just one hit by radiation on each of n sensitive targets in the cell is required for death of the cell. The shape of this survival curve is shown in Fig. 4.4b. Again, the argument can be developed using Poisson statistics,

$$p(0 \text{ hits on a specific target}) = \exp(-D/D_0)$$

Thus

$$p(\text{specific target inactivated}) = 1 - \exp(-D/D_0)$$

As there are n targets in the cell,

$$p(\text{all } n \text{ targets inactivated}) = (1 - \exp(-D/D_0))^n$$

Thus

$$p(\text{survival}) = p(\text{not all targets inactivated})$$
$$= 1 - (1 - \exp(-D/D_0))^n \qquad (4.1)$$

Figure 4.4b shows that multitarget single-hit survival curves have a shoulder whose size can be indicated by the quasi-threshold dose (D_q). This is related to n and D_0 by the relation:

$$D_q = D_0 \log_e n \qquad (4.2)$$

For the example in Fig. 4.4b, we have chosen $n = 30$ and $D_0 = 1.6$ Gy, giving $D_q = 5.4$ Gy. Such multitarget survival curves have proved useful for describing the radiation response of mammalian cells at high doses, 'off the shoulder'. They do not describe the survival response well at lower more clinically relevant doses.

4.9 THE PROBLEM WITH TARGETS

The derivation of simple cell survival relationships in terms of targets and hits, particularly the straight survival curve shown in Fig. 4.4a, is an intellectually attractive idea and it dominated radiobiological thinking for a long time. The term 'D_0' is still in common usage. The key difficulty with this concept is

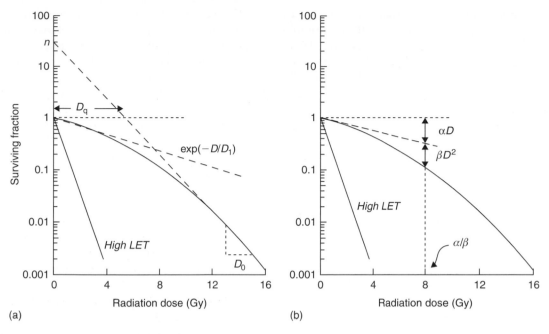

Figure 4.5 Models with non-exponential cell killing but a finite initial slope. (a) The two-component model and (b) the linear-quadratic model.

that so far the specific radiation targets have not been identified for mammalian cells, despite considerable effort to search for them. Rather, what has emerged is the key role of DNA strand breaks and their repair, with sites for such DNA damage being generally dispersed throughout the cell nucleus (see Chapter 2). An obvious shortcoming of the multitarget model is that, as shown in Fig. 4.4b, it predicts a response that is flat for very low radiation doses. This is not supported by experimental data: there is overwhelming evidence for significant cell killing at low doses and for cell survival curves that have a finite initial slope. To take account of this, the multitarget model was adjusted by adding an additional single-target component. The resulting equation for the survival curve is called the two-component model:

$$p(\text{survival}) = \exp(-D/D_1)$$
$$(1 - (1 - \exp(-D(1/D_0 - 1/D_1)))^n)$$

$$(4.3)$$

This type of survival curve is illustrated in Fig. 4.5a. In addition to the parameters n, D_0 and D_q, this curve also has a parameter D_1, which fixes an initial

slope (i.e. the dose required in the low-dose region to reduce survival from 1 to 0.37). In this example, $n = 30$ and $D_0 = 1.6\,\text{Gy}$, and $D_1 = 4.6\,\text{Gy}$. This type of curve now correctly predicts finite cell killing in the low-dose region but it still has the drawback that the change in cell survival over the range 0 to D_q occurs almost linearly. This implies that no sparing of damage should occur as dose per fraction is reduced below 2 Gy, which is usually not found to be the case either experimentally or in clinical radiotherapy (see Chapter 8, Figs 8.1 and 8.2; Chapter 10, Section 10.3). A way of overcoming this limitation would be to use a multitarget instead of single-target component as the initial slope. However, this would make the model far too complicated to be of much use in comparing survival responses. It would require at least four parameters, and would be of little value in helping to understand the fundamental mechanisms determining radiation effect.

4.10 THE LINEAR-QUADRATIC MODEL

The continually downward bending form of a cell survival can simply be fitted by a second-order polynomial, with a zero constant term to ensure that SF = 1 at zero dose. This is exactly the formulation that is termed the linear-quadratic (LQ) model. Although we can regard this as based on pure mathematics (i.e. the simplest formula which describes a curve), it has also been possible to attach radiobiological mechanisms to this model. The formula for cell survival is:

$$-\ln(S) = \alpha D + \beta D^2$$

$$p(\text{survival}) = \exp(-\alpha D - \beta D^2) \qquad (4.4)$$

and the cell survival curve is drawn in Fig. 4.5b. Although the shapes of the LQ model and the complicated two-component model are superficially similar (compare Fig. 4.5a with Fig. 4.5b), the simple LQ formula gives a better description of radiation response in the low-dose region (0–3 Gy): LQ survival curves are continuously bending with no straight portion either at low or high radiation doses. The shape (or 'bendiness') is determined by the ratio α/β.

Since the dimensions of the parameters for α are Gy^{-1} and for β are Gy^{-2}, the dimensions of α/β are Gy; as shown in Fig. 4.5b, this is the dose at which the linear contribution to damage (αD on the logarithmic scale) equals the quadratic contribution (βD^2). The response of cells to densely-ionizing radiations such as neutrons or α-particles is usually a steep and almost exponential survival curve (see Fig. 6.2). As shown in Fig. 4.5, this would be explained in the two-component model by the ratio D_1/D_0 being near to 1.0, or in the LQ model by a very high α/β ratio.

As shown in Fig. 4.5, the LQ model does not have a D_0 because the survival curve continuously bends downwards with increasing dose and so it is never completely straight. However, it is sometimes useful to be able to roughly convert between α, β and D_0; for example, if comparing two sets of research findings which have each been described with the different models. The precise mathematical description of D_0 is that it is the inverse of the first-order differential of $-\ln(S)$ with respect to dose. Applying this definition to the LQ model gives $D_0 = 1/(\alpha + 2\beta D)$. This formula shows that, in the LQ model, the effective D_0 is not constant, but decreases with increasing dose.

The LQ model is now in widespread use in both experimental and clinical radiobiology and generally works well in describing responses to radiation *in vitro* and *in vivo*. What could be its mechanistic justification? One simple idea is that the linear component [$\exp(-\alpha D)$] might result from single-track events while the quadratic component [$\exp(-\beta D^2)$] might arise from two-track events. This interpretation is supported by studies of the dose-rate effect (see Chapter 12, Section 12.3), which shows that as dose rate is reduced cell survival curves become straight and tend to extrapolate the initial slope of the high dose-rate curve: the quadratic component of cell killing disappears, leaving only the linear component. This would be expected, since at low dose rate single-track events will occur far apart in time and the probability of interaction between them will be low. Although this interpretation of the LQ equation seems reasonable, the nature of the interactions between separate tracks is still a matter of some debate. Chadwick and Leenhouts (1973) postulated that separate tracks might hit opposite strands of the DNA double helix and thus form a DSB. We now know that this is unlikely in view of the very low probability of two tracks interacting within the dimensions of the DNA molecule (diameter *c.* 2.5 nm) at a dose of a few grays. Interaction between more widely spaced regions of the complex DNA structure, or between DNA in different chromosomes, is a more plausible mechanism (see Chapter 2, Section 2.7).

4.11 THE LETHAL–POTENTIALLY LETHAL (LPL) DAMAGE MODEL

Curtis (1986) proposed the LPL model as a 'unified repair model' of cell killing. Ionizing radiation is considered to produce two different types of lesion: repairable (i.e. potentially lethal) lesions and non-repairable (i.e. lethal) lesions. The non-repairable lesions produce single-hit lethal effects and therefore give rise to a linear component of cell killing [$=\exp(-\alpha D)$]. The eventual effect of the repairable lesions depends on competing processes of repair and binary misrepair. It is this latter process that leads to a quadratic component in cell killing. As shown in Fig. 4.6, the model has

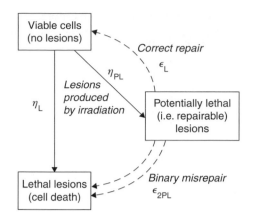

Figure 4.6 The 'lethal–potentially lethal' (LPL) damage model of radiation action.

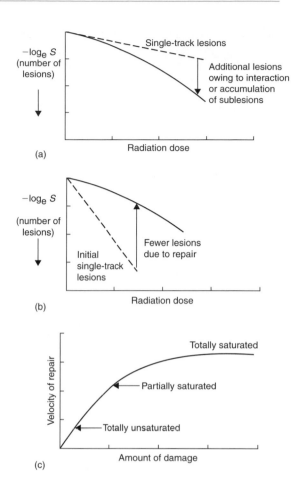

Figure 4.7 The contrast between lesion-interaction models and repair-saturation models. (a) The 'lethal–potentially lethal' (LPL) model; (b) the effect of repair becoming less effective at higher radiation doses; (c) the basic concept of repair saturation. Adapted from Goodhead (1985), with permission.

two sensitivity parameters (η_L determines the number of non-repairable lesions produced per unit dose, and η_{PL} the number of repairable lesions). There are also two rate constants (ϵ_{PL} determines the rate of repair of repairable lesions, and ϵ_{2PL} the rate at which they undergo interaction and thus misrepair).

This model produces almost identical cell survival curves to the LQ equation, down to a survival level of perhaps 10^{-2}. It can therefore be taken to provide one possible mechanistic interpretation of the LQ equation. It predicts that, as dose rate is reduced, the probability of binary interaction of potentially lethal lesions will fall and parameter values can be found that allow the model accurately to simulate cell survival data on human and animal cells irradiated at various dose rates (see Chapter 12, Sections 12.3 and 12.5).

4.12 REPAIR SATURATION MODELS

Curtis' LPL model is an example of a lesion-interaction model which also incorporates repair processes. Figure 4.7a shows how this produces the downward-bending cell survival curve: the dashed curve indicates the component of cell killing that is due to single-track non-repairable lesions. It is the extra lethal lesions produced by

the binary interaction of potentially lethal lesions which give the downward-bending curve.

Another class of models are the repair saturation models, which propose that the shape of the survival curve depends only on a dose-dependent rate of repair. Figure 4.7b,c demonstrates this idea. Only one type of lesion and single-hit killing are postulated, and in the absence of any repair these lesions produce the steep dashed survival curve in Fig. 4.7b. The final survival curve (solid line) results from repair of some of these lesions; however, if the repair enzymes become saturated (Fig. 4.7c), there

Table 4.1 Different interpretations of radiobiological phenomena by lesion-interaction and saturable-repair models

Observation	Explanation Lesion interaction	Repair saturation
Curved dose–effect relationship	Interaction of sublesions	Saturation of capacity to repair sublesions
Split-dose recovery	Repair of sublesions (sublethal damage repair)	Recovery of capacity to repair sublesions
RBE increase with LET	More non-repairable lesions at high LET	High-LET lesions are less repairable
Low dose rate is less effective	Repair of sublesions during irradiation	Repair system not saturating

LET, linear energy transfer; RBE, relative biological effectiveness.

Adapted from Goodhead (1985), with permission.

is not enough repair enzyme to bind to all damaged sites simultaneously and so the reaction velocity of repair no longer increases with increasing damage. Therefore at higher doses (more lesions), there is proportionally less repair during the time available before damage becomes fixed; this will lead to more residual damage and to greater cell kill. The mechanisms of fixation of non-repaired damage are not understood but they may be associated with the entry of cells carrying such damage into DNA synthesis or mitosis. It should be noted that an alternative 'saturation' hypothesis, leading to the same consequence, is that the pool of repair enzymes is used up during repair, so that at higher doses the repair system is depleted and is less able to repair all the induced damage.

Table 4.1 illustrates how the basic conceptual difference between the lesion accumulation/interaction models such as Curtis' LPL and the dose-dependent repair models affects the interpretation of some radiobiological phenomena (Goodhead, 1985). Both types of model predict linear-quadratic cell survival curves in the clinically relevant dose region. They also provide good explanations of split-dose recovery (see Chapter 7, Section 7.3), changing effectiveness with LET (see Chapter 6, Section 6.3) and the dose-rate effect (see Chapter 12, Section 12.2). At present, radiation scientists are uncertain whether lesion interaction or repair saturation really exist in cells but it may well be that molecular and microdosimetric studies will eventually determine which explanation (maybe both!) is correct.

4.13 THE LINEAR-QUADRATIC-CUBIC MODEL

The LQ model describes the cellular response to ionizing radiation extremely well at doses less than about 5–6 Gy and is the preferred model to use in this dose range. However, at higher doses the survival response of cells is often found to more closely resemble a linear relationship between $-\ln(S)$ and dose, as described by the models based on target theory.

A simple way of adjusting the LQ model to account for the more linear response at higher doses is to add an additional term proportional to the cube of the dose, but opposite in sign to the linear and quadratic terms. This is termed the linear-quadratic-cubic, or LQC model:

$$-\ln(S) = \alpha D + \beta D^2 - \gamma D^3$$

$$p(\text{survival}) = \exp(-\alpha D - \beta D^2 + \gamma D^3)$$

$$(4.5)$$

A comparison of the LQ and LQC models is shown in Fig. 4.8. By taking the second-order differential of $-\ln(S)$ with respect to dose, it can be shown that the survival curve can be straightened at dose D_L by choosing $\gamma = \beta/(3D_L)$. In the example of Fig. 4.8, the LQC curve becomes a straight line at a dose, D_L, of 18 Gy.

As with the two-component model, a disadvantage of the LQC model is the addition of a third parameter, but because the LQC model is a

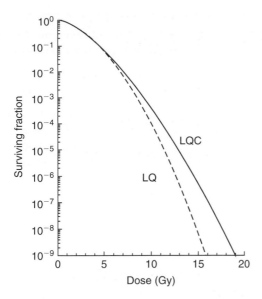

Figure 4.8 Cell survival modelled with the linear-quadratic (LQ) or linear-quadratic-cubic (LQC) equations. In this example both equations model a cell-survival response with surviving fraction at 2 Gy (SF$_2$) equal to 0.5, and an α/β ratio of 3 Gy. The value of γ in the LQC model is given by $\gamma = \beta/(3D_L)$, where D_L is the dose at which the curve becomes straight; here this dose has been chosen to be 18 Gy.

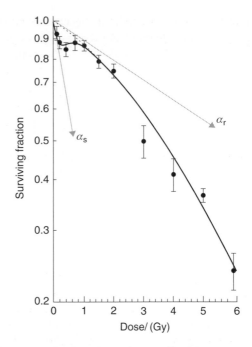

Figure 4.9 Survival of asynchronous T98G human glioma cells irradiated with 240 kVp X-rays, measured using a cell-sorter protocol (Short *et al.*, 1999). Each datum point represents 10–12 measurements. The solid line and dashed line show the fits of the induced-repair (IndRep) model and linear-quadratic (LQ) models, respectively. At doses below 1 Gy the LQ model, using an initial slope α_r, substantially underestimates the effect of irradiation and this domain is better described by the IndRep model using a much steeper initial slope α_s. Reprinted with permission of Taylor & Francis Group.

simple polynomial it is nevertheless still more mathematically manageable than the target theory models. The LQC model is actually just a third-order polynomial approximation to Curtis' LPL model, which also demonstrates a more linear relationship between $-\ln(S)$ and dose than predicted by the LQ model, at surviving fractions less than about 10^{-2}.

4.14 LOW-DOSE HYPER-RADIOSENSITIVITY

The LQ model and its mechanistic interpretations (Curtis' LPL and repair saturation) adequately describe cellular response to radiation above about 1 Gy. It has been difficult to make accurate measurements of cell killing by radiation below this dose, but this problem has been partially overcome by methods that determine exactly the number of cells 'at risk' in a colony-forming assay

(see Section 4.4). This can be achieved using a FACS to plate an exact number of cells or microscopic scanning to identify an exact number of cells after plating. Using such techniques, it can be shown that many mammalian cell lines actually exhibit the type of radiation response shown in Fig. 4.9 at doses less than 1 Gy. Below about 10 cGy, the cells show HRS, which can be characterized by a slope (α_s) that is considerably steeper than the slope expected by extrapolating back the response from high-dose measurements (α_r). The transition (over about 20–80 cGy) from a sensitive to resistant response has been termed a region of increased radioresistance (IRR). This phenomenon was originally discovered in mammalian cells by Marples and Joiner (1993) using V79 hamster fibroblasts and is thought to be caused by an increase in the extent of DNA repair of the cells in the IRR region (Joiner *et al.*, 2001). This happens because a rapid cell-cycle arrest of cells, irradiated in the G2 phase of the cell cycle, only occurs when there are enough DNA DSBs to trigger phosphorylation of the ATM damage-recognition protein. This typically starts to happen only when the average dose exceeds about 10 cGy (Marples *et al.*, 2003).

The LQ model can be modified to take account of this process and the result is called the induced repair (IndRep) model:

$$p(\text{survival})$$
$$= \exp(-\alpha_r D(1+(\alpha_s/\alpha_r-1)\exp(-D/D_c))-\beta D^2)$$

(4.6)

In this equation, D_c is around 0.2 Gy and describes the dose at which the transition from the HRS response through the IRR response starts to occur. At very high doses ($D >> D_c$), equation 4.6 tends to a LQ model with active parameters α_r and β. At very low doses ($D << D_c$), equation 4.6 tends to a LQ model with active parameters α_s and β. The IndRep model thus comprises two LQ models with different α sensitivities dependent on the dose given, merged into a single equation.

It has been proposed that this HRS phenomenon might be exploitable clinically, if it is practicable to deliver radiotherapy as a very large number of dose fractions each less than 0.5 Gy. The aim would be to take advantage of the extra radiosensitivity in the HRS region, which could improve the response of tumours that are known to be resistant to radiotherapy at doses of 2 Gy per fraction.

Key points

1. Tumour recurrence after treatment depends upon the survival of clonogenic cells, which may constitute only a small proportion of the total cells within the tumour.

2. Evaluation of the survival of clonogenic cells following treatment is an important aspect of experimental cancer therapy. In experimental situations this is relatively simple to perform, but for cells removed directly from human tumours great care is necessary in the selection and performance of the assays.

3. A number of different mathematical models adequately simulate the shape of cell-survival curves for mammalian cells.

4. Target theory proposes that a specific number of targets or DNA sites must be inactivated or damaged to kill the cell. This approach is satisfactory only if a component of single-hit killing is also introduced. To date, it has not been possible to identify the location of these vital 'targets' within the cell nucleus.

5. Lesion-interaction models explain downward-bending cell-survival curves by postulating two classes of lesion. One class is directly lethal, but the other type is only potentially lethal and may be repaired enzymatically or may interact with other potentially lethal lesions to form lethal lesions.

6. Repair-saturation models also provide a plausible explanation of cell survival phenomena.

7. Linear-quadratic equations model the shape of the cell survival curve very well at doses less than approximately 5–6 Gy. At higher doses, it may be necessary to use linear-quadratic-cubic equations to model the more linear relationship between –log (surviving fraction) and dose which is often seen.

8. The phenomenon of hyper-radiosensitivity at very low radiation doses illustrates that reactive molecular signalling and repair processes determine the balance between radiation cell killing and cell survival, and models that treat the cell only as a set of passive targets will be unlikely to describe the full spectrum of radiation response.

■ BIBLIOGRAPHY

Bosanquet AG (1991). Correlations between therapeutic response of leukaemias and *in-vitro* drug-sensitivity assay. *Lancet* **337**: 711–4.

Carmichael J, DeGraff WG, Gazdar AF, Minna JD, Mitchell JB (1987). Evaluation of a tetrazolium-based semiautomated colorimetric assay: assessment of radiosensitivity. *Cancer Res* **47**: 943–6.

Chadwick KH, Leenhouts HP (1973). A molecular theory of cell survival. *Phys Med Biol* **18**: 78–87.

Chapman JD, Peters LJ, Withers HR (eds) (1989). *Prediction of tumor treatment response.* New York: Pergamon.

Courtenay VD, Mills J (1978). An *in vitro* colony assay for human tumours grown in immune-suppressed mice and treated *in vivo* with cytotoxic agents. *Br J Cancer* **37**: 261–8.

Curtis SB (1986). Lethal and potentially lethal lesions induced by radiation – a unified repair model. *Radiat Res* **106**: 252–70.

Durand RE (1986). Use of a cell sorter for assays of cell clonogenicity. *Cancer Res* **46**: 2775–8.

Goodhead DT (1985). Saturable repair models of radiation action in mammalian cells. *Radiat Res Suppl* **8**: S58–67.

Goodwin CJ, Holt SJ, Downes S, Marshall NJ (1995). Microculture tetrazolium assays: a comparison between two new tetrazolium salts, XTT and MTS. *J Immunol Methods* **179**: 95–103.

Hill RP, Stanley JA (1975). The lung-colony assay: extension to the Lewis lung tumour and the B16 melanoma – radiosensitivity of B16 melanoma cells. *Int J Radiat Biol* **27**: 377–87.

Joiner MC, Marples B, Lambin P, Short SC, Turesson I (2001). Low-dose hypersensitivity: current status and possible mechanisms. *Int J Radiat Oncol Biol Phys* **49**: 379–89.

Klokov D, MacPhail SM, Banath JP, Byrne JP, Olive PL (2006). Phosphorylated histone H2AX in relation to cell survival in tumor cells and xenografts exposed to single and fractionated doses of X-rays. *Radiother Oncol* **80**: 223–9.

MacPhail SH, Banath JP, Yu TY, Chu EH, Lambur H, Olive PL (2003). Expression of phosphorylated histone H2AX in cultured cell lines following exposure to X-rays. *Int J Radiat Biol* **79**: 351–8.

Marples B, Joiner MC (1993). The response of Chinese hamster V79 cells to low radiation doses: evidence of enhanced sensitivity of the whole cell population. *Radiat Res* **133**: 41–51.

Marples B, Wouters BG, Joiner MC (2003). An association between the radiation-induced arrest of G2-phase cells and low-dose hyper-radiosensitivity: a plausible underlying mechanism? *Radiat Res* **160**: 38–45.

Potten CS (ed.) (1983). *Stem cells: their identification and characterization.* Edinburgh: Churchill-Livingstone.

Seymour CB, Mothersill C (1989). Lethal mutations, the survival curve shoulder and split-dose recovery. *Int J Radiat Biol* **56**: 999–1010.

Short S, Mayes C, Woodcock M, Johns H, Joiner MC (1999). Low dose hypersensitivity in the T98G human glioblastoma cell line. *Int J Radiat Biol* **75**: 847–55.

Steel GG, Adams K (1975). Stem-cell survival and tumor control in the Lewis lung carcinoma. *Cancer Res* **35**: 1530–5.

Steel GG, Stephens TC (1983). Stem cells in tumours. In: Potten CS (ed.) *Stem cells: their identification and characterization.* Edinburgh: Churchill-Livingstone.

Streffer C, van Beuningen D, Gross E, Schabronath J, Eigler FW, Rebmann A (1986). Predictive assays for the therapy of rectum carcinoma. *Radiother Oncol* **5**: 303–10.

Till JE, McCulloch CE (1961). A direct measurement of the radiation sensitivity of normal mouse bone marrow cells. *Radiat Res* **14**: 213–22.

Trott KR (1972). Relation between division delay and damage expressed in later generations. *Curr Topics Radiat Res Q* **7**: 336–7.

Wasserman TH, Twentyman P (1988). Use of a colorimetric microtiter (MTT) assay in determining the radiosensitivity of cells from murine solid tumors. *Int J Radiat Oncol Biol Phys* **15**: 699–702.

■ FURTHER READING

Alpen EL (1998). *Radiation biophysics*, 2nd edn. San Diego: Academic Press.

Douglas BG, Fowler JF (1976). The effect of multiple small doses of X rays on skin reactions in the mouse and a basic interpretation. *Radiat Res* **66**: 401–26.

Elkind MM, Sutton H (1960). Radiation response of mammalian cells grown in culture. 1. Repair of X-ray damage in surviving Chinese hamster cells. *Radiat Res* **13**: 556–93.

Elkind MM, Whitmore GF (1967). *The radiobiology of cultured mammalian cells.* New York: Gordon and Breach.

Ward JF (1990). The yield of DNA double-strand breaks produced intracellularly by ionizing radiation: a review. *Int J Radiat Biol* **57**: 1141–50.

Dose–response relationships in radiotherapy

SØREN M. BENTZEN

5.1 INTRODUCTION

Clinical radiobiology is concerned with the relationship between a given physical absorbed dose and the resulting biological response and with the factors that influence this relationship. Although the term tolerance is frequently (mis-)used when discussing radiotherapy toxicity, it is important to realize that there is no dose below which the complication rate is zero: there is no clear-cut limit of tolerance. What is seen in clinical practice is a broad range of doses where the risk of a specific radiation reaction increases from 0 per cent towards 100 per cent with increasing dose (i.e. a dose–response relationship).

An endpoint is a specific event that may or may not have occurred at a given time after irradiation. The idea of dose–response is almost built into our definition of a radiation endpoint: to classify a biological phenomenon as a radiation effect we would require that this phenomenon be never or rarely seen after zero dose and seen in nearly all cases after very high doses. Various ways to characterize normal-tissue endpoints are discussed more fully

in Chapter 13 and tumour-related end-points are described in Chapter 7.

With increasing radiation dose, radiation effects may increase in severity (i.e. grade), in frequency (i.e. incidence) or both. A plot of, say, stimulated growth hormone secretion after graded doses of cranial irradiation in children may reveal an example of severity increasing with dose. Here we will concentrate on the other type of dose–response relationship: dose–incidence curves. In the same example we can obtain a dose–incidence curve by plotting the proportion of children with growth hormone secretion below a certain threshold as a function of dose. Thus, the dependent variable in a dose–response plot is an incidence or a probability of response as a function of dose (Fig. 5.1).

In this chapter we will introduce some key concepts in the quantitative description of dose–response relationships. Many of these ideas are important in understanding the general principles of radiotherapy. Furthermore, they form the basis of most of the more theoretical considerations in radiotherapy. We will keep the mathematics to a

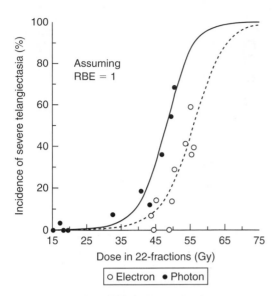

Figure 5.1 Examples of dose–response relationships in clinical radiotherapy. Data are shown on the incidence of severe telangiectasia following electron or photon irradiation. RBE, relative biological effectiveness. From Bentzen and Overgaard (1991), with permission.

minimum but a few formulae are needed to substantiate the presentation.

Empirical attempts to establish dose–response relationships in the clinic date back to the first decade of radiotherapy. In 1936 the great clinical scientist Holthusen was the first to present a theoretical analysis of dose–response relationships and this has had a major impact on the conceptual development of radiotherapy optimization. Holthusen demonstrated the sigmoid shape of dose–response curves both for normal-tissue reactions (i.e. skin telangiectasia) and local control of skin cancer. He noted the resemblance between these curves and the cumulative distribution functions known from statistics, and this led him to the idea that the dose–response curve simply reflected the variability in clinical radio-responsiveness of individual patients. This remains one of the main hypotheses on the origin of dose–response relationships and this has had a renaissance in recent years with the growing interest in patient-to-patient variability in response to radiotherapy.

5.2 SHAPE OF THE DOSE–RESPONSE CURVE

Radiation dose–response curves have a sigmoid (i.e. 'S') shape, with the incidence of radiation effects tending to zero as dose tends to zero and tending to 100 per cent at very large doses. Many mathematical functions could be devised with these properties, but three standard formulations are used: the Poisson, the logistic and the probit dose–response models (Bentzen and Tucker, 1997). The first two are most frequently used and we will concentrate on these. In principle, it is an empirical problem to decide whether one model fits observed data better than the other. In reality, both clinical and experimental dose–response data are too noisy to allow statistical discrimination between these models and in most cases they will give very similar fits to a dataset. The situation where major discrepancies may arise is when these models are used for extrapolation of experience over a wide range of dose.

The Poisson dose–response model

Munro and Gilbert (1961) published a landmark paper in which they formulated the target-cell hypothesis of tumour control: 'The object of treating a tumour by radiotherapy is to damage every single potentially malignant cell to such an extent that it cannot continue to proliferate'. From this idea and the random nature of cell killing by radiation they derived a mathematical formula for the probability of tumour cure after irradiation of 'a number of tumours each composed of N identical cells'. More precisely, they showed that this probability depends only on the average number of clonogens surviving per tumour.

Figure 5.2 shows a Monte Carlo (i.e. random number) simulation of the number of surviving clonogens per tumour in a hypothetical sample of 100 tumours with an average number of 0.5 surviving clonogens per tumour. In Fig. 5.2a each tumour is represented by one of the squares in which the figure indicates the actual number of surviving clonogens, these numbers having been generated at random. The cured tumours are those with zero surviving clonogens. In this

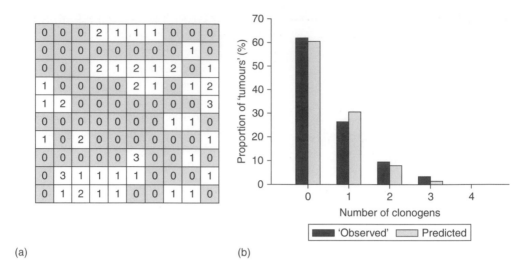

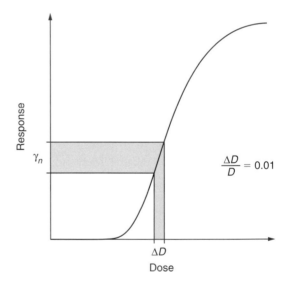

(a) (b)

Figure 5.2 Simulation of a Poisson distribution. (a) The number of clonogens surviving per tumour in a hypothetical sample of 100 tumours. The average number was 0.5 surviving clonogens per tumour. (b) Histogram shows the proportion of tumours with a given number of surviving clonogens (black bars) and this is compared with the prediction from a Poisson distribution with the same average number of surviving clonogens (grey bars).

simulation, there were 62 cured tumours. The relative frequencies of tumours with 0, 1, 2, ... surviving clonogens follow closely a statistical distribution known as the Poisson distribution, as shown in Fig. 5.2b. Many processes involving the counting of random events are (approximately) Poisson distributed, for example the number of decaying atoms per second in a radioactive sample or the number of tumour cells forming colonies in a Petri dish.

When describing tumour cure probability (TCP) it is the probability of zero surviving clonogens in a tumour that is of interest. This is the zero-order term of the Poisson distribution and if λ denotes the average number of clonogens per tumour after irradiation this is simply:

$$\text{TCP} = e^{-\lambda} \tag{5.1}$$

Munro and Gilbert went one step further: they assumed that the average number of surviving clonogenic cells per tumour was a (negative) exponential function of dose. Under these assumptions they obtained the characteristic sigmoid dose–response curve (Fig. 5.3). Thus the shape of this curve could be explained solely from the random nature of cell killing (or clonogen

Figure 5.3 Geometrical interpretation of γ. A 1 per cent dose increment (ΔD) from a reference dose D yields an increase in response equal to γ percentage points. From Bentzen (1994), with permission.

survival) after irradiation: there was no need to assume variability of sensitivity between tumours.

The Poisson dose–response model derived by Munro and Gilbert has had a strong influence on theoretical radiobiology. The simple exponential dose–survival curve was later replaced by the linear-quadratic (LQ) model (see Chapters 4.10 and 8.4) and thus we arrive at what could be called the standard model of local tumour control:

$$TCP = \exp[-N_0 \exp(-\alpha D - \beta dD)] \quad (5.2)$$

Here, N_0 is the number of clonogens per tumour before irradiation and the second exponential is simply the surviving fraction after a dose D given with dose per fraction d according to the LQ model. Thus when we multiply these two quantities we obtain the (average) number of surviving clonogens per tumour and this is inserted into the Poisson expression in equation 5.1. N_0 can easily be expressed as a function of tumour volume and the clonogenic cell density (i.e. clonogens/cm^3 of tumour tissue) and similarly it is easy to introduce exponential growth, with or without a lag time before accelerated repopulation, in this model. The immediate attraction of the Poisson model is that the model parameters appear to have a biological or mechanistic interpretation. This, however, is much less of a theoretical advantage than it appeared to be just 20 years ago. There are at least two reasons for this. First, it turns out that the model parameter estimates will be influenced by biological and dosimetric heterogeneity and therefore cannot usually be regarded as realistic measures of some intrinsic biological property of the tumour (Bentzen *et al.*, 1991; Bentzen, 1992). Second, the model parameters have no simple interpretation in case of normal-tissue effects where the radiation pathogenesis is more complex than suggested by the simple target cell model (Bentzen, 2006).

The logistic dose–response model

The logistic model is often introduced and used with more pragmatism than the Poisson model. This model has no simple mechanistic background and consequently the estimated parameters have no simple biological interpretation. Yet it is a convenient and flexible tool for estimating response probabilities after various exposures and is widely used in areas of biology other than

radiobiology. The idea of the model is to write the probability of an event (P) as:

$$P = \frac{\exp(u)}{1 + \exp(u)} \quad (5.3)$$

where, when analysing data from fractionated radiotherapy, u has the form:

$$u = a_0 + a_1 \cdot D + a_2 \cdot D \cdot d + \cdots \quad (5.4)$$

Here, D is total dose and d is dose per fraction, and the representation of the effect of dose fractionation in this way is of course reflecting the assumption of a LQ relationship between dose and effect. Additional terms, representing other patient or treatment characteristics, may be included in the model to see if they have a significant influence on the probability of effect. The coefficients $a_0, a_1, \ldots$ are estimated by logistic regression, a method that is available in many standard statistical software packages. The parameters a_1 and a_2 play a role similar to the coefficients α and β of the linear-quadratic model. But note that the mechanistic interpretation is not valid: a_1 is not an estimate of α and a_2 is not an estimate of β. What is preserved is the ratio a_1/a_2, which is an estimate of α/β.

Rearrangement of equation 5.3 yields the expression:

$$u = \ln\left(\frac{P}{1 - P}\right) \quad (5.5)$$

The ratio of P to $(1 - P)$ is called the odds of a response, and the natural logarithm of this is called the logit of P. Therefore, logistic regression is sometimes called logit analysis.

5.3 POSITION OF THE DOSE–RESPONSE CURVE

Several descriptors are used for the position of the dose–response curve on the radiation dose scale. They all have the unit of dose (Gy) and they specify the dose required for a given level of tumour control or normal-tissue complications. For tumours, the most frequently used position parameter is the TCD_{50} (i.e. the radiation dose for

50 per cent tumour control). For normal-tissue reactions, the analogous parameter is the radiation dose for 50 per cent response (RD_{50}) or in the case of rare (severe) complications RD_5, that is, the dose producing a 5 per cent incidence of complications.

5.4 QUANTIFYING THE STEEPNESS OF DOSE–RESPONSE CURVES

The most convenient way to quantify the steepness of the dose–response curve is by means of the 'γ-value' or, more precisely, the normalized dose–response gradient (Brahme, 1984; Bentzen and Tucker, 1997). This measure has a very simple interpretation, namely the increase in response in percentage points for a 1 per cent increase in dose. (Note: an increase in response from, say, 10 per cent to 15 per cent is an increase of 5 percentage points, but a 50 per cent relative increase). Figure 5.3 illustrates the definition of γ geometrically.

A more precise definition of γ requires a little mathematics. Let $P(D)$ denote the response as a function of dose, D, and ΔD a small increment in dose, then the 'loose definition' above may be written:

$$\gamma \approx \frac{P(D + \Delta D) - P(D)}{(\Delta D / D) \cdot 100\%} \cdot 100\%$$
$$= D \cdot \frac{P(D + \Delta D) - P(D)}{\Delta D} = D \cdot \frac{\Delta P}{\Delta D} \quad (5.6)$$

The second term on the right-hand side is recognized as a difference-quotient, and in the limit where ΔD tends to zero, we arrive at the formal definition of γ:

$$\gamma = D \cdot P'(D) \quad (5.7)$$

where $P'(D)$ is the derivative of $P(D)$ with respect to dose.

If we look at the right-hand side of equation 5.6, we arrive at the approximate relationship:

$$\Delta P \approx \gamma \cdot \frac{\Delta D}{D} \quad (5.8)$$

In other words, γ is a multiplier that converts a relative change in dose into an (absolute) change in response probability. Most often we insert the relative change in dose in per cent and in that case P is the (approximate) change in response rate in percentage points. This relationship is very useful in practical calculations (see Chapter 9, Section 9.10). For example, increasing the dose from 64 to 66 Gy in a schedule employing 2 Gy dose per fraction corresponds to a 3.1 per cent increase in dose. If we assume that the γ-value is 1.8, this yields an estimated improvement in local control of $1.8 \times 3.1 \approx 5.6$ percentage points.

Mathematically, equation 5.8 corresponds to approximating the S-shaped dose–response curve by a straight line (the tangent of the dose–response curve). As discussed briefly below, this will only be a good approximation over a relatively narrow range of doses; exactly how narrow depends on the response level and the steepness of the dose–response curve.

Clearly, the value of γ depends on the response level at which it is evaluated: at the bottom or top of the dose–response curve a 1 per cent increase in dose will produce a smaller increment in response than on the steep part of the curve. This local value of γ is typically written with an index indicating the response level, for example γ_{50} refers to the γ-value at a 50 per cent response level. A compact and convenient way to report the steepness of a dose–response curve is by stating the γ-value at the level of response where the curve attains its maximum steepness: at the 37 per cent response level for the Poisson curve and at the 50 per cent response level for the logistic model. From this single value and a measure of the position of the dose–response curve, the whole mathematical form of the dose–response relationship is specified (Bentzen and Tucker, 1997). In particular, the steepness at any other dose or response level can be calculated. Table 5.1 shows how the γ-value varies with the response level for logistic dose–response curves of varying steepness. Using Table 5.1, it is possible to estimate the relevant γ-value at, say, a 20 per cent response level for a curve where the γ_{50} is specified. Table 5.1 also provides a useful impression of the range of response (or dose) where the simple linear approximation in equation 5.8 will be reasonably accurate. Clearly, if we extrapolate between two response levels where the γ-value has changed markedly, the approximation of assuming a fixed value for γ will not be very precise.

Table 5.1 γ values as a function of the response level for logistic dose-response curves of varying steepness

γ_{50}	Response level (%)								
	10	20	30	40	50	60	70	80	90
1	0.2	0.4	0.7	0.9	1.0	1.1	1.0	0.9	0.6
2	0.5	1.1	1.5	1.8	2.0	2.0	1.9	1.5	0.9
3	0.9	1.7	2.3	2.8	3.0	3.0	2.7	2.1	1.3
4	1.2	2.3	3.2	3.7	4.0	3.9	3.5	2.8	1.6
5	1.6	3.0	4.0	4.7	5.0	4.9	4.4	3.4	2.0

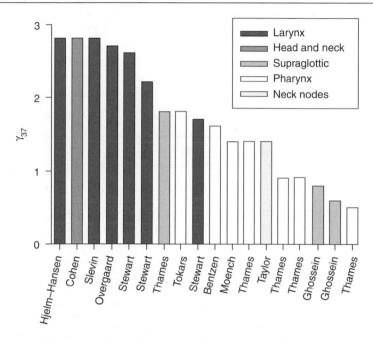

Figure 5.4 Estimated γ_{37} values from a number of studies on dose-response relationships for squamous cell carcinoma in various sites of the head and neck. From Bentzen (1994), where the original references may be found. Reprinted with permission from Elsevier.

5.5 CLINICAL ESTIMATES OF THE STEEPNESS OF DOSE–RESPONSE CURVES

Several clinical studies have found evidence for a significant dose–response relationship and have provided data allowing an estimation of the steepness of clinical dose–response curves. Clinical dose–response curves generally originate from studies where the dose has been changed while keeping either the dose per fraction or the number of fractions fixed. A further advantage of tabulating the γ-value at the steepest point of the dose–response curve is that it is independent of the

dose-fractionation details in the case of a dose–response curve generated using a fixed dose per fraction (Brahme, 1984). Figure 5.4 shows estimates of γ_{37} for head and neck tumours under the assumption of a fixed dose per fraction (Bentzen, 1994). Typical values range from 1.5–2.5. This means that, around the midpoint of the dose– response curve, for each per cent increment in dose, the probability of controlling a head and neck tumour will increase by 2 percentage points. Steepness estimates from dose–response curves for other tumour histologies have been reviewed by Okunieff *et al.* (1995), but it should be noted that data for other histologies are generally

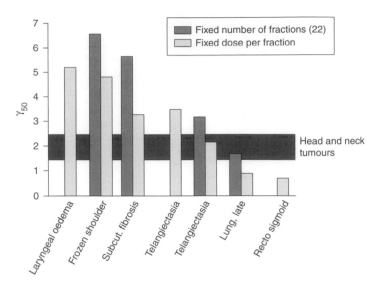

Figure 5.5 Estimated γ_{50} values for various late normal-tissue endpoints. Estimates are shown for treatment with a fixed dose per fraction and a fixed number of fractions. The shaded horizontal band corresponds to the typical γ-values at the point of maximum steepness for dose-response curves in head and neck tumours. Compare with Fig. 5.4. Data from Bentzen (1994) and Bentzen and Overgaard (1996), where the original references may be found.

more sparse than for the head and neck tumours. Also, some estimated values are obviously outliers that cannot be taken as serious estimates of the steepness of the clinical dose–response curve. These extreme values must be explained by patient selection bias or errors in dosimetry.

In the absence of other sources of variation, the maximum steepness of a tumour-control curve is determined only by the Poisson statistics of survival of clonogenic cells (Fig. 5.2), and this should roughly give rise to a value of $\gamma_{37} = 7$ (Suit *et al.*, 1992). However, values as high as this are not achieved even in transplantable mouse tumour models under highly controlled experimental conditions (Khalil *et al.*, 1997). The principal reason why dose–response curves in the laboratory and in the clinic are shallower than this theoretical limit is dosimetric and biological heterogeneity. The tendency for vocal cord tumours to have γ_{37} values at the upper end of the interval seen for other head and neck subsites probably reflects the relatively lower heterogeneity among laryngeal carcinomas treated with radiotherapy. Other patient and treatment characteristics will influence both the position and the steepness of the dose–response curve. It can be shown (Brahme,

1984) that the γ_{37} of a Poisson dose–response curve for a fixed dose per fraction depends only on the number of clonogens that have to be sterilized to cure the tumour. As mentioned in Section 5.2, many tumour and treatment variables, for example tumour volume and overall treatment time, are thought to affect the (effective) number of clonogens to be sterilized. Therefore, in a multivariate analysis, γ_{37} will depend on all the significant patient and treatment characteristics.

Figure 5.5 shows a selection of γ_{50} values for normal-tissue endpoints. Estimates are given both for treatment with a fixed dose per fraction and, where possible, also for treatment in a fixed number of fractions, in this case 22. The estimates in the latter situation are considerably higher, which is as expected from the LQ model. The explanation is that, when treating with a fixed number of fractions, increasing the dose leads to a simultaneous increase in dose per fraction, and this is associated with an increased biological effect per gray. This is another manifestation of the 'double trouble' phenomenon discussed in Chapter 9, Section 9.11. Let γ_N denote the steepness of the dose–response curve for a fixed fraction number, and γ_d the steepness for a fixed dose per fraction, then it can be shown that at a dose per fraction of d_r:

$$\gamma_N = \gamma_d \cdot \frac{(\alpha/\beta) + 2 \cdot d_r}{(\alpha/\beta) + d_r} \qquad (5.9)$$

As both α/β and d_r are positive numbers, γ_N is always larger than γ_d. In the limit of very large dose per fraction, γ_N has a limiting value of $2 \times \gamma_d$. In the limit of dose per fraction tending to zero, γ_N tends to γ_d. For more discussion of equation 5.9 and its significance for dosimetric precision requirements in radiotherapy, see Bentzen (2005).

Figure 5.5 shows a spectrum of γ_{50} values for the various endpoints. The dose–response curves for many late endpoints are steeper than for head and neck cancer. An exception is rectosigmoid complications after combined external-beam and intracavitary brachytherapy where a large dose–volume heterogeneity is present because of the steep gradients in the dose distribution from the intracavitary sources. Also, the lung data arise from a treatment technique where the dose to the lung tissue was heterogeneous. Thus it is likely that dosimetric rather than intrinsic biological factors are the main cause of the relatively low steepness seen for these endpoints.

5.6 THE THERAPEUTIC WINDOW

As with any other medical procedure, prescription of a course of radiotherapy must represent a balance between risks and benefits. The relative position and shape of the dose–response curves for tumour control and a given radiotherapy complication determine the possibility of delivering a sufficient dose with an acceptable level of side-effects. This was nicely illustrated by Holthusen, who plotted dose–response curves for tumour control and complications in the same coordinate system for two hypothetical situations: one favourable, that is with a wide therapeutic window between the two curves, and the other one less favourable. Figure 5.6 shows an example of how changing treatment parameters may affect the therapeutic window. For split-course treatment (Fig. 5.6a) the tumour and oedema curves are closer together than for conventional treatment (Fig. 5.6b) and the therapeutic window is therefore narrower. In practice, there will

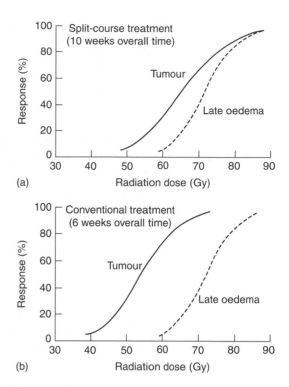

(a)

(b)

Figure 5.6 Dose–response curves for local control of laryngeal carcinoma (solid lines) and late laryngeal oedema as estimated from the data by Overgaard *et al.* (1988). Protraction of overall treatment time narrowed the therapeutic window. From Bentzen and Overgaard (1996), with permission.

be several sequelae of clinical concern and each of these will have its characteristic dose–response curve and will respond differently to treatment modifications. This complicates the simple strategy for optimization suggested by Fig. 5.6.

Several parameters are found in the literature for quantifying the effect of treatment modifications on the therapeutic window. Holthusen's proposal was to calculate the probability of uncomplicated cure, and this is still used frequently in the literature. The difficulty with this measure is that it gives equal weight to the complication in question and to tumour recurrence, which may often be fatal, and this is against common sense. A simple alternative, which is easy to interpret but not necessarily easy to estimate from an actual dataset, is to specify the tumour control probability at isotoxicity with respect to a specific end-point, as illustrated in Fig. 1.3.

5.7 METHODOLOGICAL PROBLEMS IN ESTIMATING DOSE–RESPONSE RELATIONSHIPS FROM CLINICAL DATA

An increasing number of publications are concerned with the quantitative analysis of clinical radiobiological data. Many methodological problems must be addressed in such studies and these problems may roughly be grouped as clinical, dosimetric and statistical.

- *Clinical aspects* – these include the evaluation of well-defined endpoints for tumour and normal-tissue effects. Endpoints requiring prolonged observation of the patients, such as local tumour control or late complications, should be analysed using actuarial statistical methods. Special concerns exist for evaluation, grading and reporting of injury to normal tissue and these are discussed in Chapter 13, Section 13.4. For dose–response data obtained from non-randomized studies, the reasons for variability in dose should be carefully considered. Subsets of patients treated with low/high doses may not be comparable in terms of other patient characteristics influencing the outcome. An example is where patients receive a lower total dose than prescribed because of their poor general condition, perhaps in combination with severe early reactions, or because of progressive disease during treatment.
- *Dosimetric aspects* – these involve a detailed account of treatment technique and quality assurance procedures employed. Furthermore, the identification of biologically relevant dosimetric reference points and a proper evaluation of the doses to these points are required. Modern radiation therapy techniques often give rise to a highly non-uniform dose distribution in the relevant normal tissues. This distribution will have to be converted into an equivalent dose, or similar quantity.
- *Statistical aspects* – these include the choice of valid statistical methods that are appropriate for the data type in question and which use the available information in an optimal way. Statistical tests for significance or, preferably, confidence limits on estimated parameters should be specified. When negative findings are reported, an assessment of the statistical power

of the study should be given. Finally, the censoring (i.e. incomplete follow-up) and latency should be allowed for.

For an overview of the quantitative analysis of clinical data, see Bentzen (1993) and Bentzen *et al.* (2003).

5.8 CLINICAL IMPLICATIONS: MODIFYING THE STEEPNESS OF DOSE–RESPONSE CURVES

The γ-value is not only useful as a multiplier in converting from a dose change to a change in response but may also be used as a multiplier for converting an uncertainty in dose into an uncertainty in response. If the standard deviation of the absorbed-dose distribution in a population of patients is ± 5 per cent, a γ-value of 3 would yield an estimated ± 15 per cent standard deviation on the response-probability distribution. Note that in this situation it is generally the γ for a fixed number of fractions that applies. Figure 5.5 shows that the high γ-values at the maximum steepness of the dose–response curve for normal tissues would yield a large variability in response probability for a ± 5 per cent variability in absorbed dose. This provides an indication of the precision required in treatment planning and delivery in radiotherapy.

Another field where the steepness of the dose–response curves for tumours and normal-tissue reactions plays a crucial role is in the design of clinical trials. For a discussion of this topic see Bentzen (1994).

A final issue in this chapter is the prospect for modifying the steepness of the clinical dose–response curve. Several modelling studies have shown that patient-to-patient variability in tumour biological parameters could strongly affect the steepness of the dose–response curve (Bentzen *et al.*, 1990; Bentzen, 1992; Suit *et al.*, 1992; Webb and Nahum, 1993). Compelling support for this idea also comes from experimental studies (Khalil *et al.*, 1997). A direct illustration of the effect of interpatient variability is obtained from an analysis of local tumour control in patients with oropharyngeal cancers (Bentzen, 1992). Analysing the data with the Poisson model yielded $\gamma_{37} = 1.8$. An analysis taking an assumed

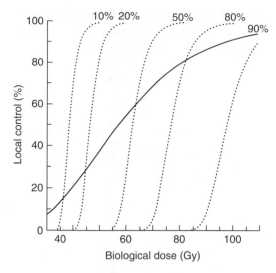

Figure 5.7 Local control of oropharyngeal carcinoma as a function of the biological dose in 2-Gy fractions. Dotted lines are theoretical dose–response curves after stratification for intrinsic radiosensitivity. These represent dose–response relationships from five homogeneous patient populations with radiosensitivity equal to selected percentiles of the radiosensitivity distribution in the total population. From Bentzen (1994), with permission.

variability in tumour cell radiosensitivity into account allowed the dose–response curve to be broken down into a series of very steep curves, each of which would apply to a subpopulation of patients stratified according to intrinsic radiosensitivity (Fig. 5.7). Clinical data on pathological response after radiotherapy analysed by Levegrün *et al.* (2002) showed how the dose–incidence curve got steeper when stratifying patients according to clinico-pathological risk group. Also, for normal-tissue effects, adjustment for patient-related risk factors leads to a steeper dose–response curve (Honore *et al.*, 2002).

This interpatient variability also has a major influence on the parameter estimates in the Poisson model (Bentzen, 1992). Fenwick (1998) proposed a closed form expression of the Poisson dose–response model that takes patient-to-patient variability explicitly into account, but this approach has only been used in a few analyses so far. For a detailed discussion of interpatient variability

and dose–response analysis, see Roberts and Hendry (2007).

Viewing these curves in relation to Fig. 5.6, it is clear that some of these subgroups could be expected to have a greater therapeutic window than others. If, by means of a reliable predictive assay, these subgroups could be identified before starting therapy, a substantial therapeutic benefit could be realized.

5.9 NORMAL TISSUE COMPLICATION PROBABILITY (NTCP) MODELS

Several dose–volume models for normal tissues have been proposed in the literature [see the recent reviews by Yorke (2001) and Kong *et al.* (2007)]. The most widely used of these is the Lyman model (Lyman, 1985). This model gives the normal tissue complication probability (NTCP), as a function of the absorbed dose, D, in a partial organ volume, V:

$$\text{NTCP}(D,V) = \frac{1}{\sqrt{2\pi}} \cdot \int_{-\infty}^{u(D,V)} \exp\left(-\frac{1}{2} \cdot x^2\right) dx$$

(5.10)

where the dependence of dose and volume is in the upper limit of the integral:

$$u(D,V) = \frac{D - D_{50}(V)}{m \cdot D_{50}(V)}$$

(5.11)

The volume dependence of the D_{50} is assumed to follow the relationship:

$$D_{50}(V) = \frac{D_{50}(1)}{V^n}$$

(5.12)

A closer inspection of these three equations shows that there are two independent variables, D and V, and three model parameters, m, $D_{50}(1)$ and n. $D_{50}(1)$ is the uniform total dose producing a 50 per cent incidence of the specific endpoint if the whole organ is receiving this dose. The volume exponent, n, is always between zero and 1 and the larger the value, the more pronounced is the volume effect. The third parameter, m, is inversely related to the steepness of the dose–response curve (i.e. smaller values of m correspond to steeper dose–response curves). The Lyman model has no simple mechanistic background but should be seen as a flexible empirical model for fitting dose–volume datasets. Attempts have been made to develop more mechanistic models but it is questionable whether the biological complexity of dose–volume effects can be encompassed in a reasonably simple mathematical model and most often these models are applied in a pragmatic way as a simple means of capturing the main effects of dose and volume.

Lyman's model only applies to fractional volumes receiving uniform doses. In practice, this is rarely (read: never!) the case. The most common way of summarizing information on a non-uniform dose distribution in an organ is the dose–volume histogram (DVH). In order to estimate the NTCP from a DVH using the Lyman model, it is necessary to reduce the DVH into a single point in dose–volume space. The most frequently used method for doing this is the effective volume method (Kutcher and Burman, 1989) whereby the DVH is transformed into an equivalent fractional volume receiving the maximum dose in the DVH. The basic assumption of this method is that each fractional volume will follow the same dose–volume relationship (described by the Lyman model) as the whole organ. The partial volume in a specific bin on the dose axis is then converted into a (smaller) volume placed at the bin corresponding to the maximum absorbed dose in the DVH.

Some caveats should be noted regarding the use of NTCP models in clinical radiotherapy. Studies have shown that models fitted to one clinical dataset may have low predictive power when applied to an independent data series (Bradley *et al.*, 2007). Also, patients receiving cytotoxic chemotherapy may require tighter dose–volume constraints in order to have a risk similar to that of patients treated with radiation alone (Bradley *et al.*, 2004). Finally, it should be noted that most models used so far have been based on analysis of the DVH alone; in other words, they do not consider the actual spatial distribution of dose in the organ at risk. One example where this analytic strategy seems to break down is the lung, where there are quite good data suggesting that the functional importance of damage to a subvolume of a given size depends on its location within the lung (Travis *et al.*, 1997; Bradley *et al.*, 2007).

Therefore, NTCP models should at present not be used in clinical decision-making and in dose-planning outside a research setting.

Key points

1. There is no well-defined 'tolerance dose' for radiation complications or 'tumouricidal dose' for local tumour control: rather, the probability of a biological effect rises from 0 per cent to 100 per cent over a range of doses.
2. The steepness of a dose–response curve at a response level of n per cent may be quantified by the value γ_n, that is the increase in response in percentage points for a 1 per cent increase in dose.
3. Dose–response curves for late normal-tissue endpoints tend to be steeper (typical γ_{50} between 2 and 6) than the dose–response curves for local control of squamous cell carcinoma of the head and neck (typical γ_{50} between 1.5 and 2.5).
4. The steepness of a dose–response curve is higher if the data are generated by varying the dose while keeping the number of fractions constant ('double trouble') than if the dose per fraction is fixed.
5. Dosimetric and biological heterogeneity cause the population dose–response curve to be more shallow.
6. Normal-tissue complication probability models, incorporating dose fractionation as well as irradiated volume, have not been validated in any clinical setting and should not be routinely used outside a research protocol.

■ BIBLIOGRAPHY

Bentzen SM (1992). Steepness of the clinical dose-control curve and variation in the *in vitro* radiosensitivity of head and neck squamous cell carcinoma. *Int J Radiat Biol* **61**: 417–23.

Bentzen SM (1993). Quantitative clinical radiobiology. *Acta Oncol* **32**: 259–75.

Bentzen SM (1994). Radiobiological considerations in the design of clinical trials. *Radiother Oncol* **32**: 1–11.

Bentzen SM (2005). Steepness of the radiation dose–response curve for dose-per-fraction escalation keeping the number of fractions fixed. *Acta Oncol* **44**: 825–8.

Bentzen SM (2006). Preventing or reducing late side effects of radiation therapy: radiobiology meets molecular pathology. *Nat Rev Cancer* **6**: 702–13.

Bentzen SM, Overgaard M (1991). Relationship between early and late normal-tissue injury after postmastectomy radiotherapy. *Radiother Oncol* **20**: 159–65.

Bentzen SM, Overgaard J (1996). Clinical normal tissue radiobiology. In: Tobias JS, Thomas PRM(eds) *Current radiation oncology.* London: Arnold, 37–67.

Bentzen SM, Tucker SL (1997). Quantifying the position and steepness of radiation dose–response curves. *Int J Radiat Biol* **71**: 531–42.

Bentzen SM, Thames HD, Overgaard J (1990). Does variation in the *in vitro* cellular radiosensitivity explain the shallow clinical dose-control curve for malignant melanoma? *Int J Radiat Biol* **57**: 117–26.

Bentzen SM, Johansen LV, Overgaard J, Thames HD (1991). Clinical radiobiology of squamous cell carcinoma of the oropharynx. *Int J Radiat Oncol Biol Phys* **20**: 1197–206.

Bentzen SM, Dorr W, Anscher MS *et al.* (2003). Normal tissue effects: reporting and analysis. *Semin Radiat Oncol* **13**: 189–202.

Bradley J, Deasy JO, Bentzen S, El-Naqa I (2004). Dosimetric correlates for acute esophagitis in patients treated with radiotherapy for lung carcinoma. *Int J Radiat Oncol Biol Phys* **58**: 1106–13.

Bradley JD, Hope A, El Naqa I *et al.* (2007). A nomogram to predict radiation pneumonitis, derived from a combined analysis of RTOG 9311 and institutional data. *Int J Radiat Oncol Biol Phys* **69**: 985–92.

Brahme A (1984). Dosimetric precision requirements in radiation therapy. *Acta Radiol Oncol* **23**: 379–91.

Fenwick JD (1998). Predicting the radiation control probability of heterogeneous tumour ensembles: data analysis and parameter estimation using a closed-form expression. *Phys Med Biol* **43**: 2159–78.

Honore HB, Bentzen SM, Moller K, Grau C (2002). Sensori-neural hearing loss after radiotherapy for nasopharyngeal carcinoma: individualized risk estimation. *Radiother Oncol* **65**: 9–16.

Khalil AA, Bentzen SM, Overgaard J (1997). Steepness of the dose–response curve as a function of volume in an experimental tumor irradiated under ambient or hypoxic conditions. *Int J Radiat Oncol Biol Phys* **39**: 797–802.

Kong FM, Pan C, Eisbruch A, Ten Haken RK (2007). Physical models and simpler dosimetric descriptors of radiation late toxicity. *Semin Radiat Oncol* **17**: 108–20.

Kutcher GJ, Burman C (1989). Calculation of complication probability factors for non-uniform normal tissue irradiation: the effective volume method. *Int J Radiat Oncol Biol Phys* **16**: 1623–30.

Levegrün S, Jackson A, Zelefsky MJ *et al.* (2002). Risk group dependence of dose–response for biopsy outcome after three-dimensional conformal radiation therapy of prostate cancer. *Radiother Oncol* **63**: 11–26.

Lyman JT (1985). Complication probability as assessed from dose–volume histograms. *Radiat Res Suppl* **8**: S13–9.

Munro TR, Gilbert CW (1961). The relation between tumour lethal doses and the radiosensitivity of tumour cells. *Br J Radiol* **34**: 246–51.

Okunieff P, Morgan D, Niemierko A, Suit HD (1995). Radiation dose–response of human tumors. *Int J Radiat Oncol Biol Phys* **32**: 1227–37.

Overgaard J, Hjelm-Hansen M, Johansen LV, Andersen AP (1988). Comparison of conventional and split-course radiotherapy as primary treatment in carcinoma of the larynx. *Acta Oncol* **27**: 147–52.

Roberts SA, Hendry JH (2007). Inter-tumour heterogeneity and tumour control. In: Dale R, Jones B (eds) *Radiobiological modelling in radiation oncology.* London: British Institute of Radiology, 169–95.

Suit H, Skates S, Taghian A, Okunieff P, Efird JT (1992). Clinical implications of heterogeneity of tumor response to radiation therapy. *Radiother Oncol* **25**: 251–60.

Travis EL, Liao ZX, Tucker SL (1997). Spatial heterogeneity of the volume effect for radiation pneumonitis in mouse lung. *Int J Radiat Oncol Biol Phys* **38**: 1045–54.

Webb S, Nahum AE (1993). A model for calculating tumour control probability in radiotherapy including the effects of inhomogeneous distributions of dose and clonogenic cell density. *Phys Med Biol* **38**: 653–66.

Yorke ED (2001). Modeling the effects of inhomogeneous dose distributions in normal tissues. *Semin Radiat Oncol* **11**: 197–209.

Linear energy transfer and relative biological effectiveness

MICHAEL C. JOINER

6.1 INTRODUCTION

Modern radiotherapy is usually given by linear accelerators producing X-rays with high-energy of 4–25 MV which have generally superseded therapy with lower energy ^{60}Co or ^{137}Cs γ-rays. X-rays and γ-rays are uncharged electromagnetic radiations, physically similar in nature to radio waves or visible light except that their wavelength is less than 10 picometres (10^{-12} m) so that the individual photons ('packets' of energy) are energetic enough to ionize molecules in tissues that they penetrate. It is this ionization that results in the biological effects seen in radiotherapy. These X- and γ-rays all have roughly the same biological effect per unit dose, although there is a small dependence on the energy with lower energies being slightly more effective. Electron beams are quantum-mechanically similar to X-rays and produce similar biological effects. Two other classes of radiations that are being increasingly adopted in radiotherapy are often referred to as:

- *Light particles* – e.g. protons, neutrons and α-particles.

- *Heavy particles* – e.g. fully stripped carbon, neon, silicon or argon ions.

These light and heavy particles may have a greater biological effect per unit dose than conventional X- and γ-rays. The charged particles have, in addition, very different depth–dose absorption profiles compared with uncharged particles (i.e. neutrons) or conventional electromagnetic radiations (X- and γ-rays) and this enables more precise dose distributions to be achieved in radiotherapy (see Chapter 24). This chapter explains the basic physics and radiobiology of these different types of radiation used in cancer therapy.

6.2 MICRODOSIMETRY

It is possible to build up a picture of the submicroscopic pattern of ionizations produced by radiation within a cell nucleus using special techniques for measuring ionization in very small volumes, together with computer simulations: this is the field of microdosimetry. Figure 6.1 shows

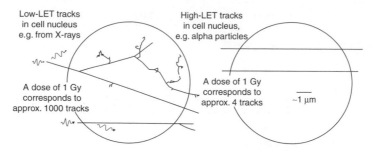

Figure 6.1 The structure of particle tracks for low-linear energy transfer (LET) radiation (left) and α-particles (right). The circles indicate the typical size of mammalian cell nuclei. Note the tortuous tracks of low-energy secondary electrons, greatly magnified in this illustration. From Goodhead (1988), with permission.

examples of microdosimetric calculations of ionization tracks from γ-rays or α-particles passing through a cell nucleus (Goodhead, 1988). At the scale of the cell nucleus, the γ-rays deposit much of their energy as single isolated ionizations or excitations and much of the resulting DNA damage is efficiently repaired by enzymes within the nucleus (see Chapter 2). About 1000 of these sparse tracks are produced per gray of absorbed radiation dose. The α-particles produce fewer tracks but the intense ionization within each track leads to more severe damage where the track intersects vital structures such as DNA. The resulting DNA damage may involve several adjacent base pairs and will be much more difficult or even impossible to repair; this is the reason why these radiations produce steeper cell survival curves and allow less cellular recovery than X-rays. At the low doses of α-particle irradiation that are encountered in environmental exposures, only some cells will be traversed by a particle and many cells will be unexposed.

Linear energy transfer (LET) is the term used to describe the density of ionization in particle tracks. LET is the average energy (in keV) given up by a charged particle traversing a distance of $1\,\mu$m. In Fig. 6.1, the γ-rays have an LET of about $0.3\,$keV/μm and are described as low-LET radiation. The α-particles have an LET of about $100\,$keV/μm and are an example of high-LET radiation.

Why are neutrons described as high-LET radiation when they are uncharged particles? Neutrons do not interact with the orbital electrons in the tissues through which they pass and they do not directly produce ionization. They do, however, interact with atomic nuclei from which they eject slow,

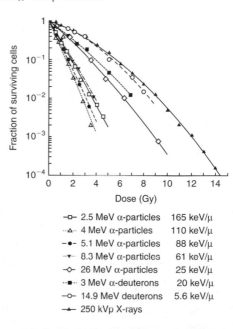

–□– 2.5 MeV α-particles	165 keV/μ
···△··· 4 MeV α-particles	110 keV/μ
–•– 5.1 MeV α-particles	88 keV/μ
–▼– 8.3 MeV α-particles	61 keV/μ
–◇– 26 MeV α-particles	25 keV/μ
···■··· 3 MeV α-deuterons	20 keV/μ
–○– 14.9 MeV deuterons	5.6 keV/μ
–▲– 250 kVp X-rays	

Figure 6.2 Survival of human kidney cells exposed *in vitro* to radiations of different linear energy transfer. From Barendsen (1968), with permission.

densely ionizing protons. It is this secondary production of knock-on protons that confers high LET.

6.3 BIOLOGICAL EFFECTS DEPEND UPON LET

As LET increases, radiation produces more cell killing per gray. Figure 6.2 shows the survival of human T1g kidney cells plotted against dose for eight different radiations, with LET varying from $2\,$keV/μm (250 kVp X-rays) to $165\,$keV/μm (2.5 MeV α-particles). As LET increases, the

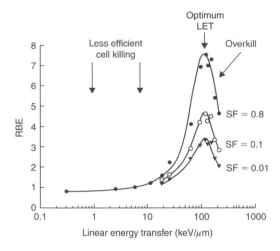

Figure 6.3 Dependence of relative biological effectiveness (RBE) on linear energy transfer (LET) and the phenomenon of overkill by very high LET radiations. The RBE has been calculated from Fig. 6.2 at cell surviving fraction (SF) levels of 0.8, 0.1 and 0.01. From Barendsen (1968), with permission.

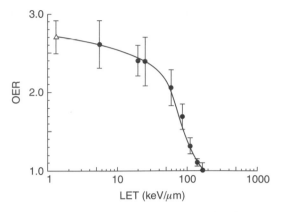

Figure 6.4 The oxygen enhancement ratio (OER) decreases with increasing linear energy transfer (LET). Closed circles refer to monoenergetic α-particles and deuterons and the open triangle to 250 kVp X-rays. From Barendsen (1968), with permission.

survival curves become steeper; they also become straighter with less shoulder, which indicates either a higher ratio of lethal to potentially lethal lesions (in lesion-interaction models; Chapter 4, Section 4.11) or that high-LET radiation damage is less likely to be repaired correctly (in repair saturation models; Chapter 4, Section 4.12). In the linear-quadratic (LQ) description, these straighter cell-survival curves have a higher α/β ratio, thus higher LET radiations usually give responses with higher α/β. For particles of identical atomic composition, LET generally increases with decreasing particle energy. However, notice that 2.5 MeV α-particles are less efficient than 4.0 MeV α-particles even though they have a higher LET; this is because of the phenomenon of overkill shown in Fig. 6.3.

The relative biological effectiveness (RBE) of a radiation under test (e.g. a high-LET radiation) is defined as:

$$\text{RBE} = \frac{\text{dose of reference radiation}}{\text{dose of test radiation}} \qquad (6.1)$$

to give the same biological effect. The reference low-LET radiation is commonly 250 kVp X-rays or ^{60}Co γ-rays since these radiations are usually available whenever RBE is being evaluated. Figure 6.3

shows RBE values for the T1g cells featured in Fig. 6.2. RBE has been calculated at cell survival levels of 0.8, 0.1 and 0.01, illustrating the fact that RBE is not constant but depends on the level of biological damage and hence on the dose level. The RBE also depends on LET, and rises to a maximum at an LET of about 100 keV/μm, then falls for higher values of LET because of overkill. For a cell to be killed, enough energy must be deposited in the DNA to produce a sufficient number of double-strand breaks (see Chapter 4, Section 4.8). Sparsely ionizing, low-LET radiation is inefficient because more than one particle may have to pass through the cell to produce enough DNA double-strand breaks. Densely ionizing, very high-LET radiation is also inefficient because it deposits more energy per cell, and hence produces more DNA double-strand breaks than are actually needed to kill the cell. These cells are 'overkilled', and per gray there is then less likelihood that other cells will be killed, leading to a reduced biological effect. Radiation of optimal LET deposits the right amount of energy per cell, which produces just enough DNA double-strand breaks to kill the cell. This optimum LET is usually around 100 keV/μm but does vary between different cell types and depends on the spectrum of LET values in the radiation beam as well as the mean LET.

As LET increases, the oxygen enhancement ratio (OER; Chapter 15, Section 15.1) decreases. The measurements shown as an example in Fig. 6.4 were also made with cultured T1g cells of human origin (Barendsen, 1968). The sharp reduction in OER occurs over the same range of LET as the sharp increase in RBE (Fig. 6.3).

6.4 RELATIVE BIOLOGICAL EFFECTIVENESS DEPENDS ON DOSE

As indicated in Fig. 6.3, the RBE is higher if measured at lower radiation doses, corresponding to higher levels of cell survival (less effect). Figure 6.5 shows in more detail the RBE for test doses of 4 MeV α-particles plotted against a reference dose of 250 kVp X-rays, for the T1g human cells irradiated *in vitro*. The data points were derived from Fig. 6.2 by reading off from the α-particle survival curve the dose required to achieve the same cell survival as obtained for each X-ray dose evaluated. The RBE for the 4.0 MeV α-particles increases with decreasing dose because the low-LET X-ray survival response is more curved and has a bigger shoulder than the high-LET survival response. If LQ equations are used to model both the low-LET (reference) and the high-LET (test) responses, RBE can be predicted mathematically as a function of the reference dose (d_R) or the test dose (d_T) using formulae containing the α/β ratios and the ratio α_T/α_R (Joiner, 1988). The formulae are:

$$\text{RBE} = \frac{K + \sqrt{K^2 + 4Kd_R(1 + d_R/V)/C}}{2(1 + d_R/V)} \quad (6.2)$$

$$\text{RBE} = \frac{-V + \sqrt{V^2 + 4VKd_T(1 + d_T/C)}}{2d_T} \quad (6.3)$$

where $K = \alpha_T/\alpha_R$, $V = \alpha/\beta$ for the reference radiation and $C = \alpha/\beta$ for the test radiation.

In Fig. 6.5, the solid line shows the prediction of equation 6.2, which gives RBE as a function of the reference dose, in this case X-rays.

The RBE can also be measured *in vivo*. In normal tissues this may be done by comparing the relationships between damage and dose for both high- and low-LET radiations. This may be done for any endpoint of damage, including tissue breakdown

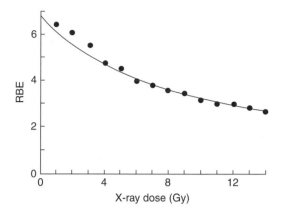

Figure 6.5 Relative biological effectiveness (RBE) of 4 MeV α-particles increases with decreasing dose for cell lines irradiated *in vitro*. RBE values were calculated from the cell survival data shown in Fig. 6.2. The full line is calculated as described in the text.

or loss of tissue function. As an example, Fig. 6.6a shows the results of an experiment to study the loss of renal function in mice after external-beam radiotherapy. This was done by measuring the increased retention of ^{51}Cr-radiolabelled ethylenediaminetetraacetic acid (EDTA) in the plasma 1 hour after injection; normally functioning kidneys completely clear this substance from the body within this time. For neutrons (in this example produced by bombarding beryllium with 4 MeV deuterons, designated d(4)-Be), fractionation makes almost no difference to the tolerance dose but for X-rays a much higher total dose is required to produce renal damage when the treatment is split into two, five or ten fractions. This difference in the fractionation response for high- and low-LET radiations *in vivo* reflects the shape of the survival curves for the putative target cells in the tissue: almost straight for neutrons with a high α/β ratio, and downwards bending for X-rays (Fig. 6.2) with a low α/β ratio. In this *in vivo* situation, RBE is calculated from the ratio of X-ray to neutron total doses required to produce the same biological effect in the same number of fractions. This is plotted against X-ray dose per fraction in Fig. 6.6b. It can be seen that, *in vivo*, RBE increases with decreasing dose per fraction in exactly the same way as RBE increases with decreasing single dose for the cells *in vitro* shown in Fig. 6.5. *In vivo*, RBE versus dose can also be modelled using equations

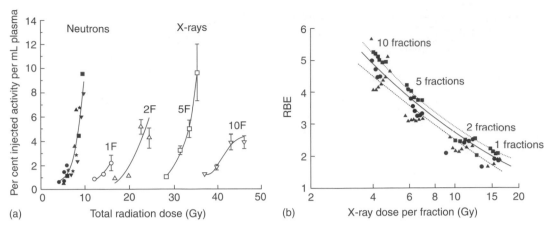

Figure 6.6 The relative biological effectiveness (RBE) for kidney damage increases with decreasing dose per fraction. The RBE values are derived from graphs similar to (a), which shows dose–effect curves for ^{51}Cr-ethylenediaminetetraacetic acid (EDTA) clearance following irradiation with 1, 2, 3, 5 and 10 fractions of neutrons or 1, 2, 5 and 10 fractions of X-rays. The RBE values in (b) were obtained with various renal-damage endpoints: isotope clearance (circles); reduction in haematocrit (squares); and increase in urine output (triangles). From Joiner and Johns (1987), with permission.

6.2 and 6.3. The solid line in Fig. 6.6b shows the mathematical fit of equation 6.2 to the data, from which it is possible to obtain $\alpha_{Neutrons}/\alpha_{Xrays}$, and α/β for X-rays and for neutrons, directly from these RBE versus dose data.

6.5 THE BIOLOGICAL BASIS FOR HIGH-LET RADIOTHERAPY

We have seen (Fig. 6.4) that the differential radiosensitivity between poorly oxygenated (more resistant) and well-oxygenated (more sensitive) cells is reduced with high-LET radiations. Therefore, tumour sites in which hypoxia is a problem in radiotherapy (some head and neck tumours and prostate cancer, for example) might benefit from high-LET radiotherapy in the same way as from chemical hypoxic-cell sensitizers (see Chapter 17, Section 17.3).

The effect of low-LET radiation on cells is strongly influenced by their position in the cell cycle, with cells in S-phase being more radioresistant than cells in G2 or mitosis (see Chapter 7, Section 7.3). Cells in stationary (i.e. plateau) phase also tend to be more radioresistant than cells in active proliferation. Both of these factors act to increase the effect of fractionated radiotherapy on

more rapidly cycling cells compared with those cycling slowly or not at all, because the rapidly cycling cells that survive the first few fractions are statistically more likely to be caught later in a sensitive phase and so be killed by a subsequent dose – a process termed 'cell-cycle resensitization'. This differential radiosensitivity due to cell-cycle position is considerably reduced with high-LET radiation (Chapman, 1980) and is a reason why we might expect high-LET radiotherapy to be beneficial in some slowly growing, X-ray-resistant tumours.

A third biological rationale for high-LET therapy is based on the observation that the range of radiation response of different cell types is reduced with high-LET radiation compared with X-rays. This is shown in Fig. 6.7, which summarizes the *in vitro* response of 20 human cell lines to photon and neutron irradiation (Britten *et al.*, 1992). This reduced range of response affects the benefit expected, which is the balance between tumour and normal-tissue responses. Thus, if tumour cells are already more radiosensitive to X-rays than the critical normal-cell population, high-LET radiation should not be used since this would reduce an already favourable differential. Possible examples are seminomas, lymphomas and Hodgkin's disease. However, if the tumour cells are more resistant to

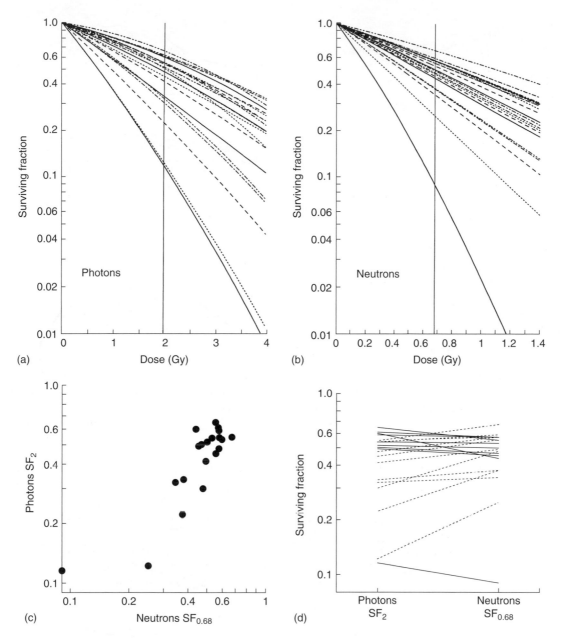

Figure 6.7 Response of 20 human tumour cell lines to (a) 4 MVp photons or (b) p(62.5)–Be neutrons. The vertical lines show the photon (2 Gy) and neutron (0.68 Gy) doses that give the same median cell survival; the average relative biological effectiveness (RBE) is therefore 2/0.68 = 2.94. (c) The range of cell survival at the reference neutron dose of 0.68 Gy (SF$_{0.68}$) is less than the range of survival at a photon dose of 2 Gy (SF$_2$). In 9/20 of the cell lines neutrons gave lower cell survival than photons at these doses (d).

X-rays than the critical normal cells, high-LET radiation might reduce this difference in radiosensitivity and thus would effectively 'sensitize' the tumour cell population relative to a fixed level of damage to normal tissue; high-LET radiation would be advantageous in this case.

In Chapter 24, we summarize the clinical experience with high-LET radiations.

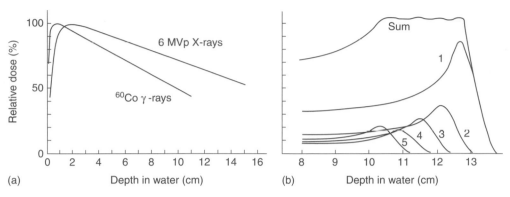

Figure 6.8 The different depth–dose characteristics of (a) photons and (b) proton beams of different intensities and ranges, achieved by passing a primary beam (1) through plastic absorbers (see text).

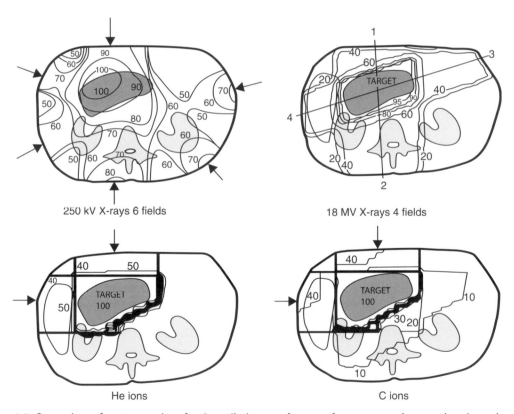

Figure 6.9 Comparison of treatment plans for the radiotherapy of a case of pancreas carcinoma using charged particle beams or photons. From Bewley (1989), with permission.

6.6 THE PHYSICAL BASIS FOR CHARGED-PARTICLE THERAPY

With conventional X-ray therapy, absorbed dose increases very rapidly within the short distance in which electronic equilibrium ('build-up') occurs,

and then decreases exponentially with increasing penetration. Figure 6.8a shows central-axis depth doses from ^{60}Co γ-rays and from X-rays generated by a 6-MV linear accelerator (Fowler, 1981). Neutrons are also uncharged and their depth–dose characteristics are similar: modern

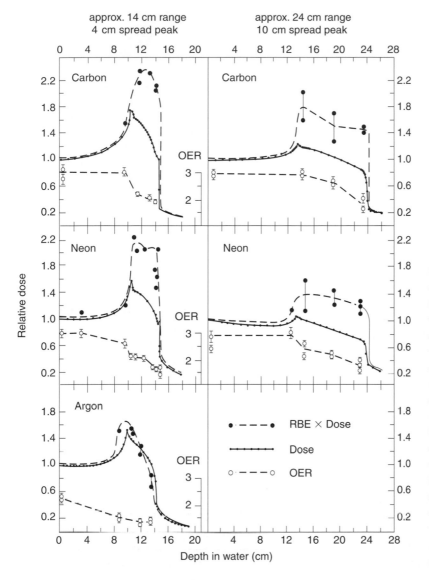

Figure 6.10 The biological effect of charged particle beams is increased further in the Bragg peak. Depth–dose curves are shown for three types of ion beam, each with a 4-cm or 10-cm spread peak. Full lines show the dose distribution; upper broken lines (full symbols) show the biologically effective dose (i.e. dose × relative biological effectiveness, RBE). The lower broken lines (open symbols) show the reduction in oxygen enhancement ratio (OER) within the spread peak. From Blakely (1982), with permission.

high-energy neutron therapy beams have a penetration that is comparable to 4 MV X-rays. The only rationale for neutron therapy is therefore radiobiological, as discussed in Section 6.5.

In contrast, ion beams (i.e. incident beams of charged particles) increase their rate of energy deposition as they slow down with increasing penetration, finally stopping and releasing an intense burst of ionization called the Bragg peak. As an example, curve 1 in Fig. 6.8b shows the depth–dose distribution of a primary beam of 160 MeV protons. The broad peak is obtained by superimposing on curve 1 four other beams of different

intensities and ranges (curves 2, 3, 4 and 5), achieved by passing the primary beam through a rotating wheel with sectors of different thickness of plastic sheet. This spread-out peak (Sum) can be adjusted to cover the tumour volume and therefore increase the ratio of tumour-to-normal-tissue dose compared with conventional photon therapy (Raju, 1980). In modern beam delivery systems, this same scanning of the Bragg peak over a range of depths is achieved by directly modulating the particle energy in variable-energy accelerators.

Figure 6.9 shows some possible treatment plans with heavy-ion beams of helium and carbon nuclei, using carcinoma of the pancreas as an example. The improvement given by the He ions over 18 MV X-rays is as dramatic as the comparison between 18 MV and 250 kVp X-rays. The mean doses to the spinal cord and kidney are almost zero for He ions, 50 per cent for 18 MV X-rays and 70 per cent for 250 kVp X-rays. Uniformity over the tumour is 2–3 per cent, 5 per cent and 15 per cent, respectively.

Carbon ions give a similar dose distribution to He ions but in addition they have a higher LET and RBE in the Bragg peak, which in suitable tumours (see above) might confer an additional radiobiological advantage. The LET of a charged particle is proportional to the square of its charge divided by the square of its velocity. Therefore, in the Bragg peak, where the particles are slowing down rapidly, heavy ions such as carbon, neon and argon have very high LET, with the potential for a greatly increased biological effect. To illustrate this, Fig. 6.10 shows depth–dose curves for beams of heavy ions accelerated to two different energies giving maximum penetrations in tissue of about 14 or 24 cm. In each case the solid line represents the pattern of dose produced by a ridge filter designed to spread out the Bragg peak to cover imaginary tumours of 4 or 10 cm, respectively. This is a similar 'peak-spreading' technique to that described in Fig. 6.8b. However, the dotted line shows the distribution of biologically effective dose, which is physical dose multiplied by RBE. The RBE values are those for Chinese hamster cells corresponding to an X-ray dose of about 2 Gy. This demonstrates that for heavy ions (not high-energy protons or helium ions) the physical advantage of better dose distribution in the spread-out Bragg peak can be further enhanced by the radiobiological advantage from the higher LET.

Figure 6.11 conveniently summarizes the relative physical and radiobiological properties of different radiations and charged particles (Fowler, 1981). Protons have excellent depth–dose distributions and have radiobiological properties similar to orthovoltage X-rays: it is highly probable that light-ion beams of protons and perhaps helium will play a key role in better radiotherapy during the next 20 years. Neutrons have no dose distribution advantage over megavoltage X-rays

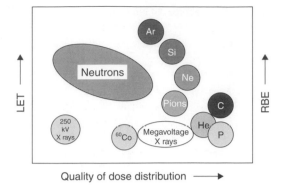

Figure 6.11 The radiations available for radiation therapy differ in the quality of beam that they produce, also in relative biological effectiveness (RBE). LET, linear energy transfer. Based on Fowler (1981).

but may be useful because of their high LET. The heavy ions give better dose distributions than X-rays and a higher LET, depending on the particle. Argon ions have a high LET but in practice they break up so readily that only limited penetration can be obtained. Carbon, neon and silicon ions are the most promising of the heavy ions at the present time and where heavy-ion therapy is adopted it will probably be with these particles (Castro, 1995).

Key points

1. Both X-rays and γ-rays are sparsely ionizing radiations with a low LET. Some particle radiations (e.g. neutrons, α-particles or heavy ions) have a high LET.
2. High-LET radiations are biologically more effective per gray than low-LET radiations. This is measured by the RBE. For most high-LET radiations at therapeutic dose levels, RBE is in the range of 2–10.
3. RBE increases as the LET increases up to about 100 keV/μm, above which RBE decreases because of cellular overkill. The OER also decreases rapidly over the same range of LET.

4. RBE increases as the dose is reduced *in vitro*, or the dose per fraction is reduced *in vivo*. In late-responding tissues, this increase occurs more rapidly than in early-responding tissues.

6. Heavy particles such as He, C and Ne ions have a high-LET and in addition they have improved physical depth–dose distributions.

7. Proton beams provide the best improvement in dose distribution for the lowest cost; their RBE is similar to low-energy photons.

■ BIBLIOGRAPHY

Barendsen GW (1968). Responses of cultured cells, tumours and normal tissues to radiations of different linear energy transfer. *Curr Topics Radiat Res Q* **4**: 293–356.

Bewley DK (1989). *The physics and radiobiology of fast neutron beams*. Bristol: Adam Hilger.

Blakely EA (1982). Biology of bevalac beams: cellular studies. In: Skarsgard LD (ed.) *Pion and heavy ion radiotherapy: pre-clinical and clinical studies*. Amsterdam: Elsevier, 229–250.

Britten RA, Warenius HM, Parkins C, Peacock JH (1992). The inherent cellular sensitivity to 62.5 MeV(p-Be) neutrons of human cells differing in photon sensitivity. *Int J Radiat Biol* **61**: 805–12.

Castro JR (1995). Results of heavy ion radiotherapy. *Radiat Environ Biophys* **34**: 45–8.

Chapman JD (1980). Biophysical models of mammalian cell inactivation by radiation. In: Meyn RE, Withers HR (eds) *Radiation biology in cancer research*. New York: Raven Press, 21–32.

Fowler JF (1981). *Nuclear particles in cancer treatment*. Bristol: Adam Hilger.

Goodhead DT (1988). Spatial and temporal distribution of energy. *Health Phys* **55**: 231–40.

Joiner MC (1988). A comparison of the effects of p(62)-Be and d(16)-Be neutrons in the mouse kidney. *Radiother Oncol* **13**: 211–24.

Joiner MC, Johns H (1987). Renal damage in the mouse: the effect of d(4)-Be neutrons. *Radiat Res* **109**: 456–68.

Raju MR (1980). *Heavy particle radiotherapy*. New York: Academic Press.

■ FURTHER READING

Alpen EL (1998). *Radiation biophysics*, 2nd edn. San Diego: Academic Press.

Conference Proceedings (1994). Nordic conference on neutrons in research and cancer therapy. Linkoping, April 29–30, 1993. *Acta Oncol* **33**: 225–327.

Engenhart-Cabillic R, Wambersie A (eds) (1998). *Fast neutrons and high-LET particles in cancer therapy. Recent results in cancer research*, Vol. 150. New York: Springer-Verlag.

Goodhead DT (1989). The initial physical damage produced by ionizing radiations. *Int J Radiat Biol* **56**: 623–34.

Noda K, Furukawa T, Fujisawa T *et al.* (2007). New accelerator facility for carbon-ion cancer-therapy. *J Radiat Res (Tokyo)* **48**(Suppl A): A43–54.

Wambersie A, Richard F, Breteau N (1994). Development of fast neutron therapy worldwide. Radiobiological, clinical and technical aspects. *Acta Oncol* **33**: 261–74.

Wambersie A, Auberger T, Gahbauer RA, Jones DT, Potter R (1999). A challenge for high-precision radiation therapy: the case for hadrons. *Strahlenther Onkol* **175**(Suppl 2): 122–8.

Withers HR, Thames HD Jr, Peters LJ (1982). Biological bases for high RBE values for late effects of neutron irradiation. *Int J Radiat Oncol Biol Phys* **8**: 2071–6.

Tumour growth and response to radiation

DANIEL ZIPS

7.1 TUMOUR GROWTH

Introduction

The growth of primary and metastatic tumours determines the clinical course of malignant disease. Tumour growth results from a disturbed tissue homeostasis, driven by functional capabilities acquired during tumourigenesis. These acquired capabilities include self-sufficiency in growth signals, insensitivity to anti-growth signals, limitless proliferative potential, evading apoptosis, and sustained angiogenesis (Hanahan and Weinberg, 2000). The speed of growth, or the growth rate, varies considerably between different tumours because of differences in cell proliferation and cell loss.

Measuring the size and growth rate of tumours

Under experimental conditions, such as with transplanted tumour models, the size of the tumour can be precisely and repeatedly measured using simple callipers. In the clinical situation, precision and feasibility of tumour size measurement depend on the anatomical site and the imaging technology. For example, only lesions of 5–10 mm or larger in diameter can be detected in the lung on chest radiographs. Advanced spiral computed tomography (CT) allows detection of nodules as small as 3 mm in diameter. From the dimensions of the lesion, the tumour volume (V) can be calculated:

$$V = \frac{\pi}{6} \times length \times width \times height$$

For experimental tumour models, a calibration curve can be obtained by plotting V against the weight of excised tumours (Steel, 1977). This procedure allows for uncertainties of external tumour volume determination resulting from, for example, irregular volumes and skin thickness.

The tumour burden and tumour growth rate can also be estimated by determination of biochemical tumour markers such as prostate specific antigen (PSA) in patients with prostate cancer (Schmid et al., 1993). Serial measurement of the tumour volume permits estimation of the growth rate. The tumour volume doubling time (VDT), for example, can be calculated by the time required for the tumour to double its volume. In untreated experimental tumours, volume doubling times have been found to be in the same range as the

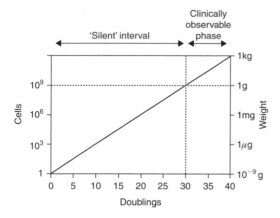

Figure 7.1 Relationship between the number of doublings from a single cell and the number of resulting cells in a tumour. To calculate the tumour weight, a cell number of 10^9 per gram was assumed. The clinically observable phase represents a minor part in the history of the tumour. Tumour weight is plotted on a logarithmic scale. If the doubling time is constant, a straight line indicates exponential tumour growth.

doubling times of tumour cell number and clonogenic tumour cell number (Jung *et al.*, 1990).

Exponential and non-exponential growth

Starting from one cell, each cell division produces two offspring resulting in 2, 4, 8, 16, 32, etc. cells after subsequent cycles of cell division. Accordingly this results in an exponential increase in cell number and volume with time, which can be expressed as:

$$V = \exp\left(\frac{time \times \ln 2}{VDT}\right)$$

Figure 7.1 illustrates that the majority of cell doublings take place before a tumour becomes detectable, which, in most clinical situations, is when the cell number approaches about 10^9. This cell number is equivalent to a tumour weight of about 1 g and a volume of about 1 cm^3. Exponential growth implies that, under constant conditions, the logarithm of tumour volume increases linearly

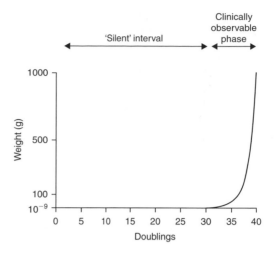

Figure 7.2 The same data as used for Fig. 7.1 but tumour weight is plotted on a linear scale. This may lead to the erroneous impression that tumour growth accelerates during the clinically observable phase.

with time. This can be seen easily from tumour growth curves if volume or weight is plotted on a logarithmic scale and therefore tumour growth is conventionally plotted in this way. Consequently, deviations from exponential growth, variability in the growth rate among different tumours and effects of treatment can be easily visualized. In contrast, plotting tumour volume on a linear scale might lead to the erroneous impression that growth accelerates with increasing volume (Fig. 7.2). Instead, the VDT actually tends to decrease with increasing volume. This effect in large tumours is caused by impairment in oxygen and nutrient supply resulting in a lower proportion of cycling cells, a prolongation of cell cycle, and/or a higher cell death rate. Such progressively slowing tumour growth has often been described by the Gompertz equation:

$$V = V_0 \exp\left[\frac{A}{B}(1 - e^{-Bt})\right]$$

Here V_0 is the volume at the arbitrary time zero and A and B are parameters that determine the growth rate. At very early time intervals (t_{small}) the equation becomes exponential:

$$V = V_0 \exp(A.t)$$

Table 7.1 Volume doubling times (VDTs) for human tumours taken from a review of early data on the growth rate of human tumours

Site and histology	Number of tumours measured	Mean VDT* (days)	Confidence limits (days)
Lung metastases			
Colon–rectum, adenocarcinoma	56	95	84–107
Breast, adenocarcinoma	44	74	56–98
Kidney, adenocarcinoma	14	60	37–98
Thyroid, adenocarcinoma	16	67	44–103
Uterus, adenocarcinoma	15	78	55–111
Head and neck, squamous cell carcinoma	27	57	43–75
Fibrosarcoma	28	65	46–93
Osteosarcoma	34	30	24–38
Teratoma	80	30	25–36
Superficial metastases			
Breast carcinoma	66	19	16–24
Primary tumours			
Lung, adenocarcinoma	64	148	121–181
Lung, squamous cell carcinoma	85	85	75–95
Lung, undifferentiated	55	79	67–93
Colon–rectum	19	632	426–938
Breast	17	96	68–134

*Geometric mean.

Data from Steel (1977).

At long time intervals $\exp(-B.t)$ becomes small compared with 1.0 and the volume tends to a maximum value of $V_0 \exp(A/B)$. The Gompertz equation is not a unique description of such growth curves. For a fuller discussion see Steel (1977).

The volume doubling time of human tumours shows a considerable variability between tumours of different histology as well as between primary and metastatic lesions (Steel, 1977) (Table 7.1). For example, primary lung tumours double their volume every 2–6 months whereas colorectal carcinomas have been found to grow at a much slower rate with a mean VDT of about 2 years. In general, metastatic lesions tend to grow faster than primary tumours. In contrast to tumours in patients, model tumours in experimental animals usually grow much faster with doubling times in the order of days.

The growth fraction and cell cycle time in tumours

The net growth rate, or the VDT, of tumours results from the balance of cell production and cell loss. Cell production is determined by the proportion of cells in the compartment of actively dividing cells (growth fraction, GF) and the time required to complete the cell cycle (cell-cycle time, T_C). Cells from the GF compartment move through the cell cycle and are distinguished from cells outside the cell cycle. Cells outside the cell cycle (in G0 phase) may enter the cell cycle (recruitment of temporarily resting cells) or remain permanently in the G0 phase (sterile or differentiated cells). Taking these parameters together, tumours grow fast if the growth fraction is high, the cell-cycle time is short, or the cell loss is low.

Table 7.2 Growth fractions determined by Ki67 labelling for different human tumour types

Tumour type and site	Mean/Median Ki67 LI (%)	Ki67 LI (% range)	Reference
Prostate	8.5	1–28.4	Taftachi *et al.* (2005)
Central nervous system:			
Meningeoma	4.4	0–58	Roser *et al.* (2004)
Astrocytoma	21.5	0–47.3	Rautiainen *et al.* (1998)
Head and neck	27.8	8.2–80.8	Roland *et al.* (1994)
Colorectal	37.2	18.9–71.4	Lanza *et al.* (1990)
Breast	31.6	0–99	Thor *et al.* (1999)
Lung (non-small cell)	36.7	0–93	Hommura *et al.* (2000)
Pancreas	29.7	0.5–82.1	Linder *et al.* (1997)
Soft-tissue sarcoma	12	1–85	Jensen *et al.* (1998)
Renal cell carcinoma	11	0–43	Haitel *et al.* (1997)
Bladder	35	3–55	Hoskin *et al.* (2004)
Oesophagus	33	6–95	Sarbia *et al.* (1996)

LI, labelling index.

The GF can be measured in tumour biopsies, for example by immunohistochemistry, using a monoclonal antibody against the cell-cycle-specific protein Ki67. Human tumours vary considerably in their Ki67 labelling index (i.e. the ratio of cells with positive staining for the Ki67 protein divided by the total cell number; Table 7.2). Clinical studies indicate a prognostic value for Ki67-labelling in some tumour types including breast cancer, soft-tissue tumours and lung cancer (Brown and Gatter, 2002). Antibodies against different cell-cycle-specific proteins also allow determination of the fractions of cells within the various phases of the cell cycle.

Determination of cell-cycle kinetics in tissues is more difficult than measuring the GF. In the past, pulsed or continuous infusion of tritiated thymidine, a radiolabelled nucleoside incorporated into the DNA during the S phase, has been widely used to estimate the duration of the cell cycle (T_C) by the per cent labelled mitosis method (Potten *et al.*, 1985). With this method the T_C for carcinomas was found to be widely scattered but averaged around 2 days (Table 7.3).

It is now possible to rapidly determine the S-phase fraction and the duration of the S phase from a single biopsy using a technique developed by Begg *et al.* (1985). In this method, thymidine

Table 7.3 Cell cycle time (T_C) for different human tumours determined by the per cent labelled mitosis method

Histology	Number of tumours measured	Mean T_C* (hours)	Range
Squamous cell carcinoma	7	43.5	14–217
Adenocarcinoma	5	34.9	25–45
Melanoma	4	102	76–144

*Geometric mean.

Data taken from Malaise *et al.* (1973).

analogues iododeoxyuridine (IdUrd) or bromodeoxyuridine (BrdUrd) are injected into a patient and are subsequently incorporated into the newly synthesized DNA in S-phase cells. A few hours after injection, a tumour biopsy is taken from which a single-cell suspension is prepared. This is stained with both a DNA-specific dye and a fluorescent-labelled antibody against BrdUrd or IdUrd. Using flow cytometry, the fraction of cells in S phase (labelling index, LI) and the duration of the S phase (T_S) can be determined. Typical values

Table 7.4 Cell kinetic parameters of human tumours derived from *in vivo* labelling with iododeoxyuridine (IdUrd) or bromodeoxyuridine (BrdUrd) and measured by flow cytometry

Site	Number of patients	LI (%)	T_S (hours)	T_{pot} (days)
Head and neck	712	9.6 (6.8–20.0)	11.9 (8.8–16.1)	4.5 (1.8–5.9)
Central nervous system	193	2.6 (2.1–3.0)	10.1 (4.5–16.7)	34.3 (5.4–63.2)
Upper intestinal	183	10.5 (4.9–19.0)	13.5 (9.8–17.2)	5.8 (4.3–9.8)
Colorectal	345	13.1 (9.0–21.0)	15.3 (13.1–20.0)	4.0 (3.3–4.5)
Breast	159	3.7 (3.2–4.2)	10.4 (8.7–12.0)	10.4 (8.2–12.5)
Ovarian	55	6.7	14.7	12.5
Cervix	159	9.8	12.8	4.8 (4.0–5.5)
Melanoma	24	4.2	10.7	7.2
Haematological	106	13.3 (6.1–27.7)	14.6 (12.1–16.2)	9.6 (2.3–18.1)
Bladder	19	2.5	6.2	17.1
Renal cell carcinoma	2	4.3	9.5	11.3
Prostate	5	1.4	11.7	28.0

Fraction of cells in S phase (LI), duration of S phase (T_S) and potential doubling time (T_{pot}) were taken from Haustermans *et al.* (1997) and Rew and Wilson (2000). Ranges (in parenthesis) represent variations in median values between studies; ranges for individual tumours are considerably larger.

for LI and T_S are shown in Table 7.4. While in most tumours the S-phase duration is about 12 hours, or approximately 25 per cent of T_C, the fraction of cells in the S phase varies widely between the different tumours.

Developments in molecular imaging, such as with radiolabelled fluorothymidine (^{18}F-FLT), may allow non-invasive assessment of tumour proliferation *in vivo*. This radiolabel is not incorporated into the DNA but it is phosphorylated by thymidine kinases (TK). While TK2 is expressed constitutively, TK1 activity is specifically regulated during the S phase. As a result, metabolites of radiolabelled ^{18}F-FLT (mono-, di- and tri-phosphates) are found preferentially in S-phase cells. The ^{18}F tracer activity can then be detected by positron emission tomography (PET).

The potential doubling time (T_{pot})

The potential doubling time (T_{pot}) of a tumour is defined as the cell doubling time without any cell loss (Steel, 1977). The T_{pot} is determined by the growth fraction (GF) and the cell-cycle time (T_C):

$$T_{pot} = T_C/GF$$

Using thymidine analogues and flow cytometry, the T_{pot} can be estimated by the duration of the S phase (T_S) and by the fraction of cells within that phase (LI) (Begg *et al.*, 1985; Terry *et al.*, 1991):

$$T_{pot} = \lambda T_S/LI$$

where λ is a parameter that corrects for the non-rectangular age distribution of growing cell populations. This parameter usually lies between 0.7 and 1.0. Using this method, T_{pot} for human tumours from different sites was found to vary between 4 days and 34 days (Table 7.4). The differences in T_{pot} are mainly attributed to the variability in LI between tumours whereas T_S appears to be relatively similar between tumours, with a value averaging about 12 hours.

To test the hypothesis that pretreatment T_{pot} reflects the effective doubling time during fractionated radiotherapy and thereby correlates with the repopulation rate of clonogenic tumour cells, treatment response of 476 patients with head and neck cancer was correlated with T_{pot} and LI (Begg *et al.*, 1999). However, multivariate analysis revealed that neither T_{pot}, nor LI, nor T_S were statistically significant determinants of local tumour control. Thus, in this large multicentre study, pretreatment cell kinetic parameters measured by

Table 7.5 Calculation of cell loss factors (CLFs) for human tumours based on labelling with radiolabelled thymidine or thymidine analogues and volume doubling times (VDTs) in separate series

Site	LI (%)	T_{pot} (days)	VDT (days)	CLF (%)
Undifferentiated bronchus carcinoma[*,1]	19.0	2.5	90	97
Sarcoma[*,1]	2.0	23.3	39	40
Childhood tumours[*,1]	13.0	3.6	20	82
Lymphoma[*,1]	3.0	15.6	22	29
Head and neck[**,2]	9.6	4.1	45	91
Colorectal[**,2]	13.1	3.9	90	96
Melanoma[**,2]	4.2	8.5	52	84
Breast[**,2,3]	3.7	9.4	82	89
Prostate[**,2,4]	1.4	28.0	1100	97

[*],[**]Labelling with radiolabelled thymidine or thymidine analogues, respectively.
[1]From Steel (1977), calculations assume $T_S = 14$ hours, $\lambda = 0.8$.
[2]Fraction of cells in S phase (LI) and potential doubling time (T_{pot}) from Haustermans et al. (1997) and Rew and Wilson (2000); calculations assume $\lambda = 0.8$ (Steel, 1977).
[3]VDT values for pulmonary metastases from Spratt et al. (1996).
[4]VDT from PSA doubling times from Schmid et al. (1993), Fowler et al. (1994) and Lee et al. (1995).

thymidine analogues and flow cytometry failed to predict outcome after radiotherapy.

Cell loss in tumours

Taking typical values for human tumours (e.g. a GF of 40 per cent and a T_C of 2 days) results in T_{pot} of 5 days. This time is obviously much shorter than the observed VDT of human tumours, which is usually in the order of months. The difference between VDT and T_{pot} is explained by the high rate of cell loss in malignant tumours. The cell loss factor (CLF) can be calculated from:

$$\text{CLF} = 1 - \frac{T_{pot}}{\text{VDT}}$$

Taking a VDT of 3 months and a T_{pot} of 5 days, the cell loss factor would be 94 per cent. Examples of cell loss factors for human tumours are listed in Table 7.5. The high cell loss factors indicate that the vast majority of newly produced cells are lost from the growth fraction, thus explaining the slow growth rate of many tumours. Cells are lost from the proliferative compartment when they enter the non-proliferative compartment (G0), for example by differentiation. The same occurs when they physically disappear from the viable tumour compartment by necrosis, apoptosis, metastasis, and exfoliation or shedding. In solid tumours, necrotic cell loss, because of insufficient oxygen and nutrient supply by the pathological tumour vasculature, appears to represent a major factor.

Transplanted tumours in experimental animals grow much faster than tumours in human patients. While T_S is comparable with tumours in patients, experimental tumour models often exhibit a higher LI, shorter T_{pot}, and a lower cell loss factor. Cell kinetic data obtained using these model systems must therefore be interpreted with caution in terms of their clinical relevance.

7.2 TUMOUR RESPONSE TO RADIATION

Introduction

Radiation effects on tumours under clinical as well as experimental conditions can be measured by different endpoints, including local tumour control, tumour regrowth delay and tumour regression. Local tumour control is the aim of curative radiotherapy. Improvements in local tumour control after radiotherapy have been shown, in many

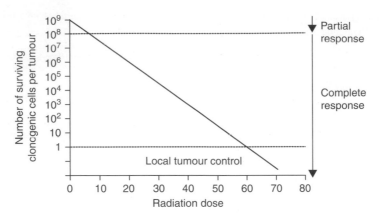

Figure 7.3 Relationship between clonogenic cell survival, radiation dose and different endpoints to assay tumour response, assuming a tumour consisting of 10^9 clonogenic cells and a surviving fraction after 2 Gy of 50 per cent.

clinical trials, to translate into the prolonged survival of cancer patients. Thus, local tumour control is conceptually the preferable endpoint for both clinical and experimental investigations on improving radiotherapy. A tumour is locally controlled when all of its clonogenic cells (i.e. cells with the capacity to proliferate and to cause recurrence after radiotherapy) have been inactivated. The probability of achieving local tumour control is radiation dose dependent and directly related to the number of surviving clonogenic tumour cells (see Chapter 5, Section 5.2). Tumour regression is a non-specific endpoint to assay radiation response. The tumour regrowth delay assay is widely used in radiobiological experiments. Tumour regrowth delay increases with radiation dose but, because of inherent methodological limitations, it is difficult or impossible to accurately estimate cell kill.

Clonogenic cell survival after irradiation

Radiotherapy is highly effective in killing clonogenic tumour cells. The quantitative relationship between radiation dose, inactivation of clonogenic cells and local tumour control is well established under clinical as well as experimental conditions (Munro and Gilbert, 1961; Wheldon *et al.*, 1977; Trott *et al.*, 1984; Rofstad *et al.*, 1986; Suit *et al.*, 1987; Hill and Milas, 1989; Baumann *et al.*, 1990;

Gerweck *et al.*, 1994; Krause *et al.*, 2006). In fractionated radiotherapy, it has been demonstrated that the logarithm of surviving clonogenic tumour cells decreases linearly with total radiation dose. If the radiation dose is high enough to sterilize all cells capable of causing a recurrence, then local tumour control is achieved. This relationship is illustrated in Fig. 7.3, which shows a theoretical clonogenic survival curve for the fractionated irradiation of a model tumour. This tumour has a diameter of about 3 cm, consisting of 10^{10} tumour cells with a clonogenic fraction of 10 per cent (i.e. the tumour consists of 10^9 clonogenic tumour cells). Assuming an intermediate radiation sensitivity, each fraction of 2 Gy inactivates 50 per cent of the clonogenic cells. In other words, after a dose of 2 Gy 50 per cent of the clonogenic cells survive, after 4 Gy 25 per cent, after 6 Gy 12.5 per cent, and so on. This results in a linear decrease of the logarithm of surviving clonogen fraction as the dose increases and is depicted by the straight line in the log-linear plot in Fig. 7.3. For this example, at doses higher than 60 Gy the number of surviving cells per tumour is less than one and local tumour control can be achieved. Clearly, this is a simplification because it neglects, for example, the possibility of changing radiosensitivity (maybe owing to changes in tumour oxygenation) and of repopulation during fractionated radiotherapy (see Chapters 10 and 15). However, it demonstrates that response parameters such as partial or complete response, which are often used as clinical descriptors, are not robust endpoints for evaluating curative radiotherapy. It is obvious that a partial response is a complete failure of the treatment because the vast majority of clonogenic cells are presumably still alive. Even if we are unable to detect the tumour with clinical imaging (in a complete response) a large number of clonogenic tumour cells may have survived the treatment and may lead to a recurrence. Thus, in studies both on patients and on experimental animals, only by following up treatment for long enough to detect all regrowing tumours can it be precisely determined whether the given treatment was effective in sterilizing all clonogenic tumour cells.

Local tumour control

If not a single tumour but a group of tumours (or patients) is considered, the local tumour control probability (TCP) as a function of radiation dose can be described statistically by a Poisson distribution of the number of surviving clonogenic tumour cells (Munro and Gilbert, 1961). It describes the random distribution of radiation-induced cell kill within a population of clonogenic cells (see Chapter 5). As an illustration, one might imagine that a given radiation dose causes a certain amount of 'lethal hits' randomly distributed within the cell population. Some cells will receive one 'lethal hit' and will subsequently die. Other cells will receive two or more 'lethal hits' and will also die. However, some cells will not be hit, will therefore survive and subsequently cause a local failure. According to Poisson statistics, a radiation dose sufficient to inflict on average one 'lethal hit' to each clonogenic cell in a tumour (number of 'lethal hits' per cell, m, = 1) will result in 37 per cent surviving clonogenic cells. The surviving fraction (SF) can be expressed as:

$$SF = \exp(-m)$$

and the number of surviving clonogenic tumour cells (N) is:

$$N = N_0 \times SF$$

where N_0 represents the initial number of clonogens. The TCP depends on the number of surviving clonogenic cells (N) and can be calculated as:

$$TCP = \exp(-N) = \exp(-N_0 SF)$$

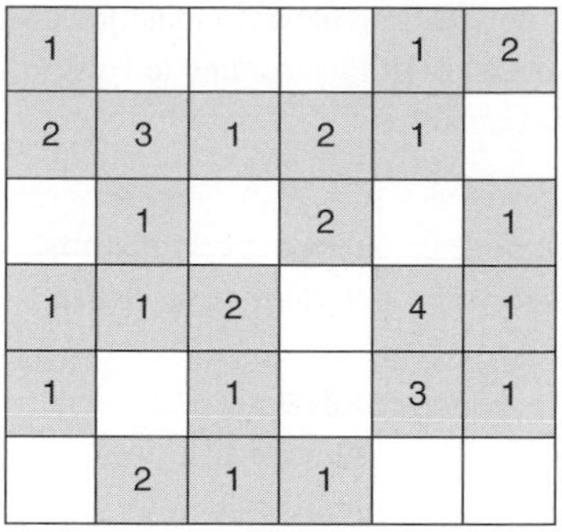

Figure 7.4 A model tumour consisting of 36 clonogenic tumour cells (each square represents one clonogenic cell) after irradiation with a dose sufficient to inflict an average of one 'lethal hit' per clonogenic cell. Owing to random distribution of the 'lethal hits' among the tumour, some clonogenic cells received one (1), two (2), three (3) or four (4) lethal hits. These cells subsequently die (grey shadow). According to Poisson statistics (SF = $exp(-m)$, see text) 37 per cent of the clonogenic cells (i.e. a total of 13 cells (received no 'lethal hit' and survived white background). The tumour control probability (TCP) after this 'treatment' can be calculated as TCP = $exp(-13)$ = 2.3 × 10^{-7}. This means that only 1 out of 23 million tumours will be locally controlled in this situation. In Table 7.6 and Fig. 7.5, the dose effects on surviving cell fraction (SF) and TCP are illustrated.

To illustrate the relationship between radiation dose, number of surviving clonogenic cells and TCP described by Poisson statistics, a model tumour consisting of 36 clonogenic cells is 'treated' (Fig. 7.4, Table 7.6). If the TCP is plotted as a function of dose (Fig. 7.5) the resulting curve shows the typical sigmoid shape. The sigmoid shape of dose–response curves for local tumour control is supported by clinical observations and has been demonstrated in numerous experiments. Application of Poisson statistics implies that, in a group of tumours with, on average, one surviving clonogenic cell per tumour, the local TCP equals 37 per cent. A TCP of 50 per cent results if, on average, 0.7 clonogenic tumour cells survive irradiation. Statistical models other than the Poisson equation, such as the logistic and probit equations, have also been used to describe dose–response relationships for local tumour control empirically (see Chapter 5, Section 5.2).

Table 7.6 Relationship between radiation dose, fraction of surviving clonogenic tumour cells (SF) and local tumour control probability (TCP) according to Poisson statistics for the 'treatment' of a model tumour consisting of 36 clonogenic tumour cells.

Radiation dose (relative units)	Number of 'lethal hits' per clonogenic cell (m)	$SF = exp^{(-m)}$ (%)	Number of surviving clonogenic tumour cells ($N = SF \times 36$)	$TCP = exp^{(-N)}$ (%)
1	36/36 = 1	37	13	<0.0001
2	72/36 = 2	14	5	1
3	108/36 = 3	5	2	17
4	144/36 = 4	1.8	0.7	52
5	180/36 = 5	0.7	0.2	78
6	216/36 = 6	0.25	0.09	91
7	252/36 = 7	0.09	0.03	97
8	288/36 = 8	0.03	0.01	99

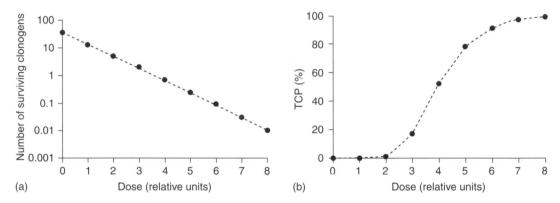

(a) Dose (relative units) (b) Dose (relative units)

Figure 7.5 Illustration of the 'treatment effects' on the model tumour consisting of 36 clonogenic cells (compare Fig. 7.4 and Table 7.6). Values for the number of surviving clonogens and tumour control probability (TCP) were taken from Table 7.6.

The quantitative relationship between radiation dose, surviving fraction of clonogenic tumour cells and TCP forms the biological basis of local tumour control as a functional assay of clonogenic tumour cell survival after irradiation (Munro and Gilbert, 1961; Wheldon *et al.*, 1977; Trott *et al.*, 1984; Rofstad *et al.*, 1986; Suit *et al.*, 1987; Hill and Milas, 1989; Baumann *et al.*, 1990; Gerweck *et al.*, 1994). In such studies, groups of transplanted tumours are irradiated with varying doses and during follow-up it is recorded whether a tumour has regrown (recurrence) or not (local control). In contrast to tumour volume measurement, which requires considerable training and is susceptible to interobserver variability, the scoring of local recurrence or local control is simple and makes the tumour control assay very robust (for comparison with other assays see Table 7.7). The rates of local tumour control at each dose level (number of controlled tumours divided by number of total tumours) are obtained and further analysed to calculate characteristic points on the dose–response curve. In the main, the TCD_{50} (i.e. the radiation dose required to control 50 per cent of the tumours) is reported (the local tumour control assay is therefore often called a TCD_{50} assay). Results from a typical experiment are shown in Fig. 7.6 and Table 7.8 in which FaDu human squamous cell carcinomas were transplanted into nude mice and irradiated with 30 fractions over 6 weeks.

Table 7.7 Comparison of different experimental assays to measure radiation effects on tumours

Assay	Advantages	Disadvantages	Comment
Local tumour control assay (TCD$_{50}$ assay)	Depends only on inactivation of clonogenic cells All clonogenic cells are assayed Response evaluated *in situ* (i.e. in the original environment) TCD$_{50}$ values can be easily obtained for comparisons with other tumour models or different treatments Data good for radiobiological modelling Endpoint scoring very simple	Labour intensive and costly Sensitive to residual immune response of the host	Most important assay for curative Effects of radiotherapy
Excision assays	Direct measurement of clonogen survival Not sensitive to host immune reaction (*in vivo/in vitro* assay) less costly and labour intensive than TCD$_{50}$ assay	Response not measured in the original environment Sensitive to effects from single-cell preparation Cannot assess clonogen survival at low levels of surviving fractions (lung colony, *in vitro/in vivo*) Effects of prolonged treatments difficult or impossible to assess	Standardized methods to assay clonogenic survival but more limitations than the TCD$_{50}$ assay
Tumour regrowth delay assay	Response evaluated *in situ* (i.e. in the original environment) Less costly and labour-intensive than TCD$_{50}$ assay Specific tumour growth delay and the use of multiple radiation dose levels may allow conclusions on clonogenic cell kill and comparisons between different tumour models	Reflects cell kill of the mass of non-clonogenic and clonogenic cells, proliferation, stromal reaction, inflammatory response. Measures the effect only in a small range of tumour cell numbers Does not necessarily reflect inactivation of clonogenic tumour cells Sensitive to experimental manoeuvres without effects on tumour cell kill	Standardized but non-specific endpoint, limited value for investigations of curative effects of radiotherapy
Tumour regression	Response is evaluated *in situ* (i.e. in the original environment) Less costly and labour intensive than other assays	Reflects cell kill, proliferation, resorption of necrosis, stromal reaction, inflammatory response, oedema Measures the effect only in a small range of tumour cell numbers. Sensitive to experimental manoeuvres without effects on tumour cell kill	Highly unspecific endpoint, not suitable for investigations of curative effects of radiotherapy

TCD$_{50}$, dose required to control 50 per cent of the tumours.

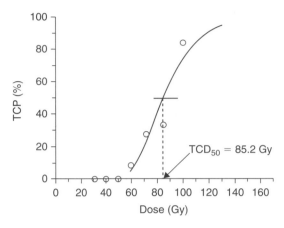

Figure 7.6 Dose–response curve for local tumour control of FaDu human squamous cell carcinoma growing in nude mice. Tumours were treated with 30 fractions over 6 weeks. Total doses ranged from 30 to 100 Gy. Treatment started for all tumours at the same tumour volume. Each symbol represents the fraction of tumours locally controlled at a given dose level (see Table 7.7). The data were fitted using a Poisson-based model and the TCD$_{50}$ (the dose required to control 50 per cent of the tumours locally) was calculated. In the experiment shown, the TCD$_{50}$ is 85.2 Gy. The error bar represents the 95 per cent confidence limit of the TCD$_{50}$. TCP, tumour control probability. Data from Yaromina et al. (2006).

Total doses ranged from 30 to 100 Gy (dose per fraction ranged from 1.0 to 3.3 Gy) and six to eight tumours per dose level were treated. Local tumour control rates were determined 120 days after the end of treatment. This follow-up period is sufficient for this tumour model to detect virtually all regrowing tumours. Careful observation in previous experiments, where animals were followed up until death (lifespan is about 2 years), revealed that 95 per cent of all recurrent FaDu tumours occur within 60 days and 99 per cent within 90 days after end of irradiation. The radiation dose–response curve for local tumour control exhibits a sigmoid shape with a threshold value. Below total doses of about 50 Gy no tumours are controlled, presumably because of the large number of clonogenic cells that survived the treatment. Above this threshold dose, local TCP increases steeply with increasing dose. The data can be fitted using a Poisson-based statistical model and the TCD$_{50}$ is calculated according to:

$$TCD_{50} = D_0 \times (\ln N_0 - \ln(\ln 2))$$

where D_0 reflects the intrinsic radiosensitivity of clonogenic cells (see Chapter 4, Section 4.8) and N_0 is the number of clonogens before irradiation. The TCD$_{50}$ value can be used to compare results obtained from different tumour models (Fig. 7.7).

Table 7.8 Results from a typical TCD$_{50}$ (dose required to control 50 per cent of the tumours) experiment

Total dose (Gy)	Number of irradiated tumours	Number of locally controlled tumours	Number of censored animals (censoring interval in days)	Observed local control rates (%)	TCP (%)
30	11	0	0	0	13.4×10^{-6}
40	11	0	0	0	12.6×10^{-3}
50	11	0	0	0	0.6
60	12	0	1 (99)	8.3	5.6
72.5	11	2	1 (119)	27.3	24.1
85	12	2	2 (55–77)	33.3	49.6
100	13	7	4 (51–116)	83.9	74.1

Human squamous cell carcinoma FaDu was transplanted subcutaneously into nude mice. At a diameter of about 7 mm, the tumours were irradiated with 30 fractions over 6 weeks. Total radiation doses ranged from 30 to 100 Gy. Local tumour control was evaluated 120 days after end of treatment. From the observed local control rates the tumour control probability (TCP) was calculated using the Poisson model. The TCD$_{50}$ is 85.2 Gy (95 per cent confidence limits 77–96 Gy).

For calculations of TCP, censored animals were taken into account according to the method described by Walker and Suit (1983).

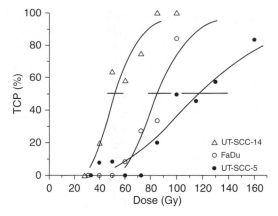

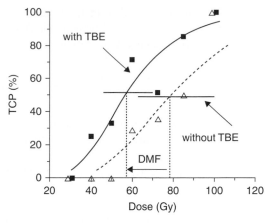

Figure 7.7 Dose-response curves for local tumour control of three different human squamous cell carcinomas growing in nude mice. Tumours were treated with 30 fractions over 6 weeks with total doses from 30 to 160 Gy. Treatment started for all tumours at the same tumour volume. The data were fitted using a Poisson-based model and the TCD_{50} (the dose required to control 50 per cent of the tumours locally) values as well as their confidence limits were calculated. The three carcinomas show clear-cut differences in radiation sensitivity with UT-SCC-14 being the most sensitive, FaDu with intermediate sensitivity and UT-SCC-5 being the most resistant. The differences in radiation sensitivity can be quantified by comparing the TCD_{50} values: 52.1 Gy (46; 59) for UT-SCC-14, 85.2 Gy (77; 96) for FaDu, and 129.8 Gy (104; 207) for UT-SCC-5. TCP, tumour control probability. Data from Yaromina et al. (2006).

The TCD_{50} assay has been used widely to investigate and quantify modifications in radiation sensitivity or number of clonogenic tumour cells (an example of a typical experiment is given in Fig. 7.8) and the data evaluation and reporting of results are well established and standardized. The effect of treatment modifications on local TCP can be quantified by calculation of a dose-modifying factor (DMF):

$$DMF = \frac{TCD_{50} \text{ (without modification)}}{TCD_{50} \text{ (with modification)}}$$

The DMF represents the relative reduction in radiation dose by a given treatment modification to achieve a certain level of TCP (isoeffect) compared with radiation without modification. In other words, DMF values larger than 1 indicate

Figure 7.8 FaDu human squamous cell carcinoma was transplanted either into unirradiated subcutaneous tissues or into pre-irradiated tissues of nude mice. Pre-irradiation of the transplantation site was performed to induce radiation damage to the supplying host tissues (tumour bed effect, TBE) as an experimental model of impaired tumour angiogenesis. At a tumour diameter of about 6 mm, tumours of both groups (with TBE and without TBE/control) were treated with 30 fractions over 6 weeks with total doses from 30 to 100 Gy. Local tumour control rates were determined 120 days after the end of fractionated irradiation. The TCD_{50} (dose required to control 50 per cent of the tumours locally) values were 56.6 Gy for the TBE group and 78.7 Gy for the control group. The effect of the pre-irradiation of the transplantation site on local tumour control after fractionated irradiation is given by the dose-modifying factor (DMF) of 1.4 ($TCD_{50,control}/TCD_{50,TBE}$). This indicates that the TBE improved local tumour control after fractionated irradiation (at the effect level 50 per cent) by a factor of 1.4. Data from Zips et al. (2001).

that the modification, for example by a new drug being tested, resulted in a greater sensitivity to radiation treatment.

Compared with other *in vivo* assays discussed below, however, the TCD_{50} assay is time-consuming and expensive. To design, perform and evaluate experiments using this local tumour-control end-point requires considerable technical knowledge and experience. Intercurrent death of animals may hamper adequate follow up, which needs to be sufficiently long to detect virtually all recurrences (i.e. mostly 4–6 months, depending on the tumour line). Small variations in the number of surviving clonogenic cells after irradiation may cause dramatic differences in local TCP. Therefore the TCD_{50} assay, particularly in xenograft models, is very sensitive to the host's immune reaction (Rofstad, 1989). Whether a tumour model evokes an immune response by the host must be therefore tested before local tumour control experiments are undertaken. Nevertheless despite these drawbacks, the local tumour control assay remains the most relevant experimental method to determine survival of clonogenic tumour cells after irradiation in their environment of treatment. Very importantly, the TCD_{50} assay is well standardized and the experimental endpoint is identical to the clinical endpoint used in curative radiotherapy.

Excision assays

Alternative experimental methods to determine clonogenic survival after irradiation include the *in vivo/in vitro* assay, the endpoint dilution assay and the lung colony assay. These assays, introduced in Chapter 4, Section 4.4, all require surgical excision of the tumours after irradiation *in situ* and the preparation of a single-cell suspension from the excised tumour using tryptic enzymes to disaggregate the tissue. For the *in vivo/in vitro* assay, different numbers of cells are seeded in culture flasks (Hill, 1987). After an incubation time of typically 7–21 days the number of colonies is counted. A colony consists of at least 50 cells and is considered to derive from a single surviving clonogenic tumour cell. As in the classical *in vitro* colony forming assay (see Chapter 4, Section 4.2), the surviving fraction is calculated from the ratio of colonies counted to the number of cells seeded. For the lung colony assay, different numbers of cells derived from a tumour irradiated *in situ* are injected intravenously (typically via a tail vein) into groups of recipient mice. Usually around 10 days later, the number of tumour-cell colonies in the lungs is counted and the surviving fraction is calculated by comparison with lung colonies that grew from cells derived from unirradiated tumours. For the endpoint dilution assay (TD_{50} assay) different numbers of cells from an irradiated tumour are inoculated into recipient animals and the frequency of tumour take (tumour growth) is scored.

Excision assays are less resource-consuming and give more rapid results than local tumour control assays. In the *in vivo/in vitro* assay, potential effects of the host immune system are also ruled out. However, a disadvantage of excision assays is that clonogen survival is not determined in the original environment of treatment. Furthermore, results may be affected by the disaggregation method used for single-cell preparation (i.e. the influence of timing, chemicals, enzymes and mechanical stress). For colony assays (in *vivo/in vitro* assay and lung colony assay) extensive background information is necessary before the experiment can start: whether the cells form colonies, how many cells at a given radiation dose need to be plated or injected and how long to incubate before counting colonies. The maximum number of cells that can be plated in Petri dishes or injected intravenously is restricted, making it difficult to detect surviving fractions accurately below about 10^{-4}. Thus, small but resistant subpopulations of clonogenic cells may be systematically overlooked particularly by colony assays. Furthermore, effects of prolonged treatment such as fractionated irradiations are difficult to assess by excision assays (Hill, 1987).

Regression

To determine tumour regression, the volumes of treated and untreated tumours at a given timepoint are compared and the ratios for treated versus control tumours (T/C ratios) are reported. The magnitude of tumour regression depends upon radiation effects on the entire cell population in a tumour, including malignant and non-malignant cells, for example endothelial cells, fibroblasts and inflammatory cells. In addition, other factors such as oedema, resorption of dead cells and proliferation of surviving cells contribute to the tumour volume after radiation. These factors differ considerably between different tumours. Whereas tumour cell kill is radiation-dose dependent, resorption, oedema and proliferation may not be. From the notion that regression increases with radiation dose one can argue that for a given tumour model the magnitude of regression reflects the radiation dose-dependent tumour cell kill. Tumour volume measurements under experimental conditions are roughly limited to a range of $1.5 \times 10^7 - 1.5 \times 10^9$ tumour cells (assuming 10^9 cells/g tumour; compare Fig. 7.1). Thus even for a given tumour model, volume measurements only assay the radiation response of a very limited proportion of all tumour cells and the response of small and possibly resistant tumour cell populations cannot be detected. In summary, tumour regression is a highly non-specific parameter and of very limited value in describing and quantifying the effect of radiation on tumours.

Tumour regrowth delay

This is a widely used assay that rapidly provides the researcher with data and can be applied in the laboratory or the clinic. The endpoint is the time to reach a certain tumour volume. Therefore, precise determination of tumour volume (e.g. by callipers for subcutaneously growing tumours or by imaging methods) is essential. In experimental studies, groups of tumours are irradiated and one group of tumours is left unirradiated (control group). Then, the volume of each individual tumour is recorded over time and a growth curve is plotted (Fig. 7.9). From this growth curve different parameters may be read, such as the time it takes for a tumour to grow (tumour growth time, TGT) to five times the treatment volume (TGT_{V5}). From the TGT values for individual tumours the average values for each treatment group ($TGT_{treated}$) and of the control group ($TGT_{control}$) are calculated. Tumour growth delay (TGD) is then calculated from:

$$TGD = TGT_{treated} - TGT_{control}$$

The specific growth delay (SGD) takes the growth rate of the tumour model into account and allows comparison between different tumour models or different treatments. The SGD is calculated from:

$$SGD = (TGT_{treated} - TGT_{control})/TGT_{control}$$

or

$$SGD = TGT/VDT_{control}$$

Tumour regrowth following irradiation depends upon the effect treatment has had on malignant and

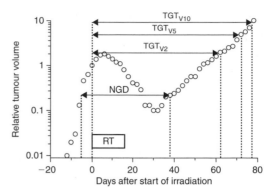

Figure 7.9 Growth curve of an individual FaDu tumour treated with 15 fractions of 2 Gy. Tumour volume was calculated using the formula for a rotational ellipsoid ($V = [\pi/6]*a*b^2$) where a is the longest tumour axis and b is the axis perpendicular to a. The parameters a and b were measured every second day using callipers. The volume is plotted as relative to the volume at the start of treatment. During the initial phase of irradiation the volume increased and later decreased to reach the lowest relative volume (nadir) on day 30 after the start of treatment. After this regression the tumour regrew at a slower rate than before radiation (the regrowth curve is shallower than the growth curve before radiotherapy) indicating the tumour bed effect. From the growth curve, different parameters of the regrowth assay can be read: tumour growth time to reach twice, five times, and ten times the starting volume (TGT_2, TGT_5, TGT_{10}). See text for explanation of NGD (net growth delay).

non-malignant cells. Radiation-induced damage to the host vascular connective tissues surrounding the tumour may result in a slower growth rate of irradiated tumours; this is called the tumour bed effect. As a consequence, SGD apparently increases with increasing tumour volume (Fig. 7.9). To correct for the tumour bed effect, the parameter net growth delay (NGD) has been suggested (Beck-Bornholdt *et al.*, 1987). Net growth delay is defined as the time between when the regrowing tumour has reached twice its minimal volume (nadir) after treatment and the time at which the tumour had the same volume before treatment. An alternative would be to choose the endpoint size as low as possible.

The TGD increases with radiation dose, reflecting the dose-dependency of cell kill (Fig. 7.10).

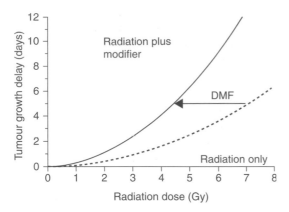

Figure 7.10 Tumour growth delay after treatment at different radiation doses with and without a treatment modifier. The modifier results in a longer tumour growth delay (TGD) per radiation dose. The effect of the modifier can be quantified as the dose-modifying factor (DMF).

The relationships found between radiation dose, the logarithm of surviving clonogenic tumour cells and the TGD suggest that the TGD is a surrogate parameter for clonogenic cell kill. However, there are several limitations. First, quantitative transplantation experiments revealed that the tumour growth rate decreases with decreasing numbers of inoculated cells (Urano and Kahn, 1987). This suggests that, at low levels of cell survival, TGD may not correlate well with the surviving number of clonogenic cells. Second, TGD depends a great deal on the radiation effect on the mass of non-clonogenic tumour cells. As a consequence, small variations in the population of clonogenic cells (number and/or sensitivity) may not be detected by the TGD assay. Third, the TGD reflects not only cell kill but also the growth rate of the regrowing tumour. Therefore, this assay is highly sensitive to variations in the proliferation rate, including pharmacological manipulations. Thus, a longer TGD does not always mean a higher cell kill. The limitations of the TGD to precisely reflect clonogenic cell kill are underlined by the observation that results from TGD assays might not correlate with results obtained from local tumour control assays (Overgaard *et al.*, 1987; Baumann *et al.*, 2003; Krause *et al.*, 2004; Zips *et al.*, 2005). This important caveat must be considered,

for example, when the TGD assay is used to evaluate radiation modifiers (see Chapter 21). Solutions to this problem include performing confirmatory local tumour control experiments or possibly obtaining TGD at different radiation dose levels (dose–response relationship) as well as calculating the growth delay per gray (i.e. the steepness of the dose–response curve; Krause *et al.*, 2006).

To quantify and report the magnitude of effect caused by radiation modifiers on TGD, the DMF or the enhancement ratio (ER) have been used. The DMF is calculated as the ratio of radiation dose with and without modifier giving the same TGD (i.e. the ratio of isoeffective radiation doses). Thus, calculation of the DMF requires the investigation of multiple radiation dose levels and the construction of dose–response curves (Fig. 7.10). Often, only one radiation dose level is investigated. In such situations the ER has been used instead of DMF to describe the effect of the modifier. The ER is the ratio of TGD with/without modifier at a given radiation dose level. Both ER and DMF depend on the position and steepness of the dose–effect curves. The ER might depend on the radiation dose and DMF might depend on the level of effect. In general, the interpretation of TGD, ER and DMF, and their relevance for clonogenic tumour cell inactivation, is complicated. Despite its apparent simplicity, the inherent methodological problems of the TGD assay (described above), the lack of consensus about data evaluation and arbitrary procedural details limit its value in reliably quantifying the radiation response of clonogenic cells. It is therefore recommended to always test the conclusions from TGD assays by undertaking local tumour control studies, before introducing novel treatments into clinical radiotherapy.

7.3 FACTORS INFLUENCING LOCAL TUMOUR CONTROL

Introduction

A number of factors can contribute to the probability of local tumour control after fractionated radiotherapy. These factors have been summarized by Withers (1975) as the four Rs of radiotherapy: recovery from sublethal damage, cell-cycle redistribution, cellular repopulation and tumour reoxygenation. Steel and colleagues have suggested intrinsic cellular radiosensitivity as a fifth 'R' to account for the different tolerance of tissues to fractionated irradiation (Steel *et al.*, 1989).

Recovery from sublethal damage

Most of the damage induced in cells by radiation is satisfactorily repaired. Evidence for this comes from studies of strand breaks in DNA, the vast majority of which disappear during the first few hours after irradiation (see Chapter 2, Sections 2.7 and 2.8). Further evidence for repair comes from the wide variety of recovery experiments that have been done, both on *in vitro* cell lines and on normal and tumour tissues *in vivo*. It is useful to draw a distinction between these two sources of evidence:

- *Repair* – refers to the process by which the function of macromolecules is restored. Rejoining of DNA strand breaks provides some evidence

for this, although the rejoining of a break does not necessarily mean that gene function is restored. Rejoining can leave a genetic defect (i.e. a mutation) and specific tests of repair fidelity are needed to detect this. The word 'repair' is often loosely used as an synonym for cellular or tissue recovery.

- *Recovery* – refers to the increase in cell survival or reduction in the extent of radiation damage to a tissue, when time is allowed for this to occur.

There are a number of experimental sources of evidence for recovery, including the following.

- *Split-dose experiments* – the effect of a given dose of radiation is less if it is split into two fractions, delivered a few hours apart. This effect has been termed 'recovery from sublethal damage' (SLD), or 'Elkind recovery' (Elkind and Sutton, 1960). The SLD recovery can be observed using various experimental endpoints: for example, using cell survival (Fig. 7.11a), tumour growth delay (Fig. 7.11c) or mouse lethality after irradiating a vital

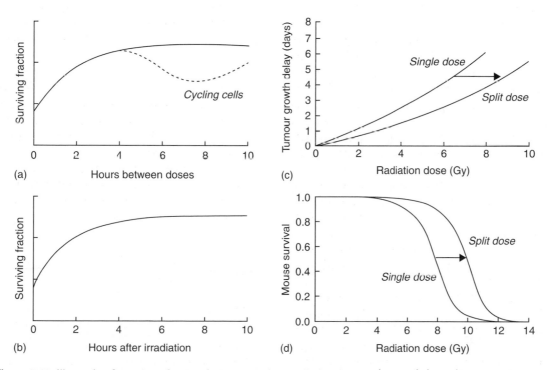

Figure 7.11 Illustrating four ways of measuring recovery from radiation damage (see text). (a, c, d) Three types of split-dose experiment; (b) the result of a 'delayed-plating experiment'. The arrows indicate the measurement of (D_2-D_1) values.

normal tissue (Fig. 7.11d). The typical timing of split-dose recovery is shown in Fig. 7.11a. Considerable recovery occurs within 15 min to 1 hour, and recovery often seems to be complete by roughly 6 hours but can be slower than this in some normal tissues such as the spinal cord (Table 9.2). When the split-dose technique is applied to cycling cells (Fig. 7.11a) there is usually a wave in the data caused by cell-cycle progression effects (see below).

- *Delayed-plating experiments* – if cells are irradiated in a non-growing state and left for increasing periods of time before assaying for survival, an increase in survival is often observed (Fig. 7.11b). During this delay the cells are recovering the ability to divide when called upon to do so. This has been termed 'recovery from potentially lethal damage' (PLD). The kinetics of PLD recovery and SLD recovery are similar.
- *Dose-rate effect* – reduction in radiation damage as dose rate is reduced to around 1 Gy/hour is primarily caused by cellular recovery (see Chapter 12).
- *Fractionation* – the sparing effect of fractionating radiation treatment within a relatively short overall time is primarily due to recovery. This is therefore the main reason why isoeffect curves slope upwards as the fraction number is increased (see Chapter 8, Figs 8.1 and 8.2).

What is the relationship between all these various ways of detecting recovery? The damage induced in cells by ionizing radiation is complex, as are the enzymatic processes that immediately begin to repair it. The various types of 'recovery experiment' listed above evaluate this complex repair process in slightly different ways. For example, the evaluation based on giving a second dose (i.e. SLD recovery) may be different from that obtained by 'asking' irradiated non-dividing cells to divide (i.e. PLD recovery).

Variation of cell killing through the cell cycle, cell-cycle delay and redistribution

The radiosensitivity of cells varies considerably as they pass through the cell cycle. This has been studied in a large number of cell lines, using cell synchronization techniques and fluorescence-activated cell sorting (FACS) to obtain cell populations in each cell-cycle phase. There is a general tendency for cells in the S phase (in particular the latter part of the S phase) to be the most resistant and for cells in very late G2 and mitosis to be the most sensitive. The reason for the resistance in S phase is thought to be homologous recombination, which is increased as a result of the greater availability of the undamaged sister template through the S phase, together with conformational changes in DNA facilitating the easier access of repair complexes during replication. Sensitivity very late in G2 and into mitosis probably results from the fact that those cells have passed a final checkpoint in G2 which occurs within minutes of radiation exposure and allows cells in early G2 to repair their damage probably using homologous recombination (see Chapter 2, Section 2.7). The classic results of Sinclair and Morton (1965) are illustrated in Fig. 7.12. They synchronized Chinese hamster cells at five different points in the cell cycle and performed cell survival experiments. The survival curves showed that it was mainly the shoulder of the curve that changed: there was little shoulder for cells in mitosis and the shoulder was greatest for cells in S phase.

The effect of this phenomenon on an asynchronous cell population is that it creates a degree of

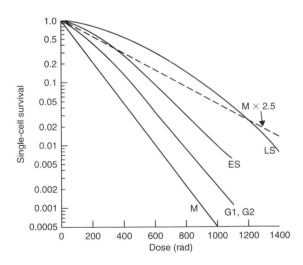

Figure 7.12 Variation of radiosensitivity through the cell cycle of Chinese hamster cells. Adapted from Sinclair and Morton (1965), with permission.

synchrony in the cells that survive irradiation. Immediately after a dose of X-rays, all the cells will still be at precisely the same point in the cell cycle as they were before irradiation, but some will have lost their reproductive integrity and it is the number that retains this which will tend to be greatest in the S phase. With increasing time after irradiation the surviving clonogenic cells will show the same distribution over the cell cycle as before irradiation. This phenomenon is called redistribution. In the 1970s there was much interest in synchronization therapy. This was an attempt to exploit cell-cycle progression phenomena by treating with a second agent (usually a cytotoxic drug) at the optimum time interval after a priming treatment with drug or radiation. Although this approach to improving tumour therapy was thoroughly researched it proved in most cases to be disappointing. One possible reason for this is that tumours tend to be very heterogeneous from a kinetic point of view: cells move at very different speeds through the phases of the cell cycle and induced cell synchrony is therefore quickly lost (Steel, 1977).

Reoxygenation

This important factor influencing local tumour control is described in Chapter 15. The clinical implications for modified fractionation are discussed in Chapters 16 and 17.

Repopulation

Each fraction during a course of fractionated radiotherapy reduces the total population of clonogenic tumour cells in a tumour (i.e. causes a depopulation of the clonogenic tumour cell compartment; Fig. 7.3). In general, clonogenic cells that survive radiation can repopulate the tumour by proliferation and/or reduced cell loss. Repopulation of clonogenic tumour cells might occur during the course of fractionated radiotherapy and thereby reduce the efficacy of treatment. If a tumour has the capacity to repopulate, any prolongation of the overall treatment time results in a higher number of clonogenic tumour cells that need to be inactivated and thereby requires a higher radiation dose to achieve local tumour

control. The so-called time factor of fractionated radiotherapy (see Chapter 10) has been largely attributed to repopulation of clonogenic tumour cells during treatment (Kummermehr et al., 1992; Thames et al., 1996; Petersen et al., 2001; Hessel et al., 2004). Accelerated repopulation describes a phenomenon that the net clonogen doubling time during or shortly after irradiation exceeds the clonogen doubling time in untreated tumours. Repopulation of clonogenic tumour cells during fractionated radiotherapy has been shown in a large variety of different experimental and clinical studies, as described in Chapter 10 and reviewed by Baumann et al. (2003). The results are most consistent for squamous cell carcinomas, but for other tumour types evidence for a time factor is also accumulating. The rate, kinetics and underlying radiobiological mechanisms of repopulation vary substantially between tumour types as well as between different tumour lines of the same tumour type. For example, FaDu human squamous cell carcinoma transplanted into nude mice repopulates rapidly with a dose of about 1 Gy recovered per day during fractionated irradiation (Baumann et al., 1994).

The kinetics and radiobiological mechanisms of repopulation have been studied in an extensive series of experiments with fractionated irradiation given to human tumour xenografts either under clamp hypoxia or under normal blood flow conditions (Petersen et al., 2001). A switch to rapid repopulation was observed after about 3 weeks of fractionated irradiation, with the clonogen doubling time decreasing from 9.8 days during the first 3 weeks to 3.4 days thereafter (Fig. 7.13). In this study, acceleration of repopulation was preceded by a decrease in tumour hypoxia after 2 weeks of fractionated irradiation, suggesting that improved tumour oxygenation might trigger repopulation in tumours either by facilitating more proliferation and/or by reducing cell loss. Increased labelling indices for BrdUrd (S-phase fraction) and Ki67 (growth fraction) during fractionated irradiation indicate that increased proliferation contributes directly to repopulation (Petersen et al., 2003). Repopulation rate was found to be lower in tumours with increased cell loss, indirectly implying that decreased cell loss might also enhance repopulation (Hessel et al., 2003). This latter

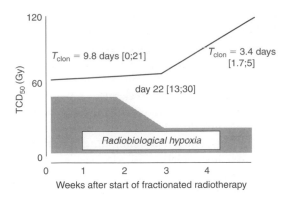

Figure 7.13 Rate, kinetics and underlying mechanism of repopulation of clonogenic tumour cells in FaDu squamous cell carcinoma growing in nude mice (data from Petersen *et al.*, 2001). As the result of repopulation, the tumour control dose (TCD$_{50}$) increases with time. Clonogenic FaDu tumour cells repopulate at a low rate during the first 3 weeks with an estimated clonogen doubling time (T_{clon}) of 9.8 days. After a switch around day 22, repopulation accelerates to a T_{clon} of 3.4 days. In this tumour model the switch in repopulation is preceded by a decrease in radiobiological hypoxia.

concept – that clonogens always proliferate at their maximum rate ('potential clonogen doubling time') but, owing to the limited supply of nutrients and oxygen, clonogens are pushed towards necrosis by the proliferative pressure from the cell layers close to supporting blood vessels – was originally postulated by Fowler (1991). Once radiotherapy has killed off enough well oxygenated tumour cells, the oxygen and nutrient supply improves and the spontaneous cell loss decreases. The effective doubling time of clonogens therefore becomes shorter and shorter during treatment and eventually the T_{pot} of clonogens is 'unmasked'.

In contrast to this concept it has been suggested, particularly for well-differentiated tumours, that an actively regulated regenerative response of surviving clonogens reminiscent of a normal epithelium represents the major mechanism of clonogen repopulation (Trott and Kummermehr, 1991; Kummermehr *et al.*, 1992; Dorr, 1997; Hansen *et al.*, 1997). Signalling via the epidermal growth factor receptor (EGFR) has been proposed as a potential molecular mechanism of this

regulated regenerative response underlying repopulation (Schmidt-Ullrich *et al.*, 1999; Petersen *et al.*, 2003; Bentzen *et al.*, 2005; Eriksen *et al.*, 2005; Krause *et al.*, 2005), as described in Chapter 21.

Tumour volume

Large tumours are more difficult to cure than small tumours. This has been known since the early years of radiotherapy (Miescher, 1929). There are several explanations for this observation. First, tumour volume is proportional to the number of clonogens per tumour. Second, hypoxia is more pronounced in large tumours than in small tumours. Third, in the clinical situation large tumours can often not be irradiated to curative doses because of the larger irradiated volume and limited tolerance of the adjacent normal tissues. Assuming a linear relationship between the number of clonogens and tumour volume, and other parameters such as density, radiosensitivity and hypoxic fraction of clonogenic tumour cells all being equal, the relationship between the tumour control probability (TCP$_2$) and the relative tumour volume (V_{rel}) can be described according to Dubben *et al.* (1998) as:

$$TCP_2 = TCP_1^{V_{rel}}$$

where TCP$_1$ represents the reference TCP when the relative tumour volume (V_{rel}) equals 1. If, for example, a TCP$_1$ of 50 per cent is chosen then the relationship between relative tumour volume and TCP can be described with the function TCP$_2$ = 50$^{V_{rel}}$ (Fig. 7.14). Over a wide range, the TCP decreases roughly linearly with the logarithm of tumour volume (or the number of clonogens), whereas at very low and very high TCPs the impact of tumour volume is less pronounced. Both experimental and clinical data lend support to this simple theory, indicating that tumour volume is indeed an important factor influencing local tumour control after radiotherapy (Baumann *et al.*, 1990; Bentzen and Thames, 1996; Dubben *et al.*, 1998). However, analysis of clinical data has also revealed that the effect of tumour volume on TCP is less than expected from Fig. 7.14 (Bentzen and Thames, 1996). This is not surprising as the

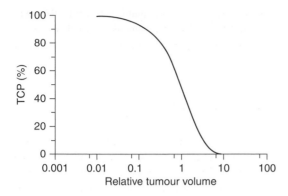

Figure 7.14 Theoretical relationship of tumour control probability (TCP) and relative tumour volume according to Dubben *et al.* (1998). A TCP of 50 per cent is arbitrarily chosen to correspond to a relative tumour volume of 1. The relationship is based on the assumption of a linear relationship between the number of clonogens and tumour volume and that all other parameters (e.g. density, radiosensitivity and hypoxic fraction of clonogenic tumour cells) are invariant. Reprinted with permission from Elsevier.

above-mentioned assumption that all other factors than volume are equal is not realistic in the clinical situation. Instead, patient-to-patient heterogeneity in a large variety of known and unknown determinants of local tumour control may interfere with the simple proportionality of TCP and tumour volume. However, as for other known prognostic factors in radiotherapy, such as stage, age, histology, etc., tumour volume should be routinely measured and reported in clinical trials as well as included into data analyses.

ACKNOWLEDGEMENT

The author gratefully acknowledges the help of A. Begg and G. Steel for allowing parts of their chapter from the previous edition of this textbook to be used.

Key points

1. Volume of growing tumours increases exponentially with time. Therefore, tumour volume should always be plotted on a logarithmic scale to facilitate evaluation of growth curves, comparison of growth rates among different tumours, and judgement of treatment effects.

2. Growth rates vary among different tumours. Primary tumours tend to grow more slowly than metastatic lesions. A volume doubling time of 3 months is typical for many primary tumours.

3. Tumour growth rate is determined by the fraction of cycling cells (growth fraction, GF), the cell cycle time (T_C) and the cell loss rate. Typical values for human tumours are 40 per cent, 2 days, and 90 per cent, respectively. However, these parameters vary considerably between tumours and even among tumours of the same histological type.

4. Potential doubling time (T_{pot}) is the theoretical volume doubling time in the absence of cell loss. Therefore, the difference between the observed volume doubling time and the T_{pot} is explained by cell loss in tumours, which exceeds 90 per cent in many histological types.

5. The faster growth of experimental tumours compared with tumours in patients results from a higher GF, shorter T_{pot} and a lower cell loss factor.

6. Response of tumours to radiation can be assayed using different endpoints, including local tumour control, tumour regrowth delay and regression.

7. Local tumour control is the aim of curative radiotherapy and therefore conceptually the most relevant endpoint to assay radiation response.

8. Local tumour control is achieved when all clonogenic tumour cells (i.e. cells with the capacity to proliferate and to cause a local recurrence) are inactivated.

9. Ionizing irradiation is highly effective in inactivating clonogenic tumour cells. The logarithm of the number of surviving clonogenic tumour cells decreases linearly with total radiation dose during fractionated radiotherapy.

10. Response criteria such as partial response or complete response are not appropriate to describe the radiation response of clonogenic tumour cells.
11. Tumour regression is a non-specific parameter of very limited value to describe and quantify radiation effects in tumours.
12. The tumour regrowth delay assay is widely used in experimental radiotherapy. Methodological problems limit the value of this assay to accurately measure the survival of clonogenic tumour cells. Thus, confirmatory local tumour control experiments are recommended.
13. Different factors influence the probability of local tumour control (five Rs of fractionated radiotherapy).
14. Repopulation of clonogenic tumour cells represents a major cause of resistance to fractionated irradiation in certain tumour types. The rate, kinetics and underlying radiobiological mechanisms vary widely among different tumours.
15. Tumour volume is an important determinant of local tumour control.

■ BIBLIOGRAPHY

Baumann M, Dubois W, Suit HD (1990). Response of human squamous cell carcinoma xenografts of different sizes to irradiation: relationship of clonogenic cells, cellular radiation sensitivity *in vivo*, and tumor rescuing units. *Radiat Res* **123**: 325–30.

Baumann M, Liertz C, Baisch H, Wiegel T, Lorenzen J, Arps H (1994). Impact of overall treatment time of fractionated irradiation on local control of human FaDu squamous cell carcinoma in nude mice. *Radiother Oncol* **32**: 137–43.

Baumann M, Krause M, Zips D *et al.* (2003). Selective inhibition of the epidermal growth factor receptor tyrosine kinase by BIBX1382BS and the improvement of growth delay, but not local control, after fractionated irradiation in human FaDu squamous cell carcinoma in the nude mouse. *Int J Radiat Biol* **79**: 547–59.

Beck-Bornholdt HP, Wurschmidt F, Vogler H (1987). Net growth delay: a novel parameter derived from tumor growth curves. *Int J Radiat Oncol Biol Phys* **13**: 773–7.

Begg AC, McNally NJ, Shrieve DC, Karcher H (1985). A method to measure the duration of DNA synthesis and the potential doubling time from a single sample. *Cytometry* **6**: 620–6.

Begg AC, Haustermans K, Hart AA *et al.* (1999). The value of pretreatment cell kinetic parameters as predictors for radiotherapy outcome in head and neck cancer: a multicenter analysis. *Radiother Oncol* **50**: 13–23.

Bentzen SM, Thames HD (1996). Tumor volume and local control probability: clinical data and radiobiological interpretations. *Int J Radiat Oncol Biol Phys* **36**: 247–51.

Bentzen SM, Atasoy BM, Daley FM *et al.* (2005). Epidermal growth factor receptor expression in pretreatment biopsies from head and neck squamous cell carcinoma as a predictive factor for a benefit from accelerated radiation therapy in a randomized controlled trial. *J Clin Oncol* **23**: 5560–7.

Brown DC, Gatter KC (2002). Ki67 protein: the immaculate deception? *Histopathology* **40**: 2–11.

Dorr W (1997). Three As of repopulation during fractionated irradiation of squamous epithelia: Asymmetry loss, Acceleration of stem-cell divisions and Abortive divisions. *Int J Radiat Biol* **72**: 635–43.

Dubben HH, Thames HD, Beck-Bornholdt HP (1998). Tumor volume: a basic and specific response predictor in radiotherapy. *Radiother Oncol* **47**: 167–74.

Elkind MM, Sutton H (1960). Radiation response of mammalian cells grown in culture. 1. Repair of X-ray damage in surviving Chinese hamster cells. *Radiat Res* **13**: 556–93.

Eriksen JG, Steiniche T, Overgaard J (2005). The influence of epidermal growth factor receptor and tumor differentiation on the response to accelerated radiotherapy of squamous cell carcinomas of the head and neck in the randomized DAHANCA 6 and 7 study. *Radiother Oncol* **74**: 93–100.

Fowler JF (1991). Rapid repopulation in radiotherapy: a debate on mechanism. The phantom of tumor treatment – continually rapid proliferation unmasked. *Radiother Oncol* **22**: 156–8.

Fowler JE, Pandey P, Braswell NT, Seaver L (1994). Prostate specific antigen progression rates after radical prostatectomy or radiation therapy for localized prostate cancer. *Surgery* **116**: 302–5.

Gerweck LE, Zaidi ST, Zietman A (1994). Multivariate determinants of radiocurability. I. Prediction of single fraction tumor control doses. *Int J Radiat Oncol Biol Phys* **29**: 57–66.

Haitel A, Wiener HG, Migschitz B, Marberger M, Susani M (1997). Proliferating cell nuclear antigen and MIB-1. An alternative to classic prognostic indicators in renal cell carcinomas? *Am J Clin Pathol* **107**: 229–35.

Hanahan D, Weinberg RA (2000). The hallmarks of cancer. *Cell* **100**: 57–70.

Hansen O, Overgaard J, Hansen HS *et al.* (1997). Importance of overall treatment time for the outcome of radiotherapy of advanced head and neck carcinoma: dependency on tumor differentiation. *Radiother Oncol* **43**: 47–51.

Haustermans KM, Hofland I, van Poppel H *et al.* (1997). Cell kinetic measurements in prostate cancer. *Int J Radiat Oncol Biol Phys* **37**: 1067–70.

Hessel F, Petersen C, Zips D *et al.* (2003). Impact of increased cell loss on the repopulation rate during fractionated irradiation in human FaDu squamous cell carcinoma growing in nude mice. *Int J Radiat Biol* **79**: 479–86.

Hessel F, Krause M, Helm A *et al.* (2004). Differentiation status of human squamous cell carcinoma xenografts does not appear to correlate with the repopulation capacity of clonogenic tumour cells during fractionated irradiation. *Int J Radiat Biol* **80**: 719–27.

Hill RP (1987). Excision assays. In: Kallman RF (eds) *Rodent tumor models in experimental cancer therapy.* New York: Pergamon Press, 67–75.

Hill RP, Milas L (1989). The proportion of stem cells in murine tumors. *Int J Radiat Oncol Biol Phys* **16**: 513–8.

Hommura F, Dosaka-Akita H, Mishina T *et al.* (2000). Prognostic significance of p27KIP1 protein and ki-67 growth fraction in non-small cell lung cancers. *Clin Cancer Res* **6**: 4073–81.

Hoskin PJ, Sibtain A, Daley FM, Saunders MI, Wilson GD (2004). The immunohistochemical assessment of hypoxia, vascularity and proliferation in bladder carcinoma. *Radiother Oncol* **72**: 159–68.

Jensen V, Sorensen FB, Bentzen SM *et al.* (1998). Proliferative activity (MIB-1 index) is an independent prognostic parameter in patients with high-grade soft tissue sarcomas of subtypes other than malignant fibrous histiocytomas: a retrospective immunohistological study including 216 soft tissue sarcomas. *Histopathology* **32**: 536–46.

Jung H, Kruger HJ, Brammer I, Zywietz F, Beck-Bornholdt HP (1990). Cell population kinetics of the rhabdomyosarcoma R1H of the rat after single doses of X-rays. *Int J Radiat Biol* **57**: 567–89.

Krause M, Hessel F, Zips D, Hilberg F, Baumann M (2004). Adjuvant inhibition of the epidermal growth factor receptor after fractionated irradiation of FaDu human squamous cell carcinoma. *Radiother Oncol* **72**: 95–101.

Krause M, Ostermann G, Petersen C *et al.* (2005). Decreased repopulation as well as increased reoxygenation contribute to the improvement in local control after targeting of the EGFR by C225 during fractionated irradiation. *Radiother Oncol* **76**: 162–7.

Krause M, Zips D, Thames HD, Kummermehr J, Baumann M (2006). Preclinical evaluation of molecular-targeted anticancer agents for radiotherapy. *Radiother Oncol* **80**: 112–22.

Kummermehr J, Dorr W, Trott KR (1992). Kinetics of accelerated repopulation in normal and malignant squamous epithelia during fractionated radiotherapy. *BJR Suppl* **24**: 193–9.

Lanza G Jr, Cavazzini L, Borghi L, Ferretti S, Buccoliero F, Rubbini M (1990). Immunohistochemical assessment of growth fractions in colorectal adenocarcinomas with monoclonal antibody Ki-67. Relation to clinical and pathological variables. *Pathol Res Pract* **186**: 608–18.

Lee WR, Hanks GE, Corn BW, Schultheiss TE (1995). Observations of pretreatment prostate-specific antigen doubling time in 107 patients referred for definitive radiotherapy. *Int J Radiat Oncol Biol Phys* **31**: 21–4.

Linder S, Parrado C, Falkmer UG, Blasjo M, Sundelin P, von Rosen A (1997). Prognostic significance of Ki-67 antigen and p53 protein expression in pancreatic duct carcinoma: a study of the monoclonal antibodies MIB-1 and DO-7 in formalin-fixed paraffin-embedded tumour material. *Br J Cancer* **76**: 54–9.

Malaise EP, Chavaudra N, Tubiana M (1973). The relationship between growth rate, labelling index and histological type of human solid tumours. *Eur J Cancer* **9**: 305–12.

Miescher G (1929). Röntgentherapie der Hautkarzinome. *Schweiz Med Wochenschr* II: 1225.

Munro TR, Gilbert CW (1961). The relation between tumour lethal doses and the radiosensitivity of tumour cells. *Br J Radiol* **34**: 246–51.

Overgaard J, Matsui M, Lindegaard JC *et al.* (1987). Relationship between tumor growth delay and modification of tumor-control probability of various treatments given as an adjuvant to irradiation. In: Kallman RF (ed.) *Rodent tumor models in experimental cancer therapy.* New York: Pergamon Press, 128–32.

Petersen C, Zips D, Krause M *et al.* (2001). Repopulation of FaDu human squamous cell carcinoma during fractionated radiotherapy correlates with reoxygenation. *Int J Radiat Oncol Biol Phys* **51**: 483–93.

Petersen C, Eicheler W, Frommel A *et al.* (2003). Proliferation and micromilieu during fractionated irradiation of human FaDu squamous cell carcinoma in nude mice. *Int J Radiat Biol* **79**: 469–77.

Potten CS, Wichmann HE, Dobek K *et al.* (1985). Cell kinetic studies in the epidermis of mouse. III. The percent labelled mitosis (PLM) technique. *Cell Tissue Kinet* **18**: 59–70.

Rautiainen E, Haapasalo H, Sallinen P, Rantala I, Helen P, Helin H (1998). Histone mRNA *in-situ* hybridization in astrocytomas: a comparison with PCNA, MIB-1 and mitoses in paraffin-embedded material. *Histopathology* **32**: 43–50.

Rew DA, Wilson GD (2000). Cell production rates in human tissues and tumours and their significance. Part II: clinical data. *Eur J Surg Oncol* **26**: 405–17.

Rofstad EK (1989). Local tumor control following single dose irradiation of human melanoma xenografts: relationship to cellular radiosensitivity and influence of an immune response by the athymic mouse. *Cancer Res* **49**: 3163–7.

Rofstad EK, Wahl A, Brustad T (1986). Radiation response of human melanoma multicellular spheroids measured as single cell survival, growth delay, and spheroid cure: comparisons with the parent tumor xenograft. *Int J Radiat Oncol Biol Phys* **12**: 975–82.

Roland NJ, Caslin AW, Bowie GL, Jones AS (1994). Has the cellular proliferation marker Ki67 any clinical relevance in squamous cell carcinoma of the head and neck? *Clin Otolaryngol Allied Sci* **19**: 13–8.

Roser F, Samii M, Ostertag H, Bellinzona M (2004). The Ki-67 proliferation antigen in meningiomas. Experience in 600 cases. *Acta Neurochir (Wien)* **146**: 37–44.

Sarbia M, Bittinger F, Porschen R *et al.* (1996). The prognostic significance of tumour cell proliferation in squamous cell carcinomas of the oesophagus. *Br J Cancer* **74**: 1012–6.

Schmid HP, McNeal JE, Stamey TA (1993). Observations on the doubling time of prostate cancer. The use of serial prostate-specific antigen in patients with untreated disease as a measure of increasing cancer volume. *Cancer* **71**: 2031–40.

Schmidt-Ullrich RK, Contessa JN, Dent P *et al.* (1999). Molecular mechanisms of radiation-induced accelerated repopulation. *Radiat Oncol Investig* **7**: 321–30.

Sinclair WK, Morton RA (1965). X-Ray and ultraviolet sensitivity of synchronized Chinese hamster cells at various stages of the cell cycle. *Biophys J* **5**: 1–25.

Spratt JS, Meyer JS, Spratt JA (1996). Rates of growth of human neoplasms: Part II. *J Surg Oncol* **61**: 68–83.

Steel GG (1977). *The growth kinetics of tumours.* Oxford: Oxford University Press.

Steel GG, McMillan TJ, Peacock JH (1989). The 5Rs of radiobiology. *Int J Radiat Biol* **56**: 1045–8.

Suit HD, Sedlacek R, Thames HD (1987). Radiation dose–response assays of tumor control. In: Kallman RF (ed.) *Rodent tumor models in experimental cancer therapy.* New York: Pergamon Press, 138–48.

Taftachi R, Ayhan A, Ekici S, Ergen A, Ozen H (2005). Proliferating-cell nuclear antigen (PCNA) as an independent prognostic marker in patients after prostatectomy: a comparison of PCNA and Ki–67. *BJU Int* **95**: 650–4.

Terry NH, White RA, Meistrich ML, Calkins DP (1991). Evaluation of flow cytometric methods for determining population potential doubling times using cultured cells. *Cytometry* **12**: 234–41.

Thames HD, Ruifrok AC, Milas L *et al.* (1996). Accelerated repopulation during fractionated irradiation of a murine ovarian carcinoma: downregulation of apoptosis as a possible mechanism. *Int J Radiat Oncol Biol Phys* **35**: 951–62.

Thor AD, Liu S, Moore DH, 2nd, Edgerton SM (1999). Comparison of mitotic index, *in vitro* bromodeoxyuridine labeling, and MIB-1 assays to quantitate proliferation in breast cancer. *J Clin Oncol* **17**: 470–7.

Trott KR, Kummermehr J (1991). Rapid repopulation in radiotherapy: a debate on mechanism. Accelerated repopulation in tumours and normal tissues. *Radiother Oncol* **22**: 159–60.

Trott KR, Maciejewski B, Preuss-Bayer G, Skolyszewski J (1984). Dose–response curve and split-dose recovery in human skin cancer. *Radiother Oncol* **2**: 123–9.

Urano M, Kahn J (1987). Some practical questions in the tumor regrowth assay. In: Kallman RF (ed.) *Rodent tumor models in experimental cancer therapy.* New York: Pergamon Press, 122–7.

Walker AM, Suit HD (1983). Assessment of local tumor control using censored tumor response data. *Int J Radiat Oncol Biol Phys* **9**: 383–6.

Wheldon TE, Abdelaal AS, Nias AH (1977). Tumour curability, cellular radiosensitivity and clonogenic cell number. *Br J Radiol* **50**: 843–4.

Withers HR. The four Rs of radiotherapy. In: Lett JT, Adler H (eds) *Advances in radiation biology.* New York: Academic Press, 1975.

Yaromina A, Zips D, Thames HD *et al.* (2006). Pimonidazole labelling and response to fractionated irradiation of five human squamous cell carcinoma (hSCC) cell lines in nude mice: The need for a multivariate approach in biomarker studies. *Radiother Oncol* **81**: 122–9.

Zips D, Eicheler W, Bruchner K *et al.* (2001). Impact of the tumour bed effect on microenvironment, radiobiological hypoxia and the outcome of fractionated radiotherapy of human FaDu squamous-cell carcinoma growing in the nude mouse. *Int J Radiat Biol* **77**: 1185–93.

Zips D, Hessel F, Krause M *et al.* (2005). Impact of adjuvant inhibition of vascular endothelial growth factor receptor tyrosine kinases on tumor growth delay and local tumor control after fractionated irradiation in human squamous cell carcinomas in nude mice. *Int J Radiat Oncol Biol Phys* **61**: 908–14.

■ FURTHER READING

Kallman RF (1987). *Rodent tumor models in experimental cancer therapy.* New York: Pergamon Press.

Steel GG (1977). *The growth kinetics of tumours.* Oxford: Oxford University Press.

Fractionation: the linear-quadratic approach

MICHAEL C. JOINER AND SØREN M. BENTZEN

8.1 INTRODUCTION

Major developments in radiotherapy fractionation have taken place during the past three decades and these have grown out of understanding in radiation biology. The relationships between total dose and dose per fraction for late-responding tissues, acutely responding tissues and tumours provide the basic information required to optimize radiotherapy according to the dose per fraction and number of fractions.

A milestone in this subject was the publication by Thames *et al.* (1982) of a survey of isoeffect curves for various normal tissues, mainly in mice. Their summary is shown in Fig. 8.1. Each of the investigations contributing to this chart was a study of the response of a normal tissue to fractionated radiation treatment using a range of doses per fraction. In order to minimize the effects of repopulation, the survey was restricted to studies in which the overall time was kept short by the use of multiple treatments per day, or 'where an effect of regeneration of target cells was shown to be unlikely'. This summary thus represents the influence of dose per fraction on response and mostly excludes the influence of overall treatment time. It was possible in each study, and for each chosen dose per fraction, to determine the total radiation dose that produced some defined level of damage to the normal tissue. These endpoints of tolerance differed from one normal tissue or experimental study to another. Each line in Fig. 8.1 is an isoeffect curve determined in this way. The dashed lines show isoeffect curves for acutely responding tissues and the full lines are for late-responding tissues. Note that fraction number increases from left to right along the abscissa and therefore the dose per fraction scale decreases from left to right. The results of this survey show that the isoeffective total dose increases more rapidly with decreasing dose per fraction for late effects than for acute effects. If the vertical axis is

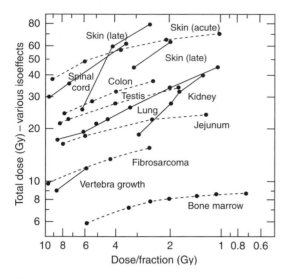

Figure 8.1 Relationship between total dose and dose per fraction for a variety of normal tissues in experimental animals. The results for late-responding tissues (unbroken lines) are systematically steeper than those for early-responding tissues (broken lines). From Thames *et al.* (1982), with permission.

8.2 HISTORICAL BACKGROUND: LQ VERSUS POWER-LAW MODELS

Two specific examples of isoeffect plots for radiation damage to normal tissues in the mouse are shown in Fig. 8.2: skin is an early-responding tissue and kidney a late-responding tissue. In each case the total radiation dose to give a fixed level of damage is plotted against dose per fraction and fraction number on a double log plot. Note that the curve for kidney is steeper than that for skin.

The solid lines in Fig. 8.2 are calculated by an equation based on the LQ model:

$$\text{Total dose} = \frac{\text{constant}}{1 + d/(\alpha/\beta)} \qquad (8.1)$$

where d is the dose per fraction (see Section 8.4 for for the derivation of this equation). The steepness and curvature of these lines are both determined by one parameter: the α/β ratio. For the skin data (Fig. 8.2a), the α/β ratio is about 10. The units of α/β are grays, so the α/β ratio in this case is 10 Gy. For the kidney data α/β is about 3 Gy.

The LQ model fits these data very well and produces curves in this type of log–log plot. Also shown in Fig. 8.2 are broken lines showing the fit of Ellis' 'Nominal Standard Dose' (NSD) model (Ellis, 1969) to both datasets. This is an example of a simple power-law relationship between total dose and number of fractions, and it and its derivatives such as TDF (time–dose–fractionation) were in clinical use for many years. The equation for NSD is:

$$\text{Total dose} = \text{NSD} \cdot N^{0.24} \cdot T^{0.11}$$

In these animal studies the overall treatment time (T) was constant. Power-law models such as NSD and TDF give straight lines in this type of plot and fit the skin data well from 4 to 32 fractions, but the data points fall below the broken line for both small and large doses per fraction. The discrepancy for doses per fraction of 1–2 Gy is important in relation to hyperfractionation (see Section 8.6). For late reactions, as illustrated by the kidney data in Fig. 8.2b, the NSD formula again does not fit as well as the LQ formula, even though the N exponent has been raised from 0.24 to 0.35 in order to

regarded as a tissue tolerance dose, it can be deduced immediately from this plot that using lower doses per fraction (towards the right-hand end of the abscissa) will tend to spare late reactions if the total dose is adjusted to keep the acute reactions constant.

The linear-quadratic (LQ) cell survival model, introduced in Chapter 4, can be used to describe this relationship between total isoeffective dose and the dose per fraction in fractionated radiotherapy. The LQ model can thus form a robust quantitative environment for considering the balance between acute and late reactions (and effect on the tumour) as dose per fraction and total dose are changed. This is one of the most important developments in radiobiology applied to therapy. In this chapter, we present the theoretical background and supporting data that have led to the wide adoption of the LQ approach to describing fractionation and we show the basic framework from which calculations can be made using this model. Examples of such calculations in a clinical setting are demonstrated practically in Chapter 9.

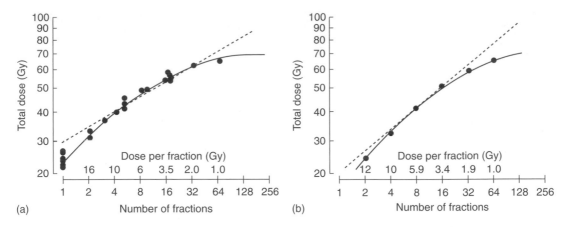

Figure 8.2 Relationship between total dose to achieve an isoeffect and number of fractions. (a) Acute reactions in mouse skin (Douglas and Fowler, 1976), with permission. (b) Late injury in mouse kidney (Stewart *et al.*, 1984), with permission. Note that the relationship for kidney is steeper than that for skin. The broken lines are nominal standard dose (NSD) formulae fitted to the central part of each dataset. The solid lines show the linear-quadratic (LQ) model, from which the guide to the dose per fraction has been calculated.

allow for the greater slope. A similar modification, but not necessarily by the same amount, must be made for all late-responding tissues if the NSD formulation is to be even approximately correct.

A crucial therapeutic conclusion is illustrated by these two sets of data. At both ends of the scale, in the region of large and small dose per fraction, power-law equations overestimate the actual tolerance dose (as shown by the experimental and clinical data). This means that the power-law models are unsafe in these regions, a conclusion that is well supported by clinical experience. At the present time it is strongly recommended that the LQ model should always be used, with a correctly chosen α/β ratio, to describe isoeffect dose relationships at least over the range of doses per fraction between 1 and 5 Gy. The LQ model is simple to use in clinical calculations and comparisons, and does not require the use of 'look-up tables'. Sections 8.4–8.8 and Chapter 9 provide a straightforward guide to LQ calculations.

8.3 CELL-SURVIVAL BASIS OF THE LQ MODEL

What is the explanation for the difference between the fractionation response of early- and late-responding tissues which is shown in Figs 8.1 and 8.2? Figure 8.3 shows hypothetical single-dose (one-fraction) survival curves for the target cells in early- and late-responding tissues, drawn according to the LQ equation (see Chapter 4, Fig. 4.5b). *E* represents the reduction in cell survival (on a logarithmic scale) that is equivalent to tissue tolerance. The total dose that would need to be given in two fractions is obtained by drawing a straight line from the origin through the survival curve at *E*/2 and measuring the intersection of this line with the dose axis. As shown by the dashed line labelled 2 in Fig. 8.3a, a dose of around 11 Gy takes the effect down to *E*/2 and (with assumed constant effect per fraction) a second 11 Gy gives the isoeffect *E*: the total isoeffect dose is approximately 22 Gy. This compares with a single dose of approximately 14 Gy to give the same isoeffect *E*, shown by the solid line. The total dose for three fractions is obtained in the same way by drawing a line through *E*/3 on the survival curve, and similarly for the other fraction numbers. Because the late-responding survival curve (Fig. 8.3b) is more 'bendy' (it has a lower α/β ratio), the isoeffective total dose increases more rapidly with increasing number of fractions than the early-responding tissue in which the survival curve bends less sharply.

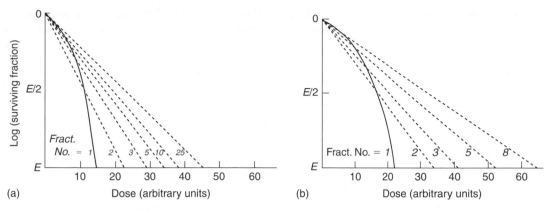

Figure 8.3 Schematic survival curves for target cells in (a) acutely responding and (b) late-responding normal tissues. The abscissa is radiation dose on an arbitrary scale. From Thames and Hendry (1987), with permission.

8.4 THE LQ MODEL IN DETAIL

The surviving fraction (SF_d) of target cells after a dose per fraction d is given in Chapter 4, Section 4.10, as:

$$SF_d = \exp(-\alpha d - \beta d^2)$$

Radiobiological studies have shown that each successive fraction in a multidose schedule is equally effective, so the effect (E) of n fractions can be expressed as:

$$E = -\log_e(SF_d)^n = -n\log_e(SF_d)$$
$$- n(\alpha d + \beta d^2)$$
$$= \alpha D + \beta dD$$

where the total radiation dose $D = nd$. This equation may be rearranged into the following forms:

$$1/D = (\alpha/E) + (\beta/E)d \qquad (8.2)$$

$$1/n = (\alpha/E)d + (\beta/E)d^2 \qquad (8.3)$$

$$D = (E/\alpha)/[1 + d/(\alpha/\beta)] \qquad (8.4)$$

The practical working of these equations may be illustrated by the results of careful fractionation experiments on the mouse kidney (Stewart *et al.*, 1984). In these experiments, functional damage to the kidneys was measured by ethylenediamine-tetraacetic acid (EDTA) clearance up to 48 weeks after irradiation with 1–64 fractions. Figure 8.4 shows the response measured as a function of total

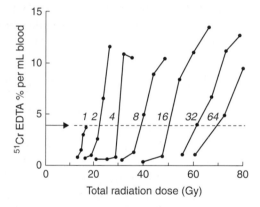

Figure 8.4 Dose–response curves for late damage to the mouse kidney with fractionated radiation exposure. Damage is indicated by a reduction in ethylenediaminetetraacetic acid (EDTA) clearance, curves determined for 1–64 dose fractions, illustrating the sparing effect of increased fractionation. From Stewart *et al.* (1984), with permission.

radiation dose for each fraction number. To apply the LQ model to this example, we first measure off from the graph the total doses at a fixed level of effect (shown by the arrow) and then plot the reciprocal of these total doses against the corresponding dose per fraction. Equation 8.2 shows that this should give a straight line whose slope is β/E and whose intercept on the vertical axis is α/E. That this is true is shown in Fig. 8.5a: the points fit a straight line well. This line cuts the *x*-axis at -3 Gy; it can be seen from equation 8.2 that this is equal to $-\alpha/\beta$, thus providing a measure of the α/β ratio for these data. The relative contributions of α and β to the α/β ratio can be judged by comparing the reciprocal total dose intercept (α/E) and the slope of the line (β/E).

An alternative way of deriving parameter values from these data is to plot the reciprocal of the number of fractions against the dose per fraction, as suggested by equation 8.3. Figure 8.5b shows that this gives the shape of the putative target-cell survival curve with the y-axis proportional to $-\log_e(SF_d)$. (Statistical note: this method combined with non-linear least-squares curve fitting is preferred over the linear-regression method shown in Fig. 8.5a for determining α/β, because the $1/n$ and the dose-per-fraction axes are independent.) Equation 8.4 shows the LQ model in the form used already to describe the relationship between total dose and dose per fraction (Fig. 8.2).

A common clinical question is: 'What change in total radiation dose is required when we change the dose per fraction?'. This can be dealt with very simply using the LQ approach. Rearranging equation 8.4:

$$E/\alpha = D[1 + d/(\alpha/\beta)]$$

For isoeffect in a selected tissue, E and α are constant. The first schedule employs a dose per fraction d_1 and the isoeffective total dose is D_1; we

change to a dose per fraction d_2 and the new (unknown) total dose is D_2. D_2 is related to D_1 by the equation:

$$\frac{D_2}{D_1} = \frac{d_1 + (\alpha/\beta)}{d_2 + (\alpha/\beta)} \tag{8.5}$$

This simple LQ isoeffect equation was first proposed by Withers *et al.* (1983). It has widely been found to be successful in clinical calculations.

8.5 THE VALUE OF α/β

Many detailed fractionation studies of the type analysed in Figs 8.2 and 8.4 have been made in animals. Table 8.1 summarizes the α/β values obtained from many of these experiments. For acutely responding tissues which express their damage within a period of days to weeks after irradiation, the α/β ratio is in the range 7–20 Gy, while for late-responding tissues, which express their damage months to years after irradiation, α/β generally ranges from 0.5 to 6 Gy. It is important to recognize that the α/β ratio is not constant and its value should be chosen carefully to match the specific tissue under consideration.

Values of the α/β ratio for a range of human normal tissues and tumours are given in Tables 9.1 and 13.2. The fractionation responses of well-oxygenated

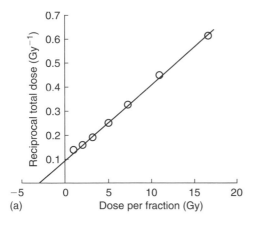

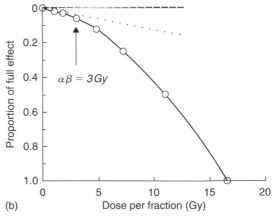

Figure 8.5 The data of Fig. 8.4 after two different transformations. (a) A reciprocal-dose plot according to equation 8.2. (b) Transformation according to equation 8.3 with the same data plotted as a proportion of full effect.

Table 8.1 Values for the α/β ratio for a variety of early- and late-responding normal tissues in experimental animals

Early reactions	α/β	References	Late reactions	α/β	References
Skin			**Spinal cord**		
Desquamation	9.1–12.5	Douglas and Fowler (1976)	Cervical	1.8–2.7	van der Kogel (1979)
	8.6–10.6	Joiner et al. (1983)	Cervical	1.6–1.9	White and Hornsey (1978)
	9–12	Moulder and Fischer (1976)	Cervical	1.5–2.0	Ang et al. (1983)
			Cervical	2.2–3.0	Thames et al. (1988)
Jejunum			Lumbar	3.7–4.5	van der Kogel (1979)
Clones	6.0–8.3	Withers et al. (1976)	Lumbar	4.1–4.9	White and Hornsey (1978)
	6.6–10.7	Tharres et al. (1981)		3.8–4.1	Leith et al. (1981)
				2.3–2.9	Amols, Yuhas (quoted by Leith et al. 1981)
Colon			**Colon**		
Weight loss	9–13	Terry and Denekamp (1984)	Weight loss	3.1–5.0	Terry and Denekamp (1984)
Clones	8–9	Tucker et al. (1983)	**Kidney**		
Testis			Rabbit	1.7–2.0	Caldwell (1975)
Clones	12–13	Tharres and Withers (1980)	Pig	1.7–2.0	Hopewell and Wiernik (1977)
			Rats	0.5–3.8	van Rongen et al. (1988)
Mouse lethality			Mouse	1.0–3.5	Williams and Denekamp (1984a,b)
30 days	7–10	Kaplan and Brown (1952)	Mouse	0.9–1.8	Stewart et al. (1984a)
30 days	13–17	Mole (1957)	Mouse	1.4–4.3	Thames et al. (1988)
30 days	11–26	Paterson et al. (1952)	**Lung**		
Tumour bed			LD$_{50}$	4.4–6.3	Wara et al. (1973)
45 days	5.6–6.8	Begg and Terry (1984)	LD$_{50}$	2.8–4.8	Field et al. (1976)
			LD$_{50}$	2.0–4.2	Travis et al. (1983)
			Breathing rate	1.9–3.1	Parkins and Fowler (1985)
			Bladder		
			Frequency, capacity	5–10	Stewart et al. (1984b)

α/β values are in grays. LD$_{50}$, dose lethal to 50 per cent.

From Fowler (1989), with permission; for references, see the original.

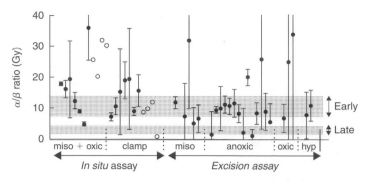

Figure 8.6 Values of α/β for experimental tumours, determined under a variety of conditions of oxygenation (see text). The stippled areas indicate the range of values for early- and late-responding normal tissues. From Williams *et al.* (1985), with permission.

carcinomas of head and neck, and lung, are thought to be similar to that of early-responding normal tissues, sometimes with an even higher α/β ratio. However, there is evidence that some human tumour types such as melanoma and sarcomas exhibit low α/β ratios, and this is also suggested for early-stage prostate and breast cancer, perhaps with α/β ratios even lower than for late normal-tissue reactions. The tumour α/β values shown in Fig. 8.6 were compiled by Williams *et al.* (1985). Values calculated from data obtained in experiments on rat and mouse tumours under fully radiosensitized conditions (marked 'miso' and 'oxic' in the Fig. 8.6) are plotted directly, and values calculated from fractionation responses under hypoxic conditions (marked 'clamp', 'anoxic' and 'hyp') are plotted after dividing by an assumed oxygen enhancement ratio (OER) of 2.7, because the α/β ratios for cells and tissues under anoxic and oxic conditions are in the same proportion as the OER. Error bars are estimates of the 95 per cent confidence interval on each value. Such experiments assayed the effect of radiation *in situ* either by regrowth delay or local tumour control or by excising the tumour from the animal and measuring the survival of cells *in vitro* (see Chapter 4, Section 4.4).

8.6 HYPOFRACTIONATION AND HYPERFRACTIONATION

Figure 8.7a shows the form of equation 8.5. Curves are shown for two ranges of α/β values: 1–4 Gy and 8–15 Gy, which, respectively, apply to most late- and acute-responding tissues. It can be seen that when dose per fraction is increased above a reference level of 2 Gy, the isoeffective dose falls more rapidly for the late-responding tissues than for the early responses. Similarly, when dose per fraction is reduced below 2 Gy, the isoeffective dose increases more rapidly in the late-responding tissues. Late-responding tissues are more sensitive to a change in dose per fraction and this can be thought to reflect the greater curvature of the underlying target-cell survival curve (Section 8.3).

Since the change in total dose is greater for the lower α/β values, so is the potential for error if a wrong α/β value is used. The α/β values should therefore be selected carefully and always conservatively when doing calculations involving changing dose per fraction. Examples of the conservative choice of α/β values and other radiobiological parameters are given in Chapter 9, Sections 9.3 (Example 1), 9.5 (Example 3) and 9.12 (Example 9).

An increase in dose per fraction relative to 2 Gy is termed hypofractionation and a decrease is hyperfractionation (this use of terms may seem contradictory but it indicates that hypofractionation involves fewer dose fractions and hyperfractionation requires more fractions). We can calculate a therapeutic gain factor (TGF) for a new dose per fraction from the ratio of the relative isoeffect doses for tumour and normal tissue. An example is shown in Fig. 8.7b where the tumour is taken to have an α/β ratio of 10 Gy. Remember that we are assuming here that the new regimen is given in the same overall time as the 2 Gy regimen and that treatment is always limited by the late

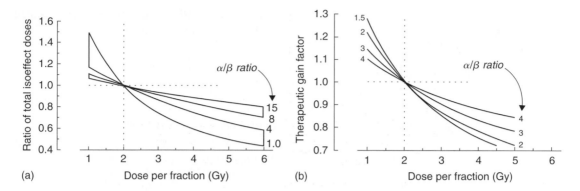

Figure 8.7 (a) Theoretical isoeffect curves based on the linear-quadratic (LQ) model for various α/β ratios. The outlined areas enclose curves corresponding to early-responding and late-responding normal tissues. (b) Therapeutic gain factors for various α/β ratios of normal tissue, assuming an α/β ratio of 10 Gy for tumours.

reactions. It can be seen from Fig. 8.7 that hyper-fractionation is predicted to give a therapeutic gain, and hypofractionation a therapeutic loss. Note, however, that hypofractionation may be used as a convenient way of accelerating treatment (i.e. shortening the overall treatment time). At least in some tumour types, this can lead to short intensive schedules that compare favourably with more protracted schedules in terms of both tumour control and late normal-tissue effects. Note, also, that the theoretical advantage of low dose per fraction would be nullified, or even reversed, for specific tumours that have low α/β ratios. If an unacceptable increase in acute normal-tissue reactions prevented the total dose from being increased to the full tolerance of the late-responding tissues, the therapeutic gain for hyperfractionation would also be less than shown in Fig. 8.7b.

8.7 EQUIVALENT DOSE IN 2-GY FRACTIONS (EQD$_2$)

The LQ approach leads to various formulae for calculating isoeffect relationships for radiotherapy, all based on similar underlying assumptions. These formulae seek to describe a range of fractionation schedules that are isoeffective. The simplest method of comparing the effectiveness of schedules consisting of different total doses and doses per fraction is to convert each schedule into an equivalent schedule in 2-Gy fractions which would give the same biological effect. This is the approach that we recommend as the method of

choice and can be achieved using a specific version of equation 8.5:

$$EQD_2 = D\frac{d + (\alpha/\beta)}{2 + (\alpha/\beta)} \qquad (8.6)$$

where EQD$_2$ is the dose in 2-Gy fractions that is biologically equivalent to a total dose D given with a fraction size of d Gy. Values of EQD$_2$ may be numerically added for separate parts of a treatment schedule. They have the advantage that since 2 Gy is a commonly used dose per fraction clinically, EQD$_2$ values will be recognized by radiotherapists as being of a familiar size. The EQD$_2$ is identical to the normalized total dose (NTD) proposed by Withers *et al.* (1983); see also Maciejewski *et al.* (1986).

8.8 INCOMPLETE REPAIR

The simple LQ model described by equations 8.1–8.6 assumes that sufficient time is allowed between fractions for complete repair of sublethal damage to take place after each dose. This full-repair interval is at least 6 hours but in some cases (e.g. spinal cord) may be as long as 1 day (see Chapter 9, Section 9.4). If the interfraction interval is reduced below this value, for example when multiple fractions per day are used, the overall damage from the whole treatment is increased because the repair (or more correctly, recovery) of damage caused by one radiation dose may not be complete

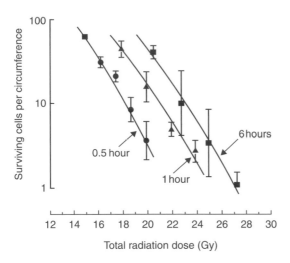

Figure 8.8 Effect of interfraction interval on intestinal radiation damage in mice. The total dose required in five fractions for a given level of effect is less for short intervals, illustrating incomplete repair between fractions. From Thames *et al.* (1984), with permission.

before the next fraction is given, and there is then interaction between residual unrepaired damage from one fraction and the damage from the next fraction. As an example of this process, Fig. 8.8 shows data from mouse jejunum irradiated with five X-ray fractions in which the number of surviving crypts per gut circumference is plotted against total dose. Much less dose is needed to produce the same effects when the interfraction interval is reduced from 6 hours to 1 hour or 0.5 hour. This process is called incomplete repair.

The influence of incomplete repair is determined by the repair halftime ($T_{1/2}$) in the tissue. This is the time required between fractions, or during low dose-rate treatment, for half the maximum possible repair to take place. Incomplete repair will tend to reduce the isoeffective dose and corrections have to be made for the consequent loss of tolerance. This can be accomplished by the use of the incomplete repair model as introduced by Thames (1985). In this model, the amount of unrepaired damage is expressed by a function H_m which depends upon the number of equally spaced fractions (m), the time interval between them and the repair halftime. For the purpose of

tolerance calculations the extra H_m term is added to the basic EQD_2 formula thus:

$$EQD_2 = D\frac{d(1 + H_m) + (\alpha/\beta)}{2 + (\alpha/\beta)}$$

(8.7; fractionated)

Once again, d is the dose per fraction and D the total dose. If repair from one day to the next is assumed to be complete, m is the number of fractions per day. Values of H_m are given in Table 8.2 for repair halftimes up to 5 hours and for two or three fractions per day given with interfraction intervals down to 3 hours. Other values can be calculated using the formulae given in the Appendix. Some clinical datasets have suggested even longer repair half-times for late reactions (Bentzen *et al.*, 1999). In that case, repair cannot be assumed to be complete in the interval between the last fraction in a day and the first fraction the following day, and a more general version of the incomplete-repair LQ model will have to be used (Guttenberger *et al.*, 1992). Table 8.4 shows values of $T_{1/2}$ for some normal tissues in laboratory animals and the available values for human normal-tissue endpoints are summarized in Table 9.2. [Advanced note: in several cases, experiments have indicated that repair has fast and slow components. The EQD_2 equation above [and biologically effective dose (BED) and total effect (TE) formulae] have to be reformulated in a more complex form to take account of these cases (Millar and Canney, 1993).]

Figure 8.9 demonstrates the fit of the incomplete repair LQ model to data for pneumonitis in mice following fractionated thoracic irradiation with intervals of 3 hours between doses (Thames *et al.*, 1984). The endpoint was mortality, expressed as the LD_{50} (radiation dose to produce lethality in 50 per cent of subjects). In these reciprocal-dose plots, incomplete repair makes the data bow upwards away from the straight line (dashed), which shows the pure LQ relationship that would be obtained when there is complete repair between successive doses, as would be the case with long time-intervals between fractions. An estimate of the repair halftime can be found by fitting data of the type shown in Figs 8.8 and 8.9 with the incomplete repair LQ model and seeking the $T_{1/2}$ value that gives the best fit.

Table 8.2 Incomplete repair factors: fractionated irradiation (H_m factors)

Repair halftime (hours)	Interval for $m = 2$ fractions per day						Interval for $m = 3$ fractions per day				
	3	4	5	6	8	10	3	4	5	6	8
0.50	0.016	0.004	0.001	0.000	0.000	0.000	0.021	0.005	0.001	0.000	0.000
0.75	0.063	0.025	0.010	0.004	0.001	0.000	0.086	0.034	0.013	0.005	0.001
1.00	0.125	0.063	0.031	0.016	0.004	0.000	0.177	0.086	0.042	0.021	0.005
1.25	0.190	0.109	0.063	0.036	0.012	0.004	0.277	0.153	0.086	0.049	0.016
1.50	0.250	0.158	0.099	0.063	0.025	0.010	0.375	0.227	0.139	0.086	0.034
2.00	0.354	0.250	0.177	0.125	0.063	0.031	0.555	0.375	0.257	0.177	0.086
2.50	0.435	0.330	0.250	0.190	0.109	0.063	0.707	0.512	0.375	0.277	0.153
3.00	0.500	0.397	0.315	0.250	0.158	0.099	0.833	0.634	0.486	0.375	0.227
4.00	0.595	0.500	0.420	0.354	0.250	0.177	1.029	0.833	0.678	0.555	0.375
5.00	0.660	0.574	0.500	0.435	0.330	0.250	1.170	0.986	0.833	0.707	0.512

Shaded cells in the table: the approximation of complete overnight repair is less precise here and this affects the precision of biological dose estimates.

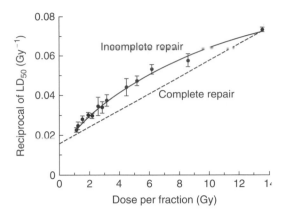

Figure 8.9 Reciprocal dose plot (compare Fig. 8.5a) of data for pneumonitis in mice produced by fractionated irradiation; the points derive from experiments with different dose per fraction (and therefore different fraction numbers), always with 3 hours between doses. The upward bend in the data illustrates lack of sparing because of incomplete repair. From Thames *et al.* (1984), with permission.

Continuous irradiation

Another common situation in which incomplete repair occurs in clinical radiotherapy is during continuous irradiation. As described in Chapter 12, irradiation must be given at a very low dose rate (below about 5 cGy/hour) for full repair to occur during irradiation. At the other extreme, a single irradiation at high dose rate may not allow any significant repair to occur during exposure. As the dose rate is reduced below the high dose-rate range used in external-beam radiotherapy, the duration of irradiation becomes longer and the induction of DNA damage is counteracted by repair, leading to an increase in the isoeffective dose. The corresponding EQD_2 formula for continuous irradiation incorporates a factor g to allow for incomplete repair:

$$EQD_2 = D\frac{dg + (\alpha/\beta)}{2 + (\alpha/\beta)} \qquad \text{(8.8; contiuous low dose rate)}$$

where D is the total dose (= dose rate × time). The parameter d is retained, as in the equation for fractionated radiotherapy, in order to deal with fractionated low dose-rate exposures. For a single

continuous exposure $d = D$. This equation assumes that there is full recovery between the low dose-rate exposures; if not, the H_m factor must also be added (see Appendix). Table 8.3 gives values of the g factor for exposure times between 1 hour and 4 days.

The simple LQ model has also been applied to, for example, permanent interstitial implants and to biologically targeted radionuclide therapy. The interested reader is referred to the book by Dale and Jones (2007) listed under Further reading.

8.9 SHOULD A TIME FACTOR BE INCLUDED?

If the overall duration of fractionated radiotherapy is increased there will usually be greater repopulation of the irradiated tissues, both in the tumour and in early-reacting normal tissues. So far, we have not discussed the change in total dose necessary to compensate for changes in the overall duration of treatment. Overall time was included in the now-obsolete NSD and TDF models but is not put into the basic LQ approach described above. The reason for this is because the time factor in radiotherapy is now perceived to be more complex than had previously been supposed. For example, Fig. 8.10 shows that the extra dose needed to counteract proliferation in mouse skin does not become significant until about 2 weeks after the start of daily fractionation. In this and other situations, the time factor in the old NSD formula (Fig. 8.10; broken line: total dose $\propto T^{0.11}$) gives a false picture because it predicts a large amount of sparing if the overall time was increased from 1 to 12 days. These wrong time factors also underestimate the dose required to compensate for planned or unplanned gaps in treatment. Thus a $T^{0.11}$ factor predicts only an 8 per cent increase in total dose for a doubling of overall time, for example from 3.5 to 7 weeks. This would correspond to a 5.6 Gy increase in the total dose for a schedule delivering, say, 70 Gy to a squamous cell carcinoma of the head and neck. Clinical data summarized in Chapter 9 suggest that in this tumour type an additional dose of 16 Gy will be required to compensate for a 3.5-week prolongation of treatment time.

The use of the LQ model in clinical practice with no time factor at all is probably the best strategy for late-reacting tissues because any extra dose

Table 8.3 Incomplete repair factors: continuous irradiation (*g* factors)

Repair halftime (hours)	Exposure time (hours)						Exposure time (days)						
	1	2	3	4	8	12	1	1.5	2	2.5	3	3.5	4
0.50	0.662	0.477	0.367	0.296	0.164	0.113	0.058	0.039	0.030	0.024	0.020	0.017	0.015
0.75	0.752	0.589	0.477	0.398	0.234	0.164	0.086	0.058	0.044	0.035	0.030	0.025	0.022
1.00	0.804	0.662	0.557	0.477	0.296	0.212	0.113	0.077	0.058	0.047	0.039	0.034	0.030
1.25	0.838	0.714	0.616	0.539	0.350	0.255	0.139	0.095	0.072	0.058	0.049	0.042	0.037
1.50	0.862	0.752	0.662	0.589	0.398	0.296	0.164	0.113	0.086	0.070	0.058	0.050	0.044
2.00	0.894	0.804	0.728	0.662	0.477	0.367	0.212	0.147	0.113	0.092	0.077	0.066	0.058
2.50	0.914	0.838	0.772	0.714	0.539	0.427	0.255	0.180	0.139	0.113	0.095	0.082	0.072
3.00	0.927	0.862	0.804	0.752	0.589	0.477	0.296	0.212	0.164	0.134	0.113	0.098	0.086
4.00	0.945	0.894	0.847	0.804	0.662	0.557	0.367	0.269	0.212	0.174	0.147	0.128	0.113
5.00	0.955	0.914	0.875	0.838	0.714	0.616	0.427	0.321	0.255	0.212	0.180	0.157	0.139

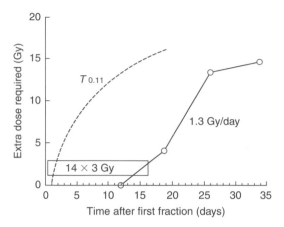

Figure 8.10 Extra dose required to counteract proliferation in mouse skin. Test doses of radiation were given at various intervals after a priming treatment with fractionated radiation. Proliferation begins about 12 days after the start of irradiation and is then equivalent to an extra dose of approximately 1.3 Gy/day. The broken line shows the prediction of the nominal standard dose (NSD) equation. Data from Denekamp (1973).

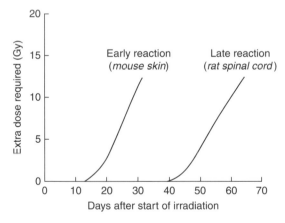

Figure 8.11 Schematic diagram showing that the extra dose required to counteract proliferation does not become significant until much later for late-responding normal tissues, such as spinal cord, beyond the 6-week duration of conventional radiotherapy. From Fowler (1984), with permission.

needed to counteract proliferation does not become significant until beyond the overall time of treatment, even up to 6 weeks. This is illustrated schematically in Fig. 8.11, which compares

the different effects of overall time in early- and late-responding tissues. Attempts have been made to include time factors in the LQ model for early-responding normal tissues and tumours, but such factors depend in a complex way on the dose per fraction and interfraction interval as well as on the tissue type, and have to take account of any delay in onset of proliferation which may depend in some way on these factors also. We therefore recommend considering the influence of changing overall time on radiotherapy as a separate problem from the effect of changing the dose per fraction, which can be done in a straightforward way using the LQ model as described here. The practical approaches to handling changes in overall time are described in Chapters 9–11.

8.10 ALTERNATIVE ISOEFFECT FORMULAE BASED ON THE LQ MODEL

Two other formulations that can be used for comparing schedules with differing doses per fraction are the concepts of extrapolated tolerance dose (ETD) introduced by Barendsen (1982) and 'total effect' (TE) described by Thames and Hendry (1987). Both of these methods are mathematically (and biologically) equivalent to the EQD_2 concept, but are mentioned here because they have found some use in the literature.

Extrapolated total dose or biologically effective dose

Both the ETD and the biologically effective dose (BED) are mathematically identical concepts. Fowler (1989) preferred the term BED because it can logically be understood to refer to levels of effect that are below normal-tissue tolerance, whereas the term ETD implies the full tolerance effect. First, we must define a particular effect, or endpoint. Although the validity of the LQ approach to fractionation depends principally on its ability to predict isoeffective schedules successfully, there is an implicit assumption that the isoeffect has a direct relationship with a certain level of cell inactivation [or final cell survival $(SF_d)^n$].

Table 8.4 Halftimes for recovery from radiation damage in normal tissues of laboratory animals

Tissue	Species	Dose delivery	$T_{1/2}$ (hours)	Source
Haemopoietic	Mouse	CLDR	0.3	Thames *et al.* (1984)
Spermatogonia	Mouse	CLDR	0.3–0.4	Delic *et al.* (1987)
Jejunum	Mouse	F	0.45	Thames *et al.* (1984)
	Mouse	CLDR	0.2–0.7	Dale *et al.* (1988)
Colon (acute injury)	Mouse	F	0.8	Thames *et al.* (1984)
	Rat	F	1.5	Sassy *et al.* (1988)
Lip mucosa	Mouse	F	0.8	Ang *et al.* (1985)
	Mouse	CLDR	0.8	Scalliet *et al.* (1987)
	Mouse	FLDR	0.6	Stüben *et al.* (1991)
Tongue epithelium	Mouse	F	0.75	Dörr *et al.* (1993)
Skin (acute injury)	Mouse	F	1.5	Rojas *et al.* (1991)
	Mouse	CLDR	1.0	Joiner *et al.* (unpublished)
	Pig	F	0.4 + 1.2*	van den Aardweg and Hopewell (1992)
	Pig	F	0.2 + 6.6*	Millar *et al.* (1996)
Lung	Mouse	F	0.4 + 4.0*	van Rongen *et al.* (1993)
	Mouse	CLDR	0.85	Down *et al.* (1986)
	Rat	FLDR	1.0	van Rongen (1989)
Spinal cord	Rat	F	0.7 + 3.8*	Ang *et al.* (1992)
	Rat	CLDR	1.4	Scalliet *et al.* (1989)
	Rat	CLDR	1.43	Pop *et al.* (1996)
Kidney	Mouse	F	1.3	Joiner *et al.* (1993)
	Mouse	F	0.2 + 5.0	Millar *et al.* (1994)
	Rat	F	1.6–2.1	van Rongen *et al.* (1990)
Rectum (late injury)	Rat	CLDR	1.2	Kiszel *et al.* (1985)
Heart	Rat	F	>3	Schultz-Hector *et al.* (1992)

Dose delivery: F, acute dose fractions, FLDR, fractionated low dose rate; CLDR, continuous low dose rate.

*Two components of repair with different halftimes.

Generally, the fraction of surviving cells associated with an isoeffect is unknown and it is customary to work in terms of a level of tissue effect, which we denote as *E*. From equation 8.4:

$$E/\alpha = D[1 + d/(\alpha/\beta)] = \text{BED}$$

BED is a measure of the effect (*E*) of a course of fractionated or continuous irradiation; when divided by α it has the units of dose and is usually expressed in grays. Note that as the dose per fraction (*d*) is reduced towards zero, BED becomes

$D = nd$ (i.e. the total radiation dose). Thus, BED is the theoretical total dose that would be required to produce the isoeffect *E* using an infinitely large number of infinitesimally small dose fractions. It is therefore also the total dose required for a single exposure at very low dose rate (see Chapter 12, Section 12.5). As with the simpler concept of EQD_2, values of BED from separate parts of a course of treatment may be added in order to calculate the overall BED value. A disadvantage of BED as a measure of treatment intensity is that it is numerically much greater than any prescribable radiation dose of fractionated radiotherapy and is therefore difficult to relate to everyday clinical practice, which is the main reason why we recommend the use of EQD_2 in this book.

Total effect

The total effect (TE) formulation is conceptually similar to BED and has also been used in the literature. In this case, we divide E by β rather than α, to get

$$E/\beta = D[(\alpha/\beta) + d] = TE$$

The units of TE are Gy^2, which again means that the TE values have no simple interpretation. The TE isoeffect formulae are similar to the EQD_2 formulae except that the denominator $(2 + \alpha/\beta)$ is omitted. This has the computational advantage that division by this factor is done only for the final TE value and not for any intermediate calculations. However, it has the disadvantage that these intermediate results are not recognizable doses, and we recommend the EQD_2 method instead as a means of making it easier to detect numerical errors in the calculation process.

8.11 LIMITS OF APPLICABILITY OF THE SIMPLE LQ MODEL, ALTERNATIVE MODELS

Uncritical application of the LQ model in clinical situations could potentially compromise the safety of a patient. Extrapolation of experience from a standard regimen to a regimen using a considerably changed overall treatment time or dose per fraction should only be attempted with great care. This is partly because of a limited precision in the radiobiological parameters of the LQ model which will be 'blown up' when extrapolation between very diverse schedules is performed. But even if the parameters of the model were known with high precision, some limitations to the use of the LQ model are suggested by laboratory experiments.

At a dose per fraction of less than 1.0 Gy, the phenomenon of low-dose hyper-radiosensitivity (HRS; see Chapter 4, Section 4.14) – provided that

it exists in the critical normal tissues and tumours in humans – would mean that using the standard LQ model could considerably underestimate the biological effect of a given total dose. This could potentially affect the estimated biological effect of some intensity-modulated radiation therapy (IMRT) dose distributions where a relatively large normal-tissue volume may be irradiated with a dose per fraction in the HRS range (Honore and Bentzen, 2006). A modified form of the LQ formula has been derived (Chapter 4, equation 4.6) but the model parameters are not yet known with any useful precision for human tissues and tumours.

Also, at very high dose per fraction the mathematical form of the LQ model is unlikely to be correct. While the LQ survival curve represents a continuously bending parabola in a plot of the logarithm of surviving fraction versus dose, a number of *in vitro* and *in vivo* datasets suggest that the empirical survival curve asymptotically approaches a straight line. Several attempts have been made to extend the LQ model to high doses per fraction as well, all of them leading to the inclusion of at least one additional parameter in the model, as described in Chapter 4, Section 4.13 (Lind *et al.*, 2003; Guerrero and Li, 2004). None of these models have found wider applications in the analysis of clinical data, at least so far, the obvious limitation being that most clinical datasets have insufficient resolution to allow the estimation of three model parameters. It is difficult to give a specific dose per fraction beyond which the simple LQ model should not be used, but extrapolations beyond 5–6 Gy per fraction are likely to lack clinically useful precision.

8.12 BEYOND THE TARGET CELL HYPOTHESIS

The target cell hypothesis dominated much of radiobiological thinking for almost half a century. As described above, this hypothesis played a key role in formulating the LQ formulae. More recently, the importance of damage processing and tissue remodelling in the pathogenesis of late effects have been recognized (see Chapter 13 and review by Bentzen, 2006). In addition, basic radiobiology studies have revealed non-targeted effects of ionizing radiation, such as the 'bystander' response induced in cells in the vicinity of a cell hit by ionizing radiation (Prise *et al.*, 2005). All of this has not restricted the clinical utility of the LQ formula. Equation 8.5 can usefully be viewed as an operational definition of α/β and a formula allowing practical correction for the change in biological effect as a function of dose per fraction. The application of this formula does not depend on the biological reality of target cells. Chapter 9 will pursue this more pragmatic or 'data-driven' approach to the LQ model in the clinic.

Key points

1. The LQ model satisfactorily describes the relationship between total isoeffective dose and dose per fraction over the range of dose per fraction from 1 Gy up to 5–6 Gy. In contrast, power-law formulae can only be made to fit data over a limited range of dose per fraction.
2. The α/β ratio describes the shape of the fractionation response: a low α/β (0.5–6 Gy) is usually characteristic of late-responding normal tissues and indicates a rapid increase of total dose, with decreasing dose per fraction and a survival curve for the putative target cells that is significantly curved.
3. A higher α/β ratio (7–20 Gy) is usually characteristic of early-responding normal tissues and rapidly-proliferating carcinomas; it indicates a less significant increase in total dose with decreasing dose per fraction and a less curved cell-survival response for the putative target cells.
4. The EQD_2 formulae provide a simple and convenient way of calculating isoeffective radiotherapy schedules, based on the LQ model. Tolerance calculations always require an estimate of the α/β ratio to be included.
5. For short interfraction intervals, a correction may be necessary for incomplete repair. When using the EQD_2 formulae to calculate schedules with multiple fractions per day or continuous low dose rate, an estimate of the repair halftime must also be included.
6. The basic LQ model is appropriate for calculating the change in total dose for an altered dose per fraction, assuming the new and old treatments are given in the same overall time. For late reactions it is usually unnecessary to modify total dose in response to a change in overall time, but for early reactions (and for tumour response) a correction for overall treatment time should be included. Although the effect of time on biological effect is complex, simple linear corrections have been shown to be of some value (see Chapters 10 and 11).

■ BIBLIOGRAPHY

Barendsen GW (1982). Dose fractionation, dose rate and iso-effect relationships for normal tissue responses. *Int J Radiat Oncol Biol Phys* **8**: 1981–97.

Bentzen SM (2006). Preventing or reducing late side effects of radiation therapy: radiobiology meets molecular pathology. *Nat Rev Cancer* **6**: 702–13.

Bentzen SM, Saunders MI, Dische S (1999). Repair halftimes estimated from observations of treatment-related morbidity after CHART or conventional radiotherapy in head and neck cancer. *Radiother Oncol* **53**: 219–26.

Denekamp J (1973). Changes in the rate of repopulation during multifraction irradiation of mouse skin. *Br J Radiol* **46**: 381–7.

Douglas BG, Fowler JF (1976). The effect of multiple small doses of X rays on skin reactions in the mouse and a basic interpretation. *Radiat Res* **66**: 401–26.

Ellis F (1969). Dose, time and fractionation: a clinical hypothesis. *Clin Radiol* **20**: 1–7.

Fowler JF (1984). The first James Kirk memorial lecture. What next in fractionated radiotherapy? *Br J Cancer* **49** (*Suppl* 6): 285–300.

Fowler JF (1989). The linear-quadratic formula and progress in fractionated radiotherapy. *Br J Radiol* **62**: 679–94.

Guerrero M, Li XA (2004). Extending the linear-quadratic model for large fraction doses pertinent to stereotactic radiotherapy. *Phys Med Biol* **49**: 4825–35.

Guttenberger R, Thames HD, Ang KK (1992). Is the experience with CHART compatible with experimental data? A new model of repair kinetics and computer simulations. *Radiother Oncol* **25**: 280–6.

Honore HB, Bentzen SM (2006). A modelling study of the potential influence of low dose hypersensitivity on radiation treatment planning. *Radiother Oncol* **79**: 115–21.

Lind BK, Persson LM, Edgren MR, Hedlof I, Brahme A (2003). Repairable–conditionally repairable damage model based on dual Poisson processes. *Radiat Res* **160**: 366–75.

Maciejewski B, Taylor JM, Withers HR (1986). Alpha/beta value and the importance of size of dose per fraction for late complications in the supraglottic larynx. *Radiother Oncol* **7**: 323–6.

Millar WT, Canney PA (1993). Derivation and application of equations describing the effects of fractionated protracted irradiation, based on multiple and incomplete repair processes. Part I. Derivation of equations. *Int J Radiat Biol* **64**: 275–91.

Nilsson P, Thames HD, Joiner MC (1990). A generalized formulation of the 'incomplete-repair' model for cell survival and tissue response to fractionated low dose-rate irradiation. *Int J Radiat Biol* **57**: 127–42.

Prise KM, Schettino G, Folkard M, Held KD (2005). New insights on cell death from radiation exposure. *Lancet Oncol* **6**: 520–8.

Stewart FA, Soranson JA, Alpen EL, Williams MV, Denekamp J (1984). Radiation-induced renal damage: the effects of hyperfractionation. *Radiat Res* **98**: 407–20.

Thames HD (1985). An 'incomplete-repair' model for survival after fractionated and continuous irradiations. *Int J Radiat Biol* **47**: 319–39.

Thames HD, Hendry JH (1987). *Fractionation in radiotherapy*. London: Taylor & Francis.

Thames HD, Withers HR, Peters LJ, Fletcher GH (1982). Changes in early and late radiation responses with altered dose fractionation: implications for dose-survival relationships. *Int J Radiat Oncol Biol Phys* **8**: 219–26.

Thames HD, Withers HR, Peters LJ (1984). Tissue repair capacity and repair kinetics deduced from multifractionated or continuous irradiation regimens with incomplete repair. *Br J Cancer* **49**(Suppl 6): 263–9.

Williams MV, Denekamp J, Fowler JF (1985). A review of alpha/beta ratios for experimental tumors: implications for clinical studies of altered fractionation. *Int J Radiat Oncol Biol Phys* **11**: 87–96.

Withers HR, Thames HD, Jr, Peters LJ (1983). A new isoeffect curve for change in dose per fraction. *Radiother Oncol* **1**: 187–91.

■ FURTHER READING

Dale RG, Jones B (eds) (2007). *Radiobiological modeling in radiation oncology*. London: British Institute of Radiology.

Joiner MC (1989). The dependence of radiation response on the dose per fraction. In: McNally NJ (ed.) *The scientific basis for modern radiotherapy* (BIR report 19). London: British Institute of Radiology, 20–6.

Thames HD, Bentzen SM, Turesson I, Overgaard M, van den Bogaert W (1990). Time-dose factors in radiotherapy: a review of the human data. *Radiother Oncol* **19**: 219–35.

APPENDIX: SUMMARY OF FORMULAE

Basic equations:

$$E = n(\alpha d + \beta d^2) = D(\alpha + \beta d)$$
$$d = \text{dose per fraction}$$
$$D = \text{total dose}$$
$$n = \text{number of fractions}$$
$$\text{SF} = \exp(-E) = \exp[-(\alpha + \beta d)D]$$

For schedules having the same E (i.e. isoeffective schedules),

$$\frac{D}{D_{\text{ref}}} = \frac{d_{\text{ref}} + (\alpha/\beta)}{d + (\alpha/\beta)} \quad \text{hence: } \text{EQD}_2 = D\frac{d + (\alpha/\beta)}{2 + (\alpha/\beta)}$$

Low dose rate:

$$\mu = \frac{\log_e 2}{T_{1/2}} \qquad T_{1/2} = \text{repair halftime}$$

$$g = 2[\mu t - 1 + \exp(-\mu t)]/(\mu t)^2$$
$$t = \text{exposure duration}$$
$$\text{EQD}_2 = D\frac{dg + (\alpha/\beta)}{2 + (\alpha/\beta)}$$

Incomplete repair correction:

$$\phi = \exp(-\mu\Delta T)$$

ΔT = interval between fractions

$$H_m = \left(\frac{2}{m}\right)\cdot\left(\frac{\phi}{1-\phi}\right)\cdot\left(m - \frac{1-\phi^m}{1-\phi}\right)$$

m = number of fractions per day

$$EQD_2 = D\frac{d(1+H_m)+(\alpha/\beta)}{2+(\alpha/\beta)}$$

Incomplete repair between low dose-rate fractions:

$$\phi = \exp(-\mu(t+\Delta T))$$

ΔT = interval between fractions

t = exposure duration per fraction

$$g = 2[\mu t - 1 + \exp(-\mu t)]/(\mu t)^2$$

$$H_m = \left(\frac{2}{m}\right)\cdot\left(\frac{\phi}{1-\phi}\right)\cdot\left(m - \frac{1-\phi^m}{1-\phi}\right)$$

m = number of fractions per day

$$C = g + 2\frac{\cosh(\mu t)-1}{(\mu t)^2}\cdot H_m$$

$$EQD_2 = D\frac{dC+(\alpha/\beta)}{2+(\alpha/\beta)}$$

For a full derivation of these equations, see Nilsson *et al.* (1990).

9

The linear-quadratic approach in clinical practice

SØREN M. BENTZEN AND MICHAEL C. JOINER

9.1 INTRODUCTION: BIOLOGICAL EFFECT ESTIMATES ADJUSTING FOR DOSE–TIME FRACTIONATION

Since the early years of radiation therapy it has been appreciated that the biological effect of a given physical absorbed dose of ionizing radiation depends on how this dose is distributed over time. For many years, the differential response of tumours and normal tissues to changes in dose–time fractionation appeared to be the most important means of improving the therapeutic ratio. Mathematical models – often referred to as bioeffect models – were first introduced in the 1920s with the aim of quantifying the biological effect of dose-fractionation schedules on tumour control and normal-tissue side-effects. As discussed in Chapter 8, the linear-quadratic (LQ) model was introduced around 1980 and has gradually become the model of choice for bioeffect estimation in radiotherapy. In the beginning, the use of the LQ model was conceptually linked to the target-cell hypothesis. However, there is increasing evidence that many late effects, and even some early effects, of radiation therapy are not directly related to simple killing of a defined population of target cells (see Chapter 13, and Bentzen, 2006). The most prevalent current view is that the LQ approach represents an approximate, pragmatic method for converting dose–time fractionation schedules into a biologically effective dose. The LQ model has a limited range of applicability, and extrapolations outside the range of available data should only be performed with the greatest care. Model parameters should be estimated from clinical observations and their statistical precision should be taken into account when used to estimate the biological effect of a given schedule.

While awareness has grown regarding the limitations to the LQ model and the dangers involved in using it uncritically, the application of this approach has also increased. There are several reasons for this. Intensity-modulated radiotherapy (IMRT) represents a convenient way of delivering radiation therapy with varying dose per fraction to multiple target volumes in a single session. At the same time, IMRT and conformal radiotherapy generally leads to non-uniform dose distributions in normal tissues and organs, delivering dose with a varying dose per fraction to various subvolumes – in contrast to parallel opposing field techniques that typically lead to partial organ irradiation with a dose per fraction close to the fraction size prescribed to the target volume. Finally, the realization that the fractionation sensitivities of at least some human tumours are in the same range as that typical of late normal-tissue effects (in contrast to what was widely assumed when the LQ model was introduced in the 1980s) has renewed the interest in the use of hypofractionation, that is, prescriptions with fraction sizes larger than 2 Gy.

9.2 QUANTITATIVE CLINICAL RADIOBIOLOGY: THE LQ FRAMEWORK

Several, mathematically equivalent, methods have been devised for performing bioeffect calculations with the LQ model as discussed in Chapter 8. The method presented in this chapter converts all phases of a treatment into the equivalent dose in 2-Gy fractions (EQD_2). This has the advantage that these doses are clinically relevant and they are measured on the scale where much of the clinical experience on dose–response relationships is available. The EQD_2 values from various parts of a fractionation schedule may be added directly. The EQD_2 is identical to the 'normalized total dose' (NTD) proposed by Withers and colleagues (1983) (see also Chapter 8).

Large fractionation studies in the laboratory, mainly conducted in rodents in the 1980s, showed the ability of the LQ model to provide a close quantitative relationship between the isoeffective

doses for schedules applying varying dose per fraction. These studies also produced a number of α/β ratio estimates for various normal-tissue endpoints (see Table 8.1). In parallel with these experimental studies, a number of clinical studies have produced α/β estimates for human endpoints and these are summarized in Table 9.1.

Bioeffect calculations should be used only as guidance for clinical decision-making. All of the formulae applied here have a limited field of applicability; the model assumptions may be violated in some circumstances, relevant parameters may not be known for human tissues and tumours and the uncertainty in parameter estimates, even when these are available, may give rise to considerable uncertainty in the biological effect estimates. A (self-)critical and cautious attitude is recommended and the health and safety of patients should not be compromised by reliance on the result of calculations of the type described in this chapter. We advocate the use of clinical parameter estimates whenever possible. If no clinical estimates are available we suggest using the values from experimental animal studies as a guide, but be well aware of the fact that these may not be valid for the clinical endpoints of interest. The use of 'generic' values, say, 3 Gy for late effects and 10 Gy for tumours, should be seen as the least evidence-based approach. There is less and less reason to believe that these values can be generalized across a wider range of human normal-tissue endpoints and tumour histologies. Therefore, calculations using these values may be seen as simply exploring the behaviour of the model – an exercise detached from the clinical reality that we should be studying. That said, a numerical estimate is often very useful when considering various therapeutic options and it is often possible to get an impression of how reliable such an estimate is, just by doing a simple calculation as illustrated in this chapter.

9.3 CHANGING THE DOSE PER FRACTION

The simplest case we will consider is when the dose per fraction is changed without change in the overall treatment time and when incomplete

Table 9.1 Fractionation sensitivity of human normal tissues and tumours

Tissue/organ	Endpoint	α/β (Gy)	95% CL (Gy)	Source
Early reactions				
Skin	Erythema	8.8	6.9; 11.6	Turesson and Thames (1989)
	Erythema	12.3	1.8; 22.8	Bentzen et al. (1988)
	Dry desquamation	~8	N/A	Chogule and Supe (1993)
	Desquamation	11.2	8.5; 17.6	Turesson and Thames (1989)
Oral mucosa	Mucositis	9.3	5.8; 17.9	Denham et al. (1995)
	Mucositis	15	−15; 45	Rezvani et al. (1991)
	Mucositis	~8	N/A	Chogule and Supe (1993)
Late reactions				
Skin/vasculature	Telangiectasia	2.8	1.7; 3.8	Turesson and Thames (1989)
	Telangiectasia	2.6	2.2; 3.3	Bentzen et al. (1990)
	Telangiectasia	2.8	−0.1; 8.1	Bentzen and Overgaard (1991)
Subcutis	Fibrosis	1.7	0.6; 2.6	Bentzen and Overgaard (1991)
Breast	Cosmetic change in appearance	3.4	2.3; 4.5	START Trialists Group (2008)
	Induration (fibrosis)	3.1	1.8; 4.4	Yarnold et al. (2005)
Muscle/vasculature/ cartilage	Impaired shoulder movement	3.5	0.7; 6.2	Bentzen et al. (1989)
Nerve	Brachial plexopathy	<3.5*	N/A	Olsen et al. (1990)
	Brachial plexopathy	~2	N/A	Powell et al. (1990)
	Optic neuropathy	1.6	−7; 10	Jiang et al. (1994)
Spinal cord	Myelopathy	<3.3	N/A	Dische et al. (1981)
Eye	Corneal injury	2.9	−4; 10	Jiang et al. (1994)
Bowel	Stricture/perforation	3.9	2.5; 5.3	Deore et al. (1993)
Bowel	Various late effects	4.3	2.2; 9.6	Dische et al. (1999)
Lung	Pneumonitis	4.0	2.2; 5.8	Bentzen et al. (2000)
	Lung fibrosis (radiological)	3.1	−0.2; 8.5	Dubray et al. (1995)
Head and neck	Various late effects	3.5	1.1; 5.9	Rezvani et al. (1991)
Head and neck	Various late effects	4.0	3.3; 5.0	Stuschke and Thames (1999)
Supraglottic larynx	Various late effects	3.8	0.8; 14	Maciejewski et al. (1986)
Oral cavity + oropharynx	Various late effects	0.8	−0.6; 2.5	Maciejewski et al. (1990)
Tumours				
Head and neck				
Various		10.5	6.5; 29	Stuschke and Thames (1999)
Larynx		14.5*	4.9; 24	Rezvani et al. (1993)
Vocal cord		~13	'wide'	Robertson et al. (1993)
Buccal mucosa		6.6	2.9; ∞	Maciejewski et al. (1989)
Tonsil		7.2	3.6; ∞	Maciejewski et al. (1989)
Nasopharynx		16	−11; 43	Lee et al. (1995)
Skin		8.5*	4.5; 11.3	Trott et al. (1984)
Prostate†		1.1	−3.3; 5.6	Bentzen and Ritter (2005)
Breast		4.6	1.1; 8.1	START Trialists Group (2008)
Oesophagus		4.9	1.5; 17	Geh et al. (2006)
Melanoma		0.6	−1.1; 2.5	Bentzen et al. (1989)
Liposarcoma		0.4	−1.4; 5.4	Thames and Suit (1986)

CL, confidence limit.

*Re-analysis of original published data.

†Several more estimates are available from comparisons of outcome after brachytherapy versus external-beam therapy.

Reference details are available from Søren Bentzen. See also Thames et al. (1990) and Table 13.2.

repair between dose fractions is negligible. We use the Withers formula to convert a total dose D delivered with dose per fraction d into the isoeffective dose in 2-Gy fractions:

$$EQD_2 = D \cdot \frac{d + (\alpha\beta)}{2 \text{ Gy} + (\alpha\beta)} \qquad (9.1)$$

Note, that the only parameter in this formula is the α/β ratio, which is a characteristic of the endpoint of interest. Any biological dose calculation will therefore start with the identification of the tumour or normal-tissue endpoint of concern in the clinical situation. For a given fractionation schedule we may, for example, be interested in EQD_2 for a squamous cell carcinoma of the lung and for lung fibrosis and we would then start by selecting appropriate α/β ratios from Tables 8.1, 9.1 or 13.2.

9.4 CHANGING THE TIME-INTERVAL BETWEEN DOSE FRACTIONS

Multiple fractions per day schedules are associated with an increase in biological effect unless the interval between fractions is sufficiently long to allow full recovery between fractions. There are data to suggest that the characteristic halftime of recovery is in the order of 4–5 hours for some human late endpoints (Bentzen *et al.*, 1999) and possibly even longer for spinal cord and brain (Dische and Saunders, 1989; Lee *et al.*, 1999). This means that recovery will not be complete even with a 6- to 8-hour interval between fractions. In this situation it is necessary to modify the simple LQ model as described in Chapter 8. Equation 8.7 can be used under the assumption that repair is complete in the long overnight interval (i.e. between the last fraction delivered in one day and the first fraction on the following day). Even this assumption starts to be problematic with repair halftimes of 4–5 hours. Guttenberger *et al.* (1992) derived a formula where unrepaired damage is allowed to accumulate throughout the fractionation course. Unfortunately, this formula is not easy to tabulate as it depends not only on the repair halftime and the dose per fraction but also on the exact arrangement of dose fractions over time.

Example 1. Converting a dose into the isoeffective dose in 2–Gy fractions

A patient with metastatic bone pain located to the 5th thoracic vertebra is considered for palliative radiotherapy using $4 \times 5 \text{ Gy}$.

Problem: What is the isoeffective dose in 2-Gy fractions for spinal cord?

Solution: First, we need to choose the value of α/β. From Table 9.1 it is seen that the upper bound on α/β from human data is 3.5 Gy. Experimental animal studies (see Table 8.1) have produced estimates around 2 Gy. We choose $\alpha/\beta = 2$ Gy, insert the values for total dose, 20 Gy, and dose per fraction, 5 Gy, in equation 9.1 and get:

$$EQD_2 = 20 \text{ Gy} \cdot \frac{5 \text{ Gy} + 2 \text{ Gy}}{2 \text{ Gy} + 2 \text{ Gy}} = 35 \text{ Gy}$$

Thus, 20 Gy delivered in 5-Gy fractions is biologically equivalent to 35 Gy in 2-Gy fractions for an endpoint with $\alpha/\beta = 2.0$ Gy.

9.5 CONTINUOUS IRRADIATION

In brachytherapy, repair takes place not only after irradiation but also during the application. In this case, the apparent dose per fraction is modified by a function of the exposure time and the repair or recovery halftime, $T_{1/2}$ (see Chapter 8, Section 8.8). Depending on the detailed dose rates, the isoeffective dose may depend strongly on $T_{1/2}$ for a given endpoint. As these halftimes are usually not known with any useful precision from clinical data, great care should be taken when interpreting the results of isoeffect calculations for continuous irradiations.

Example 2. Incomplete repair with multiple fractions per day

A patient with head and neck squamous cell carcinoma (HNSCC) is prescribed 70 Gy in 2-Gy fractions over 7 weeks. After 50 Gy, he has an intercurrent pneumonia and cannot attend radiotherapy for 1 week. In order to finish treatment on time, it is decided to give the last 20 Gy as 2×2 Gy per day on the last five treatment days.

Problem: What is the isoeffective dose in 2-Gy fractions for subcutaneous fibrosis for a 6-hour interval and an 8-hour interval?

Solution: First, we need to choose the values of α/β and $T_{1/2}$. From Table 9.1 it is seen that $\alpha/\beta = 1.7$ Gy and from Table 9.2 we get $T_{1/2} = 4.4$ hours. We now use equation 8.7:

$$EQD_2 = D \cdot \frac{d \cdot [1 + H_m(T_{1/2}; \Delta T)] + (\alpha/\beta)}{2\,\text{Gy} + (\alpha/\beta)}$$

In this case, $m = 2$ and we use Table 8.2 to look up the values of H_2. For an interfraction interval of 6 hours, we see that H_2 is between 0.35 ($T_{1/2} = 4.0$ hours) and 0.44 ($T_{1/2} = 5.0$ hours). Interpolation between these values yields

$H_2 = 0.39$ for $T_{1/2} = 4.4$ hours and therefore:

$$EQD_2(\Delta t = 6 \text{ hours}) = 50\,\text{Gy}$$
$$+ 20\,\text{Gy} \cdot \frac{2[1 + 0.39]\text{Gy} + 1.7\,\text{Gy}}{2\,\text{Gy} + 1.7\,\text{Gy}} = 74.2\,\text{Gy}$$

For an 8-hour interval the value of H_2 is between 0.25 ($T_{1/2} = 4.0$ h) and 0.33 ($T_{1/2} = 5.0$ hours). Interpolation between these values yields $H_2 = 0.28$ for $T_{1/2} = 4.4$ hours and therefore:

$$EQD_2(\Delta t = 8 \text{ hours}) = 50\,\text{Gy}$$
$$+ 20\,\text{Gy} \cdot \frac{2[1 + 0.28]\text{Gy} + 1.7\,\text{Gy}}{2\,\text{Gy} + 1.7\,\text{Gy}} = 73.0\,\text{Gy}$$

Thus, about 1.2 Gy will be spared from increasing inter-fraction intervals from 6 to 8 hours.

As mentioned above, this calculation assumes that the overnight interval is sufficiently long to assure complete repair of sublethal damage. This assumption starts to break down when $T_{1/2}$ is 4.4 hours. A calculation using the formula of Guttenberger *et al.* (1992) gives an EQD_2 for the last week of twice daily treatment of 25.2 Gy (rather than 24.2 Gy as calculated in the example) for the 6-hour interval and 24.2 Gy (rather than 23.0 Gy) for the 8-hour interval.

Table 9.2 Repair halftime ($T_{1/2}$) for human normal-tissue endpoints

Endpoint	Dose delivery*	T1/2 (hours)	95% CL (hours)	Source
Erythema, skin	MFD	0.35 and 1.2†	?	Turesson and Thames (1989)
Mucositis, head and neck	MFD	2–4	?	Bentzen *et al.* (1996)
	FLDR	0.3–0.7	?	Denham *et al.* (1995)
Laryngeal oedema	MFD	4.9	3.2; 6.4	Bentzen *et al.* (1999)
Radiation myelopathy	MFD	> 5	?	Dische and Saunders (1989)
Skin telangiectasia	MFD	0.4 and 3.5†	?	Turesson and Thames (1989)
	MFD	3.8	2.5; 4.6	Bentzen *et al.* (1999)
Subcutaneous fibrosis	MFD	4.4	3.8; 4.9	Bentzen *et al.* (1999)
Temporal lobe necrosis	MFD	> 4	?	Lee *et al.* (1999)
Various pelvic complications	HDR/LDR	1.5–2.5	?	Fowler (1997)

CL, confidence limit.

*MFD, multiple fractions per day; FLDR, fractionated low dose-rate irradiation; HDR/LDR, high dose-rate/low dose-rate comparison.

†Evidence of two components of repair with different halftimes.

Reference details are available from Søren Bentzen.

Example 3. Brachytherapy

There has been some interest in intraluminal brachytherapy combined with external-beam radiotherapy for endobronchial cancer. Fuwa *et al.* (2000) delivered external-beam radiotherapy combined with intraluminal brachytherapy: typically two or three fractions of 5 Gy in 2.5 hours delivered using a thin catheter with a ^{192}Ir wire, combined with an external-beam dose of 52 Gy.

Problem: What is the equivalent dose in 2-Gy fractions, of 5 Gy in 2.5 hours for lung fibrosis assuming two different recovery half-times, $T_{1/2}$, of 1.5 hours and 5 hours?

Solution. From Table 9.1 we find the point estimate of α/β for lung fibrosis to be 3.1 Gy. We show here the calculation for $T_{1/2} = 5$ hours. We first calculate μt, where t is the duration of one application:

$$\mu = \frac{\log_e 2}{T_{1/2}} \approx \frac{0.693}{5 \text{ hours}} \approx 0.139/\text{hour}$$

that is μt becomes $(0.139/\text{hour}) \times 2.5 \text{ hours} = 0.348$. Next, we calculate g (see equation 12.2):

$$g = \frac{2[\mu t - 1 + \exp(-\mu t)]}{(\mu t)^2}$$
$$= \frac{2[0.348 - 1 + \exp(-0.348)]}{0.348^2} \approx 0.893$$

This value is inserted into equation 8.8 (note that the total dose, D, in this case is equal to the dose per fraction, d; i.e. the dose delivered in a single application of the brachytherapy):

$$\text{EQD}_2 = D \frac{dg + (\alpha \beta)}{2 + (\alpha \beta)}$$
$$= 5 \text{Gy} \cdot \frac{5 \times 0.893 \text{Gy} + 3.1 \text{Gy}}{2 \text{Gy} + 3.1 \text{Gy}} \approx 7.4 \text{Gy}$$

For $T_{1/2} = 1.5$ hours, we get $g = 0.70$ and $\text{EQD}_2 = 6.5$ Gy, that is, roughly a 12 per cent lower equivalent dose in 2-Gy fractions than we calculated for $T_{1/2} = 5$ hours.

Example 3 shows, what we would also expect intuitively, that the effect of protracting the delivery of a dose fraction is reduced when the recovery halftime is longer (i.e. less recovery will take place during the irradiation). A 5-Gy fraction delivered with acute dose rate, that is assuming no recovery at all during delivery, would correspond to an EQD$_2$ of 7.9 Gy for $\alpha/\beta = 3.1$ Gy.

9.6 CHANGING THE OVERALL TREATMENT TIME

Very often, two fractionation schedules will differ in overall treatment time. There are good reasons to believe that overall treatment time has very little, if any, influence on late radiation effects (Bentzen and Overgaard, 1995). However, for most tumour types and for early endpoints, the biological effect of a specific dose-fractionation will decrease if overall treatment time is increased. In other words,

an extra dose will be needed to obtain the same level of effect in a longer schedule. This has traditionally been interpreted as the result of proliferation of target cells in the irradiated tissue or tumour, and many attempts have been made to include this effect in the LQ model. Experimental animal studies have shown that this is a non-linear effect as a function of time; in other words, the dose recovered per unit time will change as a function of the time since the initial trauma. At present, there is no mathematical model describing this recovery over extended intervals. Instead, the most cautious approach is to use a simple linear relationship in a fairly narrow interval around the overall time of the schedule from which it has been estimated. The magnitude of the time effect is most conveniently quantified by D_{prolif}, which is the dose recovered per day due to proliferation. However, the exact mechanism behind this recovery is not critical for this pragmatic correction. For minor changes in overall time, say, a 4-day protraction of a schedule, the

Table 9.3 Values for the dose recovered per day owing to proliferation (D_{prolif}) from clinical studies

Tissue	Endpoint	D_{prolif} (Gy/day)	95% CL (Gy/day)	$T_k{}^\dagger$ (days)	Source
Early reactions					
Skin	Erythema	0.12	−0.12; 0.22	<12	Bentzen *et al.* (2001)
Mucosa	Mucositis	0.8	0.7; 1.1	<12	Bentzen *et al.* (2001)
Lung	Pneumonitis	0.54	0.13; 0.95		Bentzen *et al.* (2000)*
Tumours					
Head and neck					
Larynx		0.74	0.30; 1.2		Robertson *et al.* (1998)
Tonsils		0.73	30		Withers *et al.* (1995)
Various		0.8	0.5; 1.1	21	Robers *et al.* (1994)
Various		0.64	0.42; 0.86		Hendry *et al.* (1996)*
Esophagus		0.59	0.18; 0.99		Geh *et al.* (2005)
Non-small cell lung cancer		0.45	N/A		Koukourakis *et al.* (1996)
Medulloblastoma		0.52	0.29; 0.75	0 or 21	Hinata *et al.* (2001)

CL, confidence limit.

*Pooled estimate from a review of studies in the literature.

†T_k is the assumed time for the onset of accelerated proliferation.

Reference details are available from Søren Bentzen.

simple estimate would then be that the EQD_2 has to be reduced by $4 \times D_{prolif}$. Using this method, the isoeffective doses in 2-Gy fractions delivered over two different times, t and T, will be related as:

$$EQD_{2,T} = EQD_{2,t} - (T - t)D_{prolif} \quad (9.2)$$

Note, that if $T > t$ then $EQD_{2,T} < EQD_{2,t}$. There is no simple rule specifying the maximum difference between the two times, T and t, where this linear correction is reasonable. For a 1-week difference this approximation would probably be reasonable whereas for a 3- to 4-week difference this would not be a safe assumption. Another concern is that D_{prolif} may depend on the intensity of the schedule; in other words, a very short intensive schedule may give rise to an increased value of D_{prolif}. A serious warning is that little is known about the value of D_{prolif} for various tumours and normal-tissue endpoints and that most of the published values only apply towards the end of a standard 6- to 8-week schedule. For tumours, the majority of available estimates are for squamous cell carcinoma of the head and neck (Table 9.3). As mentioned above, it appears safe to assume that D_{prolif} is zero for late endpoints at least for overall treatment times up to 6–8 weeks. For early reactions, a linear correction is also applicable over a limited range of treatment times, see Bentzen *et al.* (2001).

Example 4. Correcting for overall treatment time

The Danish Head and Neck Cancer Group (DAHANCA) conducted a randomized controlled trial of 66–68 Gy in 33–34 fractions randomizing between five and six fractions per week (Overgaard *et al.*, 2003). This trial, DAHANCA 6/7, comprised 1476 patients with HNSCC receiving definitive radiotherapy without chemotherapy.

Problem: What is the expected difference in biologically effective dose for HNSCC between the two arms of the trial?

Solution: Starting treatment on a Monday, 33 fractions delivered at five fractions per week will take 6 full weeks plus 3 additional treatment days (a total of 45 days). With six fractions per week the overall treatment time becomes 5 full weeks plus 3 additional treatment days (a total of 38 days). From Table 9.3 we see that D_{prolif} for HNSCC is about 0.7 Gy/day. There is no demonstrable difference in D_{prolif} among the various subsites of the head and neck region. We insert these values in equation 9.2 and get:

$$EQD_{2,38} = EQD_{2,45} - (38 - 45) \text{ days} \\ \times 0.7 \text{ Gy/day} \\ = 66 \text{ Gy} + 4.9 \text{ Gy} = 70.9 \text{ Gy}$$

Thus, 66 Gy delivered over 38 days is biologically equivalent to 70.9 Gy in 2-Gy fractions delivered over 45 days for HNSCC. This time difference will be the same for a patient receiving 68 Gy in 34 fractions with five or six fractions per week.

If the two schedules in Example 4 had employed doses per fraction that were different from 2 Gy, we would first have calculated the equivalent EQD_2 values before doing the time correction.

9.7 UNPLANNED GAPS IN TREATMENT

A problem frequently encountered in radiotherapy practice is the management of unscheduled treatment interruptions. Studies have shown that up until 1990 about a third of all patients with HNSCC experienced one or more unplanned gaps in treatment leading to a protraction of overall treatment time of more than 6 days. These interruptions were typically caused by patient-related factors (intercurrent disease, severe radiation reactions) or logistic factors (public holidays, treatment machine downtime, transport difficulties). The management of treatment gaps has been considered in some detail by a working party of the UK Royal College of Radiologists (Hendry et al., 1996). The recommendation to avoid gaps or actively modify treatment after a gap is based on the clinical evidence for a negative therapeutic effect of gaps in radiotherapy schedules. This evidence is strongest for squamous cell carcinoma (SCC) of the head and neck, non-small cell lung cancer and cancer of the uterine cervix, and it is therefore recommended that the remaining part of the treatment be modified in order to adjust for the unscheduled interruption. There is also some support for the importance of overall treatment time in SCC of the skin and vagina and in medulloblastoma. Less evidence exists for other radical treatments and there is no reason to believe that overall treatment time is a significant factor in palliative radiotherapy.

Treatment schedules may be adjusted by accelerating radiotherapy after the gap. In a planned schedule delivering one fraction per day, 5 days per week, this can be accomplished by giving more than five fractions per week, either as two fractions per day, as in Example 2 above, or preferably by treating on Saturday and/or Sunday. The idea is to deliver the planned total dose, with the prescribed dose per fraction, in as near the planned overall time as possible. If two fractions per day are delivered, these should be separated by the maximum practical interval (at least 6 hours and preferably more). Note that with long repair half-times, incomplete repair between the dose fractions may require a dose reduction if the chance of late complications is kept fixed. Alternatively, delivering the remaining part of the treatment with hypofractionation may be considered. Whether this type of adjustment will lead to increased late sequelae or decreased tumour control depends on the exact values of α/β for the relevant late normal-tissue endpoints and the tumour type in question.

9.8 ERRORS IN DOSE DELIVERY

Dosimetric errors in delivering the prescribed dose per fraction made early in a treatment can be corrected by modifying the dose per fraction and total dose given subsequent to discovery of the error, using the LQ model to calculate the correcting doses, which should be completed within the

Example 5. Change in fraction size, gap correction

A patient with colorectal cancer is planned to receive preoperative radiotherapy with five times 5 Gy from Monday to Friday (Kapiteijn *et al.*, 2001). The first two fractions are given as planned on Monday and Tuesday, but owing to a machine breakdown, no treatment could be given on Wednesday. In order to finish as planned on Friday, delivering the isoeffective tumour dose by increasing the size of the two fractions to be given on Thursday and Friday is considered. We assume that $\alpha/\beta = 10$ Gy for colorectal cancer.

Problem: What is the required dose per fraction for the last two fractions? What is the accompanying change in the risk of rectal complications from this modified fractionation schedule?

Solution: The tumour EQD_2 for the final three fractions originally planned is:

$$EQD_2 = 15\,\text{Gy} \times \frac{5\,\text{Gy} + 10\,\text{Gy}}{2\,\text{Gy} + 10\,\text{Gy}} = 18.75\,\text{Gy}$$

We want to estimate the dose per fraction, x, so that delivering two fractions of this size gives an EQD_2 of 18.75 Gy to the tumour:

$$EQD_2 = 2x \times \frac{x + 10\,\text{Gy}}{2\,\text{Gy} + 10\,\text{Gy}}$$

In the following, we remember that x will have the physical units of gray and start solving this quadratic equation:

$$18.75 = 2x \times \frac{x + 10}{2 + 10} \Leftrightarrow$$

$$18.75 \cdot 12 = 2x^2 + 20x \Leftrightarrow$$

$$2x^2 + 20x - 225 = 0$$

The solution to a quadratic equation of the form $ax + bx + c = 0$ is

$$x = \frac{-b + \sqrt{b^2 - 4ac}}{2a}$$

(Note that only the positive root produces a physically meaningful dose.) In the present case,

we get:

$$x = \frac{-20 + \sqrt{20^2 - 4 \times 2 \times (-225)}}{2 \times 2}$$

$$= \frac{-20 + \sqrt{400 + 1800}}{4} = \frac{-20 + 46.9}{4} = 6.7$$

Remember the unit: gray. In other words, we would have to give fractions of 6.7 Gy on Thursday and Friday, a total of 13.4 Gy, to achieve the same tumour effect. This is of course less than the 3×5 Gy originally planned for Wednesday to Friday, and the reason for this is the larger effect per gray deriving from the increased dose per fraction in the modified schedule.

How will this affect the risk of bowel damage? From Table 9.1, we find α/β of 4 Gy. The EQD_2 of the modified schedule to the bowel is now:

$$EQD_2 = 10\,\text{Gy} \times \frac{5\,\text{Gy} + 4\,\text{Gy}}{2\,\text{Gy} + 4\,\text{Gy}} + 2$$

$$\times 6.7\,\text{Gy} \times \frac{6.7\,\text{Gy} + 4\,\text{Gy}}{2\,\text{Gy} + 4\,\text{Gy}} = 38.9\,\text{Gy}$$

This value does not take the very short overall treatment time of 5 days into consideration and it is possible that such short schedules could involve an increased risk of consequential late reactions. Here, we focus only on the change in biological dose deriving from the change in dose fractionation and we note that the overall treatment time is unchanged in the two schedules compared here. The originally planned $\times 5$ Gy corresponds to an EQD_2 for bowel of about 37.5 Gy. Therefore, the risk of late bowel morbidity will be increased if this modification is implemented.

Clinically, one would be concerned about increasing dose per fraction from 5 to 6.7 Gy. Biologically, it may be questioned whether the use of the LQ model is safe anyway at these large doses per fraction (see Chapter 8, Section 8.11). It should also be noted that, if we use a lower α/β, for example the 1.7 Gy estimated for fibrosis, the change in EQD_2 for this endpoint is expected to be from 45 Gy to 48.5 Gy. It could be considered keeping to 5 Gy per fraction and simply accepting a 3-day protraction (i.e. finishing on Monday) or to give the fifth fraction on Saturday.

same overall time as originally prescribed. If the initial error was giving a larger dose per fraction than planned (a hypofractionated error), then the rest of the treatment should be hyperfractionated to compensate. If the initial error was giving a lower dose per fraction than planned (hyperfractionated), then the rest of the treatment should be hypofractionated to compensate.

Joiner (2004) showed how to calculate the dose per fraction used to bring the treatment back exactly to planned tolerance simultaneously for all tissues and tumour involved, following either hyperfractionated or hypofractionated errors made initially, without the need to know any α/β ratios. Defining planned treatment as p Gy per fraction to a total dose of P Gy, suppose the initial error is e Gy per fraction given to a total of E Gy. Using the LQ model to describe all isoeffect relationships between total dose and dose per fraction for the tumour and the normal tissues, then the compensating dose per fraction of d Gy to a total dose of D Gy are given by the simple formulae:

$$D = P - E \qquad (9.3)$$

$$d = \frac{P_p - E_e}{P - E} \qquad (9.4)$$

Notably, it can be seen that the total dose for the complete treatment (error plus compensation) remains as originally prescribed.

Example 6. Error in the delivered dose per fraction at the beginning of treatment

A patient is intended to receive 35×2 Gy per fraction, with five fractions per week to an overall time of 7 weeks. By error, the treatments on each of the first 2 days are given as 4 Gy per fraction.

Problem: What is the dose per fraction that should be given in the remainder of the treatment, to exactly compensate for the initial error?

Solution: The total error dose (E) is 8 Gy; therefore from equation 9.3, the total compensating dose (D) is:

70 Gy − 8 Gy = 62 Gy

The dose per fraction used for the compensation, given by equation 9.4, should be:

$$\frac{70\,\mathrm{Gy} \cdot 2\,\mathrm{Gy} - 8\,\mathrm{Gy} \cdot 4\,\mathrm{Gy}}{70\,\mathrm{Gy} - 8\,\mathrm{Gy}} = 1.74\,\mathrm{Gy} \qquad (9.4)$$

This gives 62/1.74 = 35.6 fractions for the compensating 62 Gy. Since an integral number of fractions must be given, the nearest compensating treatment is 36×1.72 Gy.

In this example, there are 33 weekday treatment days left to use in the original planned overall time, so three of the 1.72 Gy doses must be given on Saturdays, or using two fractions per day on three of the Fridays, in order not to extend overall treatment time. It must be noted that equations 9.3 and 9.4 are valid only in the absence of incomplete repair; therefore compensating treatments should not be scheduled in a way that would introduce significant incomplete repair. This favours using Saturdays to deliver the additional doses, or leaving the maximum possible time between two doses given on Fridays, but at least 6 hours.

9.9 RE-IRRADIATION

A specific problem in clinical practice is the radiotherapeutic management of patients with a new primary tumour or a loco-regional recurrence in an anatomical site that necessitates re-irradiation of a previously irradiated tissue or organ. Experimental animal data demonstrate that various endpoints differ markedly in their capacity for long-term recovery of radiation tolerance (see Chapter 19). Quantitative clinical data are sparse and it may not be safe to assume any particular value of the recovery in a clinical setting. The most reasonable approach is probably to use the LQ model to estimate the EQD_2 values for the normal-tissue endpoints of concern without any explicit recovery assumed, and then to apply a clinical assessment of the re-irradiation tolerance based in part on the experience from animal experiments. Obviously, such an assessment would also include other clinical aspects such as the life expectancy of the patient in relation to the latent period of late damage, and the prospects for long-term benefit from the re-treatment.

9.10 FROM CHANGE IN DOSE TO CHANGE IN RESPONSE RATE

Early papers on the use of the LQ model in biological dose calculations were all concerned with estimation of isoeffective doses. In practice, two dose-fractionation schedules will most often not produce exactly the same biological effect, and even if they are isoeffective with respect to a specific endpoint they will typically not be so with respect to other endpoints. In these situations, it is necessary to consider the steepness of the dose–response curve in order to estimate the associated change in the incidence of a clinical endpoint in going from one schedule to the other.

In the following, response rate refers to either a tumour control probability or a normal-tissue complication probability. If the response rate is R after a dose D, the change in response rate, in percentage points, after an increment in dose, ΔD, is approximately:

$$\Delta R \approx \frac{\Delta D}{D} \times 100\% \times \gamma_n \qquad (9.5)$$

where γ_n is the local value of the normalized dose–response gradient (see Chapter 5). The use of this formula is illustrated by the following example.

Example 7. Converting from change in dose into change in response rate

For the DAHANCA 6/7 trial, we calculated in Example 4 that the acceleration in the six fractions per week arm corresponded to an effective 4.9-Gy dose increment. Assume that the local tumour control probability (T-position alone) in the five fractions per week arm is 64 per cent (this is the actual observed control probability in this arm of the trial).

Problem: What is the expected increase in tumour control probability from the treatment acceleration?

Solution: First, we need to choose the value of γ. From Figs 5.4 and 5.5 (Chapter 5), we find that γ_{50} is around 1.8 for head and neck cancer with a trend towards higher values for vocal cord tumours. At the 64 per cent level, this value is still valid (see Table 5.1). Using this value of γ allows us to calculate the expected change in response:

$$\Delta R = \frac{4.9\,\text{Gy}}{66\,\text{Gy}} \times 100\% \times 1.8 = 13\%$$

Thus, the local tumour control probability is expected to increase by 13 per cent. The observed local tumour control rates in the trial were 64 per cent and 76 per cent in the five- and six-fraction per week arms, respectively (Overgaard *et al.*, 2003). This means that the tumour control rate increased by 12 per cent, in very good agreement with the expected increase calculated here.

9.11 DOUBLE TROUBLE

Dosimetric hot spots receive not only a higher total dose but also a higher dose per fraction. Rodney Withers (see, for example, Lee *et al.*, 1995) has called this phenomenon 'double trouble'. A hot spot could arise as a result of internal and external inhomogeneities or because of the radiation field arrangement. A special case is in the match zone between two abutted fields where, depending on the geometrical matching technique used, a small tissue volume could be markedly overdosed or underdosed.

Example 8. Double trouble

The peak absorbed dose in the match zone between two abutted photon fields is measured by film dosimetry to be 118 per cent of the dose on the central axis of one of the abutting fields. A total dose of 50 Gy is delivered in 25 fractions. The peak physical absorbed dose per fraction in the match zone is 2.36 Gy and the corresponding total dose is 25×2.36 Gy $= 59.0$ Gy.

Problem: What is the peak biologically isoeffective dose in 2-Gy fractions in the match zone for a late normal-tissue endpoint with $\alpha/\beta = 2$ Gy and for a tumour with $\alpha/\beta = 10$ Gy?

Solution: This is a straightforward application of Withers' formula (equation 9.1). For the late endpoint we get:

$$EQD_2 = 59\,Gy \times \frac{2.36\,Gy + 2\,Gy}{2\,Gy + 2\,Gy} = 64.3\,Gy$$

And for the tumour:

$$EQD_2 = 59\,Gy \times \frac{2.36\,Gy + 10\,Gy}{2\,Gy + 10\,Gy} = 60.8\,Gy$$

It is seen that the greater fractionation sensitivity of the late endpoint relative to the tumours in this example means that the biological effect of a hot spot is relatively more important for the late endpoint.

Historically, match zone overdosage of the brachial plexus has been associated with an unacceptable incidence of radiation plexopathies in patients receiving postoperative radiotherapy for breast cancer (Bentzen and Dische, 2000). These problems can largely be avoided by using a more optimal treatment technique.

Clearly, volume effects should be considered in relation to the double-trouble phenomenon.

9.12 THE UNCERTAINTY IN BIOLOGICAL EFFECT ESTIMATES

An impression of the uncertainty in biological effect estimates may be obtained simply by varying the value of α/β or D_{prolif} or γ_{50}. The idea is to insert the lower and upper 95 per cent confidence limits of the parameter in question and use these as 95 per cent confidence limits for the biological effect estimate. This technique is only straightforward if we are concerned with uncertainty in a single parameter, say, uncertainty in α/β. If we want to evaluate the effect of uncertainty in two parameters, for example D_{prolif} and γ_{50}, it is necessary to use more advanced methods. It is not a good approximation simply to insert the lower and upper confidence limits for both parameters in the calculation.

Example 9. Estimating uncertainty

We will repeat the calculation in Example 8, but this time we will use the α/β ratio for subcutaneous fibrosis from Table 9.1. In other words, we want to estimate the EQD_2 for subcutaneous fibrosis for a schedule delivering 59 Gy in 25 fractions (i.e. employing a dose per fraction of 2.36 Gy).

Problem: What is the isoeffective dose in 2-Gy fractions for subcutaneous fibrosis and the associated 95 per cent confidence limits?

Solution: Table 9.1 gives $\alpha/\beta = 1.7$ Gy with 95 per cent confidence limits 0.6 Gy and 2.6 Gy. Thus,

$$EQD_2 = 59\,Gy \times \frac{2.36\,Gy + 1.7\,Gy}{2\,Gy + 1.7\,Gy} = 64.7\,Gy$$

Similarly, for $\alpha/\beta = 2.6$ Gy, the lower 95 per cent confidence limit for EQD_2 becomes 63.6 Gy. Using $\alpha/\beta = 0.6$ Gy, the upper 95 per cent confidence limit becomes 67.2 Gy. Thus, our best estimate of EQD_2 for subcutaneous fibrosis is 64.7 Gy with 95 per cent confidence limits 63.6 Gy and 67.2 Gy.

The confidence interval in this example is atypically narrow. Most α/β values for human normal-tissue endpoints and tumours are known with poorer precision than the value for subcutaneous fibrosis. Also, when the LQ formula is used to extrapolate to doses that are further away from 2 Gy than the 2.36 Gy considered in the example, uncertainty in α/β becomes more important.

Another useful approach is to identify the main clinical concern. In Examples 8 and 9, the main concern is the added risk of complications associated with the overdosage in the match zone. In Example 5, the main concern is the possible increase of late effects after hypofractionation. In these cases, it is of course cautious to assume a low value for α/β. If, on the other hand, we want to estimate the sparing from hyperfractionation in a given patient, it would be conservative (i.e. we would not be overestimating the benefit) if we assumed a relatively high value of α/β.

A final observation is that the confidence interval for α/β derived from animal studies is generally narrower than for the corresponding human endpoint. This probably reflects that the number of subjects is often larger in the experimental studies and that dose and dose per fraction is varied more systematically and over a wider range of values. As mentioned above, we would suggest that the full calculation, including the estimation of confidence limits, is done using the parameter estimates from the human data whenever possible, and that an independent calculation is done using the animal data.

9.13 SOME CURRENT ISSUES IN THE CLINICAL APPLICATION OF THE LQ MODEL

The question whether the LQ approach has been validated can only be addressed on an endpoint-by-endpoint basis. The LQ model has been applied to datasets from quite a few clinical studies, and there has in many cases been good agreement between the predicted and observed study outcome. This gives some confidence in using the model to estimate the effects of changed dose fractionation in situations where there are clinical parameter estimates. Roughly, the dose per fraction, where use of the LQ model is supported by data, ranges from about 1.0 Gy to 5 Gy or so. As mentioned in the introduction to this chapter, even then there is often a lack of appropriate parameter estimates, or the available estimates have wide 95 per cent confidence limits. Parameter estimates for clinical endpoints remain relatively scarce. Some papers derive parameter values based on fixing one or more other parameters in the estimation. Clearly, these estimates become circular to some extent. While the clinical importance of low-dose hyper-radiosensitivity remains controversial, there is little empirical support from clinical studies for the use of the LQ model at dose per fraction of < 1.0 Gy. This is an important issue as many IMRT techniques involve irradiation of large normal-tissue volumes with dose fractions in this range. At the other end of the spectrum, techniques such as extracranial stereotactic body radiotherapy, or intraoperative radiotherapy or high dose-rate brachytherapy may deliver dose fractions of 10 Gy or more. Again, there is little empirical evidence behind the use of the simple LQ model, or any of the proposed modifications of this model, in this high-dose range. In most cases, the dose fractionation issue is intertwined with the volume effect, and in practice it is difficult to separate these effects from clinical studies where patients receive roughly similar dose distributions (see also Chapter 14).

It should also be mentioned that a number of elegant formulations of the LQ model have been developed, for example for internal emitters or permanent implants. Other formulations include relative biological effectiveness (RBE) or oxygen enhancement ratio (OER) corrections, etc. The interested reader is referred to a recent book edited by Dale and Jones (2007 – see Further reading) for an overview of many of these applications and refinements of the LQ model. From the perspective of clinical radiobiology, many of these models are over-parameterized in the sense that clinical datasets typically will not have sufficient structural resolution to allow estimation of all relevant model parameters, not to mention validating the model assumptions.

Do some tumours have low α/β ratios? Parameter estimates for malignant melanoma and liposarcoma from the late 1980s suggested that this might be the case, but this hypothesis has attracted considerable interest after Brenner and Hall (1999) derived low α/β estimates for prostate cancer from a comparison between external-beam and brachytherapy outcomes. Later studies comparing external-beam only fractionation effects have provided further support for this idea (Bentzen and Ritter, 2005; Lukka *et al.*, 2005). A number of trials are in progress that should produce valuable data allowing a rigorous test of this hypothesis (Bentzen and Ritter, 2005; Miles and Lee, 2008). There is also emerging evidence that α/β for subclinical breast cancer may be considerably less than the often assumed 10 Gy; see the report from the UK START Trialists Group (Bentzen *et al.*, 2008). A cautious attitude at present is that fractionation schedules designed to exploit these presumptive low α/β values for some cancer types should be tested in prospective clinical trials, as they could lead to major deviations from the established practice in a particular centre.

The final note here is that the move towards increasing use of combined modality therapy in many tumour types represents a further issue regarding the applicability of standard LQ modelling. The approach often taken is to perform bioeffect calculations for the radiation therapy part in isolation. This may produce valid results as long as the chemotherapy is strictly identical in the schedules being compared. However, this approach is also challenged by data suggesting that some cytotoxic and molecular targeted drugs actually modulate the dose–time fractionation response (Bentzen *et al.*, 2007). In this case, radiobiological parameters derived from radiation-alone studies may no longer be valid.

While the LQ approach 10 years ago appeared to be rather well established, a number of new developments – mainly driven by clinical and technology advances – have made bioeffect modelling an exciting and important area of clinical and experimental radiation research again.

Key points

1. The LQ approach is the model of choice for bioeffect estimation in radiotherapy and can be used for a wide range of calculations.
2. The dose range where the LQ model is well supported by data is roughly 1–5 Gy per fraction. Extrapolations made outside this range should be done with extreme caution.

3. Clinical parameter estimates should be used in calculations whenever possible. If no clinical estimates are available, values from animal studies may be used as guidance but caution should be exercised in applying the results of such calculations to the clinical situation.
4. Estimates of uncertainty in LQ calculations should always be made, based on the uncertainty in the values of the parameters used in the calculation.
5. In combined modality therapy, it may not be valid to use parameters derived from studies using radiation alone.

■ BIBLIOGRAPHY

Bentzen SM (2006). Preventing or reducing late side effects of radiation therapy: radiobiology meets molecular pathology. *Nat Rev Cancer* **6**: 702–13.

Bentzen SM, Dische S (2000). Morbidity related to axillary irradiation in the treatment of breast cancer. *Acta Oncol* **39**: 337–47.

Bentzen SM, Overgaard J (1995). Clinical normal-tissue radiobiology. In: Tobias JS, Thomas PR (eds) *Current radiation oncology*, Vol. 2, London: Arnold, 37–67.

Bentzen SM, Ritter MA (2005). The alpha/beta ratio for prostate cancer: what is it, really? *Radiother Oncol* **76**: 1–3.

Bentzen SM, Saunders MI, Dische S (1999). Repair halftimes estimated from observations of treatment-related morbidity after CHART or conventional radiotherapy in head and neck cancer. *Radiother Oncol* **53**: 219–26.

Bentzen SM, Saunders MI, Dische S, Bond SJ (2001). Radiotherapy-related early morbidity in head and neck cancer: quantitative clinical radiobiology as deduced from the CHART trial. *Radiother Oncol* **60**: 123–35.

Bentzen SM, Harari PM, Bernier J (2007). Exploitable mechanisms for combining drugs with radiation: concepts, achievements and future directions. *Nat Clin Pract Oncol* **4**: 172–80.

Bentzen SM, Agrawal RK, Aird EG *et al.* (2008). The UK Standardisation of Breast Radiotherapy (START) Trial A of radiotherapy hypofractionation for treatment of early breast cancer: a randomised trial. *Lancet Oncol* **9**: 331–41.

Brenner DJ, Hall EJ (1999). Fractionation and protraction for radiotherapy of prostate carcinoma. *Int J Radiat Oncol Biol Phys* **43**: 1095–101.

Dische S, Saunders MI (1989). Continuous, hyperfractionated, accelerated radiotherapy (CHART): an interim report upon late morbidity. *Radiother Oncol* **16**: 65–72.

Fuwa N, Ito Y, Matsumoto A, Morita K (2000). The treatment results of 40 patients with localized endobronchial cancer with external beam irradiation and intraluminal irradiation using low dose rate (192)Ir thin wires with a new catheter. *Radiother Oncol* **56**: 189–95.

Guttenberger R, Thames HD, Ang KK (1992). Is the experience with CHART compatible with experimental data? A new model of repair kinetics and computer simulations. *Radiother Oncol* **25**: 280–6.

Hendry JH, Bentzen SM, Dale RG *et al.* (1996). A modelled comparison of the effects of using different ways to compensate for missed treatment days in radiotherapy. *Clin Oncol* **8**: 297–307.

Joiner MC (2004). A simple alpha/beta-independent method to derive fully isoeffective schedules following changes in dose per fraction. *Int J Radiat Oncol Biol Phys* **58**: 871–5.

Kapiteijn E, Marijnen CA, Nagtegaal ID *et al.* (2001). Preoperative radiotherapy combined with total mesorectal excision for resectable rectal cancer. *N Engl J Med* **345**: 638–46.

Lee AW, Sze WM, Fowler JF, Chappell R, Leung SF, Teo P (1999). Caution on the use of altered fractionation for nasopharyngeal carcinoma. *Radiother Oncol* **52**: 207–11.

Lee SP, Leu MY, Smathers JB, McBride WH, Parker RG, Withers HR (1995). Biologically effective dose distribution based on the linear quadratic model and its clinical relevance. *Int J Radiat Oncol Biol Phys* **33**: 375–89.

Lukka H, Hayter C, Julian JA *et al.* (2005). Randomized trial comparing two fractionation schedules for patients with localized prostate cancer. *J Clin Oncol* **23**: 6132–8.

Miles EF, Lee WR (2008). Hypofractionation for prostate cancer: a critical review. *Semin Radiat Oncol* **18**: 41–7.

Overgaard J, Hansen HS, Specht L *et al.* (2003). Five compared with six fractions per week of conventional radiotherapy of squamous-cell carcinoma of head and neck: DAHANCA 6 and 7 randomised controlled trial. *Lancet* **362**: 933–40.

Thames HD, Bentzen SM, Turesson I, Overgaard M, van den Bogaert W (1990). Time-dose factors in radiotherapy: a review of the human data. *Radiother Oncol* **19**: 219–35.

Withers HR, Thames HD, Jr, Peters LJ (1983). A new isoeffect curve for change in dose per fraction. Radiother Oncol **1**: 187–91.

■ FURTHER READING

Dale RG, Jones B (ed.) (2007). *Radiobiological modeling in radiation oncology*. London: British Institute of Radiology.

Modified fractionation

MICHAEL BAUMANN AND VINCENT GRÉGOIRE

10.1 INTRODUCTION

The clinical evaluation and implementation of modified fractionation schedules based on biological rationales is an important focus of 'translational research' in radiation oncology. Throughout the history of radiotherapy, the optimal distribution of dose over time has been a major issue but important progress has been made in this area over the past two decades. The relationships uncovered between total dose and fraction number for late-responding normal tissues, early-responding normal tissues and tumours provide the basic information required to optimize the dose per fraction in radiotherapy. Work still needs to be done to determine the exact time of onset, the rate and the mechanisms of repopulation in tumours and normal tissues during radiotherapy, but enough is now known about time factors to support the important conclusions that: (1) the overall duration of fractionated radiotherapy should not be allowed to extend beyond the originally prescribed time; (2) a reduced overall treatment time should be considered in a number of clinical situations; and (3) inter-fraction time intervals should be made as long as possible in order to gain the full benefit from fractionation schedules employing multiple fractions per day.

This chapter summarizes the current status of modified fractionation in clinical radiotherapy.

10.2 CONVENTIONAL FRACTIONATION

Conventional fractionation is the application of daily doses of 1.8–2 Gy and five fractions per week (Monday to Friday) with a dose per week of 9–10 Gy. Depending on tumour histology, tumour size and localization, total doses ranging from 40 Gy to 70 Gy are given for macroscopic disease and lower doses when treating microscopic disease. These conventional fractionation schedules were developed on an empirical basis (Fletcher, 1988) and have been the mainstay of curative radiotherapy over the last decades in most institutions in Europe and the USA.

Radiosensitive tumours such as lymphomas and seminomas can be controlled with low doses of 45 Gy or even less and in this situation there is a low incidence of collateral normal-tissue damage. By contrast, glioblastoma multiforme is a very resistant tumour that is not controlled even after doses as high as 70 Gy. Most tumour types, including squamous cell carcinomas and adenocarcinomas, are of intermediate sensitivity. Small tumours, for example T1 or T2 carcinomas of the head and neck, are well controlled with acceptable normal-tissue damage using conventional fractionation and total doses between 60 Gy and 70 Gy. However, local tumour control rates rapidly decline for larger and more advanced tumours. As local tumour control increases with the total dose of radiotherapy, the question may be asked whether improved management of larger tumours could be gained by increasing the total dose of conventional fractionation above 70 Gy, say to doses between 80 Gy and 100 Gy. Such dose escalation is currently being tested for non-small cell lung cancer and for carcinoma of the prostate. One constraint is that not only tumour control rates but also the incidence and severity of normal-tissue damage increase with increasing total doses (see Chapter 5). This was recognized as early as 1936 when Holthusen pointed out that the uncomplicated local tumour control rate initially increases with increasing dose but then falls again because of the steep increase in the incidence of normal-tissue damage. Figure 10.1 is redrawn from one of Holthusen's papers: the frequency of 'uncomplicated tumour control' follows a bell-shaped curve. Once the optimum dose is established, further improvements in uncomplicated tumour control can only be achieved by either moving the dose–effect curve for local tumour control to lower doses or the curve for normal-tissue damage to higher doses; the latter is the objective of hyperfractionated schedules (see Section 10.3). Conformal radiotherapy is another option currently used in dose escalation protocols, reducing the volume of normal tissue irradiated to high dose and therefore also the probability of late normal-tissue damage (see Chapters 14 and 20). As dose escalation using conventional fractionation

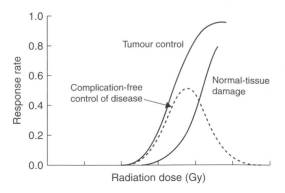

Figure 10.1 Dose–response curves for tumour control and normal-tissue damage. The uncomplicated local tumour control rate initially increases with increasing dose after which it falls again because of a steep increase in the incidence of damage to normal tissue. Adapted from Holthusen (1936).

is always associated with the prolongation of overall treatment time, some of the potential gain may be lost as a consequence of tumour-cell repopulation and this is considered in Section 10.4.

Radiotherapy is highly effective in dealing with a small number of cancer cells, as in the treatment of microscopic disease. Thus, lower doses of irradiation are also used postoperatively after complete resection of breast or head and neck cancer.

10.3 MODIFICATION OF DOSE PER FRACTION

Hyperfractionation

Hyperfractionation is the term used to describe radiotherapy with doses per fraction less than the 1.8–2.0 Gy given in conventional fractionation. The total number of fractions must be increased, hence the prefix 'hyper-'; usually two fractions are administered per day. The biological rationale of hyperfractionation is to exploit the difference between the small effect of dose per fraction on tumour control versus the larger effect of dose per fraction on the incidence and severity of late normal-tissue damage. As pointed out in Chapter 8, this differential between tumours and late-responding normal tissues is thought to be caused

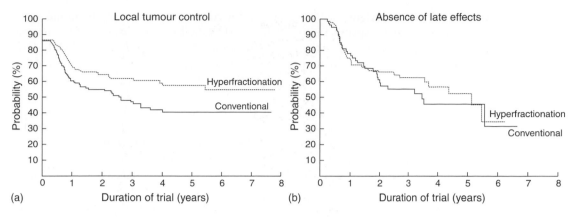

Figure 10.2 Results of the EORTC (22791) trial of dose-escalated hyperfractionation. (a) Loco-regional tumour control (log-rank $p = 0.02$); (b) patients free of late radiation effects, grade 2 or worse (log-rank $p = 0.72$). From Horiot *et al.* (1992), with permission.

by a different capacity of target cells in these tissues to recover from sublethal radiation damage between fractions.

In clinical practice hyperfractionation is usually applied to escalate the total dose compared with conventional fractionation, thereby aiming at improved tumour control rates without increasing the risk of late complications (see Fig. 8.7). Dose-escalated hyperfractionation has been tested in two large multicentre randomized clinical trials on head and neck squamous cell carcinoma [European Organisation for Cancer Research (EORTC) No. 22791 and Radiation Therapy Oncology Group (RTOG) No. 9003]. The results of the EORTC trial are shown in Fig. 10.2. In Fig. 10.2b it can be seen that hyperfractionated treatment with 70 fractions of 1.15 Gy (two fractions per day with a 4- to 6-hour interval; total dose 80.5 Gy) produced a similar incidence of pooled grades 2 and 3 late tissue damage to a conventional schedule of 35 fractions of 2 Gy (70 Gy given in the same overall time of 7 weeks). However, the larger total dose in the hyperfractionated treatment produced an increase of about 19 per cent in long-term local tumour control (Fig. 10.2a). Survival appeared higher after hyperfractionation but this difference did not reach statistical significance. In the RTOG trial (Fu *et al.*, 2000), local tumour control was increased by 8 per cent after hyperfractionation (68 fractions of

1.2 Gy, two fractions per day, 6 hours apart, total dose 81.6 Gy) compared with conventional fractionation using 2-Gy fractions to 70 Gy in the same overall time of 7 weeks. Overall survival was not significantly improved but the prevalence of grade 3 late effects was significantly increased after hyperfractionation. Both these clinical trials thus confirm the radiobiological expectation that local tumour control can be increased by dose-escalated hyperfractionation, thereby supporting a high average α/β ratio for squamous cell carcinoma of the head and neck (Table 9.1). However, while the EORTC trial supports the view that hyperfractionation allows the total dose to be increased without a simultaneous increase in late complications, the RTOG trial indicates that this is not always the case. The potential therapeutic gain from hyperfractionation is debated by Beck-Bornholdt *et al.* (1997), Baumann *et al.* (1998) and Bentzen *et al.* (1999). Factors that contribute to an increased risk of late normal-tissue damage when multiple fractions are applied per day are discussed in Section 10.5.

Hypofractionation

This is the use of doses per fraction higher than 2.0 Gy; the total number of fractions is reduced, hence the prefix 'hypo-'. As explained in Chapter 8,

Section 8.6, the radiobiological expectation is that hypofractionation will lower the therapeutic ratio between tumours and late-responding normal tissues, compared with conventional fractionation given in the same overall time. This expectation depends on the α/β ratio for the tumour being considerably higher than for late-responding normal tissues; exceptions could therefore occur for tumours that have low α/β ratios, for example some melanomas, liposarcomas and potentially early-stage prostate and breast cancer (see Table 9.1). In these cases hypofractionation may be as good or even better than conventional fractionation. For example a randomized clinical trial (Owen *et al.*, 2006), including 1410 women with invasive breast cancer who had local tumour excision, compared 50 Gy in 25 fractions, 39 Gy in 13 fractions and 42.9 Gy in 13 fractions, all given over 5 weeks. The risk of ipsilateral tumour relapse after 10 years was 12.1 per cent in the 50 Gy group, 14.8 per cent in the 39 Gy group, and 9.6 per cent in the 429 Gy group (difference between 39 Gy and 42.9 Gy groups, $p = 0.027$). The α/β ratio of breast cancer was estimated from these data to be 4.0 Gy [95 per cent confidence interval (CI) 1.0–7.8], similar to that estimated for the late adverse effects in healthy tissue from breast radiotherapy.

Single-dose irradiation or hypofractionation with only few large fractions are widely applied in palliative radiotherapy. These schedules use lower total doses than those applied in curative radiotherapy. For this reason, and because the patients have a limited life expectancy, late normal-tissue damage is of only minor concern. A number of randomized clinical trials have shown that symptom control after palliative hypofractionated schedules is comparable to that achieved with more highly fractionated schedules. Hypofractionated schedules have the advantage of being more convenient for the patient and they help spare resources.

For stereotactic radiotherapy of small tumours (e.g. in lung, where very steep dose gradients can be achieved and hence only very small volumes of surrounding normal tissue are at risk of radiation damage) single doses or hypofractionation with few large fractions are also frequently applied in clinical practice.

Moderate hypofractionation with doses per fraction up to approximately 3.5 Gy is routinely used for curative radiation therapy in many centres worldwide. To reduce the risk of late normal-tissue damage in these schedules, slightly lower total doses are applied than for conventional fractionation. For tumours with a high α/β ratio this decrease in total dose may well lead to a reduction in tumour control probability. However, some or all of this negative effect may be compensated by the shorter overall treatment times often used for this moderate hypofractionation (see Section 10.4). There is growing interest in the use of moderate hypofractionation to escalate total doses in the context of clinical trials of conformal radiation therapy. For example, using a field-in-field technique or intensity-modulated radiotherapy (IMRT), a higher dose per fraction can be applied for boosting the macroscopic tumour while potential microscopic tumour extensions are treated at conventional doses per fraction. Such hypofractionated approaches for dose escalation avoid the necessity to prolong the overall treatment time and conserve treatment resources. However, these advantages have to be carefully weighed against the increased risk of late normal-tissue injury, and clinical trials are therefore necessary to fully evaluate the therapeutic gain compared with standard approaches.

10.4 THE TIME FACTOR FOR FRACTIONATED RADIOTHERAPY IN TUMOURS

In the 1960s and 1970s the prevailing view among radiation oncologists had been that prolonged overall treatment times of fractionated irradiation did not impair local tumour control. Contrary to this general view, studies on experimental tumours were beginning to find that clonogenic cells proliferate rapidly after irradiation (see Chapter 7) so predicting that the ability of clinical radiotherapy to achieve local tumour control would actually decrease with increasing overall treatment time. Several experimental studies indicate that repopulation of clonogenic tumour cells accelerates at some point during fractionated radiotherapy (see Chapters 8 and 9). It should also be noted that other mechanisms such as long repair halftimes or increasing radiobiological

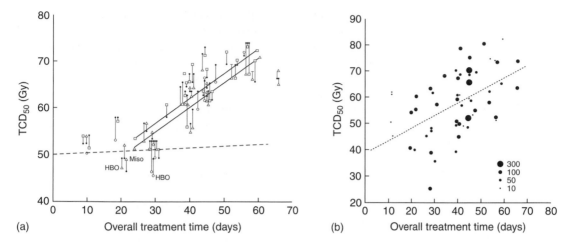

Figure 10.3 Tumour control dose (TCD$_{50}$ – dose required to control 50 per cent of the tumours) in head and neck cancer as a function of overall treatment time, normalized to a dose per fraction of 2 Gy. The same large set of clinical studies has been retrospectively summarized by (a) Withers *et al.* (1988) and (b) Bentzen *et al.* (1991). In (b) each point indicates the result of a particular trial, the size of the symbol indicating the size of the trial. There is a trend for the curative radiation dose to increase with overall treatment time, although the details of this association differ between the two studies.

hypoxia during treatment might contribute to a detrimental effect of long overall treatment times on tumour control.

The possible existence of a tumour time-factor in clinical radiotherapy became more widely acknowledged following a publication by Withers *et al.* (1988) entitled 'The hazard of accelerated tumour clonogen repopulation during radiotherapy'. This review examined the correlation between tumour control and overall treatment time for squamous cell carcinomas of the head and neck and led to the diagram shown in Fig. 10.3a: this shows the dose required to achieve tumour control in 50 per cent of cases (i.e. TCD$_{50}$ values) plotted against the overall treatment time. Since a variety of doses per fraction were used in the various original studies summarized in this plot, the linear-quadratic (LQ) model was used with an α/β ratio of 25 Gy to convert from the actual doses per fraction used into equivalent doses using 2 Gy per fraction (EQD$_2$, see Chapter 8, Section 8.7). The various studies also achieved different tumour control rates and it was therefore necessary to interpolate or extrapolate to the 50 per cent control level. This required an assumed value for the steepness of the dose–response relationship for the

tumours; it was assumed that the dose to increase control from 40 per cent to 60 per cent was 2.9 Gy. As can be seen from Fig. 10.3a, this retrospective review of head and neck cancer data found a clear trend: as overall time increased, a greater total radiation dose had been required to control these tumours. The other important conclusion was that there seemed to be an initial flat portion to this relationship (the so-called 'dog-leg'). This implied that, for treatment times shorter than 3–4 weeks, tumour proliferation had little effect and that, as shown for experimental tumours, it also takes time for accelerated repopulation to be 'switched on' in human tumours. Withers *et al.* (1988) concluded that for treatment times longer than 4 weeks, the effect of proliferation was equivalent to a loss of radiation dose of about 0.6 Gy/day.

This publication gave rise to considerable debate. Subsequent analyses of the same clinical data carried out by Bentzen and Thames (1991) and by Dubben (1994) are shown in Figs 10.3b and 10.4. The analysis of Bentzen and Thames made a different assumption about the steepness of dose–response curves for tumour control: the dose to increase control from 40 per cent to 60 per cent was taken to be 10.5 rather than 2.9 Gy, which

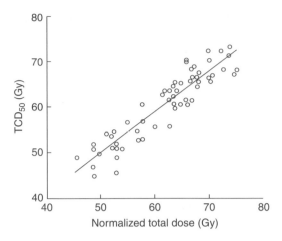

Figure 10.4 The clinical data shown in (a) and (b) of Fig. 10.3 as reanalysed by Dubben (1994). The tumour control dose (TCD) is plotted against the prescribed total dose, normalized to a dose per fraction of 2 Gy. The positive trend in these data indicates a possible prescription bias. Reprinted with permission from Elsevier.

was thought to be more clinically realistic. In addition, the data points in Fig. 10.3b were drawn to indicate the size of the patient sample from which the estimate of TCD_{50} had been made. Figure 10.3b suggests that the 'lag' period before commencement of repopulation may have been somewhat exaggerated by the plot shown in Fig. 10.3a, although this issue is still actively discussed. Furthermore, the analysis by Dubben used the same radiobiological assumptions as the review by Withers et al. (1988) and showed that the actual local tumour control rates could be replaced by random numbers without changing the conclusion of Fig. 10.3a. As shown in Fig. 10.4, the reason for this completely unexpected finding was a highly significant correlation between TCD_{50} and the prescribed total dose (normalized to 2-Gy fractions). Dubben's conclusion was that the increase of TCD_{50} with increasing treatment duration in Fig. 10.3a reflects only dose–time prescriptions and that these data neither confirm nor exclude a time factor of fractionated radiotherapy. The comparison among these three analyses of the same dataset is a good example of how difficult it is to draw reliable conclusions based on retrospective analyses of clinical data.

If we accept the data summarized in Fig. 10.3b, the slope of the line indicates that 0.48 Gy per day is recovered during fractionated radiotherapy of head and neck squamous cell carcinoma. If we further accept that this effect is caused by repopulation and assume reasonable estimates of tumour cell radiosensitivity, we can deduce a clonogen doubling time of less than 1 week, similar to the values of pretreatment potential doubling times measured in human tumours (see Tables 7.4 and 7.5). The potential doubling time (T_{pot}) is a cell kinetic parameter that indicates the rate at which cells are proliferating in an untreated tumour. Although there is much uncertainty about this, it has been suggested that during treatment the rate at which clonogenic cells within the tumour repopulate may also resemble the T_{pot} value. Thus, accelerated fractionation, which uses a reduced overall treatment time below the conventional 6–7 weeks, should increase tumour cure rates by restricting the time available for tumour cell proliferation. From Fig. 10.3b, for example, the dose in a 5-week schedule would be effectively larger than that in a 7-week schedule by a factor $0.48 \times (7 - 5) = 6.7$ Gy, or nearly 10 per cent of a 70-Gy treatment.

10.5 CLINICAL EVALUATION OF ACCELERATED RADIOTHERAPY

Through the joint activities of radiation biologists and clinicians, accelerated fractionation schedules have been developed that aim to counteract the rapid repopulation of clonogenic cells during therapy, as deduced in Section 10.4. Accelerated fractionation is defined as a shortening of the overall treatment time or, more precisely, as an increase of the average dose per week above the 10 Gy given in conventional fractionation. Early normal-tissue reactions are expected to increase using accelerated radiotherapy (see Chapter 11). In contrast, if recovery from sublethal radiation damage between fractions is complete (see Chapter 8), late normal-tissue damage is expected to remain constant for accelerated fractionation schedules using 1.8- to 2-Gy fractions and total doses comparable to conventional fractionation. If the total dose and/or the dose per fraction is reduced (sometimes termed

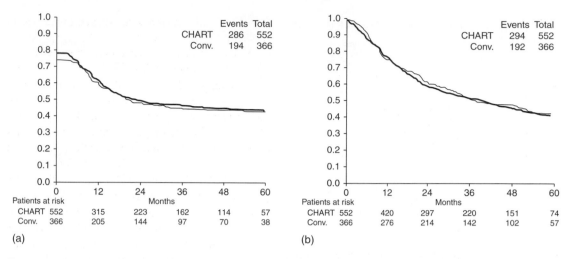

Figure 10.5 Results of a phase III randomized trial of CHART (continuous hyperfractionated accelerated radiotherapy) in squamous cell carcinoma of the head and neck. (a) Probability of loco-regional tumour control; (b) probability of overall survival of patients treated by CHART (bold line) and by conventional radiotherapy (solid line). From Dische et al. (1997), with permission.

accelerated hyperfractionation) late normal-tissue damage could even decrease.

To test these ideas, many clinical trials of accelerated radiotherapy have been set up. As of 2008, 15 trials have been reported, some of these only as abstracts. Twelve of these trials (9/11 in head and neck squamous cell carcinoma, 2/3 in non-small cell lung cancer, 1/1 in small-cell lung cancer) indicate that, for a given total dose, accelerated fractionation schedules are more effective in obtaining local tumour control than conventional fractionation schedules, or that the results are at least identical to conventional fractionation despite administering a reduced total dose in the accelerated arm. Overall, these studies on more than 7000 patients provide strong support for the existence of a significant time factor for tumours. The following paragraphs describe some of these trials of accelerated radiotherapy in more detail.

The strategy known as CHART (*c*ontinuous *h*yperfractionated *a*ccelerated *r*adio*t*herapy) is an example of strongly accelerated fractionation. This protocol applies 36 fractions over 12 consecutive days (starting on a Monday and including the following weekend), using three fractions per day with an interval of 6 hours between the fractions within each day. Dose per fraction is 1.5 Gy to a total of 54 Gy. Total dose is therefore reduced compared with conventional therapy, in order to remain within the tolerance of acutely responding epithelial tissues. Dische *et al.* (1997) have reported the results of a phase III clinical trial of CHART in 918 patients with head and neck cancer. Patients were randomized between CHART and conventional fractionation in 2-Gy fractions to 66 Gy. Figure 10.5a shows that loco-regional tumour control was identical in both treatment arms. CHART used 12 Gy less than conventional therapy in an overall time reduced by 33 days. If this dose reduction is thought to just offset repopulation, this would correspond to 0.36 Gy per day lost through tumour cell proliferation, which is somewhat lower than the 0.48 Gy per day from the data in Fig. 10.3b. This could be interpreted to mean that the lag period before onset of accelerated repopulation in head and neck carcinoma is longer than the 12-day duration of a course of CHART, but further data are required to confirm this. Overall patient survival was identical in both treatment arms (Fig. 10.5b). As expected for accelerated radiotherapy, radiation mucositis was more severe with CHART; it occurred earlier but settled sooner and was in nearly all cases healed by 8 weeks in both arms. Unexpectedly, skin reactions were less

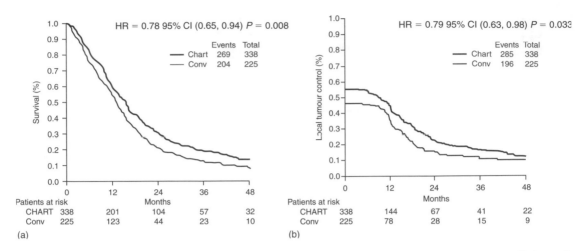

Figure 10.6 Results of a phase III randomized trial of CHART (continuous hyperfractionated accelerated radiotherapy) in non-small cell lung cancer. (a) Overall survival; (b) local tumour control of patients treated by CHART or by conventional radiotherapy (CHART results are indicated by the heavier line). HR, hazard ratio. From Saunders *et al.* (1999), with permission.

severe and settled more quickly in the CHART-treated patients. Life-table analysis showed evidence of reduced severity in a number of late morbidities in favour of CHART but the magnitude of these differences in late reactions would not allow a substantial increase in the total dose of CHART without increasing the risk of late damage over the rate observed for conventional fractionation. The overall conclusion is that CHART improved the therapeutic ratio in head and neck cancer by a small margin.

Saunders *et al.* (1997, 1999) reported the results of the CHART–Bronchus trial. A total of 563 patients with non-small cell lung cancer were randomized between CHART (as described above) and conventional fractionation to 60 Gy in 2-Gy fractions. Despite the lower total dose, survival after 2 years was significantly increased by 9 per cent, from 21 per cent in the conventional arm to 30 per cent in the CHART arm (Fig. 10.6a). Exploratory analysis revealed that this was a consequence of improved local tumour control (Fig. 10.6b) and, in squamous cell carcinoma, a reduced incidence of distant metastases. Oesophagitis occurred earlier and reached higher scores in CHART patients, but symptoms also settled earlier and were of no major concern on longer follow-up. Pneumonitis was not decreased in the CHART

arm. The overall conclusion of this study was that, compared with conventional fractionation with 60 Gy, CHART offers a significant therapeutic benefit for patients with non-small cell lung cancer.

The Danish Head and Neck Cancer Study Group (DAHANCA) trial 6 and 7 (Overgaard *et al.*, 2003) provides a typical example of weakly accelerated radiotherapy. This study was aimed at finding out whether shortening of treatment time by only 1 week by using six instead of five radiotherapy fractions per week improved the tumour response in squamous cell carcinoma of the head and neck. A total of 1476 eligible patients were randomly assigned to five ($n = 726$) or six ($n = 750$) fractions per week at the same total dose and fraction number (66–68 Gy in 33–34 fractions to all tumour sites except well-differentiated T1 glottic tumours, which were treated with 62 Gy). All patients, except those with glottic cancers, also received the hypoxic radiosensitizer nimorazole (see Chapter 17). Overall 5-year loco-regional control rates were improved by 10 per cent from 60 per cent to 70 per cent by accelerated fractionation ($p = 0.0005$). It is interesting to note that the whole benefit of shortening of treatment time was seen for primary tumour control but was non-significant for neck-node control. Disease-specific survival improved (73 vs 66 per cent for

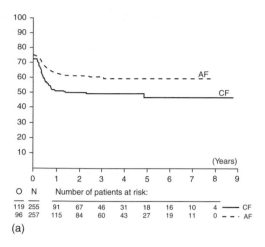
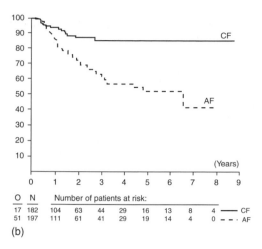

Figure 10.7 Results of the European Organisation for Cancer Research (EORTC No. 22851) trial of accelerated fractionation. (a) Loco-regional tumour control (log-rank $p = 0.02$); (b) patients free of severe radiation effects, grade 3 and 4 (log-rank $p < 0.001$). From Horiot *et al.* (1997), with permission.

six and five fractions; $p = 0.01$) but not overall survival. Acute morbidity was significantly more frequent with six than with five fractions, but was transient. The overall conclusion of this study is that shortening of overall treatment time by increasing the weekly number of fractions is beneficial in patients with head and neck cancer. Very importantly, the DAHANCA trial as well as some other clinical studies clearly shows that not only large differences in overall treatment time but also a comparably small difference of only 1 week influences substantially the probability of achieving local tumour control.

In the EORTC trial No. 22851 (Horiot *et al.*, 1997) 512 patients with head and neck cancer were randomized to receive their treatment either conventionally in a median overall time of 54 days (using 1.8–2 Gy per fraction each day, total 35–40 fractions, treatment on 5 days per week) or accelerated in a median of 33 days (using 1.6 Gy per fraction three times per day with 4 hours minimum inter-fraction interval, total 45 fractions, treatment on 5 days per week, overall time allocated to 8 days radiotherapy, 12–14 days gap and 17 days radiotherapy). The report of this EORTC trial indicates that patients who received the accelerated treatment showed a 13 per cent increase in loco-regional tumour control from 46 per cent to

59 per cent at five years (Fig. 10.7a); there was no increase in survival compared with patients receiving conventional treatment. Early radiation effects, particularly mucositis, were much more pronounced in the accelerated arm. Thirty-eight per cent of patients had to be hospitalized for acute toxicity compared with only 7 per cent of the patients in the conventional arm. Fig. 10.7b shows that grades 3 and 4 late damage (according to the EORTC/RTOG scale) also occurred significantly more frequently after the accelerated fractionation than after conventional fractionation ($p < 0.001$). The probability of being free of severe late damage at 3 years was 85 per cent in the conventional arm but only 63 per cent in the accelerated arm. With increasing follow-up this difference is even greater. Most of the difference in late effects has been attributable to late damage to connective tissues and mucosal sequelae.

In summary, accelerated fractionation has been shown in randomized clinical trials to counteract the time factor in head and neck and lung cancer. Some of the trials indicate an improved therapeutic ratio compared with conventional fractionation. However, one of the most intriguing biological observations from the clinical trials on accelerated fractionation is that sparing of late normal-tissue morbidity compared with conventional fractionation was much less than anticipated. In fact, late damage in the EORTC trial was even higher than after conventional fractionation. Possible reasons for these unexpected findings are discussed below.

10.6 COMPARISON BETWEEN HYPERFRACTIONATION AND ACCELERATED FRACTIONATION

Bourhis *et al.* (2006) have reported a meta-analysis of hyperfractionation and accelerated radiotherapy in patients with head and neck tumours. This analysis included 15 randomized trials with a total of 6515 patients. In all of these trials, patients had been randomized between conventional radiotherapy and hyperfractionated or accelerated radiotherapy. The majority of patients had stage III or IV oropharyngeal or laryngeal squamous cell carcinoma and were monitored with a median follow-up of 6 years. When all the trials were put together, a 3–4 per cent significant increase in overall survival (hazard ratio 0.92, 95 per cent CI 0.86–0.97; $p = 0.003$) was found. There was a significant benefit for loco-regional control in favour of altered fractionation (6.4 per cent at 5 years, $p < 0.0001$), which was particularly important for local control (Table 10.1). No effect was observed with altered fractionation on distant metastasis. The survival advantage was more pronounced with hyperfractionation (8 per cent at 5 years) than with accelerated fractionation (2 per cent for regimens without dose reduction and 1.7 per cent for regimens with dose reduction). Interestingly, the survival advantage observed with altered fractionation regimens is of the same order of magnitude seen with concomitant chemo-radiotherapy regimens (see Chapter 18), indicating that the debate on the relative merits of these two strategies is likely to continue.

10.7 SPLIT-COURSE RADIOTHERAPY

Intentional gaps in radiation therapy have sometimes been introduced in order to allow recovery of early-responding normal tissues. However if such gaps prolong the overall treatment time then local tumour control rates are expected to decrease. As discussed for the DAHANCA 6 and 7 trial (see Section 10.5) not only differences in the overall treatment time by several weeks but also for only 1 week may significantly change the chance for local tumour control. These data imply that even small prolongations of overall treatment times in the order of one or few days should be avoided. If this is not possible, appropriate compensation has to be applied. Studies on experimental tumours suggest that, for a given overall treatment time, the magnitude of the time factor is the same for continuous fractionation or for fractionation protocols including gaps (Baumann *et al.*, 2001). This supports the current clinical guidelines for the compensation of unscheduled treatment gaps that are discussed in Chapter 9.

Table 10.1 Hazard ratio of altered fractionated radiotherapy versus conventional radiotherapy on overall population and by type of radiotherapy for loco-regional, local, regional and metastatic control

	Hyperfractionation	Accelerated radiotherapy (no dose reduction)	Accelerated radiotherapy (dose reduction)	Overall	*p*
Loco-regional	0.76 (0.66–0.89)*	0.79 (0.72–0.87)	0.90 (0.80–1.02)	0.82 (0.77–0.88)	<0.0001
Local	0.75 (0.63–0.89)	0.74 (0.67–0.83)	0.83 (0.71–0.96)	0.77 (0.71–0.83)	<0.0001
Regional	0.83 (0.66–1.03)	0.90 (0.77–1.04)	0.87 (0.72–1.06)	0.87 (0.79–0.97)	0.01
Metastatic	1.09 (0.76–1.58)	0.93 (0.74–1.19)	0.95 (0.68–1.32)	0.97 (0.82–1.15)	0.75

Number of patients, $n = 7073$.

*The 95 per cent confidence intervals are given in parenthesis.

Reproduced from Bourhis *et al.* (2006), with permission.

10.8 REASONS FOR INCREASED LATE NORMAL-TISSUE DAMAGE AFTER MODIFIED FRACTIONATION

Hyperfractionation and accelerated radiotherapy both require multiple radiation treatments per day. In the case of hyperfractionation this is because in order to give an adequate number of small fractions, one per day, the overall treatment time would have to be very long. In the EORTC and RTOG trials mentioned above the fraction number was increased to 68–70, which would require once-daily treatment over 14 weeks; this would be unacceptable in view of the time factor for tumour-cell repopulation. In the case of accelerated radiotherapy, shortening the overall time but still giving one fraction per day would require an increase in dose per fraction; this would be expected to lead to an increase in late effects although hypofractionation is clinically acceptable in some situations (see Section 10.3).

A radiobiological constraint in giving multiple fractions per day is that these should not be given too close together because of incomplete repair (see Chapter 8). As indicated in Chapter 7, Section 7.3, the damage inflicted by radiation is very largely repaired in most cell types, both normal and malignant. The repair of normal-tissue stem cells is vital for their tolerance to radiation therapy and if fractions are given so close together that repair is incomplete, tissue tolerance will be reduced. Repair halftimes for many tumours and normal tissues are in the region of 0.5–2 hours (Table 9.2). Assuming exponential decay of radiation damage, it takes six halftimes for the damage to decay to 1/64 (i.e. 1–2 per cent of its initial value). The problem is that, as shown in Table 9.2, some late-responding normal tissues appear to have long repair halftimes. These tissues will therefore be especially disadvantaged by radiotherapy given with multiple fractions at a short inter-fraction interval: the therapeutic index will be impaired and the total radiation dose will have to be lowered in order to remain within tolerance. Most current schedules with multiple fractions per day employ inter-fraction times of at least 6 hours; in some situations even this gap may be too short.

Evidence on the clinical impact of incomplete repair comes from an analysis by Bentzen *et al.* (1999) of data from the CHART head and neck trial. As noted above, several late-damage end-points were significantly reduced after CHART, compared with conventional treatment. The reduction was much less than expected on the basis of LQ calculations and analysis of these data yielded repair halftimes in the range of 4–5 hours for the three late morbidities investigated: laryngeal oedema, skin telangiectasia and subcutaneous fibrosis. Even the lower ends of the confidence intervals were around 3 hours. This suggests that even 6 hours between dose fractions in multiple-fractions-per-day-schedules may be too short for complete repair in some situations. Long repair halftimes for late effects in human normal tissues therefore pose a significant problem for the development of novel fractionation schedules.

Consequential late effects (see Chapter 13) may also contribute to greater than expected late morbidity after modified fractionation. Compared with conventional fractionation the dose per week is increased, both in accelerated radiotherapy and in hyperfractionation. This is expected to produce an increase in early normal-tissue damage such as mucositis and more severe or more prolonged early damage may then lead to more pronounced consequential late effects.

10.9 IS THE SAME MODIFIED FRACTIONATION SCHEDULE OPTIMAL FOR ALL PATIENTS?

Figure 10.8 summarizes the results of experiments testing different modified fractionation schedules in two experimental squamous cell carcinoma xenografts (FaDu and GL) in mice. For a constant number of 30 fractions in FaDu tumours, the TCD_{50} increased by roughly 0.6 Gy for each day of prolongation for overall treatment times up to 40 days but more steeply for longer times (Fig. 10.8a); this effect was much less pronounced (0.28 Gy/day) in GL squamous cell carcinomas. In contrast, when the number of fractions was increased from 12 to 60 in a constant overall treatment time of 6 weeks (Fig. 10.8b), the TCD_{50} in FaDu tumours appeared to be constant while in GL tumours the TCD_{50} increased with increasing fraction number. Both dose-escalated hyperfractionation and accelerated

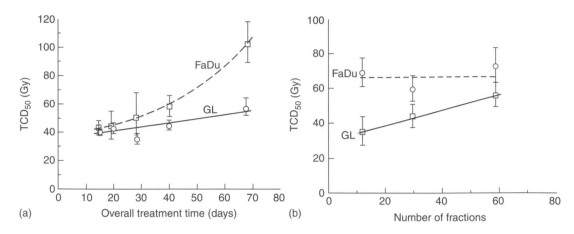

Figure 10.8 Tumour control dose (TCD) in two experimental squamous cell carcinoma xenografts (FaDu, GL) as a function of overall treatment time for irradiation with 30 fractions (a) or as a function of number of fractions in a constant overall treatment time of 6 weeks (b). There are considerable differences in the response of these tumours to modification of the fractionation schedule. See Baumann *et al.* (2001) for sources.

fractionation (using constant or reduced total doses) would be advantageous in human tumours that behave like FaDu. In contrast, for tumours like GL, dose-escalated hyperfractionation would at best yield identical control rates, while after accelerated fractionation with reduced total dose such tumours would do worse than with conventional radiotherapy. These results show that the response of experimental tumours to modified fractionation may be variable and it may well be that such heterogeneity also exists between tumours in patients. There is a clear need for research on how to best select patients for modified fractionation schedules.

Results from clinical studies always reflect the average effect of a treatment modification. For example, after the accelerated CHART treatment the local control rates of head and neck cancer were identical to those obtained after conventional fractionation with a 12-Gy higher total dose (see Section 10.5). Under the assumption of inter-tumour heterogeneity this would mean that some tumours with a small time-factor that would have been controlled after conventional treatment to 66 Gy recurred after CHART treatment because of the reduction in total dose. This negative effect may have been compensated by additional local control achieved in tumours that showed greater repopulation and a more pronounced time factor (i.e. tumours in which the dose recovered per day

was higher than the average value of 0.36 Gy). To further improve the results of modified fractionation we need to identify subgroups of patients who are likely to benefit from a particular modification, and thus to individualize treatment. Considerable efforts have been made to develop predictive tests, for example for the rate of tumour-cell repopulation; so far these investigations have not identified strong predictors that could be employed in clinical practice.

Key points

1. Hyperfractionation is the use of a reduced dose per fraction over a conventional overall treatment time, employing multiple fractions per day. A therapeutic advantage is thought to derive from the more rapid increase in tolerance with decreasing dose per fraction for late-responding normal tissues than for tumours.
2. Accelerated radiotherapy is the use of a reduced overall treatment time with a conventional dose per fraction, achieved using multiple fractions per day. The aim is to reduce the protective effect of tumour-cell repopulation during radiotherapy.

3. Hypofractionation is the use of doses per fraction higher than 2.0 Gy, which will increase late-responding normal tissue damage compared with conventional fractionation. Hypofractionation is routinely applied for palliation, but for certain curative situations hypofractionation may also be an option.

4. Multiple fractions per day should be given as far apart as possible and certainly not closer than 6 hours.

■ BIBLIOGRAPHY

Baumann M, Bentzen SM, Ang KK (1998). Hyperfractionated radiotherapy in head and neck cancer: a second look at the clinical data. *Radiother Oncol* **46**: 127–30.

Baumann M, Petersen C, Wolf J, Schreiber A, Zips D (2001). No evidence for a different magnitude of the time factor for continuously fractionated irradiation and protocols including gaps in two human squamous cell carcinoma in nude mice. *Radiother Oncol* **59**: 187–94.

Beck-Bornholdt HP, Dubben HH, Liertz-Petersen C, Willers H (1997). Hyperfractionation: where do we stand? *Radiother Oncol* **43**: 1–21.

Bentzen SM, Thames HD (1991). Clinical evidence for tumor clonogen regeneration: interpretations of the data. *Radiother Oncol* **22**: 161–6.

Bentzen SM, Saunders MI, Dische S (1999). Repair halftimes estimated from observations of treatment-related morbidity after CHART or conventional radiotherapy in head and neck cancer. *Radiother Oncol* **53**: 219–26.

Bourhis J, Overgaard J, Audry H *et al.* (2006). Hyperfractionated or accelerated radiotherapy in head and neck cancer: a meta-analysis. *Lancet* **368**: 843–54.

Dische S, Saunders M, Barrett A, Harvey A, Gibson D, Parmar M (1997). A randomised multicentre trial of CHART versus conventional radiotherapy in head and neck cancer. *Radiother Oncol* **44**: 123–36.

Dubben HH (1994). Local control, TCD$_{50}$ and dose–time prescription habits in radiotherapy of head and neck tumours. *Radiother Oncol* **32**: 197–200.

Fletcher GH (1988). Regaud Lecture: perspectives on the history of radiotherapy. *Radiother Oncol* **12**: 253–71.

Fu KK, Pajak TF, Trotti A *et al.* (2000). A Radiation Therapy Oncology Group (RTOG) phase III randomized study to compare hyperfractionation and two variants of accelerated fractionation to standard fractionation radiotherapy for head and neck squamous cell carcinomas: first report of RTOG 9003. *Int J Radiat Oncol Biol Phys* **48**: 7–16.

Holthusen H (1936). Erfahrungen über die verträglichkeitsgrenze für röntgenstrahlen und deren nutzanwendung zur verhütung von schäden. *Strahlenther Onkol* **57**: 254–69.

Horiot JC, Le Fur R, N'Guyen T *et al.* (1992). Hyperfractionation versus conventional fractionation in oropharyngeal carcinoma: final analysis of a randomized trial of the EORTC cooperative group of radiotherapy. *Radiother Oncol* **25**: 231–41.

Horiot JC, Bontemps P, van den Bogaert W *et al.* (1997). Accelerated fractionation (AF) compared to conventional fractionation (CF) improves loco-regional control in the radiotherapy of advanced head and neck cancers: results of the EORTC 22851 randomized trial. *Radiother Oncol* **44**: 111–21.

Overgaard J, Hansen HS, Specht L *et al.* (2003). Five compared with six fractions per week of conventional radiotherapy of squamous-cell carcinoma of head and neck: DAHANCA 6 and 7 randomised controlled trial. *Lancet* **362**: 933–40.

Owen JR, Ashton A, Bliss JM *et al.* (2006). Effect of radiotherapy fraction size on tumour control in patients with early-stage breast cancer after local tumour excision: long-term results of a randomised trial. *Lancet Oncol* **7**: 467–71.

Saunders M, Dische S, Barrett A, Harvey A, Gibson D, Parmar M (1997). Continuous hyperfractionated accelerated radiotherapy (CHART) versus conventional radiotherapy in non-small-cell lung cancer: a randomised multicentre trial. CHART Steering Committee. *Lancet* **350**: 161–5.

Saunders M, Dische S, Barrett A, Harvey A, Griffiths G, Palmar M (1999). Continuous, hyperfractionated, accelerated radiotherapy (CHART) versus conventional radiotherapy in non-small cell lung cancer: mature data from the randomised multicentre trial. CHART Steering committee. *Radiother Oncol* **52**: 137–48.

Withers HR, Taylor JM, Maciejewski B (1988). The hazard of accelerated tumor clonogen repopulation during radiotherapy. *Acta Oncol* **27**: 131–46.

■ FURTHER READING

Baumann M, Bentzen SM, Dörr W *et al.* (2001). The translational research chain: is it delivering the goods? *Int J Radiat Oncol Biol Phys* **49**: 345–51.

Thames HD, Withers HR, Peters LJ, Fletcher GH (1982). Changes in early and late radiation responses with altered dose fractionation: implications for dose–survival relationships. *Int J Radiat Oncol Biol Phys* **8**: 219–26.

Thames HD, Peters LJ, Withers HR, Fletcher GH (1983). Accelerated fractionation vs hyperfractionation: rationales for several treatments per day. *Int J Radiat Oncol Biol Phys* **9**: 127–38.

Withers HR, Maciejewski B, Taylor JMG (1989). Biology of options in dose fractionation. In: McNally NJ (ed.) *The scientific basis of modern radiotherapy.* London: The British Institute of Radiology, 27–36.

Time factors in normal-tissue responses to irradiation

WOLFGANG DÖRR

11.1 INTRODUCTION

The radiation exposure of normal tissues must be considered over a wide range of overall treatment durations (Fig. 11.1). First, on a short scale of minutes to hours, incomplete recovery of sublethal damage may reduce the radiation tolerance of a tissue. Second, over a range of days to weeks (i.e. during a course of fractionated radiotherapy with varying overall treatment times) radiation-induced tissue regeneration ('repopulation') may modulate radiation tolerance. This radiation-induced regeneration response is seen in early-responding tissues. Third, over a range of months to years, long-term restoration can occur in some tissues, which renders them more resistant to re-irradiation. Also, long-term progression of the damage can occur in other tissues, which causes decreased re-irradiation tolerance.

The impact of incomplete recovery within short time-intervals is covered in the chapters on fractionation and the linear-quadratic (LQ) approach (see Chapters 8 and 9). The changes in radiation tolerance that may occur in intervals that are clearly longer than the general duration of a radiotherapy course are discussed in Chapter 19 on retreatment tolerance. Therefore, this chapter describes the impact of repopulation processes on early radiation effects.

Repopulation is the term used to describe the regeneration response of early-reacting tissues to fractionated irradiation, which results in an increase in radiation tolerance with increasing overall treatment time. The biological basis of repopulation is a complex restructuring of the proliferative organization of the tissue. A number of clinical and experimental observations can assist in illuminating the biological mechanisms underlying the repopulation processes. The majority of investigations have been performed in oral mucosa as the dose-limiting early side-effect in head and neck cancer radiotherapy, and hence this tissue will be mainly used as a model for the description of radiation-induced repopulation in early-responding normal tissues.

11.2 CLINICAL OBSERVATIONS

A number of clinical studies with accelerated radiotherapy protocols (i.e. with a shortened overall treatment time) have resulted in an aggravation of early radiation side-effects. The most prominent example is the CHART (continuous

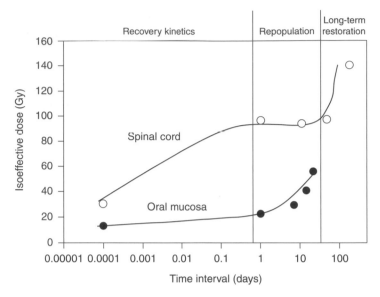

Figure 11.1 Changes in normal tissue tolerance with time. The figure compiles data for mouse oral mucosa (Dörr and Kummermehr, 1990; Dörr *et al.*, 1993) and for rat spinal cord (Ruifrok *et al.*, 1992; Landuyt *et al.*, 1997). From the original data, isoeffective doses in 3-Gy fractions have been calculated using α/β ratios of 2 Gy for spinal cord and 11 Gy for oral mucosa. Note the log scale of the abscissa. At short durations of radiation exposure (<1 day), increasing completeness of recovery from sublethal damage increases tissue tolerance. At intermediate intervals from 1 day to several weeks (i.e. the duration of radiotherapy) tolerance increases by repopulation in early-responding tissues such as oral mucosa but not in late-responding tissues such as spinal cord. For long intervals clearly beyond the overall treatment time in radiotherapy, an increase in radiation tolerance by long term restoration is seen in some (e.g. spinal cord), but not all, late-responding tissues.

hyperfractionated accelerated radiation therapy) head and neck trial, where a total dose of 54 Gy was administered in 36 fractions in only 12 days, compared with 66 Gy given in 33 fractions in 6.5 weeks in the control arm (Dische *et al.*, 1997). A significant shift of oral mucosal effects towards more severe, confluent reactions was observed, resulting in an incidence of 73 per cent with CHART versus 43 per cent with the conventional fractionation. Similarly, the EORTC 22851 trial, comparing 72 Gy in 5 weeks with 70 Gy given conventionally in 7 weeks, resulted in a clear increase in the rate of confluent mucositis during as well as 6 weeks after the end of radiotherapy in the accelerated arm (Horiot *et al.*, 1997).

Oral mucositis heals in a much higher proportion of patients during the last treatment weeks compared with earlier times, when doses below 2 Gy are administered (Fletcher *et al.*, 1962). This indicates a time delay before repopulation becomes effective. Furthermore, these data show that the

repopulation capacity is limited by the daily or weekly radiation dose. Oral mucositis has also been studied in split-course regimens (Maciejewski *et al.*, 1991). In a first radiotherapy series with 32 Gy in 12 days, 90 per cent of the patients developed confluent reactions. After a split of 9–13 days, which was introduced to allow for healing of mucositis, a second series of radiotherapy (34–38 Gy/12–14 days) was administered. None of the same patients developed confluent mucosal reactions in the second series, despite the higher dose. This again indicates that the onset of repopulation occurs within the first weeks after the start of radiotherapy.

11.3 EXPERIMENTAL OBSERVATIONS

Changes in radiation tolerance with increasing overall treatment time have been studied in a number of early-responding tissues, such as

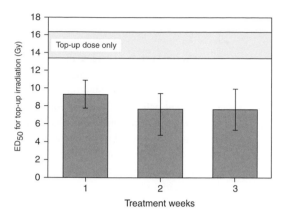

Figure 11.2 Changes in mucosal radiation tolerance with overall treatment time. Mouse tongue mucosa was irradiated with 5 × 3 Gy/week over 1, 2 or 3 weeks, followed by graded test doses (Dörr and Kummermehr, 1990). Irradiation over 1 week decreased the ED_{50} (dose at which mucosal ulceration occurs in 50 per cent of the animals) from about 15 Gy in control animals to 9.3 Gy, the difference reflecting the biological effect of 5 × 3 Gy. Despite administration of a further 15 Gy per week, the ED_{50} after 2 weeks was only slightly lower (7.7 Gy) and no further reduction was found after the third treatment week (ED_{50} = 7.6 Gy). Error bars indicate 95% confidence intervals. Reprinted with permission from Elsevier.

mouse epidermis, rat epidermis, pig epidermis, mouse lip mucosa and mouse tongue mucosa (Dörr, 2003a; Hopewell *et al.*, 2003). One example is illustrated in Fig. 11.2 in which oral mucosa was irradiated with 5 × 3 Gy/week over 1, 2 or 3 weeks (Dörr and Kummermehr, 1990). Irradiation over 1 week clearly decreased the ED_{50} (dose, at which a response, i.e. ulceration, is expected in 50% of the animals) for the terminating test irradiation, which reflects residual tissue tolerance. However, despite ongoing irradiation in weeks 2 and 3, no further reduction in the test ED_{50} was found.

A similar pattern of the time-course of the changes in radiation tolerance during radiotherapy was found in most other tissues studied (Fig. 11.3). Tolerance remained constant within the initial treatment period, and subsequently increased almost linearly. The time of onset of this increase was tissue dependent at 5–7 days in mouse oral mucosa and skin, and 20–30 days in rat and pig skin (Hopewell *et al.*, 2003). The initial drop at short treatment intervals can be related to changes in

the capacity for recovery of sublethal damage, which have been reported for these early-responding tissues (Dörr *et al.*, 2000).

The capacity for repopulation, once these compensatory processes have started, was estimated by (Dörr, 2003a) in terms of the dose (number of 2-Gy fractions) compensated per day. In human oral mucosa, 0.5–1.0 fractions are counteracted per day, thus confirming the clinical results on mucositis healing despite ongoing radiotherapy (see above). These experimental data indicate similar numbers – close to one fraction of 2 Gy/day – for most tissues, with a few possible exceptions (e.g. mouse epidermis; Denekamp, 1973), which could be related to experimental design. In some experiments, where various weekly doses were applied, a dependence of the repopulation rate on the dose intensity (Gy/week) was observed.

In oral mucosa, the functional measurements of radiation tolerance have been supplemented by detailed histological assessments of changes in mucosal cell density and proliferation (Dörr and Kummermehr, 1990; Dörr, 1997). A reduction in cell number to approximately 70 per cent occurred during the first week of daily fractionated treatment. Subsequently, constant to increasing cell numbers were found, despite continuing irradiation at the same dose intensity. In good agreement with this, mucosal proliferation was significantly suppressed during the first week, but subsequently returned to subnormal to near-normal values (Dörr, 1997). Similar observations have been made in other tissues (Shirazi *et al.*, 1995). In human oral mucosa, a reduction of cell production and consequently a steep decline in cell numbers were observed over the initial week of radiotherapy (Dörr *et al.*, 2002). Subsequently, proliferation rates were partly restored and cell depletion was significantly slower.

11.4 MECHANISMS OF REPOPULATION

Three important observations have been made in both clinical and experimental studies:

1. dose is compensated with increasing overall treatment time once repopulation has become effective;

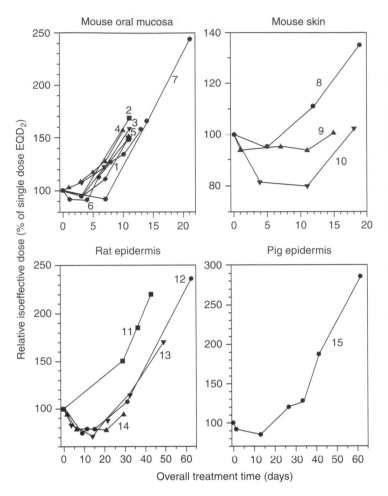

Figure 11.3 Time-course of repopulation: experimental results. From reports in the literature of studies with variations in overall treatment time, the isoeffective EQD$_2$ (equivalent dose in 2 Gy fractions) has been calculated for the individual overall treatment times using an α/β ratio of 10 Gy. Note the different time scales of the abscissae. Treatment protocols and references are: 1, 2F (Ang et al., 1985); 2, 2 × 5F (Ang et al., 1985); 3, 10F (Ang et al., 1985); 4, 13 Gy + 1F (Dörr and Kummermehr, 1990); 5, 10 Gy + 1F (Dörr and Kummermehr, 1990); 6, 8 Gy + 1F (Dörr and Spekl, unpublished); 7, 5 × 3 Gy/week (Dörr and Kummermehr, 1990); 8, 5 × 3 Gy/wk (Shirazi et al., 1995); 9, 5 × 3 Gy/week (Denekamp, 1973); 10, 2F (Ang et al., 1984); 11, 5 × 3 Gy/week (van Rongen and Kal, 1984); 12, 10F (Moulder and Fischer, 1976); 13, 3F/week (Moulder and Fischer, 1976); 14, 5F/week (Moulder and Fischer, 1976); 15, 2F (van den Aardweg et al., 1988).

2. the rate at which this compensation occurs is in the range of 5 × 2 Gy/week;
3. the loss of cells is counteracted after the lag phase before repopulation starts, resulting in more or less constant cell numbers.

In general, the mechanisms of repopulation that can explain these observations can be described by the following three As: *asymmetry loss, acceleration*, and *abortive divisions* (Dörr, 1997).

Asymmetry loss

According to the stem cell concept (see Chapter 13), the radiation tolerance of a tissue is defined by the number of tissue stem cells and their intrinsic radiosensitivity. Hence, radiation tolerance must decrease during fractionated irradiation according to the daily stem cell kill. This is clearly seen during the time lag before the onset of repopulation. However, after repopulation has started, the effect of at least part of the radiation dose is counteracted. This indicates that new stem cells must be produced to replace those sterilized by the irradiation.

In unperturbed tissues, stem cells divide on average into one new stem cell and one differentiating cell (see Chapter 13). These divisions are called asymmetrical because two different cells are generated. In this setting, the number of stem cells in each cell generation remains constant, independent of the proliferation rate. For additional production of new stem cells, as postulated on the basis of dose compensation during repopulation, stem cell divisions must result in two stem cell daughters, a pattern that is depicted as symmetrical division.

Therefore, an asymmetry loss of stem cell divisions is one essential mechanism underlying repopulation in normal tissues. This loss can be complete, with two stem cell daughters from each division, or incomplete, with, on average, less than two, but more than one, stem cell generated per stem cell division. A fraction of these divisions, presumably of cells with gross radiation-induced chromosomal damage, are abortive and can be observed histologically as abnormal mitotic figures (Dörr, 1997). These result in binucleate or multinucleate cells.

Acceleration of stem cell proliferation

As illustrated earlier, human oral mucosa and other tissues are able to compensate weekly doses of about five times 0.5–1.0 fractions of 2 Gy. For this to occur, assuming the surviving fraction of the stem cells after each radiation fraction to be about 0.5, five symmetrical divisions are needed within 7 days. This requires an average cell-cycle time of 1.4 days. Compared with cell-cycle times of at least 3.5 days in unperturbed tissue (Dörr, 1997), this indicates clear acceleration of stem cell proliferation as the second mechanism of repopulation. Cell-cycle times must be even shorter if the asymmetry loss is incomplete, or if higher doses (more stem cell kill) are compensated. The detailed interrelation between surviving fraction, number of symmetrical divisions between fractions and the proportion of symmetrical divisions is discussed in Dörr (1997).

The degree to which the stem cell proliferation is accelerated is highly dependent on the radiation dose administered (i.e. on the daily or weekly stem cell kill; Dörr, 2003a). For example, in oral mucosa irradiated with 5 × 3.5 Gy/week, this dose was completely counteracted by repopulation in weeks 2 and 3 (Dörr and Kummermehr, 1990). However, during treatment with 5 × 2.5 Gy/week, repopulation was exactly adjusted to compensate this lower dose, despite the clearly higher regenerative capacity.

In the vast majority of tissues, no specific marker yet exists that would allow for the specific identification of stem cells. Therefore, cell kinetic studies can only assess proliferation of the entire cell population. After the lag phase of repopulation, stem cells constitute only a minor fraction of the general population, and hence such studies are not suitable to identify the acceleration at the stem cell level. However, in the intestinal crypts, which have well-defined localization of the stem cell population, a significant shortening of the stem cell-cycle time after irradiation has indeed been described (Withers, 1970), which reflects accelerated repopulation, albeit after single doses.

Abortive divisions

After the onset of repopulation, the overall cell number in the tissue remains at a near-constant, although reduced level. In contrast, it has been shown that differentiation and cell loss (e.g. at the surface of mucosal tissues) continue at a normal, physiological rate (Dörr et al., 1996). Also, cell production, which can be directly measured, continues, which is indirectly reflected by the lack of change in cell numbers (Dörr et al., 1994). Hence the question arises of whether this cell production can be based only on the surviving stem cells.

In unperturbed mucosa, with a relative stem cell number of 100 per cent, the cells proliferate with a cell cycle time of at least 3.5 days (Dörr et al., 1994). A dose of 5 × 2 Gy during the first treatment week, before repopulation sets in, reduces the stem cell number to clearly below 10 per cent. Hence, to result in the same number of cells as in controls, the remaining stem cells would have to proliferate with a cycle time of only a few hours (Dörr et al., 1994; Dörr, 1997). This is extremely unlikely on the basis of epithelial biology, which indicates a minimum cell-cycle time of 10–12 hours. Therefore, cells must be produced from other sources.

It has been shown in vitro (see Chapter 3) that 'sterilized' cells can undergo a limited number of divisions even after high doses of radiation. It can therefore be assumed, and indirectly concluded from experimental studies (Dörr et al., 1996), that similar, so-called abortive, divisions of sterilized or doomed cells can also occur in vivo. This limited proliferative activity results in cells that undergo near-normal differentiation, and hence counteract the ongoing cell loss. Quantitatively, in oral mucosa, the radiation-sterilized cells on average have to undergo two or three abortive divisions each to account for the cell production measured.

11.5 REGULATION OF REPOPULATION

The time at which repopulation processes become effective, is tissue-specific (Fig. 11.3) and we may assume that it correlates with the turnover time of the tissue, and therefore the rate at which cells are lost. Reduced cell numbers may result in changes in intercellular communication or altered cell–matrix interactions (see Chapter 13). This correlation between tissue turnover and lag time of repopulation, however, is only weak (Dörr, 2003a), so other factors must also be important.

It has been demonstrated that the lag time before repopulation begins is shorter, if the radiation dose is higher (Dörr and Kummermehr, 1990; Dörr, 2003a). This suggests that the rate at which stem cells are depleted may regulate the onset of repopulation. Autoregulatory processes within the stem cell compartment have also been suggested for intestinal crypts (Paulus et al., 1992). The reduction in stem cell numbers can result in (still unidentified) intercellular signalling, which eventually prevents the daughter cells of the stem cell divisions from undergoing differentiation.

The regulation of the asymmetry loss is a very precise and rapidly responding mechanism. During short treatment breaks, even during weekends, the overall cell production clearly increases (Dörr et al., 1994). However, the radiation tolerance of the tissue during these breaks remains almost constant, indicating that the cells that are produced are not stem cells (Dörr, 2003a). Hence, despite stimulated symmetrical stem cell divisions during the daily fractionated treatment, the stem cells quickly return to asymmetrical divisions if one radiation fraction is missing.

Acceleration of stem cell divisions may be caused by overall cell depletion and by impairment of the epithelial barrier function (Dörr et al., 1994; Shirazi et al., 1995), which may increase the normal signals that physiologically regulate proliferation. This hypothesis is supported by increased proliferation rates after chemical ablation of superficial mucosal material, which has been observed in mice and humans, or after mechanical ablation ('tape stripping') in rodents. However, this increased proliferation rate is not associated with increased tolerance to single-dose irradiation (i.e. increased stem cell numbers). This indicates that acceleration has occurred independently of the asymmetry loss. It must be assumed that sterilized cells initially continue to proliferate at

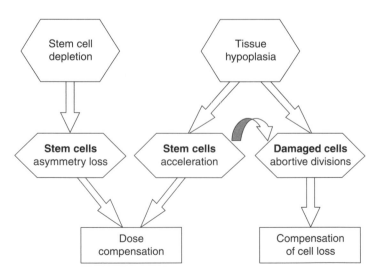

Figure 11.4 Regulation of repopulation. Stem cell depletion, via autoregulatory processes, results in the loss of the division asymmetry of the stem cells. Tissue hypoplasia controls the acceleration of stem cell division and presumably also the rate of abortive division, which is indirectly also defined by the proliferation rate of the stem cells. Asymmetry loss and acceleration of stem cell division account for compensation of dose, while abortive divisions of sterilized cells counteract the overall cell loss to maintain tissue function.

nearly the rate of the stem cell divisions before chromosomal damage accumulates and decreases the proliferation rate.

In combination with the asymmetry loss (e.g. by fractionated irradiation) artificially increased stem cell proliferation rates may shorten the lag time before repopulation becomes effective. This has been demonstrated for chemical ablation in oral mucosa (Maciejewski *et al.*, 1991). A similar mechanism has been suggested for the increase in mucosal radiation tolerance after administration of keratinocyte growth factor (KGF, palifermin) in preclinical and clinical studies as reviewed in Dörr (2003b), and summarized in Chapter 22.

In conclusion (Fig. 11.4), the asymmetry loss in the stem cell compartment is regulated independently of the acceleration of proliferation, presumably by autoregulatory processes on the basis of stem cell depletion. Acceleration of the stem cell divisions is controlled by tissue hypoplasia. The stem cell proliferation rate then translates into the initial rate of abortive divisions of sterilized cells. However, the doomed cells may also directly respond to paracrine signals released owing to tissue hypoplasia.

11.6 CONSEQUENTIAL LATE EFFECTS

Consequential late effects are chronic normal-tissue complications, which are influenced by the extent (i.e. severity and/or duration, of the early response in the same tissue or organ; Dörr and Hendry, 2001), as explained in Chapter 13. As the early response depends on the overall treatment time on the basis of repopulation processes, the same is therefore true for the corresponding consequential late effects. This has been demonstrated in experimental studies for intestinal fibrosis, and in clinical studies for skin telangiectasia, and for late (mucosa related) side-effects after head and neck irradiation, as reviewed in Dörr and Hendry (2001).

11.7 CONCLUSIONS

Repopulation processes that occur in early-responding normal tissues follow a very complex biology. The major mechanisms are asymmetry loss and acceleration of stem cell division, as well as abortive divisions of sterilized cells. A number of parameters that modulate the repopulation response, such as dose intensity (weekly dose), have been identified. However, the precise regulatory mechanisms of tissue repopulation during fractionated radiotherapy still remain largely unclear. These regulatory signals would be attractive targets for biologically based modulation of radiation effects in early-responding normal tissues.

Taking into consideration all the underlying biology of repopulation indicates that a time factor, in the sense of compensated dose, should be included in mathematical models of normal-tissue complications only with great care and caution, as these models currently do not include the dominating repopulation-modifying factors.

Key points

1. The radiation tolerance of early-responding normal tissues increases with increasing overall treatment time.
2. This phenomenon is depicted as repopulation.
3. Repopulation starts after a tissue-specific lag time.
4. The biological basis is a complex restructuring of the proliferative tissue organization.
5. This includes asymmetry loss and acceleration of stem cell proliferation.
6. Abortive divisions of doomed cells significantly contribute to cell production.
7. Tissue hypoplasia controls stem cell acceleration and abortive divisions, while the asymmetry loss is regulated by stem cell depletion.

■ BIBLIOGRAPHY

Ang KK, Landuyt W, Rijnders A, van der Schueren E (1984). Differences in repopulation kinetics in mouse skin during split course multiple fractions per day (MFD) or daily fractionated irradiations. *Int J Radiat Oncol Biol Phys* **10**: 95–9.

Ang KK, Xu FX, Vanuytsel L, van der Schueren E (1985). Repopulation kinetics in irradiated mouse lip mucosa: the relative importance of treatment protraction and time distribution of irradiations. *Radiat Res* **101**: 162–9.

Denekamp J (1973). Changes in the rate of repopulation during multifraction irradiation of mouse skin. *Br J Radiol* **46**: 381–7.

Dische S, Saunders M, Barrett A, Harvey A, Gibson D, Parmar M (1997). A randomised multicentre trial of CHART versus conventional radiotherapy in head and neck cancer. *Radiother Oncol* **44**: 123–36.

Dörr W (1997). Three As of repopulation during fractionated irradiation of squamous epithelia: asymmetry loss, acceleration of stem-cell divisions and abortive divisions. *Int J Radiat Biol* **72**: 635–43.

Dörr W (2003a). Modulation of repopulation processes in oral mucosa: experimental results. *Int J Radiat Biol* **79**: 531–7.

Dörr W (2003b). Oral mucosa: response modification by keratinocyte growth factor. In: Nieder C, Milas L, Ang KK (eds) *Modification of radiation response: cytokines, growth factors and other biological targets.* Berlin: Springer-Verlag, 113–22.

Dörr W, Hendry JH (2001). Consequential late effects in normal tissues. *Radiother Oncol* **61**: 223–31.

Dörr W, Kummermehr J (1990). Accelerated repopulation of mouse tongue epithelium during fractionated irradiations or following single doses. *Radiother Oncol* **17**: 249–59.

Dörr W, Breitner A, Kummermehr J (1993). Capacity and kinetics of SLD repair in mouse tongue epithelium. *Radiother Oncol* **27**: 36–45.

Dörr W, Emmendorfer H, Haide E, Kummermehr J (1994). Proliferation equivalent of 'accelerated repopulation' in mouse oral mucosa. *Int J Radiat Biol* **66**: 157–67.

Dörr W, Emmendorfer H, Weber-Frisch M (1996). Tissue kinetics in mouse tongue mucosa during daily fractionated radiotherapy. *Cell Prolif* **29**: 495–504.

Dörr W, Brankovic K, Hartmann B (2000). Repopulation in mouse oral mucosa: changes in the effect of dose fractionation. *Int J Radiat Biol* **76**: 383–90.

Dörr W, Hamilton CS, Boyd T, Reed B, Denham JW (2002). Radiation-induced changes in cellularity and proliferation in human oral mucosa. *Int J Radiat Oncol Biol Phys* **52**: 911–7.

Fletcher GH, MacComb WS, Shalek RJ (1962). *Radiation therapy in the management of cancer of the oral cavity and oropharynx.* Springfield: Charles Thomas.

Hopewell JW, Nyman J, Turesson I (2003). Time factor for acute tissue reactions following fractionated irradiation: a balance between repopulation and enhanced radiosensitivity. *Int J Radiat Biol* **79**: 513–24.

Horiot JC, Bontemps P, van den Bogaert W *et al.* (1997). Accelerated fractionation (AF) compared to conventional fractionation (CF) improves loco-regional control in the radiotherapy of advanced head and neck cancers: results of the EORTC 22851 randomized trial. *Radiother Oncol* **44**: 111–21.

Landuyt W, Fowler J, Ruifrok A, Stuben G, van der Kogel A, van der Schueren E (1997). Kinetics of repair in the spinal cord of the rat. *Radiother Oncol* **45**: 55–62.

Maciejewski B, Zajusz A, Pilecki B *et al.* (1991). Acute mucositis in the stimulated oral mucosa of patients during radiotherapy for head and neck cancer. *Radiother Oncol* **22**: 7–11.

Moulder JE, Fischer JJ (1976). Radiation reaction of rat skin. The role of the number of fractions and the overall treatment time. *Cancer* **37**: 2762–7.

Paulus U, Potten CS, Loeffler M (1992). A model of the control of cellular regeneration in the intestinal crypt after perturbation based solely on local stem cell regulation. *Cell Prolif* **25**: 559–78.

Ruifrok AC, Kleiboer BJ, van der Kogel AJ (1992). Reirradiation tolerance of the immature rat spinal cord. *Radiother Oncol* **23**: 249–56.

Shirazi A, Liu K, Trott KR (1995). Epidermal morphology, cell proliferation and repopulation in mouse skin during daily fractionated irradiation. *Int J Radiat Biol* **68**: 215–21.

van den Aardweg GJ, Hopewell JW, Simmonds RH (1988). Repair and recovery in the epithelial and vascular connective tissues of pig skin after irradiation. *Radiother Oncol* **11**: 73–82.

van Rongen E, Kal HB (1984). Acute reactions in rat feet exposed to multiple fractions of X-rays per day. *Radiother Oncol* **2**: 141–50.

Withers HR (1970). Cellular kinetics of intestinal mucosa after irradiation. In: Burdette WJ (ed.) *Carcinoma of the colon and antecedent epithelium.* Springfield: Charles Thomas, 243–57.

■ FURTHER READING

Bentzen SM (1994). Radiobiological considerations in the design of clinical trials. *Radiother Oncol* **32**: 1–11.

Denekamp J (1975). Changes in the rate of proliferation in normal tissues after irradiation. In: Nygaard OF, Adler HI, Sinclair WK (eds) *Radiation research. Biomedical, chemical and physical perspectives.* New York: Academic Press, 810–25.

Denham JW, Walker QJ, Lamb DS *et al.* (1996). Mucosal regeneration during radiotherapy. Trans Tasman Radiation Oncology Group (TROG). *Radiother Oncol* **41**: 109–18.

Trott KR, Kummermehr J (1993). The time factor and repopulation in tumors and normal tissues. *Semin Radiat Oncol* **3**: 115–25.

The dose-rate effect

ALBERT J. VAN DER KOGEL

12.1 INTRODUCTION

Low dose-rate irradiation is the ultimate form of fractionation, equivalent to multiple infinitely small fractions being given without radiation-free intervals, and thereby damage induction and repair take place at the same time. In clinical radiotherapy, continuous low dose-rate (CLDR) is widely used in brachytherapy either by permanent or temporary implantation of radioactive sources (e.g. ^{125}I, ^{103}Pd) into tumours. By utilizing remote afterloading of medium or high dose-rate sources, notably ^{192}Ir, various combinations of dose-rate and fractionation can also be chosen, such as pulsed dose-rate (PDR) and high dose-rate (HDR) brachytherapy. With external-beam treatments using intensity-modulated radiotherapy (IMRT), the dose-rate effect may also have some impact as the longer treatment times per session, which can be needed in more complex plans, may lead to a reduction in effectiveness.

12.2 MECHANISMS UNDERLYING THE DOSE-RATE EFFECT

The dose rates used for most radiobiological studies on cells and tissues tend to be in the range

1–5 Gy/min, as are dose rates used clinically for external-beam radiotherapy. Exposure times for a dose of, for example, 2 Gy are therefore no more than a couple of minutes. Within this time, the initial chemical (i.e. free radical) processes that are generated by radiation can take place but such exposure times are not long enough for the repair of DNA damage or for any other biological processes to occur significantly. As the dose rate is lowered, the time taken to deliver a particular radiation dose increases; it then becomes possible for a number of biological processes to take place during irradiation and to modify the observed radiation response. These processes have classically been described by the four Rs of radiobiology: recovery (or repair), redistribution in the cell cycle, repopulation (proliferation), and reoxygenation (see Chapter 7, Section 7.3).

Figure 12.1 illustrates the operation of these processes in producing the dose-rate effect. The range of dose rates over which each process has an effect depends upon its speed. Intracellular repair is the fastest of these processes (half-time <1 hour) and when the exposure duration is of the order of 1 hour considerable repair will take place. Calculations show that repair at this speed will modify radiation effects over the dose-rate range from around 1 Gy/min down to about 0.1 cGy/min

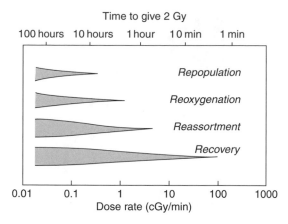

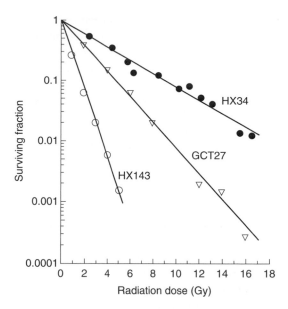

Figure 12.1 The range of dose rates over which repair, reassortment and repopulation modify radiosensitivity depends upon the speed of these processes. From Steel *et al.* (1986), with permission.

Figure 12.3 Cell-survival curves for three human tumour cell lines irradiated at the low dose-rate of 1.6 cGy/min. HX143, neuroblastoma; GCT27, germ-cell tumour of the testis; HX34, melanoma. From Steel (1991), with permission.

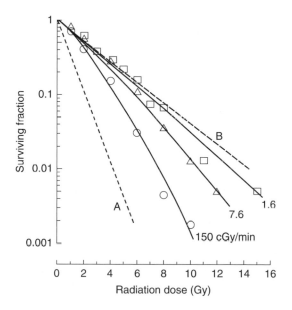

Figure 12.2 Cell-survival curves for a human melanoma cell line irradiated at dose rates of 150, 7.6 or 1.6 cGy/min. The data are fitted by the 'lethal–potentially lethal' (LPL) model, from which the lines A and B are derived (see text). From Steel *et al.* (1987), with permission.

tumours or normal tissues cannot be less than 1 day; the range is probably very wide – from a few days to weeks (Table 7.1). Only when the exposure duration exceeds about a day will significant repopulation occur during a single radiation exposure. Repopulation, in either tumours or normal tissues, will therefore influence cellular response over a much lower range of dose rates, below say 2 cGy/min, depending upon the cell proliferation rate. Redistribution (i.e. cell-cycle progression) will modify response over an intermediate range of dose rates, as will reoxygenation in tumours. The kinetics of reoxygenation are variable among tumour types and may involve various mechanisms (see Chapter 15, Section 15.5, and Table 15.3); this could, nevertheless, be a significant factor reducing the effectiveness of brachytherapy given over a short overall time.

12.3 EFFECT OF DOSE RATE ON CELL SURVIVAL

As the radiation dose rate is lowered in the range 1 Gy/min down to 1 cGy/min, the radiosensitivity

(Figs 12.2 and 12.3). Even in the range of clinical external-beam dose rates, small effects on tolerance may arise from changes in dose rate. In contrast, repopulation is a much slower process. Doubling times for repopulation in human

of cells decreases and the shouldered cell-survival curves which are observed at high dose-rates gradually become straighter. This is illustrated in Fig. 12.2. At 150 cGy/min, the survival curve has a marked curvature; at 1.6 cGy/min it is almost straight (on the semi-log plot) and seems to extrapolate the initial slope of the high dose-rate curve. The amount of sparing associated with the dose-rate reduction can be expressed by reading off the radiation doses that give a fixed surviving fraction, for example 0.01: these values are 7.7 Gy at 150 cGy/min and 12.8 Gy at 1.6 cGy/min. The ratio of these doses ($12.8/7.7 = 1.6$) is called the dose-recovery factor (DRF). The data at all three dose rates in Fig. 12.2 have been simultaneously fitted by Curtis' 'lethal–potentially lethal' (LPL) model (see Chapter 4, Section 4.11), a model that is particularly useful for describing the dose-rate effect. This allows an estimate to be made of the halftime for cellular recovery (0.16 hours) and it also predicts cell survival under conditions of no repair (line A) or full repair (line B). Three further examples of low dose-rate survival curves in human tumour cell lines are shown in Fig. 12.3: they well illustrate the linearity of low dose-rate survival curves.

For four selected human tumour cell lines (Fig. 12.4), cell-survival curves are shown at two dose rates (150 cGy/min and 1.6 cGy/min). These four sets of data have been chosen to illustrate the dose-rate effect and the range of radiosensitivities seen among human tumour cells (Steel *et al.*, 1987). At high dose-rate there is a range of approximately 3 in the radiation dose that gives a survival of 0.01, the $D_{0.01}$. At low dose-rate the curves fan out and become straight or nearly so: the range of $D_{0.01}$ values is now roughly 7. This illustrates an important characteristic of low dose-rate irradiation: it discriminates better than high dose-rate irradiation between cell lines of differing radiosensitivity.

12.4 DOSE-RATE EFFECT IN NORMAL TISSUES

Most normal tissues show considerable sparing as the dose rate is reduced. An example is shown in Fig. 12.5. The thorax of conscious mice was irradiated with ^{60}Co γ-rays and damage to the lung was measured using a breathing-rate assay (Down

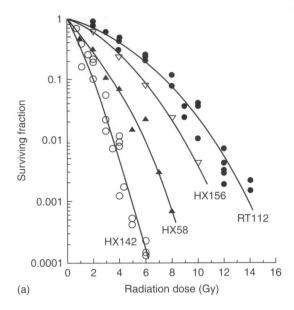

(a)

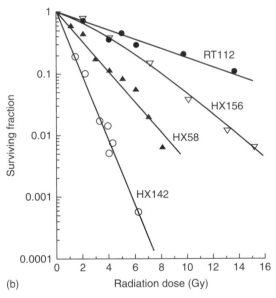

(b)

Figure 12.4 Cell-survival curve for four representative human tumour cell lines irradiated (a) at high dose-rate (150 cGy/min) or (b) at low dose-rate (1.6 cGy/min). HX142, neuroblastoma; HX58, pancreas; HX156, cervix; RT112, bladder carcinoma. From Steel (1991), with permission.

et al., 1986). The radiation dose that produced early pneumonitis in 50 per cent of the mice (i.e. the ED_{50}) was 13.3 Gy at 100 cGy/min but it increased to 34.2 Gy at the lowest dose-rate of

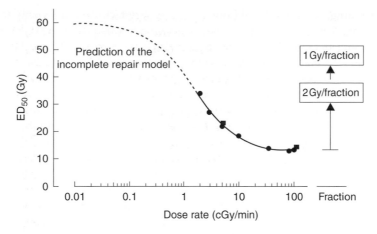

Figure 12.5 The dose-rate effect for pneumonitis in mice. The full line fitted to the data was calculated on the basis of the incomplete repair model; the broken line shows its extrapolation to very low dose-rates. The boxes on the right show the ED_{50} (effect dose–50 per cent) values for fractionated irradiation. From Down *et al.* (1986), with permission.

2 cGy/min (DRF = 2.6). Note that a similar degree of sparing could be achieved (in studies of other investigators) by fractionated high dose-rate irradiation using 2 Gy per fraction, and even more sparing at 1 Gy per fraction. Note also that at 2 cGy/min the curve is still rising rapidly. It was not possible in these experiments to go down to dose rates below 2 cGy/min because of the difficulty of immobilizing the mice for long periods of time.

The data in Fig. 12.5 have been fitted by the incomplete repair model (Thames, 1985) as explained in Chapter 8.8. This model simulates the effect of recovery (repair) on tissue sensitivity; it does not take account of cell proliferation during irradiation. The model fits the data well and it also allows extrapolation down to low dose-rates. It predicts, in this example, that dose-sparing due to recovery will continue to increase down to about 0.01 cGy/min at which the ED_{50} is 59 Gy and the recovery factor (i.e. DRF value) is 4.4. Proliferation of putative stem cells in the lung may lead to even greater sparing at very low dose-rates.

The comparison between a single low dose-rate exposure (2 cGy/min) and fractionated high dose-rate irradiation (2 Gy per fraction) allows an important conclusion to be drawn. If the fractions are delivered once per day then the overall time to deliver an ED_{50} dose of 34 Gy is 17 days. The same effect is produced by a single low dose-rate treatment in 28 hours. Continuous low dose-rate

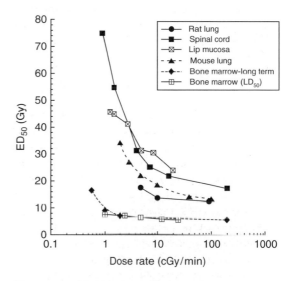

Figure 12.6 The dose-rate effect in various rodent normal tissues: lung, spinal cord, lip mucosa and bone marrow.

exposure is thus the most efficient way of allowing maximum tissue recovery in the shortest overall time. It minimizes the effects of cell proliferation, which is an advantage in terms of damage to tumour cells but a disadvantage for the tolerance of those early-responding normal tissues that rely more on proliferation than (intra)cellular recovery.

Figure 12.6 shows some examples of other studies of the dose-rate effect on normal tissues in rodents: lip mucosa, lung, spinal cord and bone-marrow. When comparing two typical late-responding tissues (lung and spinal cord) with an early-responding tissue (lip mucosa in the mouse) the patterns of recovery are very similar, with the largest sparing in the spinal cord. This is to be expected for the central nervous system as this tissue shows the largest increase in tolerance when decreasing the fraction size (low α/β ratio). For early-responding epithelial tissues such as the lip mucosa the dose-rate effect is less pronounced, but for overall times longer than 1–2 days proliferation adds to a rapid increase in tolerance, in contrast to late-responding tissues.

The two bone marrow endpoints, lethality owing to bone marrow syndrome and long-term repopulation of haemopoietic stem cells, show only a minimal recovery for dose rates as low as 1 cGy/min. This is predominantly due to the high sensitivity of the bone marrow, as a LD_{50} (radiation producing lethality in 50 per cent of a population) dose in the range of 6–9 Gy is even at 1 cGy/min delivered in a total time of only 10–15 hours. It is of interest to note that a slow proliferating haemopoietic stem cell population showed a significant recovery when lowering the dose rate to approximately 0.5 cGy/min, in agreement with a low α/β ratio (van Os *et al.*, 1993).

12.5 ISOEFFECT RELATIONSHIPS BETWEEN FRACTIONATED AND CONTINUOUS LOW DOSE-RATE IRRADIATION

A variety of theoretical descriptions of the dose-rate effect have been made but for clinical application the most widely used is the incomplete repair model of Thames (1985). The calculations of Dale and Deehan (2007) make the same basic assumptions, although the formulation is slightly different. The basic equation of the incomplete repair model for continuous irradiation is:

$$E = \alpha D + \beta D^2 g \qquad (12.1)$$

where E is the level of effect, α and β are parameters of the linear-quadratic equation, D is the total dose and g is a function of the duration of continuous exposure. Note that the time-dependent

recovery factor modifies only the quadratic term in the linear-quadratic (LQ) equation, a feature that is supported by experimental data (Steel *et al*, 1987; Fig. 12.2). Note also that repopulation is ignored in these calculations.

The value of g depends upon the halftime for recovery ($T_{1/2}$) and the duration of continuous exposure (t) according to the relation:

$$g = 2[\mu t - 1 + \exp(-\mu t)]/(\mu t)^2 \qquad (12.2)$$

where $\mu = 0.693/T_{1/2}$. Values of g for a wide range of $T_{1/2}$ and t are given in Table 8.3.

This model allows isoeffect relationships to be calculated and, as shown in Fig. 12.5, it is successful in describing experimental data over a range of dose rates. Further examples of calculated curves are shown in Fig. 12.7. The purely fractionated case is shown in Fig. 12.7a, with high dose-rate irradiation, described by the LQ model. The line in this chart corresponds to equation 8.5 (Chapter 8) with $D_1 = 60$ Gy, $d_1 = 2$ Gy and $\alpha/\beta = 10$ Gy. The inter-fraction intervals have here been assumed to be long enough to allow complete recovery between fractions. Figure 12.7b shows isoeffect curves for a single continuous exposure at any dose rate, calculated using equation 12.1 and with values of the halftime for recovery of 1.0, 1.5 or 2.0 hours. The three curves are slightly different and this illustrates the dependence of the isoeffect curve for continuous exposure on the speed of recovery: the curve shifts laterally to lower dose rates as the halftime is prolonged. Unfortunately, recovery halftime is not well known in clinical situations, which limits the value of calculations of this sort.

The curves in Fig. 12.7a–c are mutually isoeffective. They are calculated for the same effect level and for the same values of α and β (the α/β ratio is 10 Gy), chosen to give an extrapolated dose of 72 Gy at infinitely small doses per fraction or infinitely low dose-rate, which corresponds to an equivalent dose in 2-Gy fractions (EQD_2) of 60 Gy. This example illustrates the equivalence that is predicted by the mathematical models between a particular continuous dose rate and a corresponding dose per fraction. For the parameters assumed here (as shown by the vertical arrows), a dose rate of around 1–2 cGy/min (roughly 1 Gy/hour) is equivalent to fractionated

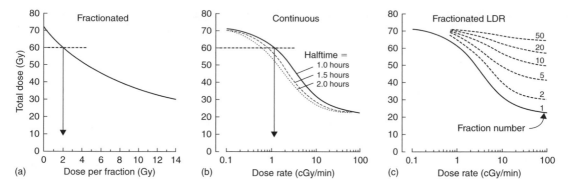

Figure 12.7 Isoeffect curves calculated with the incomplete repair model (Thames, 1985) for fractionated, continuous, or fractionated low dose-rate radiation exposure (a–c are mutually isoeffective). Repopulation is ignored. The α/β ratio is 10 Gy and the EQD$_2$ (equivalent dose in 2-Gy fractions) is 60 Gy. Adapted from Steel (1991) and Steel *et al.* (1989), with permission.

treatment with approximately 2 Gy per fraction, for both of which the isoeffective dose is 60 Gy.

A further important conclusion can be drawn from calculations of the type shown in Fig. 12.7. In Chapter 8, Section 8.6 (see Fig. 8.7), we have seen how the use of large fraction sizes leads to a therapeutic disadvantage in tumours with a high α/β ratio, relative to late normal-tissue injury. The same is true for high continuous dose rate treatments. By drawing further horizontal lines between Fig. 12.7a and Fig. 12.7b it can be seen that a dose rate of 5 cGy/min is equivalent to around 6–8 Gy per fraction and 10 cGy/min to over 10 Gy per fraction.

Figure 12.7c shows the results of model calculations for fractionated low dose-rate irradiation. Once again using the incomplete repair model isoeffect curves were calculated for treatment with 2–50 fractions, each given at the dose rate shown on the abscissa and with full recovery between fractions. Again, repopulation is ignored. This diagram indicates the basic feature of fractionated low dose-rate exposure: as we increase the number of fractions the dose-rate effect is reduced (i.e. the curves become flatter), and as we lower the dose rate the effect of fractionation is reduced (as seen by the vertical spread between the curves). This results from a simple principle. As we protract irradiation it is cellular recovery that produces all these effects and there is a limit to how much recovery the cells can accomplish. If we

allow recovery between fractions then there is less to be recovered during each fraction, and vice versa.

An alternative approach to the description of the dose-rate effect is the LPL model of Curtis (1986). This is a mechanistic model that is described in Chapter 4, Section 4.11. It has theoretical advantages for studies that seek to describe the cellular mechanisms of radiation cell killing but is less appropriate for clinical calculations than the empirical equations of Thames and Dale referred to above.

Effect of cell proliferation

The effect of proliferation at very low dose-rates is graphically illustrated in Fig. 12.8. These calculations are made for a hypothetical cell population with an α/β ratio of 3.7 Gy and a repair halftime of 0.85 hour. Cell proliferation is assumed to occur with the doubling times shown in the figure and no account has been taken of radiation effects on the rate of proliferation (if this occurred it would reduce the effect of proliferation at the higher dose-rates). For these parameter values there is no effect of proliferation at dose rates above 1 cGy/min but as the dose rate is lowered to 0.1 cGy/min the isoeffective dose rises very steeply. The implication for brachytherapy is that above 1 cGy/min repopulation effects can be ignored, but below this dose rate

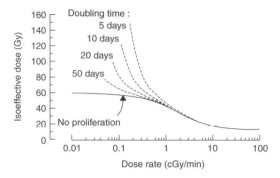

Figure 12.8 Illustrating the effect of cell proliferation as a function of dose rate. Isoeffect curves are shown for no proliferation or with the doubling times indicated. The calculations are based on a simple model of exponential growth, ignoring radiation effects on the rate of cell proliferation.

they will be substantial, both in tumours and in early-responding normal tissues.

The inverse dose-rate effect

Although in situations affecting clinical practice it is a general rule that cellular sensitivity decreases with decreasing dose rate, exceptions to this rule have been noted. Mitchell and Bedford in early studies of cell killing in mammalian cell lines occasionally found a slight inversion which they attributed to a lower dose rate allowing cells to progress though the cell cycle into more sensitive phases, thus suffering greater damage. The mechanism of the inverse dose-rate effect has been elucidated further in more recent experimental work related to the 'low-dose hyper-radiosensitivity' (HRS) process discovered by Joiner and colleagues (see Chapter 4, Section 4.14). In cell lines showing a pronounced HRS response below doses of 0.4 Gy, a reversal of the usual sparing at low dose-rates can also be observed at dose rates below 1.5 cGy/min. An example of this HRS-driven inverse dose rate effect is shown in Fig. 12.9 (Mitchell *et al.*, 2002). It is possible that this phenomenon could be a factor promoting the effectiveness of low dose-rate permanent[125] implants, for example in the treatment of prostate cancer and glioblastoma, where exposure rates over much of the target volume are generally less than 1 cGy/min.

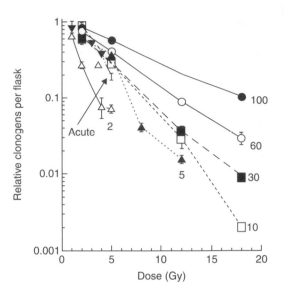

Figure 12.9 Survival curves obtained after exposure of asynchronously growing T98G glioblastoma cells to low dose-rate ^{60}Co γ radiation. Curve labels indicate the dose rate of radiation exposure in cGy/hour. Relative clonogens per flask was calculated by multiplying the surviving fraction by the relative cell yield following irradiation. Each datum point is plotted as the mean ± SEM. The acute dose rate was 33 Gy/hour. This cell line is an example of those which demonstrate an inverse dose-rate effect on cell survival at dose rates below 100 cGy/hour, whereby a decrease in dose rate results in an increase in cell killing per unit dose. Analysis of the cell cycle indicates that these inverse dose-rate effects are not caused by accumulation of cells in G2/M phase or by other cell-cycle perturbations, but result from the process of low-dose hyper-radiosensitivity (see Chapter 4, Section 4.14). From Mitchell *et al.* (2002), with permission.

12.6 RADIOBIOLOGICAL ASPECTS OF BRACHYTHERAPY

The principal reasons for choosing interstitial or intracavitary radiotherapy in preference to external-beam treatment relate to dose delivery and dose distribution rather than to radiobiology. Irradiation from an implanted source within a tumour carries a distinct geometrical advantage for sparing the surrounding normal tissues that will inevitably tend to receive a lower radiation dose. Brachytherapy thus exploits the volume effect in normal tissues (see Chapter 14). Normal tissues will also often be exposed to a lower dose-rate, which gives the additional advantage of 'negative double trouble' (i.e. 'double benefit', see Chapter 9, Section 9.11).

Variation in cell killing around an implanted radioactive source

The non-uniformity of the radiation field around an implanted source has important radiobiological consequences. Close to the source the dose rate is high and the amount of cell killing will be close to that indicated by the acute-radiation survival curve. As we move away from the source, two changes take place: cells will be less sensitive at the lower dose-rates, and within a given period of implantation the accumulated dose will also be less. These two factors lead to a very rapid change in cell killing with distance from the source. Within tissues (tumour or normal) that are close to the source the level of cell killing will be so high that cells of virtually any radiosensitivity will be killed. Further out, the effects will be so low that even the most radiosensitive cells will survive. Between these extremes there is a critical zone in which differential cell killing will occur. As shown by Steel *et al.* (1989), for cells of any given level of radiosensitivity model calculations imply that there will be cliff-like change from high to low local cure probability, taking place over a radial distance of a few millimetres (Fig. 12.10). The distance of the 'cliff' from the source is determined by the radiosensitivity of the cells at low dose-rate – nearer for radioresistant cells and further away for radiosensitive cells (Steel, 1991).

Is there a radiobiological advantage in low dose-rate radiotherapy?

The question of whether low dose-rate irradiation itself carries a therapeutic advantage is an interesting one. There is a considerable volume of literature on the dose-rate effect, both in tumours and in normal tissues, on the basis of which it would be difficult to claim that under all circumstances low dose-rate treatment would have the best therapeutic index. As shown in Fig. 12.4, cells that

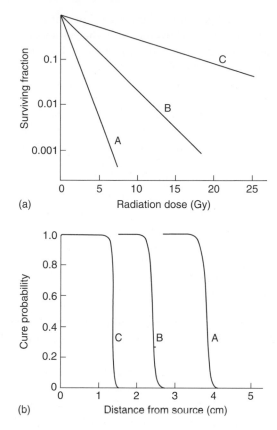

(a)

(b)

Figure 12.10 The likelihood of local tumour control varies steeply with distance from a point radiation source. The radius at which failure occurs depends upon the steepness of the survival curve at low dose-rate (a). From Steel *et al.* (1989), with permission.

are the least sensitive to radiation and have the largest shoulder on the cell-survival curve will show the greatest degree of dose-sparing. These are not necessarily cell lines of low α/β ratio, for Peacock *et al.* (1992) have shown that a range of human tumour cell lines, including those shown in Fig. 12.4, have similar α/β ratios: radioresistant tumour cells tend to have both a lower α and a lower β than more sensitive cells. In a particular therapeutic situation we could make a calculation comparing the relative DRF between tumour and critical normal tissues. This would tell us whether the normal tissues might be spared more or less than the tumour cells if we were to lower the dose rate. However, this does not answer the therapeutic question, because to treat with one large high dose-rate fraction has for a long time not been a clinical option. However, with the advances in functional imaging and combination of positron emission tomography (PET)/computed tomography (CT) with high-precision IMRT, hypofractionation and even large single doses for treatment of metastases are now coming back into the realm of modern radiation oncology. This is similar to comparing hypofractionation with the use of conventional or reduced dose per fraction (see Fig. 10.2). The appropriate clinical question is whether a single continuous low dose-rate treatment is better than using a conventional fractionation schedule.

As illustrated in Fig. 12.7, there is, on the basis of the incomplete repair model, an equivalence between dose per fraction in fractionated radiotherapy and dose rate for a single continuous exposure. Roughly speaking, for a given level of cell killing the total dose required at a continuous dose-rate of 1 Gy/hour is similar to that required by acute fractionated treatment with 2 Gy per fraction. This equivalence depends upon the half-time for recovery but it is relatively independent of the α/β ratio (Fowler, 1989). In radiobiological terms, these two treatments should be equally effective. Lowering the (fractionated) dose per fraction will spare late-responding normal tissues whose α/β ratio is low, as will lowering the dose rate (continuous) below 1 Gy/hour.

The success of intracavitary therapy may result from two factors: (1) the lower volume of normal tissue irradiated to a dose that discriminates between tissue sensitivities; and (2) the practical and radiobiological benefits of short treatment times. The clearest advantage for low dose-rate irradiation is that for a given level of cell killing, and without hazarding late-responding normal tissues, this treatment will be complete within the shortest overall time (see Section 12.4). Tumour cell repopulation will therefore be minimized. This could confer a therapeutic advantage for the treatment of rapidly repopulating tumours.

A potential disadvantage of low dose-rate irradiation is that because of the short overall treatment time there may be inadequate time available for the reoxygenation of hypoxic tumour cells and therefore greater radioresistance because of hypoxia.

Pulsed brachytherapy

The availability of computer-controlled high dose-rate afterloading systems provides the opportunity to deliver interstitial or intracavitary radiotherapy in a series of pulses (PDR). The gaps between pulses allow greater freedom for the patient and increased safety for nursing staff, as well as technical advantages, for example in allowing corrections for the decay of the radioactive source that minimize effects on the quality of treatment.

In principle, any move away from continuous exposure towards treatment with gaps carries a radiobiological disadvantage. This is because the dose rate within each pulse is higher and this allows less opportunity for repair of radiation damage. Slowly-repairing tissues will therefore be disadvantaged and, as argued in Chapter 10, Section 10.8, there will be a loss of therapeutic index between tumour tissues that repair quickly and those late-responding normal tissues that repair more slowly. The magnitude of this effect was considered by Brenner and Hall (1991), who concluded that for gaps between pulses of up to 60 min the radiobiological deficit may be an acceptable trade-off for the increase in dosimetric localization to the target volume. During the ensuing years there has been much theoretical discussion of the guidelines for safe treatment with pulsed brachytherapy. Extensive laboratory studies comparing PDR and CLDR with cells *in vitro* have been carried out in Oslo by the group of Pettersen (Hanisch *et al.*, 2007). They concluded that in some cell lines PDR had a greater than predicted effect. This could not be explained by the inverse dose-rate effect (see Section 12.5). Cell lines that showed an inverse dose-rate effect did so similarly under both CLDR and PDR conditions.

Theoretical studies have examined the effect of halftimes for repair in normal and tumour tissues, including the evidence for multiple halftime components within each tissue (Fowler and van Limbergen, 1997). Brachytherapy studies on laboratory animals are technically difficult, not least because of the differences in scale between rats and humans, but detailed studies of effects in the rat spinal cord have been carried out (Pop *et al.*, 2000).

Clinical experience in the use of pulsed brachytherapy is increasing and the availability of equipment that allows a single high-intensity source to be 'stepped' through the treatment field provides an important degree of control. The method does, however, need to be applied with care because there are penalties in terms of the quality of treatment when pulse sizes are allowed to be too large or when time between pulses is increased much above 1 hour. High dose-rate afterloading systems create the temptation to shorten the overall time and, as indicated above, this could lead to increased early reactions to radiotherapy and greater tumour radioresistance owing to inadequate reoxygenation. A prospective clinical trial comparing CLDR and PDR for cervical cancer was carried out in the Princess Margaret Hospital in Toronto (Bachtiary *et al.*, 2005). No statistical difference was observed in survival or late toxicity, and the authors concluded that PDR has the advantage of a better dose optimization. The use of PDR as a boost in combination with IMRT might yield the best options for dose escalation, as high doses are obtained within the target volume (Pieters *et al.*, 2008).

IMRT and dose rate

Intensity-modulated radiotherapy, one of the highest precision implementations of external-beam radiotherapy, is generally accepted as the best tool to allow dose-escalation with conventional photons in the target volume while sparing the surrounding normal tissues. This higher precision is achieved by a more complex technology, including a high number of separate segments and thereby often longer delivery times of the complete dose fraction of up to 30 min. Thus, part of the escalated dose may be biologically lost by repair during the treatment. Various investigators have addressed this question by *in vitro* cell culture experiments. A recent series of experiments, along with a review of the literature, concluded that in general the effectiveness in terms of cell kill decreases by up to 20 per cent for treatment times of 20–30 min (Bewes *et al.*, 2008). An important observation is that these figures differ for various cell lines, and are more dependent on the rate of repair than the α/β ratio, as also predicted by the 'incomplete repair' or the LPL model (see

Chapters 4 and 8). To date, no indications of a reduced effectiveness of IMRT treatments have been reported, and it should be realized that the outcome of therapy is not determined only by the intrinsic sensitivity of tumour cells. Of interest in this respect is an experimental study comparing *in vitro* radiosensitivity with *in vivo* tumour response in the same cell line (Tomita *et al.*, 2008), which showed that the loss of effect due to lower cell kill was compensated *in vivo* by rapid reoxygenation.

Key points

1. Low dose-rate irradiation is the ultimate form of fractionation which allows the maximal amount of recovery in the shortest overall treatment time.
2. The dose-rate effect results primarily from repair of sublethal damage, while repopulation may play a role for treatment times longer than 1–2 days.
3. Cell-survival curves become straighter at low dose-rates and approach the initial slope of the survival curve.
4. An inverse dose-rate effect, the reversal of sparing at dose rates less than *c.* 1 cGy/min, is observed in cell lines showing the phenomenon of low-dose HRS.
5. PDR provides the same radiobiological advantage as continuous low dose-rate with the added benefit of optimized dose distributions and patient logistics.
6. IMRT given in 20–30 min per fraction may be intrinsically less effective owing to lower cell kill, but this may be compensated in tumours by rapid reoxygenation.

■ BIBLIOGRAPHY

Bachtiary B, Dewitt A, Pintilie M *et al.* (2005). Comparison of late toxicity between continuous low-dose-rate and pulsed-dose-rate brachytherapy in cervical cancer patients. *Int J Radiat Oncol Biol Phys* **63**: 1077–82.

Bewes JM, Suchowerska N, Jackson M, Zhang M, McKenzie DR (2008). The radiobiological effect of intra-fraction dose-rate modulation in intensity modulated radiation therapy (IMRT). *Phys Med Biol* **53**: 3567–78.

Brenner DJ, Hall EJ (1991). Fractionated high dose rate versus low dose rate regimens for intracavitary brachytherapy of the cervix. I. General considerations based on radiobiology. *Br J Radiol* **64**: 133–41.

Curtis SB (1986). Lethal and potentially lethal lesions induced by radiation – a unified repair model. *Radiat Res* **106**: 252–70.

Dale RG, Deehan C (2007). Brachytherapy. In: Dale RG, Jones B (eds) *Radiobiological modelling in radiation oncology*. London: The British Institute of Radiology, 113–37.

Down JD, Easton DF, Steel GG (1986). Repair in the mouse lung during low dose-rate irradiation. *Radiother Oncol* **6**: 29–42.

Fowler JF (1989). Dose rate effects in normal tissues. In: Mould RF (ed.) *Brachytherapy 2, proceedings of the 5th International Selectron Users' Meeting 1988* . Leersum: Nucletron International BV, 26–40.

Fowler JF, van Limbergen EF (1997). Biological effect of pulsed dose rate brachytherapy with stepping sources if short half-times of repair are present in tissues. *Int J Radiat Oncol Biol Phys* **37**: 877–83.

Hanisch PH, Furre T, Olsen DR, Pettersen EO (2007). Radiobiological responses for two cell lines following continuous low dose-rate (CLDR) and pulsed dose rate (PDR) brachytherapy. *Acta Oncol* **46**: 602–11.

Mitchell CR, Folkard M, Joiner MC (2002). Effects of exposure to low-dose-rate ^{60}Co gamma rays on human tumor cells *in vitro*. *Radiat Res* **158**: 311–18.

Peacock JH, Eady JJ, Edwards SM, McMillan TJ, Steel GG (1992). The intrinsic alpha/beta ratio for human tumour cells: is it a constant? *Int J Radiat Biol* **61**: 479–87.

Pieters BR, van de Kamer JB, van Herten YR *et al.* (2008). Comparison of biologically equivalent dose-volume parameters for the treatment of prostate cancer with concomitant boost IMRT versus IMRT combined with brachytherapy. *Radiother Oncol* **88**: 46–52.

Pop LA, Millar WT, van der Plas M, van der Kogel AJ (2000). Radiation tolerance of rat spinal cord to pulsed dose rate (PDR-) brachytherapy: the impact of differences in temporal dose distribution. *Radiother Oncol* **55**: 301–15.

Steel GG (1991). The ESTRO Breur lecture. Cellular sensitivity to low dose-rate irradiation focuses the problem of tumour radioresistance. *Radiother Oncol* **20**: 71–83.

Steel GG, Down JD, Peacock JH, Stephens TC (1986). Dose-rate effects and the repair of radiation damage. *Radiother Oncol* **5**: 321–31.

Steel GG, Deacon JM, Duchesne GM, Horwich A, Kelland LR, Peacock JH (1987). The dose-rate effect in human tumour cells. *Radiother Oncol* **9**: 2 99–310.

Steel GG, Kelland LR, Peacock JH (1989). The radiobiological basis for low dose-rate radiotherapy. In: Mould RF (ed.) *Brachytherapy 2, Proceedings of the 5th International Selectron Users' Meeting 1988*. Leersum: Nucletron International BV, 15–25.

Thames HD (1985). An 'incomplete-repair' model for survival after fractionated and continuous irradiations. *Int J Radiat Biol* **47**: 319–39.

Tomita N, Shibamoto Y, Ito M *et al.* (2008). Biological effect of intermittent radiation exposure *in vivo*: recovery from sublethal damage versus reoxygenation. *Radiother Oncol* **86**: 369–74.

van Os R, Thames HD, Konings AW, Down JD (1993). Radiation dose-fractionation and dose-rate relationships for long-term repopulating hemopoietic stem cells in a murine bone marrow transplant model. *Radiat Res* **136**: 118–25.

■ FURTHER READING

Dale RG, Deehan C (2007). Brachytherapy. In: Dale RG, Jones B (eds) *Radiobiological modelling in radiation oncology*. London: The British Institute of Radiology, 113–37.

Pathogenesis of normal-tissue side-effects

WOLFGANG DÖRR

13.1 INTRODUCTION

Despite optimum conformation of the treatment fields to the tumour and precise treatment planning and application, the target volume in curative radiotherapy necessarily includes a substantial amount of normal tissue, for several reasons. First, malignant tumours infiltrate microscopically into normal structures, which hence must be included into the high-dose volume as a tumour margin. Second, normal tissues within the tumour, such as soft tissue and blood vessels, are exposed to the full tumour dose. Third, normal structures in the entrance and exit channels of the radiation beam may be exposed to clinically relevant doses. Therefore, effective curative radiotherapy is unavoidably associated with an accepted risk for early and late radiation side-effects ('adverse events') in order to achieve adequate tumour cure rates.

The optimum radiation dose in curative radiotherapy is defined as the dose that is associated with a certain low incidence of sequelae of a defined severity in cured patients ('complication-free healing'). The manifestation of side-effects is hence an indicator for optimum treatment and maximum tumour cure probability; side-effects cannot, a priori, be considered as a consequence of incorrect treatment.

Early (acute) side-effects are observed during or shortly after a course of radiotherapy. In contrast, late (chronic) side-effects become clinically manifest after latent times of months to many years. The cut-off time to distinguish early from late effects has arbitrarily been set to 90 days after the onset of radiotherapy. This classification is based exclusively on the time-course (i.e. the time of first diagnosis of the pathological changes). However, early and late effects have specific (radio)biological features which distinguish them.

Early effects are usually found in tissues with a high proliferative activity that counteracts a permanent cell loss (turnover tissues), such as bone marrow, epidermis or mucosae of the upper and lower intestinal tract. The acute symptoms are based on radiation-induced impairment of cell production in the face of ongoing cell loss, which is usually independent of the treatment. The consequence is progressive cell depletion. This response is regularly accompanied by inflammatory changes, which either can be directly induced by the radiation exposure or secondary to the changes in the turnover compartment of the tissue. Healing, which is usually complete, is based on the proliferation of surviving tissue stem cells within the irradiated volume or migration of stem cells in from unirradiated tissue.

Late radiation side-effects are basically found in all organs. In contrast to the development of early side-effects, which are characterized by cell depletion as a leading mechanism, the pathogenetic pathways of chronic side-effects are more complex. The dominating processes occur in the parenchyma of the organs (i.e. in the tissue-specific compartments) but also in the connective and vascular tissues. Regularly, the immune system (macrophages, mast cells) contributes to the tissue reaction. Late radiation effects hence represent a multifaceted, orchestrated response with various components (Dörr et al., 2005b; Bentzen, 2006).

Late radiation sequelae, in contrast to early effects, with few exceptions, are irreversible and progressive, with increasing severity occurring with longer follow-up times. Therefore, the longer the survival times of the patients (i.e. the better the radiation therapy) the higher is the number of patients at risk for late reactions. A risk for the manifestation of a chronic reaction remains throughout the life of the patient (Jung et al., 2001).

Early and late radiation effects are independent with regard to their pathogenesis and, in general, conclusions from the severity of early reactions on the risk of late effects cannot be drawn. However, in particular situations, interactions between acute and chronic reactions can occur within one organ, resulting in consequential late effects (CLE). This is the case when the early-responding tissue compartments (e.g. epithelia) have a protective function against mechanical and/or chemical exposure. This barrier function is impaired during the acute radiation reaction because of cell depletion. In consequence, secondary traumata can impact on the target structures of the late sequelae (connective tissue, vasculature) in addition to the direct effects of radiation, which can then aggravate the late radiation response (Dörr and Hendry, 2001). Consequential late effects have been demonstrated for intestine, urinary tract, oral mucosa and particularly stressed skin localizations (Dörr and Hendry, 2001), as well as for lung (Dörr et al., 2005a).

In this chapter, after a description of the general pathogenesis of early and late radiation effects, specific effects in clinically relevant organs and tissues will be described. This latter part also includes side-effects that follow an atypical pathogenesis, such as late cardiovascular changes or radiation cataract induction. This chapter does not include systemic sequelae such as fatigue or nausea and emesis. Moreover, responses to high single doses or a few large fractions, as administered in stereotactic radiotherapy, which may be based on different pathogenetic pathways, are excluded.

13.2 EARLY RADIATION EFFECTS

Radiation effects in skin and epidermis were dose-limiting during the orthovoltage era, with peak doses occurring near the entrance sites of the beam. In contrast, with modern treatment techniques, distributions of high doses within the body can, in general, be achieved without severe epidermal toxicity.

However, early radiation effects are still relevant even in face of the progress in the physical application of radiotherapy. Early reactions significantly affect the quality of life of the patients. Some early responses are dose-limiting, such as oral mucositis in radiotherapy of advanced head and neck tumours, and hence reduce the chance for tumour cure. Moreover, early reactions can result in consequential late effects (Dörr and Hendry, 2001). In addition, the costs of supportive care are an important socio-economic factor.

Additional traumas can significantly aggravate early radiation responses. Chemotherapy is one prominent example. Moreover, in epithelial tissues, mechanical stress can influence early complications, such as epidermal irritation by clothing or in skin folds, or oral mucosal trauma through dental prostheses or sharp-edged food components. Similarly, chemical exposure, such as smoking, alcohol or spicy diet in oral mucosa, can intensify the response. Such exacerbating factors should be avoided during radiotherapy.

Precise knowledge of the pathogenesis and radiobiology of acute radiation effects forms the essential basis for the development of selective, biology-based interventions. One example is radiation-induced leukopenia after bone marrow irradiation, which can be treated by haematopoietic growth factors such as granulocyte colony-stimulating

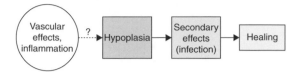

Figure 13.1 Components of early radiation effects. Early radiation effects usually start with vascular changes, clinically visible as erythema, accompanied by inflammatory changes. The depletion of functional cells, based on insufficient cellular supply in the face of ongoing differentiation and cell loss, is the dominating response to irradiation. The interaction of this phase with the vascular response is unclear. Progressive hypoplasia promotes secondary reactions (e.g. infections owing to oral mucositis, moist skin desquamation or leukopenia). Eventually healing occurs, based on surviving stem cells within the irradiated volume or stem cells migrating in from outside the irradiated volume.

factor (G-CSF) or granulocyte/macrophage colony-stimulating factor (GM-CSF) (see Chapter 22).

Phases of early radiation reactions

Different pathogenetic phases and components can be distinguished for early radiation responses in normal tissues (Sonis, 2004; Dörr et al., 2005b), as illustrated schematically in Fig. 13.1. Regularly a 'humoral' response is observed, based on the release of paracrine active substances, for example by vascular endothelial cells and macrophages, but also by fibroblasts or parenchymal cells such as epithelial keratinocytes. The associated changes in the functions of the target cells are accompanied by inflammatory changes. This phase usually precedes the clinically dominating reaction (i.e. the reduction in the number of functional cells). This hypoplasia is seen, for example, as epidermal or mucosal epitheliolysis or as leukopenia. Based on the breakdown of epithelial structures, which normally constitute a protective barrier function, secondary infections are frequently seen, which can even progress into septicaemia. Eventually, with the exception of very severe reactions, healing occurs, based on surviving stem cells within the irradiated volume or on migrating stem cells,

for example bone marrow stem cells from the circulation or epidermal/mucosal stem cells migrating from the margins into the irradiated area.

CHANGES IN CELLULAR FUNCTION

Early after the onset of radiotherapy, after the first or the first few fractions, increased protein expression is observed (e.g. in endothelial cells, vascular smooth muscle cells or macrophages). These proteins are predominantly pro-inflammatory, such as interleukin-1a (IL-1a) and other interleukins, tumour necrosis factor-α (TNF-α), or cyclooxygenase-2 (COX-2). Similarly, the activity of inducible nitric oxide synthase (iNOS) is increased (e.g. Rubin et al., 1995; Sonis, 2004). These are only a few examples.

The paracrine, intercellular communication is modified by the induction of cytokines, their receptors, adhesion molecules and components of the cell–matrix interaction (Dörr et al., 2005b). For example, keratinocytes of the epidermis and oral mucosa show an increased expression of epidermal growth factor (EGF), its receptor (EGFR) or the intercellular adhesion molecule-1 (ICAM-1). The EGFR is subsequently internalized and translocated into the nucleus, and can act as a transcription factor and modulate DNA repair (Dittmann et al., 2005).

Initiation and regulation of these processes – because of their early onset – cannot exclusively be attributed to the release of mediators during the disintegration of damaged cells or to tissue hypoplasia. However, the signals underlying these very early changes in cellular function are unclear and are the focus of current research projects. Their relevance for the pathophysiology of the early radiation effects is similarly indistinct. An impact on the clinical symptoms, such as pain, is obvious, and modification of the tissue response (e.g. of the regeneration processes – repopulation, see Chapter 11) is likely. The available data, however, do not yet allow us to distinguish which of the intracellular, paracrine or humoral aspects are causally involved in the pathogenesis, and which are epiphenomena.

CELLULAR DEPLETION

The cellular depletion phase, like leukopenia after bone marrow irradiation or epitheliolysis in

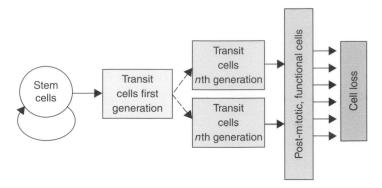

Figure 13.2 Proliferative organization of turnover tissues. Typical early reactions occur in turnover tissues. The entire cell production is based on tissue stem cells, which generate, on average, one stem cell and one transit cell in asymmetrical divisions (see also Fig. 13.3). Transit cells can undergo a limited number of divisions, which increase the cell yield per stem cell division. The cells undergo maturation and differentiation and are eventually lost. The turnover time from the initial stem cell division to cell loss is tissue specific.

epidermis and mucosa, is the clinically most relevant component of early radiation responses. As mentioned above, these changes are found in turnover tissues, with a precisely regulated equilibrium between permanent cell loss from the functional compartment and cell production in the germinal compartment. The hierarchical proliferative organization of these tissues is illustrated in Fig. 13.2.

The entire cell production takes place in the germinal components of the tissue (e.g. the basal and suprabasal layers of epithelia, intestinal crypts, or bone marrow sinuses). The basis are tissue stem cells. With very few exceptions, no cellular markers, such as surface antigens, have so far been identified that would allow for differentiation between stem cells and other proliferating cells. Therefore, the stem cell concept must be regarded as strictly functional: the stem cell population consists of cells that can completely and correctly restore the integrity and structure of a tissue after an insult. Hence, the radiation tolerance of a tissue is defined by the number and the intrinsic radiosensitivity of the stem cells.

The equilibrium between cell production and cell loss is based on the division pattern of the stem cells. On average, each stem cell division results in one cell that remains in the stem cell pool, and one cell which eventually differentiates (Dörr, 1997). This pattern, with two different daughter cells, is called asymmetrical division.

Daughter cells which are not stem cells (transit or precursor cells) can undergo a limited number (e.g. up to 10 in bone marrow) of transit divisions, which substantially increases the yield of cells per stem cell division. The regulation of these processes remains unclear. The number of functional cells seems to feed back on the general proliferation activity. However, the number of stem cells itself seems to modulate stem cell proliferation, indicating an (additional) autoregulation within this compartment (see also Chapter 11).

In most turnover tissues, transit cells by far dominate the proliferative cell population; the relationship between the numbers of transit and stem cells depends on the number of transit divisions. Hence, studies into the proliferative activity, such as S-phase labelling with BrdUrd, Ki67-labelling or mitotic counts, are dominated by transit-cell proliferation and cannot accurately assess the proliferation parameters in the stem-cell compartment. The post-mitotic cells arising from the last transit division usually undergo several steps of maturation before they reach a terminal differentiation state and are eventually lost. Their lifespan is tissue-specific, but can vary markedly between different tissues, from a few days in the epithelia of the upper and lower alimentary tract to several months in the urothelium of the urinary bladder. The overall turnover time (i.e. the time in which all cells are renewed once) defines the time-course of the early radiation response (Fig. 13.3).

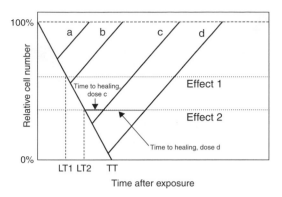

Figure 13.3 Radiation-induced cell depletion and clinical manifestation of early radiation effects. Radiation exposure of turnover tissues results in an impairment of cell production, while cell loss continues independent of the treatment. The rate at which cells are lost is determined by the tissue turnover time (TT). If the residual proliferation of sterilized cells (abortive divisions) is not taken into consideration, then a complete loss of cells would be observed after one turnover time. A defined clinical effect 1, which is associated with a specific reduction of the cell number, can occur dependent on the dose (dose level b, c or d), and is not observed at lower radiation doses (dose level a). The latent time to clinical manifestation, however, is independent of dose. A more severe effect level 2 is based on a higher reduction in cell numbers, and hence is observed only at higher doses (c and d). Compared with effect 1, the latent time is longer, but is also independent of dose. In contrast, the time to clinical healing is longer with higher doses (d versus c).

The radiosensitivity of the cells decreases during their differentiation process. Therefore, radiation doses administered in radiotherapy are predominantly lethal for stem cells, while transit cells are only minimally affected, and no effect is seen on post-mitotic cells. Some studies in experimental models have demonstrated with specific assays that the stem cell inactivation by radiation follows a dose–effect relationship, which corresponds in its shape to a typical cell survival curve *in vitro* (see Chapter 4). Such studies have been performed with micro- or macro-colony-forming assays in intestinal epithelium and skin (Withers and Elkind, 1970), or with spleen colony assays for surviving bone marrow stem cells (Potten and Hendry, 1983). However, despite qualitative similarities in cell survival, there are significant quantitative differences between the *in vivo* and the *in vitro* situations.

The reduction of proliferation in the stem cell compartment results in a lack of support to the transit population, with the consequence of a decline in overall cell production. Furthermore, depending on the dose, direct effects on transit proliferation are also possible, which further affect the amplifying function of the transit compartment. Hence, increasing radiation doses result in a progressive decline in the number of precursor cells available for differentiation into post-mitotic cells. In contrast, despite the radiation exposure, differentiation and cell loss continue almost physiologically in qualitative and quantitative terms (Dörr, 1997). The radiation-induced imbalance between cell production and cell loss results in progressive hypoplasia, which becomes clinically manifest after a threshold cell depletion is reached (Fig. 13.3). Different grades of severity of an early reaction, such dry and moist desquamation in skin, are based on different degrees of cell depletion, as illustrated by different threshold levels in Fig. 13.3. As the cell loss rate depends on the turnover time of the tissue, and is independent of the treatment, the latent time until a clinical response is reached is tissue-dependent but independent of dose.

Usually, the turnover times are shorter than the latent time to complete cell depletion. For example, the turnover time in human and murine oral mucosa is in the range of 5 days (Dörr, 1997), but it takes about 10 days for ulceration to develop in mouse mucosa after single dose of irradiation (Dörr and Kummermehr, 1991) and about 9 days after a (fractionated) dose of 20 Gy in human mucosa (van der Schueren *et al.*, 1990). This prolongation is due to the residual proliferative capacity (abortive divisions) of sterilized cells even after high doses (see also Chapter 11).

In epithelial tissues, the progressive cell depletion is associated with an exudative response, which results in the formation of a pseudomembrane consisting of fibrin and cellular remnants, which covers the ulcerative lesion. Healing of acute radiation effects is based on stem cells surviving within the irradiated volume or migrating in from outside. For the restoration of the stem cell population, symmetrical divisions, with the generation of two stem cell daughters, are required (see also Chapter 11). It is likely that this process is regulated via the local environment, which does not provide the signals that allow the daughter cells to differentiate. This is depicted as a differentiation block, which results in the recruitment of both daughter cells into the stem cell pool. The generation of transit cells through asymmetrical divisions recurs only when a sufficient number of stem cells have been produced.

The higher the dose, the fewer stem cells survive the treatment. Therefore, the clinically manifest response persists over a longer time with higher doses. This is illustrated by the EORTC (European Organization for Research and Treatment of Cancer) 22851 study in head and neck tumours (Horiot *et al.*, 2006), where accelerated fractionation (and hence a biologically more effective treatment) resulted in clearly increased oral mucositis rates even at 6 weeks after the treatment (see Chapter 11). Also, complete restoration of cell numbers and tissue architecture takes longer with higher doses (Fig. 13.3), which should be considered if treatment breaks are introduced in clinical protocols for healing of early effects.

13.3 CHRONIC RADIATION EFFECTS

Tissue organization models have been developed that define late-responding tissues as flexible or F-type tissues. In these tissues, in contrast to early-responding hierarchical tissues (see Section 13.2), no clear separation can be made between proliferating and functional cells. Proliferating cells are recruited into the functional population on demand, and vice versa. It is assumed that the clinical manifestation of late radiation effects is based on a defined, critical depletion of functional cells (such as for early reactions). The compensatory proliferation of the surviving parenchymal cells, which were originally functional cells, results in mitotic death and hence accelerates cell loss and therefore shortens the time to the loss of organ function. The higher the initial cell depletion (i.e. the higher the dose) the more relevant this mechanism becomes. Hence, this model predicts a dose-dependent shortening of the latent time to the clinical manifestation of the effect, which is indeed a general clinical observation.

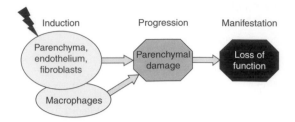

Figure 13.4 Pathogenesis of late radiation effects. Chronic radiation effects are based on complex pathophysiological processes. These involve radiation-induced changes in organ-specific parenchymal cells (cell death), fibroblasts (differentiation) and vascular endothelial cells (loss of capillaries). All these cells, as well as macrophages, interact through a variety of cytokines and growth factors. This orchestrated response results in progressive parenchymal damage and eventually in loss of function within the irradiated volume. The clinical consequences depend on the architecture of the organ and the volume irradiated (see Chapter 14).

An alternative model (Withers *et al.*, 1988) assumes that, in late-responding tissues, structures with stem cell-like characteristics, so-called tissue rescuing units (TRU) or functional subunits (FSU) exist. Their radiation-induced inactivation results in the clinical radiation responses seen. For some tissues or organs, relatively independent structures can be defined, such as nephrons in the kidney, or bronchioli in the lung, which may represent TRU.

Undoubtedly, parenchymal cells in any organ are inactivated by radiation exposure. However, it is also accepted that, in addition to the parenchyma of the organs and the organ-specific cells, further tissue structures and cell populations are involved in the pathogenesis of late effects (Fig. 13.4). These are predominantly vascular endothelial cells, mainly in small blood vessels and capillaries, and connective tissue fibroblasts. Endothelial cell death, by apoptosis or as delayed mitotic death, is induced by radiation exposure. In contrast, mitotic fibroblasts are triggered into differentiation to post-mitotic fibrocytes, with the consequence of a drastically increased collagen synthesis and deposition (Rodemann and Bamberg, 1995). Moreover macrophages, irradiated or recruited into the tissue after irradiation, are also known to contribute to the pathogenesis of late radiation reactions. Reactive oxygen and nitrogen species, chronically produced by various cell populations, in combination with chronic hypoxia, and a perpetual cascade of cytokines (Rubin *et al.*, 1995; Dörr and Herrmann, 2003), seem to play an essential role in the pathogenesis of chronic radiation sequelae (Bentzen, 2006). The interactive response of the individual components of late radiation reactions results in progressive parenchymal damage and eventually in loss of function within the irradiated volume (Fig. 13.4). The clinical consequences depend on the architecture of the organ and the volume irradiated (see Chapter 14).

Each of the participating cellular components of a late effect responds to radiation exposure with a specific dose-dependence, which, in an orchestrated response, then defines the overall dose–response for the different clinical endpoints of the entire tissue. Hence, it is unlikely that the radiation sensitivity of one single cellular component can be used as a predictor of the sensitivity of the whole organ. For different organs, the relevance of the different pathogenetic components can differ (see Section 13.5). For example in the liver, the radiation response of the parenchymal cells (hepatocytes) is less important for the clinical symptoms (i.e. veno-occlusive disease; Dörr *et al.*, 2005b). In the lung, type II pneumocytes (a slow turnover H-type tissue), endothelial cells and fibroblasts seem to contribute similarly to radiation-induced fibrosis (Dörr and Herrmann, 2003). In contrast, late fibrotic changes in the bladder are secondary to the functional impairment, which is predominantly based on urothelial and endothelial changes, and is not primarily radiation-induced (Dörr *et al.*, 2005b).

Vasculature and endothelial cells

Irradiation causes changes in the function of the endothelial cells (Schultz-Hector, 1992; Dörr *et al.*, 2005b). Endothelial cell vacuolization and foci of endothelial detachment are regularly seen. Also, transudation of serum components into the vessel wall and subendothelial oedema have been observed, and formation of thrombi and occlusion of capillaries have been reported (Fajardo *et al.*, 2001). Leukocyte adhesion and infiltration into the vessel wall is regularly observed. Based on all

these changes, irradiation eventually results in a progressive loss of capillaries, associated with a 'sausage-like' appearance of the arterioles, indicating substantial impairment of perfusion. The detailed interrelation of the individual changes described above with the eventual capillary loss remains unclear. Delayed mitotic death, based on the long turnover times of the endothelium, may contribute. The role of radiation-induced endothelial apoptosis, which occurs at early times after irradiation, is currently being discussed. As a result of the insufficient supply of oxygen and nutrients, atrophy of the downstream parenchyma develops. The morphological and functional consequences of this atrophy differ between the organs.

Telangiectasia (i.e. pathologically dilated capillaries) are observed in all irradiated tissues and organs. The pathogenesis is unclear but it is assumed that endothelial cell damage is involved. The loss of smooth muscle cells surrounding larger capillaries and veins may also contribute to the development of telangiectasia. In the intestine, the urinary system or the central nervous system (CNS), telangiectasia can be clinically relevant because of the tendency for capillary haemorrhage. In the skin, telangiectasia can be a cosmetic problem, but has also been used as a quantitative endpoint for radiobiological studies (see Section 13.5). In arterioles, progressive sclerosis of the tunica media is observed, which also results in impaired supply of the downstream parenchyma. The bases are presumably direct radiation effects on the cells in the media layer, in combination with endothelial changes.

Studies on the pathogenesis of late radiation effects have been performed in various experimental animal models, and predominantly with high single doses or few large fractions. Hence, no clear conclusions on the correlation of the individual changes described above and their time-course after fractionated radiotherapy can be drawn, although it can be assumed that similar changes occur.

Fibroblasts

In living organisms, a balance between mitotic fibroblasts and post-mitotic fibrocytes exists.

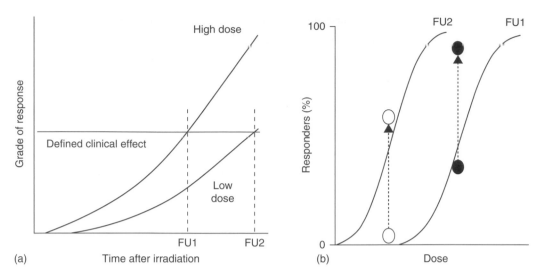

Figure 13.5 Time-course and dose dependence of late radiation sequelae. Late radiation effects are progressive in nature. The latent time for a specific clinical effect as well as the progression rate are dependent on dose (a). In consequence, an increasing number of individuals presenting with the effect (responders) is found in the individual dose groups with prolongation of the follow-up time, i.e. from follow-up 1 (FU1) to follow-up 2 (FU2). Therefore, a shift of the dose–effect curve to lower doses is found with increasing follow-up (b).

Irradiation results in stimulation of the differentiation of fibroblasts into fibrocytes, with the consequence of substantially increased collagen synthesis and deposition (Rodemann and Bamberg, 1995), which affects organ function. This process is modulated by the synthesis and release of transforming growth factor-β (TGF-β) from various cell populations, which further triggers fibroblast differentiation (Hakenjos *et al.*, 2000). Increased expression of TGF-β at the mRNA and protein level can be observed over long time intervals in various cell populations (Bentzen, 2006).

Latent times

The latent time for chronic radiation effects, as well as the rate at which the severity of the clinical changes progresses, is inversely dependent on dose (Fig. 13.5). This dose-dependence results from several processes: with higher doses, more endothelial cells are damaged and the progression of the loss of capillaries is faster. Therefore, less time is required until tissue function is lost. Similarly, higher doses trigger more fibroblasts into differentiation, which results in a higher synthesis rate of collagen, and the collagen level

associated with loss of tissue function is reached earlier. Parenchymal radiation effects contribute to these processes in an organ-specific manner. As a consequence of the dose-dependence of latent time and progression rate, with increasing follow-up time responses are also seen at lower dose levels (Fig. 13.5). Hence, the isoeffective doses for a defined clinical response decrease with increasing follow-up time. In consequence, the definition of tolerance doses for late effects always requires information about the follow-up time on which the estimate is based.

13.4 DOCUMENTATION AND ASSESSMENT OF NORMAL-TISSUE EFFECTS

Two aspects must be considered for the documentation and quantification of normal tissue complications: the frequency of assessment and the scoring system used. Early reactions can undergo considerable changes in their clinical manifestation in short periods. For example, oral mucositis can change from a slight erythema response to confluent epithelial denudation over just a few days, particularly if additional damage is inflicted

Table 13.1 Systems for documentation of side-effects, with examples for oral mucositis

Grade	General	RTOG/EORTC	CTCAE v3	WHO
0	No change	No change	No change	No change
1	Mild	Erythema, mild soreness, painless erosions	Erythema; normal diet	Soreness, erythema
2	Moderate/clear	Painful erythema, oedema or ulcers; can eat	Patchy ulceration; can eat and swallow modified diet	Erythema, ulcers; can eat solids
3	Severe/significant	Painful erythema, oedema or ulcers; cannot eat	Confluent ulcerations, bleeding with minor trauma; unable to adequately aliment or hydrate orally	Ulcers; requires liquid diet only
4	Life-threatening	Requires parenteral or enteral support	Tissue necrosis; significant spontaneous bleeding	Alimentation not possible
5	Death owing to side-effects	Death owing to side-effects	Death owing to side-effects	Death owing to side-effects

RTOG/EORTC, Radiation Therapy and Oncology Group and the European Organisation for Research and Treatment of Cancer; CTCAE v3, the Common Terminology Criteria for Adverse Events, version 3; WHO, World Health Organization.

by spicy food, etc. In contrast, chronic radiation sequelae develop slowly and, more importantly, are usually irreversible. In conclusion, detailed assessment of early reactions requires scoring at least on a weekly basis during and for some weeks after radiotherapy. For studies on oral mucositis, even more frequent assessment is recommended. Late effects should be scored at intervals of several months after the end of radiotherapy, in order to assess the dynamics of their development, and may, at later time points, be documented at annual intervals. It must be emphasized that, for some chronic reactions, such as in the heart or the urinary bladder (see Section 13.5), the time to clinical manifestation of the reaction, particularly after low radiation doses (see Section 13.3), can be in the range of decades. Hence, life-long follow-up of patients is recommended.

Standardized classification systems have been established for documentation of normal-tissue reactions suitable for comparison between investigators, institutions and studies. In general, complications are graded from 0 (no response) to 5 (lethal), as shown in Table 13.1:

- Grade 1 reactions (mild) are reversible and heal spontaneously without any specific therapeutic intervention or interruption of the oncological treatment.

- Grade 2 reactions (moderate/clear) can be treated on an outpatient basis and do not require a radiation dose reduction or treatment interruption.
- Grade 3 effects (severe, pronounced) frequently require hospitalization and intense supportive care, and often necessitate interruption of the treatment and/or dose modifications.
- Grade 4 reactions are life-threatening, require immediate hospitalization and intense therapeutic interventions, plus cessation of radiotherapy.

The most widely used classification systems in radiation oncology (see the references in the Further reading section) are:

- RTOG/EORTC classification, jointly developed by the Radiation Therapy and Oncology Group and the European Organisation for Research and Treatment of Cancer;
- CTCAE v3, the Common Terminology Criteria for Adverse Events, version 3, developed by the National Cancer Institute (NCI);
- WHO (World Health Organization) classification;
- LENT/SOMA system (Late Effects in Normal Tissue/Subjective Objective Management Analytic) was developed specifically for scoring late sequelae resulting from oncological treatment.

In principle, all these classification systems are comparable, and the scores from one system may be translated into the scores for another protocol (Table 13.1), but with exceptions. This translation is definitely precluded if sum scores are calculated, as has been suggested for LENT/SOMA, where the information on individual symptoms is lost; this method cannot, therefore, be recommended.

In addition to these scores, more detailed protocols, or systems specifically designed for side-effects in certain organs, for example OMAS (Oral Mucositis Assessment Scale), have been suggested. For clinical reports on side-effects, the scoring protocol applied must be described in detail, particularly if modified versions of the original protocols are applied.

13.5 RADIATION EFFECTS IN SPECIFIC TISSUES AND ORGANS

In this section the response and tolerance of some clinically important dose-limiting normal tissues will be summarized. In general, an overview of clinical symptoms and consequences for the various radiation sequelae can be found in the classification protocols (see Section 13.4). As a guideline for clinical treatment planning, Table 13.2 provides estimated tolerance dose levels for various endpoints, and corresponding α/β values. However, the numbers in this table should be used with considerable caution, as they are influenced by a number of factors, particularly the irradiated volume (see Chapter 14).

Skin

The sequence of events in skin during radiotherapy is illustrated in Fig. 13.6 (page 182). Skin erythema is closely related to radiation effects in vessels, with intermittent phases of vasodilation. In contrast, epidermal changes are based on the radiation-induced impairment of cell production, as described in Section 13.2. The clinical manifestation is dry desquamation (radiodermatitis sicca), followed by moist desquamation. According to the turnover time of human epidermis of 20–45 days, this phase is usually seen at 2–3 weeks after the onset of radiotherapy. The skin reaction displays a significant area effect (see Chapter 14, Section 14.5). Any variation in overall treatment time can have a large influence on skin tolerance: as an approximation, skin tolerance doses decrease by about 3–4 Gy/week when treatment duration is shortened from the standard 6–8 weeks.

Chronic subcutaneous fibrosis, clinically manifest as induration, is based on an increase in collagen fibres and a reduction of fatty tissue (see Section 13.3). The development of skin telangiectasia (Fig. 13.7, page 182) illustrates the progression of vascular injury in the dermis. The corresponding latent time distribution and the cumulative incidence for various grades of the response are shown in Fig. 13.8 (page 182). With high-energy X-rays, in contrast to orthovoltage radiotherapy, the maximum dose is deposited below the surface and late damage may therefore occur without preceding early reactions.

Skin appendices

After a cumulative dose of 12 Gy, a loss in the function of sebaceous glands is observed, and at slightly higher doses the perspiratory glands also respond, both resulting in a typical dry skin. In hair follicles, single doses of 4 Gy or 10 Gy result in transient or permanent hair loss. In fractionated protocols, significantly higher doses up to 40 Gy still allow hair regrowth within 1 year, but regrowth is frequently associated with discoloration.

Oral mucosa and oesophagus

Oral mucositis is the most severe and frequently dose-limiting early side-effect of radio(chemo)therapy for head and neck tumours. Erythema, focal and confluent mucositis/ulceration are the lead symptoms (Table 13.1). Almost all patients with curative radiotherapy in this region develop some form of mucositis, with usually more than 50 per cent confluent reactions (depending of the definition of 'confluency'). The latter typically develop during the third to fourth week of a conventionally fractionated protocol with 5×2 Gy/week. Oral mucosa is most sensitive to changes in dose intensity (i.e. weekly dose) and overall treatment time. Accelerated protocols regularly result in earlier onset, an aggravation of the response, and/or an

Table 13.2 Tolerance doses and fractionation response (α/β ratio) for acute and late organ damage in humans

Organ	Endpoint	Time to manifestation during/after irradiation	α/β ratio (Gy)	Tolerance dose for total volume (Gy)	Comments
Cartilage, growing	Growth arrest	Next growth spurt	6	20	Associated with vascular damage
Cartilage, adult	Necrosis	Months–years		70	
Bone, adult	Osteoradionecrosis	Years–decades	60	Mandible: 40–50	Vascular damage and trauma
Connective tissue	Fibrosis	9 months–years	2	60	Most frequent late reaction
Capillaries	Capillary changes/loss	6 months–years	3	60	Contribute to a variety of (late) radiation effects
Large vessels	Wall changes, stenosis	Years		70	Resembles atherosclerotic changes
Heart	ECG-changes, arrhythmia	During RT	3	20	Reversible
	Cardiomyopathy (pericarditis)	Months–years		40	Late myocardial infarction
Skin	Erythema	During RT	9–10		Varies with localization (additional mechanical/chemical stress)
	Dry radiodermatitis	During RT	10	40 (100 cm^2)	
	Moist radiodermatitis	During RT	10	60 (100 cm^2)	
	Gangrene, ulcer		3	55 (100 cm^2)	Vasculature!
Hair follicles	Hair loss	During RT (4th week)	7	40	Discoloration!
Sebaceous glands	Dry skin	During RT (2nd week)		12	Transient loss of function
Perspiratory glands	Dry skin, loss of transpiration	During RT (4th week)		30–40	Long-lasting or permanent loss of function
Oral mucosa	Ulcerative mucositis	During RT (2nd to 3rd weeks)	10	20	Early mucositis
Salivary glands	Atrophy/fibrosis			60–70	
	Transient loss of function – xerostomia	During RT (2nd week)		10–20	'Radiation sickness'
	Permanent loss of function – xerostomia	Continuous development from the early response	3	25	One-third capacity is sufficient for saliva production
Oesophagus	Dysphagia	During RT–months		40–45	
	Ulcer–fistula	During RT		55	
Stomach	Atony	Months	4	20	
	Ulcer	During RT	8	50	
Small intestine	Malabsorption			30	Reduced tolerance due to fixation of intestinal loops, e.g. postoperative
	Ulcer/obstruction	Months	4	40	

(Continued)

Table 13.2 (Continued)

Organ	Endpoint	Time to manifestation during/after irradiation	α/β ratio (Gy)	Tolerance dose for total volume (Gy)	Comments
Large intestine	Diarrhoea, pain	During–post RT		10–20	Ileus symptoms possible
	Ulcer/obstruction	Months–years		45	
Rectum	Proctitis	During RT		50	
	Chronic inflammation, ulcer	Months–years	5	60	Partial irradiation of the circumference increases tolerance
Liver	Veno-occlusive disease (VOD)	2–3 weeks		30	Lethal after total organ irradiation. Hence late effects only after partial organ irradiation
Biliary tract	Fibrosis	Months–years			
	Stenosis/stricture	Months–years	1		
Pancreas	Fibrosis	Months–years		50–60	No early symptoms known, included in 'radiation sickness'?
Kidney	Nephropathy	9 months–years	2	20	Vascular effects, potential interaction with surgery
Ureter	Stricture	2 years		60–70	
Urinary bladder	Cystitis	During RT	10	20–35	Uncommon pathophysiology, no urothelial depletion
Urethra	Shrinkage, ulceration	Years–decades	5–10	50	Strong consecutive component
	Stricture	Months–years		60–70	Reduced tolerance after transurethral resection of the prostate (TURP)
Larynx	Oedema	During RT	2–4	45	Permanent changes in voice quality, necrosis after decades
	Chronic oedema, necrosis	Months		70	
Lung	Pneumonitis	2–6 weeks	5	12–14	Single-dose irradiation
	Pneumonitis	4–6 weeks	5	45	
	Fibrosis	6 months–2 years	4		
Testis	Permanent sterility	Weeks–months		1.5	Negative fractionation effect
Ovary	Permanent sterility	Weeks–months		2.5	Strong inverse age dependence
Uterus	Atrophy	Months–years		100	
Vagina	Mucositis	During RT		30	
	Ulcer, fibrosis	Months–years		50	
Breast, child	Growth arrest	At puberty		10	

Organ/tissue	Endpoint	Time to manifestation			Comments
Breast, adult	Fibrosis/atrophy	Years	2–3	60	
Adrenal glands	Loss of function	Months–years		90	
Pituitary gland/diencephalon (children)	Growth hormone deficit	Months–years		18–24	Growth retardation
Cerebrum, child	Somnolence syndrome	During–post RT		24	Specific response in children
Cerebrum, adult	Necrosis	Months–years		55	
Spinal cord	Lhermitte syndrome	Weeks–months		35	Reversible
Cervical/thoracic	Radiation myelopathy	6 months–2 years	2	55	
Thoracic/lumbar	Radiation myelopathy	6 months–2 years	2	55	
Peripheral nerves	Functional impairment	Months–years		60	Frequently associated with connective tissue fibrosis
Eye lens[1]	Cataract	Months–years	1–2[1]	5[1]	Surgical management
Lachrymal system	Dry eye, ulceration	Weeks–months	3	40	Most critical radiation effect in the eye
Retina	Retinopathy	Weeks–months		45	
Optic nerve	Neuropathy	Months–years	2	55	
Chiasma opticum	Loss of vision	Months–years	2	55	
Conjunctiva	Kerato–conjunctivitis	During–post RT		50	Reversible
Ear	Serous otitis	During–post RT		30	
Ear	Inner ear injury	During RT plus; months		30	Slight hearing loss (15 dB) frequently not recognized by patients; overlap with age effects
Taste	Taste impairment, loss	During RT plus; months		30	Reversible
Lymph nodes	Permanent atrophy	Months–years		70	
Lymphatic vessels	Sclerosis	Months–years		90	Frequently associated with connective tissue fibrosis
Bone marrow	Transient hypoplasia	During RT	10	2	Total body irradiation
	Lethal aplasia (1 year)		5	4	Total body irradiation
	Permanent aplasia	During–post RT			Compensation by unirradiated parts; post-irradiation homing of circulating stem cells possible

[1]Tolerance doses for the eye lens are currently under discussion and may be significantly lower (1/10th) than usually estimated.

Time to manifestation: relative to irradiation with 5 × 2 Gy/week. Times after the treatment relate to the last fraction.

α/β value: see also Chapters 8 and 9. Missing values indicate that no valid estimates are possible. RT, radiotherapy.

Tolerance dose total organ relates to irradiation of large volumes that include the entire organ or, for ubiquitous tissues (connective tissue, capillaries, etc.), to larger volumes. For partial organ irradiation, see Chapter 14. Early reaction/late reaction, see Section 13.1.

Adapted from Herrmann et al. (2006), with permission.

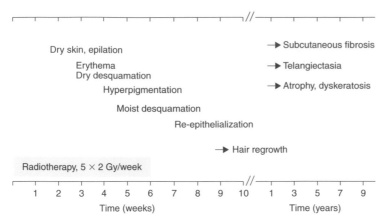

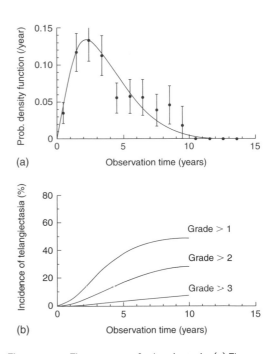

Figure 13.6 Sequence of radiation effects in skin and appendices. Shown are the time-courses of early and late skin reactions induced by conventional radiotherapy with 5 × 2 Gy per week over 6 weeks, if the same skin area is exposed to the maximum dose of 2 Gy at each dose fraction. The duration of radiotherapy is indicated on top of the abscissa.

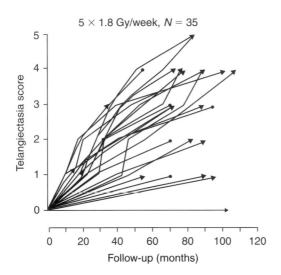

Figure 13.7 Clinical manifestation of skin telangiectasia. Progression of skin telangiectasia in individual patients treated with five fractions of 1.8 Gy per week to a total of 35 fractions. Note the pronounced differences between patients and the continuous increase in severity even up to 8 years. From Turesson (1990), with permission.

Figure 13.8 Time-course of telangiectasia. (a) The latent time distribution for any grade of telangiectasia as observed in 174 treatment fields with an intermediate probability of developing any response. The probability density function may be interpreted as the fraction of patients who developed the response within a specific year after irradiation. (b) The cumulative incidence of telangiectasia as a function of time for various grades, after radiotherapy with 44.4 Gy in 25 fractions. The model calculations are based on observations in 401 treatment fields. From Bentzen *et al.* (1990), with permission.

increase in the frequency of patients with severe reactions (Fig. 13.9, page 183). Repopulation processes have been most intensely studied in this tissue (see Chapter 11).

Chronic effects of radiotherapy include mucosal atrophy and ulceration, and telangiectasia, which render the epithelium vulnerable. Any additional trauma may secondarily result in osteonecrosis. The early radiation response of the oesophagus

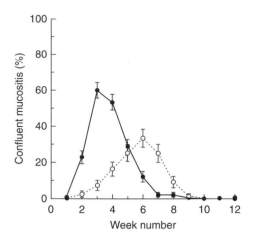

Figure 13.9 Prevalence of confluent mucositis. The percentage of patients presenting with confluent mucositis within a given treatment week after onset of radiotherapy was plotted for accelerated radiotherapy: CHART (continuous hyperfractionated accelerated radiotherapy; filled circles) or conventional radiotherapy (open circles). From Bentzen *et al.* (2001), with permission.

mirrors that of the oral mucosa and in the chronic phase, strictures may develop.

Teeth

Radiation caries, with a very fast manifestation, is a frequent complication of radiotherapy in adults. The response is based on both direct radiation effects at the dentine–enamel border zone, and indirectly on radiation effects in the salivary glands (xerostomia, see below) and the associated changes in the oral micromilieu. Rigorous pretreatment dental restoration or extractions are of major importance, because of the risk of osteoradionecrosis, if extractions are required after radiotherapy. In order to avoid dose peaks in the mucosa around metallic dental implants, mucosal retractors should be used to displace the mucosa by about 3 mm.

Salivary glands

Salivary glands are sensitive to radiation exposure: after the first week of therapy (accumulated dose of 10–15 Gy) saliva production is significantly reduced, frequently after a transient phase of hypersalivation. After total doses in excess of 40 Gy to both parotid glands, saliva production practically stops after about 4 weeks and does not recover at all after doses over 60 Gy. Volume effects are very pronounced, and sparing of partial volumes usually leads to recovery of function.

Chronic xerostomia has a major impact on the quality of life of the patients. It depends not only on reduced serous fluid production in the parotid glands, but also on the reduced amount of mucin from the submandibular glands, and reduced function of the small salivary glands. The submandibular glands produce most of the mucinous components of the saliva; by their water-binding capacity they keep the mucous membranes hydrated and have a barrier function.

Stomach

Functional impairment, with a prolongation of the time for gastric emptying, and a reduction in HCl secretion are frequently seen. The symptoms are equivalent to those of gastritis. Ulceration, mainly based on vascular effects, can develop as a late effect at doses of 25–40 Gy.

Intestine

'Fixed' intestinal loops (e.g. through postoperative adhesions) are particularly at risk as these may be permanently located within a high-dose volume, in contrast to mobile loops. The same is true for the rectum.

The sequence of radiation-induced events in the intestine includes:

- initial increase in motility, followed by an atonic phase
- loss of epithelium and villi owing to proliferative impairment in the crypts, with the consequence of:
  - water electrolyte and protein loss into the lumen, resulting in diarrhoea
  - changed resorption (including increased resorption of some substances, which must be considered if drugs are administered orally)
- risk of sepsis.

Late effects include chronic ulcers, based on an orchestrated response of all intestinal wall components, plus mechanical/chemical stress from faeces, as well as infections. Fibrotic remodelling may result in stenosis and ileus. Frequently, telangiectasia are found, which may result in bleeding.

It has been demonstrated experimentally by inhibition of pancreatic secretion by somatostatin analogues that pancreatic enzymes contribute to the manifestation of the early effect. Interestingly, this treatment also reduces late fibrosis, underlining the consequential nature of chronic changes in the intestine.

Liver

The liver is radiosensitive, with a tolerance dose of around 30 Gy in 2-Gy fractions. However, liver tolerance is only dose-limiting when the whole organ is irradiated (see Chapter 14, Section 14.5). An example is total-body irradiation preceding bone marrow transplantation. In this situation, the lung is well known as a dose-limiting organ, but liver and kidney are also at risk, especially after regimes equivalent to single doses of 10 Gy or higher.

Two phases of radiation hepatopathy are recognized, with acute radiation hepatitis being the more dominant. This acute phase develops approximately 2–6 weeks after irradiation, with signs of liver enlargement and ascites. Liver function tests during this period are abnormal. Acute hepatitis usually presents as veno-occlusive disease (VOD), characterized by central vein thrombosis whereby occlusion of the centrilobular veins causes atrophy and loss of the surrounding hepatocytes. Total liver VOD is usually lethal.

Chronic hepatopathy, which obviously can develop only after partial organ irradiation, has a variable latency ranging from 6 months to more than a year post-irradiation, and shows progressive fibrotic changes in both centrilobular and periportal areas. These alterations are accompanied by blood-flow redistribution through recanalization or newly formed veins, and regenerative proliferation of hepatocytes and bile ducts.

Upper respiratory tract

The mucosa of nose, paranasal sinuses and trachea respond to irradiation similarly to oral epithelium, but appear to be slightly more radioresistant.

Early changes in the larynx are oedema and perichondritis. Doses above 50 Gy may result in a long-lasting impairment of the quality of the voice, which must be considered in patients depending on their voice in their professional life.

Lung

In the lung, two separate radiation syndromes can be distinguished clinically: early pneumonitis, usually observed at 4–6 weeks after the end of radiotherapy, and fibrosis, which develops slowly over a period of several months to years. The lung is among the most sensitive of late-responding organs, but with a pronounced volume effect (see Chapter 14). In addition to a reduction in irradiated volume, reduced doses per fraction are most effective in avoiding severe (clinically manifest) lung reactions.

Clinical signs or symptoms of radiation pneumonitis are reduced pulmonary compliance, progressive dyspnoea, decreased gas exchange and dry cough. When there is insufficient functional reserve, cardiorespiratory failure may occur within a short time. The development of chronic radiation pneumopathy (i.e. lung fibrosis) follows the general pathways described in Section 13.3. The complexity of the signalling cascades is illustrated in Fig. 13.10. Local fibrotic responses must be expected in all patients with early reactions, indicating a strong consequential component of the late reaction (Dörr et al., 2005a). Higher age and tamoxifen treatment significantly increase the incidence of early pneumopathy.

Kidney

The kidney is among the most sensitive of the late-responding critical organs. Radiation damage develops very slowly and may take years to be recognized. Radiation nephropathy usually manifests as proteinuria, hypertension and impairment in urine concentration. Anaemia is usually present, and has been attributed both to haemolysis and to a decreased production of erythropoietin. A mild form of nephritis, presenting only as a sustained proteinuria, may be observed over a period of many years. Parts of one or both kidneys can

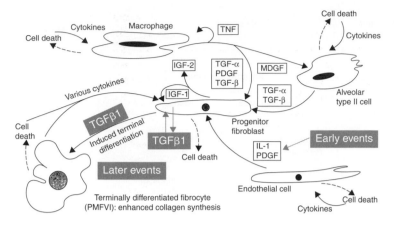

Figure 13.10 Possible cellulae interactions and events after irradiation of lung tissue. IGF, insulin-like growth factor; IL-1, interleukin 1; MGDF, megakaryocyte growth and development factor; PDGF, platelet-derived growth factor; TNF, tumour necrosis factor. Modified from Rodemann and Bamberg (1995), with permission.

receive much higher doses without affecting excretory function. However, after partial kidney irradiation hypertension may develop after a latent period of up to or beyond 10 years.

The fractionation sensitivity of the kidney is high (i.e. the α/β ratio is low). The dose tolerated by the kidney does not increase with increasing time after radiotherapy, but declines because of a continuous progression of damage, after doses well below the threshold for induction of functional deficit, which usually precludes re-irradiation (see Chapter 19, Section 19.3).

The pathogenesis of radiation nephropathy is complex. Most studies suggest glomerular endothelial injury as the start of a cascade leading to glomerular sclerosis and later tubulo-interstitial fibrosis. Several experimental studies have shown the importance of the renin–angiotensin system in the induction of glomerular sclerosis via upregulation of plasminogen activator inhibitor 1 (PAI-1) and enhanced fibrin deposition. Owing to loss of tubular epithelial cells, fibrin may then leak into the interstitium causing the onset of tubulo-interstitial fibrosis.

Urinary bladder

In patients, two phases of radiation-induced changes in the urinary bladder are observed, with both a reduction in bladder storage capacity and a consequential increase in micturition frequency. An early phase occurs 2–6 weeks after the start of

fractionated irradiation, which is characterized morphologically by hyperaemia and mucosal oedema. Experimentally, in mice, two waves of early injury have been observed. Mechanistically, the first phase seems to be related to direct radiation-induced changes of the prostaglandin metabolism (which regulates the tone of the bladder wall), as suggested by the beneficial effect of aspirin when administered during this phase. The second early phase is associated with changes in urothelial barrier function, but without epithelial cell depletion (which is not expected at this time because of the very long turnover time of the urothelium). Infection may complicate this early response, which then may progress to desquamation and ulceration.

A chronic phase develops with latent times that are inversely dose-dependent and can range up to 10 years or longer. The morphological correlate in the initial late phase is a progressive mucosal breakdown, ranging from superficial denudation to ulceration and even the formation of fistulae. The urothelial changes are accompanied by urothelial areas of compensatory hyperproliferation. Vascular changes and signs of local ischaemia have been described. These processes progress into secondary fibrosis of the bladder wall. Telangiectasia can result in severe bleeding episodes.

The early changes clearly correlate with the chronic radiation sequelae, illustrating a strong consequential component. A schematic illustration of the sequence of events leading to late fibrosis, as concluded from animal studies, is given in Fig. 13.11.

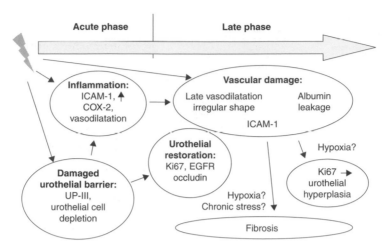

Figure 13.11 Pathogenesis of radiation effects in the urinary bladder. The individual processes have been studied in mouse urinary bladder after single dose irradiation. Morphological changes were related to functional impairment as assessed by transurethral cystometry. COX-2, cyclooxygenase-2; EFGR, epidermal growth factor receptor; ICAM-1, intercellular adhesion molecule-1; UP-III, uroplakin III. Modified with permission from Jall (2006).

Nervous system

The nervous system is less sensitive to radiation injury than some other late-responding tissues such as the lung or kidney. However, damage to this organ results in severe consequences such as paralysis: although tolerance doses are often quoted at the 5 per cent complication level (TD5) they generally are chosen to include a wide margin of safety.

A schematic outline of the development of various delayed lesions in the CNS as studied in animals is given in Fig. 13.12.

BRAIN

The most important radiation syndromes in the CNS develop a few months to several years after therapy. The often-used separation into early or late delayed injury is not very useful, as different types of lesions with overlapping time-distributions occur. Some reactions occurring within the first 6 months comprise transient demyelination ('somnolence syndrome') or the much more severe leukoencephalopathy. The more typical radiation necrosis may also occur by 6 months, but even after as long as 2–3 years. Histopathologically, changes that occur within the first year are mostly

restricted to the white matter. For times beyond 6–12 months, the grey matter usually also shows changes along with more pronounced vascular lesions (telangiectasia and focal haemorrhages). Radionecrosis of the brain with latent times between 1 and 2 years usually shows a mixture of histological characteristics.

The brain of children is more sensitive than in adults. Functional deficits, such as a reduction in IQ, can at least partly be attributed to radiotherapy.

SPINAL CORD

Radiation-induced changes in the spinal cord are similar to those in the brain in terms of latent period, histology and tolerance dose. Among the relatively early syndromes, the Lhermitte sign is a frequently occurring, usually reversible type of demyelinating reaction, which develops several months after completion of treatment and lasts for a few months to more than a year. It may occur at doses as low as 35 Gy in 2-Gy fractions, well below tolerance for permanent radiation myelopathy, when long segments of cord are irradiated, and does not predict for later development of permanent myelopathy.

As in the brain, the later types of myelopathy include two main syndromes. The first, occurring

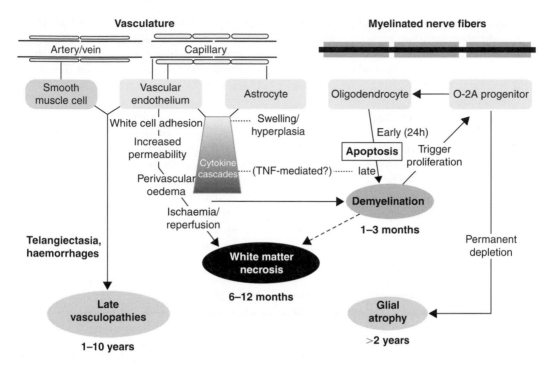

Figure 13.12 Schematic outline of tissue components and cell types and their potential role in the pathophysiology of radiation-induced lesions in the central nervous system. From van der Kogel (1991), with permission.

from about 6–18 months, is mostly limited to demyelination and necrosis of the white matter, whereas the second (with a latency of usually 1 to >4 years) is mostly a vasculopathy. The tolerance dose of the spinal cord largely depends on the size of the dose per fraction: variations in overall treatment time up to 10–12 weeks have a negligible effect in conventional schedules using one fraction per day (see Chapter 11). For longer times or intervals, substantial recovery occurs which has important implications for retreatment (see Chapter 19, Section 19.3).

PERIPHERAL NERVES

Radiation effects in peripheral nerves, mainly plexuses and nerve roots, are probably more common than effects in the spinal cord but are less well documented. Peripheral nerves are often quoted as being more resistant to radiation than the cord or the brain, but this view is not well supported by clinical data. As is the case for all nervous tissues, a dose of 60 Gy in 2-Gy fractions is associated with a less than 5 per cent probability

of injury, but this probability rises steeply with increasing radiation dose.

The brachial plexus is often included in treatments of the axillary and supraclavicular nodes in breast cancer patients. Clinically, plexopathy is characterized by mixed sensory and motor deficits, developing after a latent period ranging from 6 months to several years. The pathogenesis involves progressive vascular degeneration, fibrosis and demyelination with loss of nerve fibres.

Heart

In the heart, low doses can result in reversible functional changes in electrocardiogram (ECG), which are not predictive for late radiation sequelae. At higher doses, morphological changes can be observed. The most common type of radiation-induced heart effect is pericarditis with a variable degree of pericardial effusion. This complication has a relatively early onset (about 50 per cent occurrence within the first 6 months, remainder within 2 years). It is asymptomatic and clears spontaneously in the majority of patients.

Radiation-induced cardiomyopathy is another form of complication that presents either as reduced ventricular ejection or conduction blocks and develops slowly over a period of 10–20 years. Current estimates of doses giving a 50 per cent complication probability are approximately 50 Gy in 2-Gy fractions. With long-term follow-up of patients treated for Hodgkin's disease or breast cancer, the enhanced risk of ischaemic heart disease after periods in excess of 10 years has increasingly been reported. The large variation in risk estimates reported in different studies suggests that volume effects are important, but also that sensitive substructures are present. In this respect the heart auricles and the proximal parts of the coronary arteries have been suggested to be particularly sensitive to radiation damage.

Histopathologically, late damage to the myocardium is characterized predominantly by diffuse interstitial and perivascular fibrosis, and loss of cardiomyocytes. Vascular radiation effects also contribute significantly to myocardial infarction after radiation exposure of the heart. However, the (molecular) pathophysiology of these effects at present remains unclear.

Cartilage and bone

Growing cartilage (epiphysial plate) is extremely radiosensitive; single doses of 4–7 Gy are sufficient to induce changes in chondrocytes within a few days, with a loss of the columnar structure and a reduction in cellular density. The reduced cell production translates into (bone) growth impairment, which is more pronounced at earlier age. In contrast, adult cartilage (e.g. in joints, larynx or trachea), as well as adult bone, is relatively radiation resistant. However, late effects in these structures, including osteoradionecrosis, must be considered as an interaction with vascular radiation effects.

Sense organs

EYE

Inclusion of the eye into the high-dose volume results in keratoconjunctivitis, which, however, resolves soon after the end of radiotherapy. In the eye lens, epithelial degeneration in the equator zone, where proliferation occurs physiologically, is observed after low radiation doses. The damaged fibres develop vacuolization and partly retain their nuclei. Eventually, a usually posterior subcapsular radiation cataract develops in varying degrees. The latent times are inversely related to dose, and range from 6 months to several decades (hence frequently preventing evaluation by the radiation oncologist). The tolerance doses usually reported are in the range of 4–5 Gy for fractionated irradiation and around 1 Gy for single-dose exposure. However, more recent epidemiological studies indicate a clearly lower tolerance. A fractionation effect seems to be pronounced for the eye lens, but no long-term restoration can be expected.

As cataracts can readily be treated with modern surgical techniques (although with significant postoperative complication rates), late effects in the lachrymal glands (loss of function) and consequently in the cornea, depicted as 'dry eye', are becoming more important and dose-limiting. After moderate radiation doses, these can result in chronic corneal ulceration and loss of the eye.

EAR

The most frequent early radiation effect in the ear is a serous inflammation (otitis media), which affects hearing function. In addition, doses >30 Gy result in direct effects in the inner ear, with the consequence of permanent hearing impairment.

TASTE

Radiation effects on taste acuity are a multifactorial process, including direct changes (cell loss) in taste buds, xerostomia with reduced cleansing of the buds and changes in smelling ability. Taste impairment is usually observed after doses of around 30 Gy. Usually, the changes in the individual taste qualities resolve after radiotherapy, in intervals up to 1 year, but a general increase in threshold concentration may remain.

Key points

1. Early radiation effects, developing in turnover tissues, are dominated by tissue hypoplasia.
2. The latent time of early effects is largely independent of dose, while severity and duration are dose dependent.
3. Additional trauma aggravates early reactions.
4. Healing of early responses, based on surviving stem cells, is usually complete.
5. Late radiation sequelae, observed after months to years after therapy, are progressive and irreversible.
6. Late effects are based on an interactive response of parenchymal cells, vascular endothelium and fibroblasts, with a contribution of macrophages and other cells.
7. The latent time of chronic reactions is inversely dependent on dose.

■ BIBLIOGRAPHY

Bentzen SM (2006). Preventing or reducing late side effects of radiation therapy: radiobiology meets molecular pathology. *Nat Rev Cancer* **6**: 702–13.

Bentzen SM, Turesson I, Thames HD (1990). Fractionation sensitivity and latency of telangiectasia after postmastectomy radiotherapy: a graded-response analysis. *Radiother Oncol* **18**: 95–106.

Bentzen SM, Saunders MI, Dische S, Bond SJ (2001). Radiotherapy-related early morbidity in head and neck cancer: quantitative clinical radiobiology as deduced from the CHART trial. *Radiother Oncol* **60**: 123–35.

Dittmann K, Mayer C, Rodemann HP (2005). Inhibition of radiation-induced EGFR nuclear import by C225 (Cetuximab) suppresses DNA-PK activity. *Radiother Oncol* **76**: 157–61.

Dörr W (1997). Three As of repopulation during fractionated irradiation of squamous epithelia: Asymmetry loss, Acceleration of stem-cell divisions and Abortive divisions. *Int J Radiat Biol* **72**: 635–43.

Dörr W, Hendry JH (2001). Consequential late effects in normal tissues. *Radiother Oncol* **61**: 223–31.

Dörr W, Herrmann T (2003). Pathogenetic mechanisms of lung fibrosis. In: Nieder C, Milas L, Ang KK (eds) *Biological modification of radiation response*. Berlin: Springer, 29–36.

Dörr W, Kummermehr J (1991). Proliferation kinetics of mouse tongue epithelium under normal conditions and following single dose irradiation. *Virchows Arch B Cell Pathol Incl Mol Pathol* **60**: 287–94.

Dörr W, Bertmann S, Herrmann T (2005a). Radiation induced lung reactions in breast cancer therapy. Modulating factors and consequential effects. *Strahlenther Onkol* **181**: 567–73.

Dörr W, Herrmann T, Riesenbeck D (eds) (2005b). *Prävention und therapie von nebenwirkungen in der strahlentherapie*. Bremen: UNI-MED Science.

Fajardo LF, Berthrong M, Anderson RE (2001). *Radiation pathology*. New York: Oxford University Press.

Hakenjos L, Bamberg M, Rodemann HP (2000). TGF-beta1-mediated alterations of rat lung fibroblast differentiation resulting in the radiation-induced fibrotic phenotype. *Int J Radiat Biol* **76**: 503–9.

Herrmann T, Baumann M, Dörr W (2006). *Klinische strahlenbiologie – kurz und bündig*, 4th edn. Munich: Elsevier.

Horiot JC, Bontemps P, van den Bogaert W *et al.* (2006). Accelerated Fractionation (AF) compared to Conventional Fractionation (CF) improves loco-regional control in the radio therapy of advanced head and neck cancers: results of the EORTC 22851 randomized trial. *Radiother Oncol* **44**: 111–21.

Jaal J (2006). *Radiation effects in the urinary bladder (mouse): histopathologic features and modification by recombinant human keratinocyte growth factor*, Thesis, Technische Universität Dresden.

Jung H, Beck-Bornholdt HP, Svoboda V, Alberti W, Herrmann T (2001). Quantification of late complications after radiation therapy. *Radiother Oncol* **61**: 233–46.

Potten CS, Hendry JH (eds) (1983). *Cytotoxic insults to tissues: effects on cell lineages*. Edinburgh: Churchill-Livingstone.

Rodemann HP, Bamberg M (1995). Cellular basis of radiation-induced fibrosis. *Radiother Oncol* **35**: 83–90.

Rubin P, Johnston CJ, Williams JP, McDonald S, Finkelstein JN (1995). A perpetual cascade of cytokines postirradiation leads to pulmonary fibrosis. *Int J Radiat Oncol Biol Phys* **33**: 99–109.

Schultz-Hector S (1992). Radiation-induced heart disease: review of experimental data on dose response and pathogenesis. *Int J Radiat Biol* **61**: 149–60.

Sonis ST (2004). A biological approach to mucositis. *J Support Oncol* **2**: 21–32.

Turesson I (1990). Individual variation and dose dependency in the progression rate of skin telangiectasia. *Int J Radiat Oncol Biol Phys* **19**: 1569–74.

van der Kogel AJ (1991). Central nervous system radiation injury in small animal models. In: Gutin PH, Leibel SA, Sheline GE (eds) *Radiation injury to the nervous system*. New York: Raven Press, 91–111.

van der Schueren E, van den Bogaert W, Vanuytsel L, van Limbergen E (1990). Radiotherapy by multiple fractions per day (MFD) in head and neck cancer: acute reactions of skin and mucosa. *Int J Radiat Oncol Biol Phys* **19**: 301–11.

Withers HR, Elkind MM (1970). Microcolony survival assay for cells of mouse intestinal mucosa exposed to radiation. *Int J Radiat Biol* **17**: 261–7.

Withers HR, Taylor JM, Maciejewski B (1988). Treatment volume and tissue tolerance. *Int J Radiat Oncol Biol Phys* **14**: 751–9.

Brown JM, Mehta MP, Nieder C (eds) (2006). *Multimodal concepts for integration of cytotoxic drugs and radiation therapy*. Berlin: Springer.

Dörr W (ed.) (2001). *Growth factors in the pathogenesis of radiation effects in normal tissues*. Munich: Urban and Vogel.

Dörr W (2006). Skin and other reactions to radiotherapy – clinical presentation and radiobiology of skin reactions. *Front Radiat Ther Oncol* **39**: 96–101.

Grötz KA, Riesenbeck D, Brahm R *et al.* (2001). Chronic radiation effects on dental hard tissue (radiation caries). Classification and therapeutic strategies. *Strahlenther Onkol* **177**: 96–104.

National Cancer Institute, Washington DC, USA (2006). *Common terminology criteria for adverse events v3.0 (CTCAE)*. http://ctep.cancer.gov/forms/CTCAEv3.pdf

Pavy JJ, Denekamp J, Letschert J *et al.* (1995). EORTC Late Effects Working Group. Late effects toxicity scoring: the SOMA scale. *Radiother Oncol* **35**: 11–5.

■ FURTHER READING

Bentzen SM, Dörr W, Anscher MS *et al.* (2003). Normal tissue effects: reporting and analysis. *Semin Radiat Oncol* **13**: 189–202.

The volume effect in radiotherapy

WOLFGANG DÖRR AND ALBERT J. VAN DER KOGEL

14.1 INTRODUCTION

Volume specifications in radiotherapy (Fig. 14.1) are described in publications 50 and 62 of the International Commission on Radiation Units and Measurements (ICRU, 1999). Even the smallest volume, the gross tumour volume (GTV), contains normal tissue elements (e.g. blood vessels and normal connective tissue) within the tumour. In addition, the clinical target volume (CTV) encompasses a relevant number of normal parenchymal cells of the respective organ, intermingled between the suspected tumour cells. The volume difference between the CTV and the treated volume (TV) – the volume enclosed by a surface of the clinically effective isodose – is exclusively composed of normal tissue. In all these normal cells and structures, radiation side-effects may be induced. However, all the normal tissues within the TV are unavoidably exposed to the entire tumour dose, which therefore may be limited by the normal tissue volume, depending on the size of the TV.

In contrast, the irradiated volume (IV), which receives a dose that is considered significant with regard to normal tissue tolerance, is dependent on the physical parameters of the radiation delivery, for example the type and quality of the radiation (photons, electrons, protons, energy), mode of radiotherapy (brachytherapy, conformal teletherapy, intensity-modulated radiotherapy) and treatment planning (number of fields, etc.). Technological improvements in the physical administration of radiotherapy have led to increasing conformation of the TV with the planning target volume (PTV) and of the IV with the TV. In this process of improvement of the quality of radiotherapy, the volumes of organs at risk exposed to significant doses has significantly decreased, resulting in increased inhomogeneities in the dose distributions within these organs. This has increased the importance of identifying volume effects in normal tissues.

The volume of tissue irradiated can be an important determinant of clinical tolerance without having any influence on tissue sensitivity per unit volume. An example of this is skin or mucosal ulceration. If this occurs over a large area, the ulcer will lead to pain and will heal only slowly. A small area of ulceration, by contrast, may lead only to minor discomfort and will heal more rapidly. In

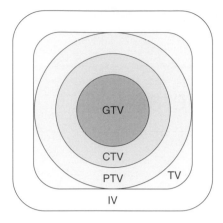

Figure 14.1 Volume definitions in radiotherapy according to the International Commission on Radiation Units and Measurements (ICRU, 1999) Report 62 (ICRU, 1999). GTV, gross tumour volume (detectable tumour volume); CTV, clinical target volume (GTV plus volumes with expected subclinical spread); PTV, planning target volume (CTV plus safety margin for movements or deformations of CTV, technical uncertainties, etc.); TV, treatment volume (receiving the prescribed dose); IV, irradiated volume (that is exposed to significant doses with regard to normal tissue tolerance).

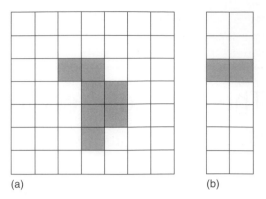

Figure 14.2 (a) Parallel and (b) serial organization of functional subunits (FSUs) in normal tissues. In parallel organized tissues (a), a critical number of functional subunits must be damaged before a clinical response (i.e. loss of function) becomes manifest (threshold volume), although structural damage may be diagnosed in individual FSUs. In contrast, in serial organs (b), failure of only one FSU results in a loss of function of the entire organ. Adapted from Withers et al. (1988), with permission from Elsevier.

this situation the clinical tolerance is strongly dependent on irradiated volume although structural tolerance is not. There is very little evidence for any increase in cellular radiosensitivity when the irradiated volume is increased, either in skin or in other tissues. However, the pathology underlying the same clinical changes may change with dose, as has been demonstrated for lung (Novakova-Jiresova et al., 2007).

14.2 TOLERANCE DOSE IN RELATION TO TISSUE ARCHITECTURE

Withers et al. (1988) originally introduced the concept of tissue radiation tolerance based on functional subunits (FSUs), which may be considered as anatomical structures such as bronchioli, or simply as tissue stem cells. Per definition, a FSU is the largest tissue volume, or unit of cells, that can be regenerated from a single surviving clonogenic cell. Functional subunits are sterilized independently by irradiation. This results in structural damage within the exposed volume. The number of FSUs that are sterilized, and hence the severity of the damage, depends on their intrinsic radiosensitivity, and on dose and other radiobiological parameters, such as fractionation (see Chapter 5) or overall treatment time (see Chapter 11). With suitable procedures (e.g. radiological imaging) the changes can be diagnosed.

However, the clinical consequences are dependent on the arrangement of the FSU within the exposed organ (Fig. 14.2). Similar to the connection of elements in an electrical circuit, the FSU can be arranged either in parallel or in series. In organs with a parallel structure (Fig. 14.2a), FSUs function independently. Hence, a clinical radiation effect is observed only if the number of surviving FSUs is too low to sustain the physiological organ function. Hence, a threshold volume must be considered in treatment planning, which must not be exceeded but within which large doses may be administered. The risk of complications depends on the distribution of the total dose within the organ rather than on individual 'hot spots'. Examples of organs with a (predominantly) parallel architecture are lung, kidney, and liver.

In contrast, in organs with a serial (or 'tubular') architecture (Fig. 14.2b), the function of the entire organ depends on the function of each individual FSU; inactivation of only one FSU results in clinical side-effects in a binary response. In these organs, the risk of complications is highly dependent on 'hot spots', while the dose distribution within the entire organ is less relevant. Examples of (mainly) serially structured organs are spinal cord, intestine and oesophagus.

The purely parallel or serial organization of an organ, however, represents the extreme cases. In reality, no organ is organized simply as a chain of FSUs. Moreover, as described in Chapter 13, Section 13.3, one component of late radiation effects is the response of the (micro)vasculature, and individual small vessels may be considered as serially arranged, which introduces a serial factor into parallel arranged tissues. This has led to the concept of a variable seriality factor of organs, which has been incorporated into the mathematical modelling of volume effects (Källman et al., 1992). The modelling of volume effects on the basis of their serial or parallel organization is useful and explains the apparent paradox that relatively radiosensitive organs, such as kidney and lung, can sustain the loss of more than half their total mass without significant loss of function, whereas relatively radioresistant tissues such as spinal cord can be functionally inactivated by the irradiation of only a small volume.

The relative seriality model, as well as other models for the definition of normal tissue complication probabilities (NTCP), does not take into account the influence of cellular migration and regeneration from outside the irradiated area (Section 14.3) or other factors such as regional differences in radiation sensitivity within one organ, which have been demonstrated in lung, urinary bladder or parotid gland. Therefore, these models should be used with caution.

Many organs, such as the brain, are better described by an intermediate type of organizational structure which is neither serial/tubular nor parallel. Specific areas of the brain perform specific functions. The clinical tolerance of brain tissue is therefore much more dependent on which area of brain is irradiated than the total volume irradiated. Damage to even a small area may lead to permanent loss of the particular function controlled by that area, since the undamaged parts of the brain are unable to take over these functions, although other brain functions may be unaffected. Similarly, the eye is an organ with many very different tissues and structures, and hence displays volume characteristics similar to those of the brain.

14.3 MATHEMATICAL MODELLING OF VOLUME EFFECTS

Theoretical models have been developed to estimate NTCP for partial-volume irradiations and inhomogeneous dose distributions. Models using power-law functions were the earliest and were followed by models with a more biophysical basis.

In the model of Lyman (1985), a power-law relationship was assumed between the tolerance dose for uniform whole- or partial-organ irradiation, where the parameter n (the exponent of the partial volume) describes the volume dependence of the tolerance dose. When $n \to 1.0$ then the volume effect is large and the tolerance dose increases steeply with decreasing volume, and when $n \to 0$ then the volume effect is small. The Lyman model has been extended to inhomogeneous irradiation by converting the original dose–volume histogram (DVH) into an equivalent DVH for uniform irradiation, usually by the effective-volume method (Kutcher and Burman, 1989). The resulting so-called Lyman–Kutcher–Burman (LKB) model is currently one of the most commonly used models for predicting normal-tissue complication probability.

Intermediate between the purely empirical and more biophysically based models is the *relative seriality model* of Källman et al. (1992). In this model, an extra parameter, s (the 'degree of seriality'), is introduced to describe the functional organization of a tissue (Section 14.2). A near-zero value of s represents a parallel structure and an s value close to unity represents an organ with a serial organization.

The first model, which assumed that an organ can be divided into physiologically discrete compartments or FSUs, was the integral response model (Withers et al., 1988). This model allows for the spatial distribution of FSUs in the tissue to be non-uniform. The radiation response of each independent FSU is determined by Poisson statistics and the functional architecture of FSUs determines the organ's response to partial volume irradiation (see Section 14.2).

In the concept of the equivalent uniform dose (EUD), inhomogeneous dose distributions within one organ are converted to a homogeneous dose, which would result in the same cell survival. Hence, the concept is dependent on survival parameters of tissue stem cells, clonogenic cells, or tissue-rescuing units. This might be applicable for early radiation effects. However, late radiation effects are based on a variety of target cells (see Chapter 13, Section 13.3), and the estimates of EUD must hence be considered to be empirical rather than biology-based.

Clinical application of dose–volume models

Modern developments in the high-precision delivery of radiation, particularly intensity-modulated radiotherapy (IMRT) and tomotherapy, or administration of protons or heavy ions, have stimulated clinical trials on dose escalation, notably in lung and prostate. Data are now available for tolerance to partial-organ irradiation at doses well above the levels that were previously established. The new data obtained from prospective dose-escalation studies, combined with precise knowledge of dose-distributions and dose–volume histograms, should in the future allow the derivation of more realistic parameters and a validation of mathematical models used for describing volume effects. However, there are many limitations and uncertainties in current multiparameter models and it seems unlikely that the biologically based models will quickly replace the relatively simple empirical models such as the LKB probability model.

With the rapid implementation of conformal three-dimensional radiation therapy (3D-RT), dose–volume histograms have proved useful as a tool for the evaluation and comparison of treatment plans. However, despite ample clinical data for some organs, it remains unclear which of the

DVH-derived parameters is optimal for the prediction of NTCP, as has recently been demonstrated for lung by Rodrigues *et al.* (2004). Moreover, the loss of information on the spatial dose-distribution in a DVH is a serious constraint in determining the relationship between local tissue damage and overall morbidity. A high-dose region in the histogram may represent a single hot-spot in the volume of interest or a number of smaller hot-spots from contiguous regions or from different regions. These could have quite different implications for tissue tolerance. Dose–volume histograms also do not differentiate between functionally or anatomically different subregions or compartments within an organ, such as in brain or eye (Section 14.2). This becomes particularly relevant if variations in radiosensitivity and/or functional consequences within the organ are evident, such as in lung, kidney, urinary bladder, parotid gland, or particularly in the eye and the brain.

The models are based on tissue-specific tolerance doses and fractionation parameters, such as the α/β ratio or even halftimes for recovery of sublethal damage. For tolerance doses the compilation by Emami *et al.* (1991) is frequently used; However, the numbers in this paper are not wholly based on clinical or even experimental data, but on 'opinions and experience of the clinicians from four universities', and hence even now require validation in clinical studies. The fractionation parameters for various endpoints in human tissues, as well as for experimental endpoints (see Chapters 8 and 9), usually have been defined with broad confidence intervals (i.e. with a significant uncertainty), which is not considered in the models. If a parameter for the overall treatment time is included, this does not take into account the complexity of the underlying processes and their consequences (see Chapter 11), for example the dose-dependence of dose compensation, and the time to onset of repopulation and its dynamics. Moreover, none of the models yet considers out-of-field effects.

Importantly, the NTCP models also do not account for the functional status of the unirradiated organ volume. For example, lung function in heavy smokers can be substantially impaired, and the usually accepted tolerance limits should thus be significantly lowered. Similar effects can occur with impaired liver function, or with haemorrhoids that may influence the radiation tolerance of the rectum. In general, previous or additional chemotherapy also has a potential to impair the function of the unirradiated organ volume. Consideration of the impact of functional impairment of unirradiated tissue on the tolerance limits for radiotherapy must be subject to the experience and expert knowledge of the responsible radiation oncologist. Similar to functionally inoperable patients, 'functionally unirradiatable' patients can be identified.

The available models, which are even being integrated into some treatment-planning systems, should therefore be used with great caution and with a clear understanding of all their pitfalls and drawbacks. They should be regarded as an aid to the evaluation and comparison of clinical data using different treatment set-ups, rather than giving accurate predictions of clinical outcome.

14.4 EFFECT OF TISSUE STEM CELLS OUTSIDE THE TREATMENT VOLUME

An important factor in the influence of irradiated volume on radiation effects is the migration of unirradiated clonogenic cells. The most prominent example is the bone marrow. After complete sterilization of the stem and precursor cells in a fraction of active marrow, this volume – provided that the supportive structures are regenerated can be repopulated by haematopoietic stem cells that are present in the circulation, or recruited from unirradiated bone marrow. Other examples are epithelial tissues with a high cellular migratory capacity, such as skin, oral mucosa or intestinal epithelium, which exhibit a steep increase in tolerance as the irradiated field-size decreases to small areas (see Section 14.5). This type of volume effect is also seen in some other tissues with a relatively linear or tubular structural organization (e.g. spinal cord). However, none of the existing NTCP models incorporates such effects and hence is capable of adequately describing the volume effect data, the spinal cord being a good example.

Repopulation from neighbouring subunits is much less likely in tissues with a parallel type of arrangement of the FSUs with long migratory distances between FSUs, and has not been demonstrated in kidney or lung.

14.5 EXPERIMENTAL AND CLINICAL DATA FOR VOLUME EFFECTS IN INDIVIDUAL ORGANS

In this section, volume effects will be described for selected organs: lung, spinal cord, kidney, liver, intestinal tract, parotid gland and skin. Preclinical studies of the volume effect, if available, will be summarized for these organs. The literature on clinical dose–volume effects is expanding rapidly and examples of relevant clinical data will be cited where possible.

Lung

The influence of irradiated lung volume on structural and functional damage has been investigated experimentally in mice, rats, dogs and pigs. Most of these studies have focused on pneumonitis as the endpoint, and hence the data may not be wholly applicable to lung fibrosis. All studies demonstrate a pronounced volume effect for total lung function, with little or no symptomatic pneumonitis for partial irradiated volumes below 50 per cent. These volume effects depend on the compensatory capacity of the unirradiated tissue, which enables overall function to be maintained despite destruction of a substantial part of one lung (Herrmann et al., 1997). In contrast, local structural lung damage, assessed by radiography, histology or collagen content, is independent of the volume irradiated (Fig. 14.3). This indicates that cellular radiosensitivity is not influenced by the size of the irradiated volume, although the consequence of cell death for lung function is strongly dependent on volume.

Several prospective clinical studies have described the influence of a change in irradiated lung volume on local lung damage and on NTCP (reviewed in Mehta, 2005). Local structural and functional lung damage can be quantified using computed tomography (CT)-based lung-density distributions and single-photon emission

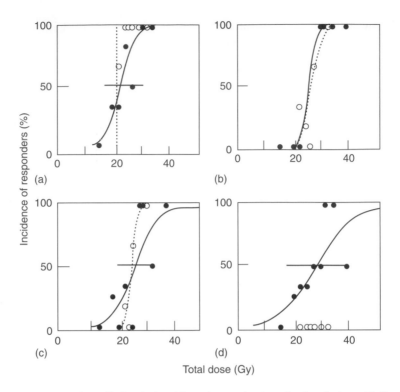

Figure 14.3 Dose–response curves for radiation-induced lung damage in pigs after irradiation with five fractions, given to half of the right lung (open circles) or to the whole right lung (filled circles). Damage was assessed from radiographic (X-ray) changes (a), histological evidence of fibrosis (b), elevated hydroxyproline (collagen) levels (c), or increased breathing rate (d). Only the functional endpoint demonstrated a volume effect. From Herrmann *et al.* (1997), with permission.

computed tomography (SPECT) ventilation and perfusion distributions. By matching pre- and post-treatment SPECT scans to the 3D dose distributions in the lung, changes in perfusion and ventilation can be quantified in relation to the locally delivered radiation dose (Fig. 14.4). For patients with malignant lymphoma and breast cancer, well-defined dose–response relationships have been determined for local changes in lung function per SPECT voxel (6 mm³ volume) in the irradiated areas, relative to the low-dose or un-irradiated regions (Fig. 14.5). These and other studies demonstrate that the magnitude of local, structural pulmonary changes is independent of the irradiated volume but does depend on patient-related factors such as concurrent chemotherapy, smoking and age.

In an extension of these studies, the observed incidence of radiation-induced pneumonitis can be related to the DVH for the irradiated lung. For this analysis, the complex 3D physical dose distribution is converted into a mean biological dose to the whole lung, after a normalization procedure using the linear-quadratic (LQ) model with α/β ratios of 2.5–3 Gy. This parameter, the 'mean normalized total lung dose', which does not include any critical-volume parameter, correlates well with the incidence of pneumonitis, as for example shown in a large series of 540 patients treated for malignant lymphoma, lung or breast cancer. Results on pneumonitis in 264 patients treated for lymphoma, lung and breast cancer from one institute are displayed in Fig. 14.6. Further studies have focused on other, simple parameters such as the

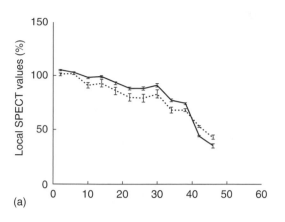

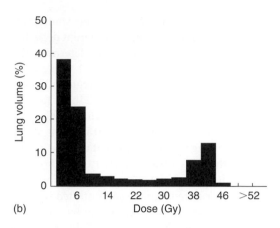

(a)

(b)

Figure 14.4 Dose–effect relationship for local lung perfusion (solid line) and ventilation (dashed line) at 3–4 months after irradiation, as a percentage of the pretreatment value, in a patient treated for malignant lymphoma (a). The corresponding dose–volume histogram of the three-dimensional dose distribution to the lung of this patient is shown in (b). From Boersma *et al.* (1994), with permission.

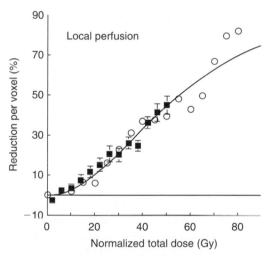

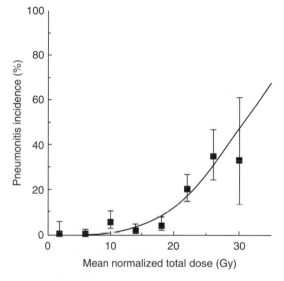

Figure 14.5 Dose–effect relationships for the average change in local lung function (i.e. perfusion) as a function of the normalized total dose. Data are shown from functional studies carried out at Duke University (circles) and The Netherlands Cancer Institute (squares). From Theuws *et al.* (1998) and including data from Marks *et al.* (1997), with permission from Elsevier.

Figure 14.6 Incidence of radiation pneumonitis as a function of mean normalized total dose to the whole lung. Pooled data are shown from a group of 264 patients with lung cancer, breast cancer or malignant lymphoma, treated in five different centres. The absolute number of patients contributing to each dose level is indicated. From Kwa *et al.* (1998), with permission from Elsevier.

percentage of total lung volume irradiated with defined doses (i.e. 20 Gy or 30 Gy), which hence incorporate a critical-volume component. These parameters can be used to predict the probability of radiation pneumonitis. In a comprehensive

review, Rodrigues *et al.* (2004) demonstrated that the ideal parameter for estimation of the NTCP for pneumonitis from DVH, despite ample data and studies, has not yet been identified. This raises serious doubts of whether further studies on patients treated with a range of different dose distributions will ever be sufficient to determine the best approach.

A few studies have investigated regional differences in radiation sensitivity of the lung. Experiments in mice demonstrate that functional damage is more prevalent after irradiation of the base of the lung than an equivalent volume irradiation of the apex (Travis *et al.*, 1997). This may indicate that functional subunits are not homogeneously distributed, but are concentrated in basal areas. Cytokine release from partial liver irradiation, included in the basal lung field, may also contribute to these field localization effects. However, studies in pigs have not demonstrated differences in cellular damage in apical versus basal parts of the lung. Data from clinical studies are controversial.

In summarizing the clinical data available (Bentzen *et al.*, 2000), tolerance limits for unaffected lung may be defined by the ratio of total volume of both lungs (V_{tot}) to the volume exposed to doses >25 Gy (V_{25}). If this ratio, V_{25}:V_{tot} is greater than 50 per cent, then pneumonitis can be dose limiting, or pneumonitis is not relevant. The mean lung dose for a 5 per cent incidence of pneumonitis is in the order of 15 Gy. No conclusive data are available for fibrotic reactions.

Spinal cord

LENGTH OF IRRADIATED SPINAL CORD

A marked volume effect for irradiation of very short lengths of spinal cord (<1 cm), and less pronounced or no volume effects for cord lengths <2 cm, have been demonstrated in rats, pigs, monkeys and dogs. This suggests migration of tissue-restoring cells, with only a limited migration distance, from outside the irradiated volume (Section 14.4).

In rat spinal cord, a very steep rise in ED_{50} (i.e. the radiation dose at which white-matter necrosis and myelopathy are expected in 50 per cent of treated animals) was observed when the irradiated cord length was reduced below 10 mm (Fig. 14.7). For irradiation of cord lengths between 10 and

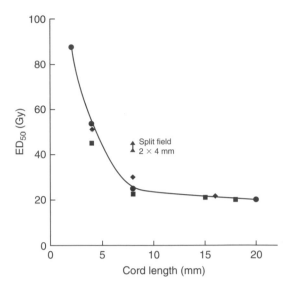

Figure 14.7 The influence of field size on biological response in rat spinal cord after single-dose irradiation with small fields. A steep rise in ED_{50} occurs as field size is reduced below 10 mm, with very little change in ED_{50} for larger field-sizes. The single fields were centred around C4, the two concomitant 4-mm fields were at C1/C2 and C7/T1, separated by approximately 10 mm. Data show the ED_{50} for induction of white-matter necrosis. From Hopewell and Trott (2000) and Bijl *et al.* (2002, 2006), with permission.

30 mm, little change in ED_{50} was found. This observation has been confirmed by more detailed studies, exploiting a high-precision proton beam for irradiation (Bijl *et al.*, 2003): rats were irradiated with either a single field of 8 mm or two fields of 4 mm, separated by an unirradiated length of cord of 8 mm or 12 mm (Fig. 14.8). The ED_{50} for myelopathy with 2×4 mm fields was 42–45 Gy, which is less than 54 Gy for a single field of 4 mm, but considerably greater than the ED_{50} for 1×8 mm (25 Gy).

Single radiation doses given to 2.5-, 5- and 10-cm lengths of pig spinal cord showed only a small (*c.* 1 Gy) decrease in ED_{50} for induction of white-matter necrosis with increasing field size. At low probabilities of injury, which are clinically relevant, this difference was no longer significant (van den Aardweg *et al.*, 1995), similar to the results in the kidney (see below). The irradiated cord length

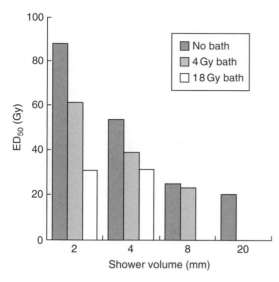

Figure 14.8 The influence of a surrounding low dose on the tolerance of a small high-dose volume ('bath and shower' irradiations) in the rat cervical spinal cord. The high-dose volumes of 2, 4 or 8 mm ('shower') were centred at C5, while the remainder of the 20-mm cervical cord was irradiated with a 'bath' dose of 4 Gy or 18 Gy. From Bijl *et al.* (2003, 2006), with permission from Elsevier.

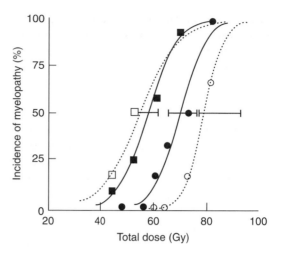

Figure 14.9 Influence of change in field size on spinal cord damage in dogs. Increasing the field size from 4 cm (circles) to 20 cm (squares) had a more marked influence on the development of neurological signs of injury (dotted lines) than on the occurrence of severe pathological lesions (solid lines). Redrawn from Powers *et al.* (1998), with permission.

also influenced the incidence of myelopathy in monkeys given fractionated irradiation (Schultheiss *et al.*, 1994). The incidence of myelopathy after a total dose of 70.2 Gy (2.2 Gy per fraction) increased from 15 per cent, to 20 per cent to 37.5 per cent for field sizes of 4, 8 and 16 cm, respectively.

In an extensive study in dogs (Powers *et al.*, 1998), irradiation of 4- and 20-cm lengths of spinal cord were compared using a fractionated schedule of 4 Gy per fraction. For functional, neurological symptoms, such as thoracic pain or paresis, a large increase in ED_{50} from 54 Gy for the large field to 78 Gy for the small field was found. In contrast, a much less pronounced increase was observed for morphological, necrotic lesions (Fig. 14.9). This again indicates the relevance of the endpoint studied for volume effects.

INFLUENCE OF DOSE SURROUNDING THE HIGH-DOSE VOLUME

The marked volume effect for irradiation of only very short lengths of spinal cord is clearly compromised when a small dose is given to the surrounding tissue. This has been demonstrated for rat spinal cord in 'bath-and-shower' experiments (Bijl *et al.*, 2003), where graded subtolerance doses ('bath') were given to a large segment (20 mm) of spinal cord and a high dose ('shower') was given to small segments of 2–8 mm in the centre of the low dose volume. The ED_{50} for a 4-mm field given 53 Gy alone was reduced to 39 Gy with a bath dose of only 4 Gy. For a 2-mm high-dose segment, the ED_{50} was reduced from 88 Gy to 61 Gy. Paralysis was based on necrotic lesions in the high-dose region whereas no histological changes were seen in the bath volume. The hypothesis to describe these observations was that migration of presumptive stem cells into the high-dose region was compromised by the bath dose.

In further experiments with the same model (Bijl *et al.*, 2003), the shower dose was placed at the edge rather than the centre of the low-dose segment. Assuming migration phenomena, the tolerance in this setup should be similar to that with high-dose irradiation alone (88 Gy) for a 2-mm shower segment. However, the observed ED_{50} was intermediate, at 69 Gy, indicating additional mechanisms underlying the volume effect for small cord lengths. It is important to note that none of the existing NTCP models take these non-local effects into account.

LATERAL DOSE DISTRIBUTION

With conformal radiotherapy, variations not only in the length of spinal cord irradiated but also in the lateral distribution of the dose can occur. These effects have also been studied in rats irradiated with high-precision proton beams (Bijl *et al.*, 2005). The left lateral half of the spinal cord was irradiated with a penumbra (20–80 per cent isodose) of 1.1 mm or 0.8 mm, or the midline of the cord with a penumbra of 0.8 mm. The irradiated length of spinal cord was 20 mm in all experiments. The resulting ED_{50} values for paralysis were 29 Gy and 33 Gy for lateral irradiation, respectively, and 72 Gy for midline irradiation; the corresponding homogeneous irradiation of a 20-mm cord segment resulted in an ED_{50} of 20 Gy. Hence, the grey matter is highly resistant to radiation as no lesions observable by light microscopy were induced, even after a single dose as high as 80 Gy; all lesions were restricted to white matter structures.

In a recent analysis of clinical data from single-dose radiosurgery of 230 vertebral column metastases in 177 patients (Ryu *et al.*, 2007), an average dose of 9.8 ± 1.5 Gy to 10 per cent of the spinal cord volume, given in single-dose radiosurgery, was associated with only one spinal cord injury in 86 patients surviving more than 1 year.

In summary, there is a clear volume effect for severe lesions in the spinal cord which lead to irreversible signs of myelopathy; this is most pronounced at high levels of injury. At low probabilities of injury (< 5 per cent), which usually define clinical tolerance doses, a volume effect may not be detectable and should have minimal impact on the clinical practice of maintaining spinal cord dose below 55 Gy. However, when clinical conditions require the choice of higher dose levels closer to tolerance, such as in a re-irradiation situation, the existence of a volume effect might be taken into consideration. The volume effect in the spinal cord is complex, with an impact of the surrounding dose as well as of the lateral dose distribution across the tissue. It must be emphasized that none of the existing NTCP models take this complexity into account.

Kidney

Volume effects in the irradiated kidney are strongly influenced by the duality of this organ and by its parallel organization, with a large reserve capacity. Unirradiated parts of one kidney and the contralateral kidney are able to undergo drastic post-irradiation hypertrophy and increase their performance to compensate for functional impairment within another part of the organ and thus maintain renal function.

Experiments in pigs (Robbins and Hopewell, 1988) have demonstrated that the individual function of a kidney after unilateral irradiation can actually be poorer than after irradiation of both kidneys with the same dose. Total renal function is, however, much less reduced after irradiation of only one kidney (Fig. 14.10). Interestingly, if the unirradiated kidney is removed after unilateral irradiation, the previously non-functional, irradiated kidney may be capable of partial restoration of glomerular filtration rate and effective renal plasma flow to maintain a viable level of total renal function. These experiments demonstrate that the functional response of a unilaterally irradiated kidney depends on the compensatory response in the unirradiated, contralateral organ. The presence and increased function of the unirradiated kidney may actually promote functional impairment, or inhibit functional recovery, in the irradiated kidney.

A pronounced volume effect was also observed in scintigraphic studies in 91 patients who received abdominal irradiation with various doses and to varying volumes (Köst *et al.*, 2002), but only at higher incidence levels for the loss of kidney function. The dose for a 5 per cent incidence was in the range of 3–6 Gy, independent of volume, owing to uncertainties in the dose–effect analysis. However, the doses estimated for a 50 per cent incidence clearly increased with decreasing kidney volume, from approximately 8 Gy for 100 per cent to 27 Gy for 10 per cent of the volume.

In a study in 44 patients receiving radio-chemotherapy for gastric cancer (Jansen *et al.*, 2007), where the left kidney was included in the

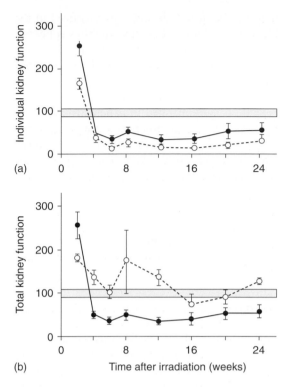

(a)

(b)

Time after irradiation (weeks)

Figure 14.10 Time-related changes in glomerular filtration rate in pigs in which one (open circles) or both (filled circles) kidneys were irradiated with a single dose of 12.6 Gy. (a) The change in individual kidney function, as a percentage of control values; (b) the total renal function in the same pigs. Redrawn from Robbins and Hopewell (1988), with permission from Elsevier.

high-dose radiotherapy volume, the V_{20} (left kidney) and mean left kidney dose were identified as parameters associated with decreased kidney function.

Liver

The liver is usually regarded as a prime example of a parallel-type organ, with liver acini as FSUs. Similar to lung, structural damage (i.e. loss of function within the irradiated volume) can be demonstrated with scintigraphy and other methods. Whole-liver irradiation with doses around 30 Gy (2 Gy per fraction) is generally associated

with the induction of 5–10 per cent hepatitis. Until the introduction of 3D treatment planning, the relationship between tolerance dose and partial volume irradiation was very conservatively interpreted. However, extensive clinical data on liver tolerance to partial organ irradiation has now been accumulated at the University of Michigan for more than 200 patients (Dawson and Ten Haken, 2005). LKB–NTCP analyses resulted in a large volume–effect parameter (the n-exponent in the power law function) of 0.97, demonstrating that the liver indeed behaves as a parallel-type organ with a large reserve capacity. No cases of radiation-induced liver disease grade 3 according to RTOG/EORTC (Radiation Therapy and Oncology Group and the European Organisation for Research and Treatment of Cancer) were observed when the mean liver dose was <31 Gy. Estimates of tolerance doses associated with 5 per cent risk of liver disease after uniform irradiation to partial volumes were 47 Gy for two-thirds and >90 Gy for one-third of the total volume. A negligible complication risk, regardless of dose, is associated with irradiation of a partial volume of ≤25 per cent. A recent analysis by Kim *et al.* (2007) in 105 patients with hepatocellular carcinoma revealed that the total liver volume receiving ≥30 Gy also appears to be a useful dose–volumetric parameter for predicting the risk of hepatic toxicity and should be limited to ≤60 per cent.

The tolerance of patients with primary liver cancer is lower than that of patients with liver metastases or without liver tumours (Dawson and Ten Haken, 2005). However, the functionality of the unirradiated liver volume, which may be impaired by chemotherapy, alcohol consumption or other trauma, has to be taken into consideration. The presence of liver cirrhosis is known to be the predominant risk factor for hepatic toxicity following radiotherapy.

Intestinal tract

The results of several trials have been published for treatment of prostate, rectal or cervical cancer, relating the bowel volume irradiated, i.e. various DVH parameters, to the incidence of complications. Restricting dose conformation to the PTV can substantially decrease the normal tissue volumes exposed to significant doses. For example, a study from the Royal Marsden Hospital in London showed that the volume of small bowel irradiated to >90 per cent of the prescribed dose could be reduced from 24 per cent using conventional fields to 18 per cent for 3D conformal therapy and 5–8 per cent for IMRT, depending on the number of fields used. For the rectum, the high-dose irradiated volumes could be reduced from 89 per cent to 51 per cent and 6–16 per cent, respectively (Nutting et al., 2000). It should be noted that early complications in the intestine result in an increased incidence of late effects, thus representing a consequential component (see Chapter 13). Therefore, volume–effect studies on late complications may be affected by a varying influence of early effects.

ORAL MUCOSA

The clinical consequences of oral mucositis are closely related to the localization where the reaction occurs. For example, complications can be significantly reduced if the lips are excluded from the irradiated volume. Also, changes in taste acuity can be prevented by a reduction of the tongue volume included in the high-dose volume.

OESOPHAGUS

A study on 215 patients treated for non-small cell lung cancer (Wei et al., 2006) revealed that acute oesophageal symptoms were dominated by DVH parameters, such as the mean dose, or the relative volume treated to doses above 20 Gy (rV_{20}), but were independent of clinical factors.

SMALL BOWEL

The mobility of the small intestine largely prevents irradiation of the same segment or loop during subsequent fractions. Hence, the dose to individual loops can vary over wide ranges, and usually is lower than the dose to the target volume. However, previous surgery, related or independent of the oncological disease, as well as inflammatory changes in the abdominal cavity, can compromise mobility and hence significantly

increase the dose to bowel segments fixed in the high-dose volume. These uncertainties appear to be one of the reasons for the conflicting data for a correlation of dose and volume with the incidence of small bowel symptoms.

Volume effects for small bowel obstruction have been demonstrated in patients treated with extended field radiotherapy (bowel volumes >800 cm³), as reviewed by Letschert et al. (1994). No volume effects for bowel obstruction were observed in patients receiving postoperative radiotherapy for rectal carcinoma. In these patients, the incidence of chronic diarrhoea was 31 per cent for volumes <77 cm³, compared with 42 per cent for volumes >328 cm³. The type of surgery was a strong influence on the incidence of chronic diarrhoea and malabsorption.

RECTUM

The incidence of late rectal bleeding and other chronic changes has generally been found to correlate with irradiated volume exposed to high doses, as quantified by DVH parameters. Some studies have demonstrated a significant dose–volume relationship for late rectal bleeding using a single cut-off value for the rectal volume irradiated to certain doses (Fig. 14.11). Other studies describe a more complex relationship with several cut-off levels which significantly discriminated between a high or low risk of severe rectal bleeding, or a continuous relationship between rectal bleeding and dose–volume parameters. A study on rectal mucosal changes assessed by rectoscopy using a specific score in 35 patients receiving external–beam radiotherapy and high dose-rate brachytherapy for carcinoma of the cervix revealed ED_{50} values for irradiated volumes of 2 cm³, 1 cm³ or 0.1 cm³ of 68 Gy, 73 Gy and 84 Gy (Fig. 14.12). The corresponding doses for changes according to LENT/SOMA were 73 Gy, 78 Gy and 97 Gy.

One aspect to be considered for highly conformal radiotherapy, particularly for the rectum, is the dose distribution through the cross-section of the organ. Gross clinical symptoms are observed only if a larger part or the entire circumference is exposed to significant doses. In rats, it was demonstrated that shielding of half the circumference completely prevented late bowel obstruction, which occurred

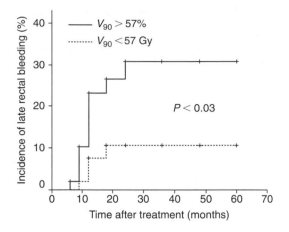

Figure 14.11 Actuarial incidence of rectal bleeding in patients with rectal volumes (V_{90}) irradiated to at least 90 per cent of the isodose (approximately 60 Gy) of greater than 57 per cent or less than 57 per cent. From Wachter *et al.* (2001), with permission from Elsevier.

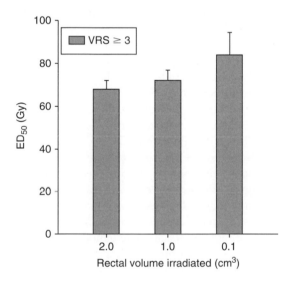

Figure 14.12 The ED_{50} values for rectoscopic mucosal changes [Vienna Rectoscopy Score (VRS) $\geqslant$3] in patients receiving teletherapy and brachytherapy for cervical cancer in rectal volumes of 2 cm^3, 1 cm^3 or 0.1 cm^3. Data from Georg *et al.* (unpublished), with permission of the authors.

with increasing dose in animals with irradiation of the entire rectal wall. The incidence (but not the area) of mucosal ulceration was similar in both groups. Similarly, an intrarectal balloon can be

applied for displacement of the posterior rectal wall and hence for a reduction in dose to this part, which results in a decrease in side-effects. In contrast, emptying of the rectum before irradiation increases dose homogeneity and reduces variations of DVH parameters for the PTV, but may increase the risk of rectal complications.

As with other organs, such as the lung (see above), the functional status of the rectum can influence the volume tolerance. Huang *et al.* (2002) demonstrated that an individual history of haemorrhoids clearly correlated with the incidence of rectal bleeding at a given volume irradiated.

Parotid gland

The parotid glands are important dose-limiting organs in treatment of the head and neck with conventional radiation techniques, as they often cannot be spared. Doses above 40–50 Gy lead to permanent loss of function contributing to xerostomia (parotid glands produce *c.* 60 per cent of the saliva) and impairment of quality of life. One of the major advantages of the introduction of 3D-conformal techniques in the head and neck area is the possibility of limiting the irradiated volume to parts of the parotids and this has resulted in a reduction of permanent xerostomia. A DVH-based prospective trial showed complete recovery of salivary flow at 1 year after mean doses to the parotid of around 26 Gy (Eisbruch *et al.*, 1999). The anatomical organization in acini as FSUs was clearly reflected in the outcome of modelling the partial-volume data, as derived from the DVH. The LKB model showed the volume-effect parameter *n* to be close to 1.0, which indicates a nearly parallel behaviour, whereby the mean dose determines NTCP. In these studies partial-volume thresholds were (approximately) 45 Gy for 25 per cent, 30 Gy for 50 per cent and 15 Gy for 67 per cent of the total volume.

Rat studies (Konings *et al.*, 2006) have demonstrated significant regional variations in radiation sensitivity in the parotid gland. The dose effect for late changes in saliva production, but not for early changes, was different for the cranial and caudal part of the glands, with a substantially higher radiosensitivity of the cranial part. The reduction in saliva output after a single dose of 30 Gy was 65 per cent for irradiation of the cranial and 25 per cent for irradiation of the caudal 50 per cent volume of the gland, and 100 per cent after irradiation of the entire organ. Histological studies showed that irradiation of the cranial 50 per cent volume also caused late development of secondary damage in the shielded caudal part at late time-points.

Skin

The skin shows an 'area' effect similar to oral mucosa. In studies in pig skin (Hopewell *et al.*, 1986), no effect of the irradiated area was observed for acute epidermal changes when the field diameter was larger than 20 mm, and for late effects when the diameter was larger than 10 mm. At smaller diameters, a steep rise in isoeffective doses was found (Fig. 14.13). In the orthovoltage era, this area effect of small fields used to be exploited by using a 'sieve technique', where part of the skin was shielded with the bridges of a lead sieve, and hence tolerable reactions occurred only in the small irradiated fields, but did not achieve confluency. This allowed for curative tumour doses despite the unfavourable depth-dose distribution of these low-energy X-rays.

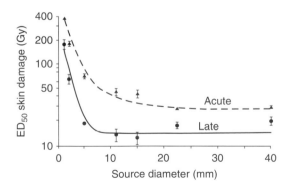

Figure 14.13 The influence of field-diameter on the dose required to induce acute and late skin reactions in 50 per cent of pigs after single-dose irradiation with small fields. A steep rise in ED_{50} is seen below a diameter of 20 mm for early reactions and 10 mm for late sequelae, respectively. At larger field-sizes, the ED_{50} is independent of the area exposed. From Hopewell and Trott (2000), with permission.

Key points

1. Structural tissue tolerance depends on cellular radiation sensitivity and is independent of volume irradiated. Functional tolerance depends on tissue organization and functional reserve capacity.

2. Tissues with a parallel organization (e.g. lung) have a large reserve capacity and show a pronounced volume effect, with a threshold volume below which functional damage does not occur. The risk of developing a complication depends on dose distribution throughout the whole organ rather than the maximum dose to a small area.

3. Tissues with a serial organization (e.g. spinal cord) have little or no functional reserve and the risk of developing a complication is less dependent on volume irradiated than for tissues with a parallel organization. The risk of complication is strongly influenced by high-dose regions and hot-spots.

4. Migration of surviving clonogenic cells into the edge of irradiated fields can lead to a steep increase in tissue tolerance for field diameters up to 20 mm in some tissues (e.g. spinal cord, intestine, skin).

5. Theoretical models have been developed to estimate NTCP for partial-volume irradiations and inhomogeneous dose distributions. Simple power-law and probability models have been expanded to incorporate parameters relating to tissue architecture and reserve capacity. These models need to be validated against clinical data emerging from conformal treatment schedules.

■ BIBLIOGRAPHY

Bentzen SM, Skoczylas JZ, Bernier J (2000). Quantitative clinical radiobiology of early and late lung reactions. *Int J Radiat Biol* **76**: 453–62.

Bijl HP, van Luijk P, Coppes RP, Schippers JM, Konings AW, van der Kogel AJ (2002). Dose-volume effects in the rat cervical spinal cord after proton irradiation. *Int J Radiat Oncol Biol Phys* **52**: 205–11.

Bijl HP, van Luijk P, Coppes RP, Schippers JM, Konings AW, van der Kogel AJ (2003). Unexpected changes of rat cervical spinal cord tolerance caused by inhomogeneous dose distributions. *Int J Radiat Oncol Biol Phys* **57**: 274–81.

Bijl HP, van Luijk P, Coppes RP, Schippers JM, Konings AW, van Der Kogel AJ (2005). Regional differences in radiosensitivity across the rat cervical spinal cord. *Int J Radiat Oncol Biol Phys* **61**: 543–51.

Bijl HP, van Luijk P, Coppes RP, Schippers JM, Konings AW, van der Kogel AJ (2006). Influence of adjacent low-dose fields on tolerance to high doses of protons in rat cervical spinal cord. *Int J Radiat Oncol Biol Phys* **64**: 1204–10.

Boersma LJ, Damen EM, de Boer RW *et al.* (1994). Dose-effect relations for local functional and structural changes of the lung after irradiation for malignant lymphoma. *Radiother Oncol* **32**: 201–9.

Dawson LA, Ten Haken RK (2005). Partial volume tolerance of the liver to radiation. *Semin Radiat Oncol* **15**: 279–83.

Eisbruch A, Ten Haken RK, Kim HM, Marsh LH, Ship JA (1999). Dose, volume, and function relationships in parotid salivary glands following conformal and intensity-modulated irradiation of head and neck cancer. *Int J Radiat Oncol Biol Phys* **45**: 577–87.

Emami B, Lyman J, Brown A *et al.* (1991). Tolerance of normal tissue to therapeutic irradiation. *Int J Radiat Oncol Biol Phys* **21**: 109–22.

Herrmann T, Baumann M, Voigtmann L, Knorr A (1997). Effect of irradiated volume on lung damage in pigs. *Radiother Oncol* **44**: 35–40.

Hopewell JW, Trott KR (2000). Volume effects in radiobiology as applied to radiotherapy. *Radiother Oncol* **56**: 283–8.

Hopewell JW, Coggle JE, Wells J, Hamlet R, Williams JP, Charles MW (1986). The acute effects of different energy beta-emitters on pig and mouse skin. *Br J Radiol Suppl* **19**: 47–51.

Huang EH, Pollack A, Levy L *et al.* (2002). Late rectal toxicity: dose-volume effects of conformal radiotherapy for prostate cancer. *Int J Radiat Oncol Biol Phys* **54**: 1314–21.

ICRU (1999). *Prescribing, recording and reporting photon beam therapy*. ICRU report 62. Oxford: Oxford University Press.

Jansen EP, Saunders MP, Boot H *et al.* (2007). Prospective study on late renal toxicity following postoperative chemoradiotherapy in gastric cancer. *Int J Radiat Oncol Biol Phys* **67**: 781–5.

Källman P, Agren A, Brahme A (1992). Tumour and normal tissue responses to fractionated non-uniform dose delivery. *Int J Radiat Biol* **62**: 249–62.

Kim TH, Kim DY, Park JW *et al.* (2007). Dose-volumetric parameters predicting radiation-induced hepatic toxicity in unresectable hepatocellular carcinoma patients treated with three-dimensional conformal radiotherapy. *Int J Radiat Oncol Biol Phys* **67**: 225–31.

Konings AW, Faber H, Cotteleer F, Vissink A, Coppes RP (2006). Secondary radiation damage as the main cause for unexpected volume effects: a histopathologic study of the parotid gland. *Int J Radiat Oncol Biol Phys* **64**: 98–105.

Köst S, Dörr W, Keinert K, Glaser FH, Endert G, Herrmann T (2002). Effect of dose and dose-distribution in damage to the kidney following abdominal radiotherapy. *Int J Radiat Biol* **78**: 695–702.

Kutcher GJ, Burman C (1989). Calculation of complication probability factors for non-uniform normal tissue irradiation: the effective volume method. *Int J Radiat Oncol Biol Phys* **16**: 1623–30.

Kwa SL, Lebesque JV, Theuws JC *et al.* (1998). Radiation pneumonitis as a function of mean lung dose: an analysis of pooled data of 540 patients. *Int J Radiat Oncol Biol Phys* **42**: 1–9.

Letschert JG, Lebesque JV, Aleman BM *et al.* (1994). The volume effect in radiation-related late small bowel complications: results of a clinical study of the EORTC Radiotherapy Cooperative Group in patients treated for rectal carcinoma. *Radiother Oncol* **32**: 116–23.

Lyman JT (1985). Complication probability as assessed from dose-volume histograms. *Radiat Res Suppl* **8**: S13–9.

Marks LB, Munley MT, Spencer DP *et al.* (1997). Quantification of radiation-induced regional lung injury with perfusion imaging. *Int J Radiat Oncol Biol Phys* **38**: 399–409.

Mehta V (2005). Radiation pneumonitis and pulmonary fibrosis in non-small-cell lung cancer: pulmonary function, prediction, and prevention. *Int J Radiat Oncol Biol Phys* **63**: 5–24.

Novakova-Jiresova A, van Luijk P, van Goor H, Kampinga HH, Coppes RP (2007). Changes in expression of injury after irradiation of increasing volumes in rat lung. *Int J Radiat Oncol Biol Phys* **67**: 1510–8.

Nutting CM, Convery DJ, Cosgrove VP *et al.* (2000). Reduction of small and large bowel irradiation using an optimized intensity-modulated pelvic radiotherapy technique in patients with prostate cancer. *Int J Radiat Oncol Biol Phys* **48**: 649–56.

Powers BE, Thames HD, Gillette SM, Smith C, Beck ER, Gillette EL (1998). Volume effects in the irradiated canine spinal cord: do they exist when the probability of injury is low? *Radiother Oncol* **46**: 297–306.

Robbins ME, Hopewell JW (1988). Effects of single doses of X-rays on renal function in the pig after the irradiation of both kidneys. *Radiother Oncol* **11**: 253–62.

Rodrigues G, Lock M, D'Souza D, Yu E, van Dyk J (2004). Prediction of radiation pneumonitis by dose-volume histogram parameters in lung cancer – a systematic review. *Radiother Oncol* **71**: 127–38.

Ryu S, Jin JY, Jin R *et al.* (2007). Partial volume tolerance of the spinal cord and complications of single-dose radiosurgery. *Cancer* **109**: 628–36.

Schultheiss TE, Stephens LC, Ang KK, Price RE, Peters LJ (1994). Volume effects in rhesus monkey spinal cord. *Int J Radiat Oncol Biol Phys* **29**: 67–72.

Theuws JC, Kwa SL, Wagenaar AC *et al.* (1998). Prediction of overall pulmonary function loss in relation to the 3-D dose distribution for patients with breast cancer and malignant lymphoma. *Radiother Oncol* **49**: 233–43.

Travis EL, Liao ZX, Tucker SL (1997). Spatial heterogeneity of the volume effect for radiation pneumonitis in mouse lung. *Int J Radiat Oncol Biol Phys* **38**: 1045–54.

van den Aardweg GJ, Hopewell JW, Whitehouse EM (1995). The radiation response of the cervical spinal cord of the pig: effects of changing the irradiated volume. *Int J Radiat Oncol Biol Phys* **31**: 51–5.

Wachter S, Gerstner N, Goldner G, Potzi R, Wambersie A, Potter R (2001). Rectal sequelae after conformal radiotherapy of prostate cancer: dose-volume histograms as predictive factors. *Radiother Oncol* **59**: 65–70.

Wei X, Liu HH, Tucker SL *et al.* (2006). Risk factors for acute esophagitis in non-small-cell lung cancer patients treated with concurrent chemotherapy and three-dimensional conformal radiotherapy. *Int J Radiat Oncol Biol Phys* **66**: 100–7.

Withers HR, Taylor JM, Maciejewski B (1988). Treatment volume and tissue tolerance. *Int J Radiat Oncol Biol Phys* **14**: 751–9.

■ FURTHER READING

Deasy JO, Niemierko A, Herbert D *et al.* (2002). Methodological issues in radiation dose-volume outcome analyses: summary of a joint AAPM/NIH workshop. *Med Phys* **29**: 2109–27.

Kong FM, Pan C, Eisbruch A, Ten Haken RK (2007). Physical models and simpler dosimetric descriptors of radiation late toxicity. *Semin Radiat Oncol* **17**: 108–20.

Sundar S, Symonds P, Deehan C (2003). Tolerance of pelvic organs to radiation treatment for carcinoma of cervix. *Clin Oncol* **15**: 240–7.

The oxygen effect and fractionated radiotherapy

MICHAEL R. HORSMAN, BRADLY G. WOUTERS,
MICHAEL C. JOINER AND JENS OVERGAARD

15.1 THE IMPORTANCE OF OXYGEN

The response of cells to ionizing radiation is strongly dependent upon oxygen (Gray *et al.*, 1953; Wright and Howard-Flanders, 1957). This is illustrated in Fig. 15.1 for mammalian cells irradiated in culture. Cell surviving fraction is shown as a function of radiation dose administered either under normal aerated conditions or under hypoxia, which can generally be achieved by flowing nitrogen gas over the surface of the cell suspensions for a period of 30 min or more. The enhancement of radiation damage by oxygen is dose-modifying (i.e. the radiation dose that gives a particular level of cell survival is reduced by approximately the same factor at all levels of survival). This allows us to calculate an oxygen enhancement ratio (OER):

$$\text{Oxygen enhancement ratio} = \frac{\text{Radiation dose in hypoxia}}{\text{Radiation dose in air}}$$

for the same level of biological effect. For most cell types, the OER for X-rays is around 3.0. However, some studies suggest that at radiation doses of

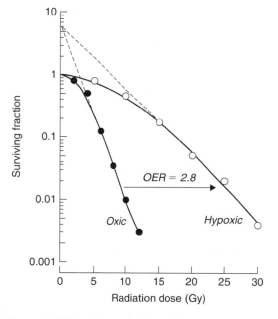

Figure 15.1 Survival curves for cultured mammalian cells exposed to X-rays under oxic or hypoxic conditions, illustrating the radiation dose-modifying effect of oxygen. Note that the broken lines extrapolate back to the same point on the survival axis ($n = 6$). OER, oxygen enhancement ratio.

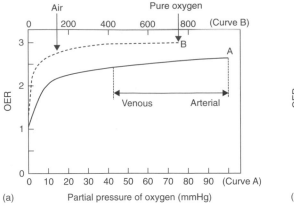
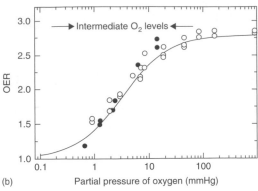

Figure 15.2 Variation of oxygen enhancement ratio (OER) with oxygen partial pressure scaled linearly in (a) and logarithmically in (b). In (a), the horizontal arrows indicate the range of physiological blood oxygen tensions on the lower scale (to convert mmHg to kPa, multiply by 0.133). (b) Published OER values at different oxygen partial pressures adapted from Koch *et al.* (1984) (closed circles) and Whillans and Hunt (1982) (open circles). (a) Adapted from Denekamp (1989), with permission; (b) from Wouters and Brown (1997), with permission.

3 Gy or less the OER can be reduced (Palcic and Skarsgard, 1984). This is an important finding because this is the dose range for clinical fractionation treatments.

It has been demonstrated from rapid-mix studies that the oxygen effect occurs only if oxygen is present either during irradiation or within a few milliseconds thereafter (Howard-Flanders and Moore, 1958; Michael *et al.*, 1973). The dependence of the degree of sensitization on oxygen tension is shown in Fig. 15.2. By definition, the OER under anoxic conditions is 1.0. As the oxygen tension increases there is a steep increase in radiosensitivity (and thus in the OER) which Fig. 15.2a shows against a linear scale of oxygen tension. In Fig. 15.2b, oxygen tension is scaled logarithmically to demonstrate that cells below 0.15 mmHg (0.02 per cent) are maximally resistant to radiation and the OER starts to rise significantly above 1.0 only when the oxygen tension exceeds this level and then the greatest change occurs from about 0.5 to 20 mmHg. A further increase in oxygen concentration, up to that seen in air (155 mmHg) or even to 100 per cent oxygen (760 mmHg), produces a much smaller though definite increase in radiosensitivity. Also shown in Fig. 15.2a are the oxygen partial pressures typically found in arterial and venous blood. Thus

from a radiobiological standpoint most normal tissues can be considered to be well oxygenated, although it is now recognized that moderate hypoxia is a feature of some normal tissues such as cartilage and skin.

The mechanism responsible for the enhancement of radiation damage by oxygen is generally referred to as the oxygen-fixation hypothesis and is illustrated in Fig. 15.3. When radiation is absorbed in a biological material, free radicals are produced. These radicals are highly reactive molecules and it is these radicals that break chemical bonds, produce chemical changes and initiate the chain of events that result in biological damage. They can be produced either directly in the target molecule (usually DNA) or indirectly in other cellular molecules and diffuse far enough to reach and damage critical targets. Most of the indirect effects occur by free radicals produced in water, since this makes up 70–80 per cent of mammalian cells. It is the fate of the free radicals ultimately produced in the critical target, designated as R$^{\bullet}$ in Fig. 15.3, that is important. These R$^{\bullet}$ molecules are unstable and will react rapidly with oxygen, if present, to produce RO$_2^{\bullet}$, which then undergoes further reaction ultimately to yield ROOH in the target molecule. Thus we have a stable change in the chemical composition of the target and the

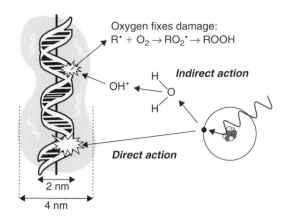

Figure 15.3 The oxygen fixation hypothesis. Free radicals produced in DNA by either a direct or indirect action of radiation can be repaired under hypoxia but fixed in the presence of oxygen. Adapted from Hall (1988), with permission.

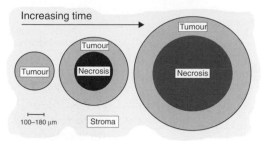

Figure 15.4 Simplified description of the development of microscopic regions of necrosis in tumours. Conclusions by Thomlinson and Gray from studies on histological sections of human bronchial carcinoma showing the development of necrosis beyond a limiting distance from the vascular stroma. Adapted from Hall (1988), with permission.

damage is said to be chemically 'fixed'. Subsequently, this damage is recognized by biological pathways that participate in the DNA damage response (DDR) to invoke enzymatic processing of the lesions and perhaps their successful repair (see Chapter 2). In the absence of oxygen, or in the presence of reducing species, the unstable $R^\bullet$ molecules have a longer half-life and can react with H^+, thus chemically restoring its original form without the need for biological and enzymatic intervention.

15.2 THE TUMOUR MICROENVIRONMENT

For most solid tumours to grow they need to develop their own blood supply. This new vasculature is formed from the already established normal-tissue vessels by a process which is referred to as angiogenesis. However, the formation of the neo-vasculature usually lags behind the more rapidly increasing number of neoplastic cells; the tumours are said to 'outgrow' their blood supply. As a result, the neo-vasculature is unable to meet the increasing nutrient demands of the expanding tumour mass. The vasculature that is formed is also very primitive in nature and, like the cancerous tissue it supplies, is morphologically and

functionally abnormal. All these factors combine to result in the development of microregional areas within tumours that are nutrient deprived, acidic and oxygen deficient, yet the hypoxic cells existing in these areas may still be viable, at least for a limited time (see also Chapter 16).

The first clear indication that hypoxia may be present in tumours was made by Thomlinson and Gray (1955) from their observations on histological sections of fresh specimens from human carcinoma of the bronchus; this is summarized schematically in Fig. 15.4. They observed viable tumour regions surrounded by vascular stroma from which the tumour cells obtained their nutrient and oxygen requirements. As these regions expanded, areas of necrosis appeared at the centre. The thickness of the resulting cylindrical shell of viable tissue (100–180 μm) was found to be similar to the calculated diffusion distance of oxygen in respiring tissues; it was thus hypothesized that as oxygen diffused from the stroma it was consumed by the cells and, while those cells beyond the diffusion distance were unable to survive, cells immediately bordering on the necrosis might be viable yet hypoxic.

Tannock (1968) made similar observations in mouse mammary tumours. The extent of necrosis in these tumours was much greater and each patent blood-vessel was surrounded by a cord of viable tumour cells outside which was necrosis. This 'corded' structure is also seen in other solid

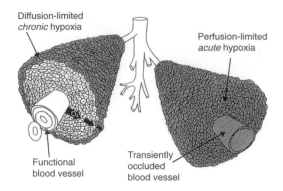

Figure 15.5 Representation of diffusion-limited chronic hypoxia and perfusion-limited acute hypoxia within tumour cords. From Horsman (1998), with permission.

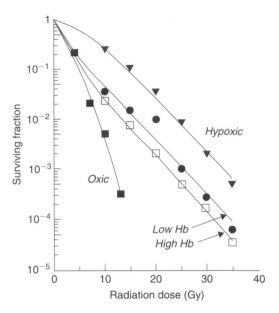

Figure 15.6 Cell survival curves for KHT mouse sarcoma cells irradiated under aerobic or hypoxic conditions. The hypoxic data were obtained by killing the mice shortly before irradiation. Two sets of data for tumours in air-breathing mice are shown, with high and low haemoglobin levels. The oxic curve represents the survival of aerobic cells irradiated *in vitro*. From Hill *et al.* (1971), with permission.

tumours and is illustrated in Fig. 15.5. Cells at the edge of the cords are thought to be hypoxic and are often called 'chronically hypoxic cells'. Tannock showed, however, that since the cell population of the cord is in a dynamic state of cell turnover these hypoxic cells will have a short lifespan, being continually replaced as other cells are displaced away from the blood vessel and in turn become hypoxic. More recently it was shown that some tumour blood vessels may periodically open and close, leading to transient or acute hypoxia (Fig. 15.5). The mechanisms responsible for intermittent blood flow in tumours are not entirely clear. They might include: the plugging of vessels by blood cells or by circulating tumour cells; temporary collapse of vessels in regions of high tumour interstitial pressure; or spontaneous vasomotion in incorporated host arterioles affecting blood flow in downstream capillaries.

15.3 HYPOXIA IN EXPERIMENTAL TUMOURS

Since hypoxic cells are resistant to radiation, their presence in tumours can be critical in determining the response of tumours to treatment, especially with large doses of radiation. The presence of such treatment limiting cells in experimental tumours can easily be demonstrated, as shown in Fig. 15.6. This shows the cell survival response of

KHT mouse sarcomas, irradiated *in situ* in air-breathing mice, or in nitrogen-asphyxiated (i.e. hypoxic) mice; or as a single-cell suspension *in vitro* under fully oxic conditions. The studies in air-breathing mice were made under both normal and anaemic conditions. Cell survival was estimated immediately after irradiation using a lung colony assay (see Chapter 7, Section 7.2). The survival curves for tumours irradiated in air-breathing mice are biphasic. At low radiation doses the response is dominated by death of the aerobic cells and the curves are close to the response of cells under well-oxygenated conditions. At larger radiation doses the presence of hypoxic cells begins to influence the response and the survival curve eventually becomes parallel to the response of cells under hypoxic conditions. At this level all of the aerobic cells have been killed and thus the response is determined solely by the initial fraction of hypoxic cells. The proportion of hypoxic cells (the hypoxic fraction) can thus be calculated from the vertical separation between the hypoxic and air-breathing survival curves in the region where they are parallel. In this mouse sarcoma the hypoxic fraction was calculated to be 0.06 in mice with a high haemoglobin level (*c.* 16.5 g per cent) and 0.12 in anaemic mice (haemoglobin level *c.* 9.5 g per cent). These data thus illustrate not only the presence of hypoxic cells in these tumours but also the influence of oxygen transport.

Two other techniques are routinely used to estimate hypoxia in animal tumours. These are the so-called 'clamped tumour growth-delay assay', which involves measuring the time taken for tumours to grow to a specific size after irradiation, and the 'clamped tumour-control assay', in which the percentage of animals showing local tumour control at a certain time after treatment is recorded. For both techniques it is necessary to produce full radiation dose–response curves under normal and clamped conditions and the hypoxic fractions can then be calculated from the displacement of these curves. It is important to recognize that these techniques assay the fraction of viable radiation-resistant hypoxic cells. This is commonly referred to as the radiobiological hypoxic fraction and can be very different from the fraction of hypoxic cells measured using other methods (described in Section 15.4). The radiobiological hypoxic fraction is a very relevant value for radiotherapy since it directly measures cells that can contribute to treatment failure. Using these assays, and the paired survival-curve assay described above, it has been demonstrated that most experimental solid tumours contain radiation-resistant hypoxic cells, with estimates of the radiobiological hypoxic fractions ranging from below 1 per cent to well over 50 per cent of the total viable cell population.

15.4 HYPOXIA IN HUMAN TUMOURS

Attempts to estimate the level of hypoxia in human tumours have proven more difficult. A major reason is that the experimental procedures that have just been described are not directly applicable to the human situation. Instead, it is

Table 15.1 Potential methods for measuring the oxygenation status of human tumours

Tumour vascularization
    Intercapillary distance
    Vascular density
    Distance from tumour cells to nearest vessel

Haemoglobin–oxygen saturation
    Cryospectroscopy
    Near-infrared spectroscopy

Tumour metabolic activity
    Biochemical/HPLC analysis
    Bioluminescence
    NMR/PET

DNA damage
    Comet assay
    Alkaline elution

Hypoxic markers
    Immunohistochemistry (e.g. PIMO/EF5)
    ^{18}F-Fluoromisonidazole
    ^{123}I-Iodoazomycin arabinoside

Oxygen partial pressure distributions
    Polarographic oxygen electrodes
    ^{19}F-NMR spectroscopy

Miscellaneous
    ESR spectroscopy
    Tumour interstitial pressure
    Phosphorescence imaging
    Hypoxic stress proteins

ESR, electron spin resonance; EF5, a fluorinated derivative of etanidazole; HPLC, high-pressure liquid chromatography; NMR, nuclear magnetic resonance; PET, positron emission tomography; PIMO, pimonidazole.

From Horsman *et al.* (1998) with permission.

necessary to rely on more indirect approaches, as listed in Table 15.1. The endpoints have included:

- measurements of tumour vascularization because the oxygenation status of tumours is strongly dependent on vascular supply;
- haemoglobin–oxygen saturation, because this controls oxygen delivery to tumours;
- tumour metabolic activity, which changes under hypoxic conditions;
- estimating the degree of DNA damage, since hypoxic cells are likely to show less DNA damage than aerobic cells for a given radiation dose;

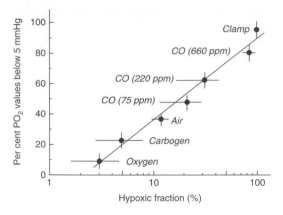

Figure 15.7 Relationship between partial pressure of oxygen (PO$_2$) electrode measurements and the hypoxic fraction in a C3H mouse mammary carcinoma. Results were obtained from normal air-breathing mice, in clamped tumours, and in mice allowed to breathe oxygen, carbogen or various concentrations of carbon monoxide (CO). From Horsman *et al.* (1993), with permission.

- hypoxic markers, based on the observations that certain nitro-aromatic compounds are reduced, under hypoxic conditions, to reactive species that subsequently bind to hypoxic cells and then can be identified;
- estimates of tumour oxygen partial pressure (PO$_2$) distributions.

A technique that has received considerable attention has been the use of polarographic oxygen electrodes for measuring tumour PO$_2$. The popularity of this approach came about with the development of the Eppendorf histograph. This differed from older oxygen electrodes in employing more robust and re-usable electrodes plus an automatic stepping motor, thus making it possible to obtain large numbers of oxygen measurements along several tracks within a short period. Using this machine a direct relationship between electrode estimates of tumour oxygenation and the actual percentage of hypoxic clonogenic (i.e. viable) cells was found. This is illustrated in Fig. 15.7 in which the radiobiological hypoxic fraction, determined using a clamped tumour-control assay, was altered in a C3H mouse mammary carcinoma by allowing the mice to breathe different gas mixtures. A strong correlation was found between radiobiological hypoxic fraction and the percentage of measured PO$_2$ values that were equal to or less than 5 mmHg.

Note, however, that these measurements are within a single-tumour model and thus do not demonstrate that the relationship between oxygen electrode measurements and radiobiological hypoxia will be the same in all tumours. For example, cells from one tumour may be less tolerant to hypoxia than those from another tumour and thus have reduced viability. In this case, the amount of hypoxia measured by oxygen electrodes could be the same in two tumours, whereas the amount of radiobiological hypoxia could be different (since one tumour is less tolerant of hypoxia). The tolerance of cells to hypoxia is determined by several oxygen-sensitive biological pathways that are discussed further in Chapter 16. However, oxygen electrodes have been used to measure PO$_2$ distributions in human tumours and in at least two sites (cervical cancers and tumours of the head and neck region) the PO$_2$ measurements have been related to outcome after radiation therapy (Table 15.2). In general, good correlations between treatment outcome and pretreatment PO$_2$ measurements were observed for both tumour types, with the less well-oxygenated tumours showing the poorest results.

Evidence that hypoxia exists in human tumours and can influence radiation response also comes from clinical trials in which some form of hypoxic modification has been attempted and found to improve tumour response. Using hyperbaric oxygen, chemical radiation sensitizers or techniques to improve oxygen supply, a significant improvement in local tumour control has been seen, particularly in head and neck cancers (see Chapter 17). This is also illustrated in Fig. 15.8, in which local–regional control of tumours is expressed as a function of pretreatment haemoglobin concentration in male or female patients treated with radiotherapy for squamous cell carcinoma of the larynx and pharynx. Local tumour control was lower in those patients with reduced haemoglobin concentrations. Such a reduction in haemoglobin would make less oxygen available to the tumour and thus increase the level of tumour hypoxia.

15.5 REOXYGENATION

The time-course of changes in the radiobiological hypoxic fraction of a tumour before and after

Table 15.2 Clinical studies in which Eppendorf estimates of pretreatment partial pressure of oxygen have been related to radiotherapy outcome

Study (source)	Number of patients	Influence of hypoxia
Head and neck cancer		
Adam *et al.* (*Laryngoscope*, 1998)	25	No
Brizel *et al.* (*Int J Radiat Oncol Biol Phys*, 1998)	43	Yes
(*Radiother Oncol*, 1999)	63	Yes
Eschewege *et al.* (*Int J Radiat Oncol Biol Phys*, 1997)	35	No
Nordsmark *et al.* (*Radiother Oncol*, 1996)	35	Yes
(*Radiother Oncol*, 2000)	66	Yes
Rudat *et al.* (*Radiother Oncol*, 2001)	41	Yes
Stradler *et al.* (*Int J Radiat Oncol Biol Phys*, 1997)	59	Yes
Cancer of the uterine cervix		
Fyles *et al.* (*Radiother Oncol*, 1998)	74	Yes
Hoeckel *et al.* (*Cancer Res*, 1996)	89*	Yes
Knocke *et al.* (*Radiother Oncol*, 1999)	51	Yes
Sundfor *et al.* (*Radiother Oncol*, 2000)	40	Yes

*Forty-seven patients received surgery as the primary treatment with adjuvant chemotherapy with or without radiation.

From M. Nordsmark (unpublished data).

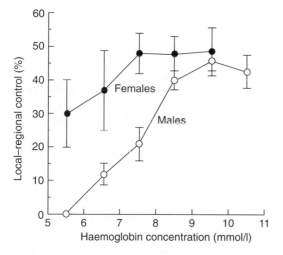

Figure 15.8 Local–regional tumour control as a function of gender and pretreatment haemoglobin value in 1112 patients treated with radiotherapy for squamous cell carcinoma of the larynx and pharynx. From Overgaard (1988), with permission.

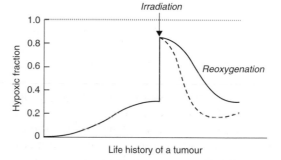

Figure 15.9 The time-course of changes in the hypoxic fraction during the life history of a tumour. Small lesions are well oxygenated but as the tumour grows the hypoxic fraction rises perhaps in excess of 10 per cent. A large, single dose of radiation kills oxic cells and raises the hypoxic fraction. The subsequent fall is termed reoxygenation.

irradiation is illustrated in Fig. 15.9. Tumours less than 1 mm in diameter have been found to be fully oxygenated (Stanley *et al.*, 1977). Above this size they usually become partially hypoxic. If tumours

are irradiated with a large single dose of radiation, most of the radiosensitive aerobic cells in the tumour will be killed. The cells that survive will predominantly be hypoxic and therefore the radiobiological hypoxic fraction immediately after irradiation will be close to 100 per cent (note that the oxygenation status of cells in the tumour has not

Table 15.3 Mechanisms and time-scales of tumour reoxygenation

Mechanism	Time
Recirculation through temporarily closed vessels	Minutes
Reduced respiration rate in damaged cells	Minutes to hours
Ischaemic death of cells without replacement	Hours
Mitotic death of irradiated cells	Hours
Cord shrinkage as dead cells are resorbed	Days

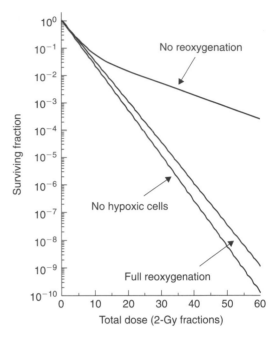

Figure 15.10 Calculated cell survival curves following repeated 2-Gy fractions of radiotherapy for tumours initially containing 90 per cent well-oxygenated cells and 10 per cent hypoxic cells (upper and middle lines) compared with no hypoxic cells (lower line). The upper line shows the progressive depletion of oxic and hypoxic cells in the absence of reoxygenation. The middle line assumes that, after each dose fraction, full reoxygenation restores the hypoxic fraction to its pre-treatment level. A surviving fraction at 2 Gy (SF$_2$) of 0.47 for oxic cells has been assumed with an OER of 2.8 relative to fully hypoxic cells.

been changed at this point: selective abolition of colony-forming ability has led to survivors having a raised hypoxic fraction). Subsequently, the radiobiological hypoxic fraction falls and approaches its initial starting value. This phenomenon is termed reoxygenation and refers specifically to changes in the hypoxic status of the remaining viable cells (i.e. radiobiological hypoxic fraction). The process of reoxygenation has been reported to occur in a variety of tumour systems, although the speed of reoxygenation varies widely, occurring within a few hours in some tumours and taking several days in others. Furthermore, the final level of hypoxia after reoxygenation can also be higher or lower than its value before irradiation.

The mechanisms underlying reoxygenation in tumours are not fully understood. A number of contributing processes are listed in Table 15.3. If reoxygenation occurs rapidly then it may be caused by either recirculation of blood through vessels that were temporarily closed or decreased cellular respiration (which will increase the oxygen diffusion distance). Reoxygenation occurring at longer intervals is probably the result of cell death leading to tumour shrinkage and a reduction in intercapillary distances, thus allowing oxygen to reach hypoxic cells.

Reoxygenation has important implications for successful clinical fractionated radiotherapy. Figure 15.10 illustrates the hypothetical situation in a tumour following fractionated radiation treatments. In this example (Wouters and Brown, 1997), 90 per cent of the viable tumour cells are

considered well oxygenated and 10 per cent are initially hypoxic. The responses of oxic and hypoxic cells to repeated dose fractions of 2 Gy are illustrated. In this example model, SF$_2$ (surviving fraction at 2 Gy) of 0.47 for the oxic cells has been assumed with an OER of 2.8 relative to fully hypoxic cells. If no reoxygenation occurs, then each successive dose of radiation would be expected to kill fewer and fewer cells with increasing total dose, because the surviving cell population becomes dominated by hypoxic cells after only about six fractions. At the end of a 60-Gy treatment, the tumour response, measured by $-\ln(SF)$, is only about one-third of the response that would be obtained in the absence of hypoxic cells. However, if reoxygenation occurs between fractions then the radiation killing of initially hypoxic cells will be greater and the hypoxic cells then have less impact on response. In the model shown in Fig. 15.10, if full reoxygenation takes place so that the radiobiological hypoxic fraction returns to 10 per cent before each 2-Gy fraction, the tumour response achieved, measured by −ln(SF), exceeds 90 per cent of the response that would be obtained in the absence of hypoxic cells. The existence of extensive reoxygenation during clinical radiotherapy is supported by the fact that local control can be achieved in a variety of tumours given fractionated radiotherapy with 30–35 fractions of 2 Gy. However, the study of Wouters and Brown (1997) has shown that cells at intermediate levels of oxygenation (i.e. those with an intermediate OER) can also cause significant radioresistance during fractionated radiotherapy despite extensive reoxygenation. These cells do not influence the response to large single doses, which is determined solely by the most resistant fraction of hypoxic cells. However, they do contribute significantly to the response to clinically relevant doses and therefore may play an additional important role in determining the outcome of fractionated treatment.

15.6 DRUG RESISTANCE

The presence of hypoxic cells in tumours not only has a significant impact on radiation therapy, there are also strong indications that these same cells may be responsible for tumour resistance to certain types of chemotherapy. Evidence from animal studies has shown that drugs such as bleomycin, 5-fluorouracil, methotrexate and *cis*-platinum are less effective at killing tumour cells when they are hypoxic than when they are well oxygenated (Grau and Overgaard, 1992). Whether this is a consequence of hypoxia *per se* or because hypoxic cells are normally distant from blood vessels, thus creating problems for drug delivery, or because such cells are typically non-cycling and exist in areas of low pH (both of which can influence drug activity) has never been fully established. It is likely that all of these mechanisms contribute to resistance *in vivo*.

Key points

1. Hypoxic cells are much less sensitive to radiation than well-oxygenated cells.
2. Hypoxic cells occur in most animal and human tumours; they are believed to be an important cause of treatment failure after radiotherapy, especially using a small number of large-dose fractions.
3. Hypoxia in tumours can be chronic or acute, for which the underlying mechanisms differ. Attempts to eliminate radioresistant tumour cells require treatments that are effective against each of these types of hypoxia.
4. Reoxygenation has been shown to occur in animal tumours; some tumours reoxygenate rapidly, others more slowly. The evidence for reoxygenation in human tumours is less direct.
5. Hypoxic cells in tumours are also known to be resistant to certain chemotherapeutic agents.

■ BIBLIOGRAPHY

Denekamp J (1989). Physiological hypoxia and its influence on radiotherapy. In: Steel GG, Adams GE, Horwich A (eds) *The biological basis of radiotherapy*, 2nd edn. Amsterdam: Elsevier, 115–34.

Grau C, Overgaard J (1992). Effect of etoposide, carmustine, vincristine, 5-fluorouracil, or methotrexate on radiobiologically oxic and hypoxic cells in a C3H mouse mammary carcinoma *in situ*. *Cancer Chemother Pharmacol* **30**: 277–80.

Gray LH, Conger AD, Ebert M, Hornsey S, Scott OC (1953). The concentration of oxygen dissolved in tissues at the time of irradiation as a factor in radiotherapy. *Br J Radiol* **26**: 638–48.

Hall EJ (1988). *Radiobiology for the radiologist*, 3rd edn. Philadelphia: Lippincott.

Hill RP, Bush RS, Yeung P (1971). The effect of anaemia on the fraction of hypoxic cells in an experimental tumour. *Br J Radiol* **44**: 299–304.

Horsman MR (1998). Measurement of tumor oxygenation. *Int J Radiat Oncol Biol Phys* **42**: 701–4.

Horsman MR, Khalil AA, Nordsmark M, Grau C, Overgaard J (1993). Relationship between radiobiological hypoxia and direct estimates of tumour oxygenation in a mouse tumour model. *Radiother Oncol* **28**: 69–71.

Horsman MR, Nordsmark M, Overgaard J (1998). Techniques to assess the oxygenation of human tumors – state of the art. *Strahlenther Onkol* **174**(Suppl 4): 2–5.

Howard-Flanders P, Moore D (1958). The time interval after pulsed irradiation within which injury to bacteria can be modified by dissolved oxygen. I. A search for an effect of oxygen 0.02 second after pulsed irradiation. *Radiat Res* **9**: 422–37.

Koch CJ, Stobbe CC, Bump EA (1984). The effect on the K_m for radiosensitization at 0°C of thiol depletion by diethylmaleate pretreatment: quantitative differences found using the radiation sensitizing agent misonidazole or oxygen. *Radiat Res* **98**: 141–53.

Michael BD, Adams GE, Hewitt HB, Jones WB, Watts ME (1973). A posteffect of oxygen in irradiated bacteria: a submillisecond fast mixing study. *Radiat Res* **54**: 239–51.

Overgaard J (1988). The influence of haemoglobin concentration on the response to radiotherapy. *Scand J Clin Lab Invest* **48**(Suppl 189): 49–53.

Palcic B, Skarsgard LD (1984). Reduced oxygen enhancement ratio at low doses of ionizing radiation. *Radiat Res* **100**: 328–39.

Stanley JA, Shipley WU, Steel GG (1977). Influence of tumour size on hypoxic fraction and therapeutic sensitivity of Lewis lung tumour. *Br J Cancer* **36**: 105–13.

Tannock IF (1968). The relation between cell proliferation and the vascular system in a transplanted mouse mammary tumour. *Br J Cancer* **22**: 258–73.

Thomlinson RH, Gray LH (1955). The histological structure of some human lung cancers and the possible implications for radiotherapy. *Br J Cancer* **9**: 539–49.

Whillans DW, Hunt JW (1982). A rapid-mixing comparison of the mechanisms of radiosensitization by oxygen and misonidazole in CHO cells. *Radiat Res* **90**: 126–41.

Wouters BG, Brown JM (1997). Cells at intermediate oxygen levels can be more important than the 'hypoxic fraction' in determining tumor response to fractionated radiotherapy. *Radiat Res* **147**: 541–50.

Wright EA, Howard-Flanders P (1957). The influence of oxygen on the radiosensitivity of mammalian tissues. *Acta Radiol* **48**: 26–32.

■ FURTHER READING

Brown JM (1979). Evidence for acutely hypoxic cells in mouse tumours, and a possible mechanism of reoxygenation. *Br J Radiol* **52**: 650–6.

Bussink J, Kaanders JH, van der Kogel AJ (2003). Tumor hypoxia at the micro-regional level: clinical relevance and predictive value of exogenous and endogenous hypoxic cell markers. *Radiother Oncol* **67**: 3–15.

Chaplin DJ, Durand RE, Olive PL (1986). Acute hypoxia in tumors: implications for modifiers of radiation effects. *Int J Radiat Oncol Biol Phys* **12**: 1279–82.

Chapman JD (1984). The detection and measurement of hypoxic cells in solid tumors. *Cancer* **54**: 2441–9.

Horsman MR, Bohm L, Margison GP *et al.* (2006). Tumor radiosensitizers – current status of development of various approaches: report of an International Atomic Energy Agency meeting. *Int J Radiat Oncol Biol Phys* **64**: 551–61.

Kallman RF, Rockwell S (1977). Effects of radiation on animal tumor models. In: Becker FF (eds) *Cancer: a comprehensive treatise*, Vol. 6. New York: Plenum Press, 225–79,

Moulder JE, Rockwell S (1984). Hypoxic fractions of solid tumors: experimental techniques, methods of analysis, and a survey of existing data. *Int J Radiat Oncol Biol Phys* **10**: 695–712.

Overgaard J (1989). Sensitization of hypoxic tumour cells – clinical experience. *Int J Radiat Biol* **56**: 801–11.

Vaupel P, Kallinowski F, Okunieff P (1989). Blood flow, oxygen and nutrient supply, and metabolic microenvironment of human tumors: a review. *Cancer Res* **49**: 6449–65.

The tumour microenvironment and cellular hypoxia responses

BRADLY G. WOUTERS AND MARIANNE KORITZINSKY

16.1 OXYGENATION PATTERNS OF TUMOURS

The steady-state oxygen concentration in tissues is determined by the balance between oxygen supply and demand. Oxygen is supplied from the blood, mainly in a form that is bound to haemoglobin in red blood cells and is consumed by cells primarily through a process called oxidative phosphorylation. In this process, mitochondria use oxygen as the terminal electron acceptor in a cascade of reactions called the electron transport chain. Here, nutrients are oxidized to produce the cellular energy currency ATP (adenosine triphosphate). Oxidative phosphorylation plays a very important role in energy production by extracting the maximum amount of energy from cellular nutrients. For example, a molecule of glucose can produce as much as 38 molecules of ATP under conditions where oxygen is present (oxidative respiration) but only two molecules of ATP when oxygen is absent (anaerobic glycolysis). The consumption of oxygen in this process gives rise to a

limited ability of oxygen to diffuse through unvascularized tissues. Estimates of the oxygen diffusion distance ranges from 75 to 200 μm depending on the actual respiration rate (oxygen consumption rate) of the tissue in question.

The oxygen concentration of most normal tissues is stably maintained at around 5–7 per cent. When oxygen concentrations drop to 3 per cent or below, the tissue is considered hypoxic. Below this value, oxygen deprivation then leads to the activation of several different biological pathways that serve to alter the behaviour or 'phenotype' of the cell. Many of these pathways are activated to allow adaptation of the cell or the tissue to the stress associated with oxygen deprivation. For example, these pathways can increase the capacity for anaerobic glycolysis (to maintain energy production), mediate changes in blood flow, and stimulate angiogenesis (new blood vessel growth) to increase the oxygen supply to the tissue. For the most part, these pathways operate both in normal tissues and in tumours. Numerous studies have demonstrated the presence of hypoxic cells in human tumours and, furthermore, show that oxygenation patterns are highly heterogeneous (Magagnin *et al.*, 2006).

Two distinct mechanisms cause tumour hypoxia

The rapid and uncontrolled proliferation of tumour cells often results in a demand for oxygen that exceeds the capacity of the vascular network. Although the resulting hypoxia may stimulate tumour angiogenesis (through mechanisms described below), the developing vessels are often still unable to provide adequate oxygenation for the rapidly proliferating tumour. Thus, although angiogenesis becomes a 'hallmark' of cancer, hypoxic tumour areas remain a common feature throughout the lifetime of the tumour. The lack of sufficient numbers of tumour blood vessels gives rise to one of the two main causes of hypoxia in human tumours known as 'chronic' or 'diffusion-limited' hypoxia. In this type of hypoxia, individual perfused vessels are characterized by a gradient of oxygenation surrounding them. Diffusion-limited hypoxia in tumours was first documented in 1955 (Thomlinson and Gray, 1955; see Chapter 15) and its presence indicates the existence of cells at all possible oxygen concentrations ranging from anoxia at distal locations to normal values next to the vessels.

In some situations, hypoxic cells can also be found much closer to blood vessels than would be expected from diffusion limitations. This observation reflects the poor functionality of tumour vasculature, which is characterized by being highly tortuous and poorly organized (Fig. 16.1). Tumour vessels are often immature, leaky, lack smooth muscle cells, and have structural abnormalities including blind ends and arterial–venous shunts that together result in unstable blood flow, the cause of what is termed 'acute' or 'perfusion-limited' hypoxia. Perfusion-limited hypoxia is characterized by rapidly changing oxygen concentrations in areas where blood flow through the vessel is unstable (Lanzen *et al.*, 2006). As a result, cells may be exposed to oxygen concentrations that vary transiently between normal (well perfused) and anoxia (complete vessel blockage) and anywhere in between. Examples of perfusion (acute) and

diffusion (chronic) hypoxia observed in experimental tumour models are shown in Fig. 16.2.

16.2 THE HETEROGENEITY OF TUMOUR HYPOXIA

Heterogeneity in severity (oxygen concentration)

Limitations in diffusion and in perfusion give rise to tumour cells at widely different oxygen levels. As cells are pushed away from blood vessels by the proliferation of cells close to the vessel, they experience a steady decline in oxygen availability. Eventually, these cells may reach distances where the oxygen concentration drops to zero and they can then die and contribute to the necrotic areas in the tumour. Diffusion-limited hypoxia, therefore, is characterized by an oxygen gradient where cells exist at all possible oxygen concentrations from normoxic to anoxic. Similarly, the limitations in perfusion that give rise to acute hypoxia can be complete or partial, resulting in surrounding tumour cells at varying oxygen tensions. As a result, both mechanisms of tumour hypoxia are expected to produce cells at a wide range of oxygen concentrations. Consistent with this prediction, direct measurements made in patients using polarographic oxygen electrodes have demonstrated the presence of a large range of oxygen concentrations. Vaupel and Hoeckel were among the first to use this technique in the clinic and an example of their data from a series of breast cancers and normal tissues is shown in Fig. 16.3. Immunohistological staining of tumour sections also reveals variable degrees of staining intensities that reflect the presence of cells at a wide range of oxygen concentrations (Fig. 16.2).

The fact that tumours contain cells at many different oxygen concentrations is an important factor to consider when assessing the consequences of tumour hypoxia. In fact, the term 'hypoxia' is rather ill-defined and can refer to different cell populations in different contexts. As discussed in Chapter 15, hypoxia-associated radioresistance results from the participation of oxygen in radiochemical events that take place immediately after irradiation. Thus, we can think

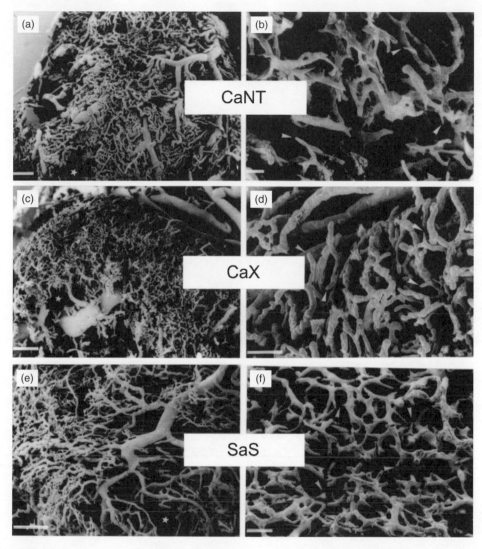

Figure 16.1 Scanning electron micrographs of vascular corrosion casts of murine carcinomas (CaX and CaNT) and sarcoma (SaS) grown subcutaneously in mice. Photomicrographs on the left represent low magnifications (bars = 500 μm) and photomicrographs on the right represent high magnifications (bars = 100 μm). From Konerding *et al.* (1999), with permission. See colour plate section for full colour images.

of 'radiobiological hypoxia' as oxygen concentrations below those causing maximum resistance to radiation, about 0.02 per cent. However, oxygen also influences a number of biological responses that are controlled by several distinct molecular pathways. The sensitivity of these molecular pathways to oxygen deprivation can be very different from the relationship between oxygen concentration and radiosensitivity. For example, activation of some molecular pathways reaches a maximum at much more moderate hypoxia (around 1–2 per cent O_2). These biological responses may in turn affect many tumour properties that are important for treatment outcome, including the response to radiation. Therefore, the relevant fraction of hypoxic cells may be considerably different from the radiobiological hypoxic fraction.

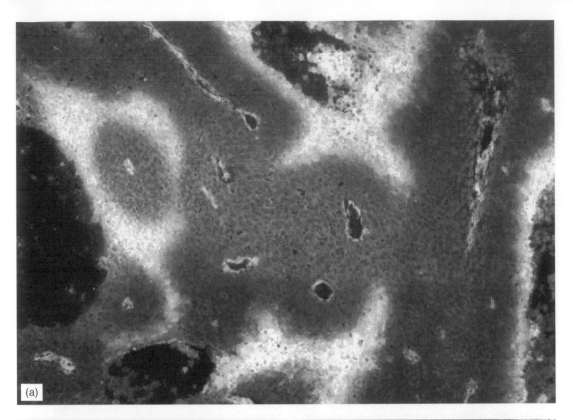

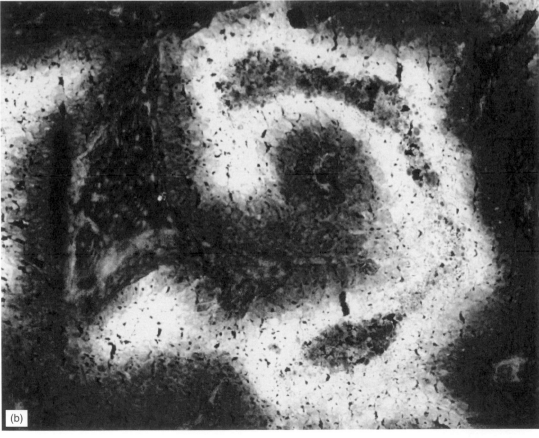

Despite this confusion about the definition of hypoxia, it has become commonplace in clinical situations to try to define the level of tumour hypoxia by a single number, the so-called hypoxic fraction. In Chapter 15, we emphasized the importance of considering cell viability and we

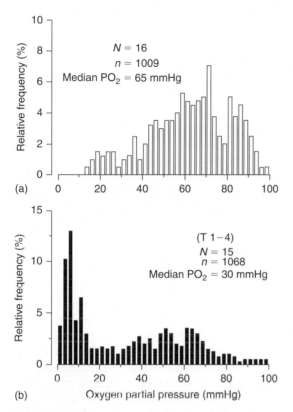

(a)

(b)

Figure 16.3 Frequency distributions of oxygen partial pressures for normal breast tissue (a) and breast cancers (b). Measurements were performed with a polarographic O_2-sensitive needle electrode with multiple recordings along three tracks for each patient. N, number of patients; n, number of measurements. From Vaupel *et al.* (1991), with permission.

defined the radiobiological hypoxic fraction as the fraction of viable radiation-resistant hypoxic cells. For assessments made by oxygen electrodes, the hypoxic fraction is usually defined as the fraction of measurements below some arbitrary low value of oxygen partial pressure, often 5 or 10 mmHg. For immunohistochemical detection with hypoxic markers (e.g. the nitroimidazoles), the hypoxic fraction is typically calculated as the fraction of cells that reach a certain threshold of staining intensity. In either case, the values arrived at are typically interpreted as a surrogate for the radiobiological hypoxic fraction. It is important to realize that because these thresholds are arbitrary and do not distinguish clonogenic from non-clonogenic cells, these two techniques will not necessarily give similar results and may not even correlate with each other. Furthermore when used in this way, both of these methods ignore potentially important hypoxic cells that lie above the threshold and, perhaps even more importantly, the variation in oxygen concentrations found within the tumour.

Heterogeneity in space

Hypoxia arising from either diffusion or perfusion limitations also gives rise to substantial intra-tumour heterogeneity in space. This spatial heterogeneity exists at the cellular level and is beautifully illustrated in immunologically stained tumour sections that cover a large area of the tumour (see Fig. 16.2, 16.4 and 16.11). This staining demonstrates the existence of steep oxygen gradients over distances of only a few cell diameters, contrasting with the common misconception that hypoxia is found mainly in the 'cores' of large tumours. In reality, hypoxia has the potential to exist around every blood vessel in the tumour and thus has no

Figure 16.2 (a) Multimarker greyscale image of human mucoepidermoid carcinoma MEC82 grown as xenograft, with vasculature (white), Hoechst 33342 (blue) staining nuclei of cells adjacent to perfused vessel, first hypoxia marker (pimonidazole, green), and second hypoxia marker (CCI-103F, red). Spatial co-localization of both markers (red and green) appears as yellow. At an injection interval of 2 hours, most of the hypoxic cells were labelled by both the first and second hypoxia markers. Acute (or transient) hypoxia is illustrated as an area that was not hypoxic at the time of the injection of the first marker but had become hypoxic at the time of the second hypoxia marker injection (red only). From Ljungkvist *et al.* (2007), with permission. (b) Grayscale image of C38 murine colon carcinoma, showing vessels (red) and hypoxia stained by pimonidazole (green). From van Laarhoven *et al.* (2004), with permission from Elsevier. See colour plate section for full colour images.

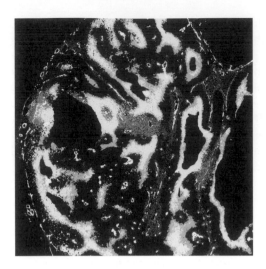

Figure 16.4 Composite binary image of a larger tumour area of the same tumour shown in Fig. 16.2a. See colour plate section for full colour image.

association with tumour size. The misconception of 'central tumour hypoxia' may stem from the common observation of central necrotic regions in human tumour xenografts grown in mice. However, in human tumours, hypoxia typically exists throughout the tumour volume, albeit at greater levels in certain tumour regions.

The extent of spatial oxygen heterogeneity also has implications for the way in which tumour hypoxia is evaluated in the clinic. It is important to obtain a sufficient number of measurements in different parts of the tumour in order to get a picture of the overall level of hypoxia and its variation, a task that is difficult with immunohistochemical techniques that are often limited to small biopsies. In this situation, one is forced to assume that the biopsy is representative of the overall tumour. This may often not be the case, as demonstrated by non-invasive imaging of positron emission tomography (PET) labelled hypoxia probes (e.g. misonidazole) that are able to assess the entire tumour volume. These PET images often show macroscopic 'hot spots' where hypoxia is more common.

Measurements in the clinic using oxygen probes are performed along more than one track in the tumour, with several samplings along each track. This gives rise to a frequency histogram that should reasonably reflect the overall distribution of oxygen

values. However, a word of caution is appropriate here since not only does this technique lose all spatial information, but each measurement made by the oxygen electrode represents an average concentration over a volume that contains several hundred cells. It is likely that oxygen gradients exist even within these volumes. Consequently, the actual cellular oxygen concentration will not be the same as that measured by the electrode. This 'averaging' problem is even greater with non-invasive techniques to image hypoxia. In this case, each imaging voxel can contain thousands or millions of cells. The limitations of all methods to reflect the true spatial heterogeneity (microscopic or macroscopic) is something that needs to be considered in the ongoing efforts to target radiotherapy specifically to hypoxic areas in tumours. Although areas with a larger proportion of hypoxic cells can receive higher doses, it will never be possible to specifically target all hypoxic tumour cells.

Heterogeneity in time

The biological consequences of hypoxia are influenced not only by the severity of oxygen deprivation, but also by the length of time that cells are exposed to this stress. If we consider diffusion-limited hypoxia, the oxygen concentration is expected to decrease as a function of distance away from the vessel. Owing to cellular proliferation in well-oxygenated areas close to the vessel, individual cells within a diffusion-limited gradient experience a slow decline in oxygen concentration over time as they are gradually pushed away from the vessel. The rate at which cells move through this gradient, and thus the length of exposure to various oxygen concentrations, is determined by the rate of cell proliferation. This can vary dramatically from one tumour to another, and even within different regions of the same tumour. Consequently, the lifetime of hypoxic tumour cells ranges from hours to days.

Much more rapid and dramatic oxygen fluctuations can occur as a result of limited perfusion as a vessel shuts down or reopens. Transient hypoxia has been convincingly demonstrated using several different methods in experimental tumours. For example, serial administration of two different

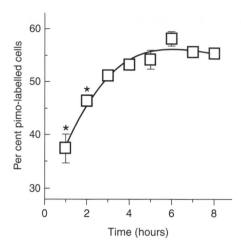

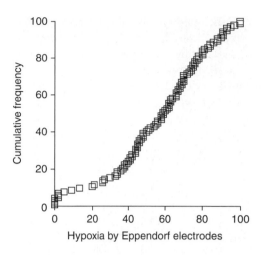

Figure 16.5 Percentage of SiHa tumour cells (human cervical squamous carcinoma) labelled with pimonidazole (pimo) as a function of labelling time. Tumours were grown subcutaneously in mice which were administered pimo by i.p. injection hourly before tumour excision. Tumours were processed to a single-cell suspension and the pimonidazole signal detected by flow cytometry. From Bennewith and Durand (2004), with permission.

Figure 16.6 Cumulative frequency of tumour oxygenation in 105 patients with primary uterine cervical cancer. Measurements were performed with a polarographic O_2-sensitive needle electrode with multiple recordings along three tracks for each patient. The percentage of measurements $\leqslant 5$ mmHg (HP$_5$) was used as a parameter for tumour oxygenation status. Adapted from Nordsmark et al. (2006), with permission.

hypoxia-specific markers analysed by immunohistochemistry identifies cells that stain for only one of the two markers (Fig 16.2 and Fig 16.4). This indicates that these cells were sufficiently hypoxic at one of the times to stain for hypoxia, but not at the other. Similarly, if a hypoxia marker is administered in a short pulse (1 hour), a much smaller number of cells are labelled than when it is given for a longer period of time (Fig. 16.5). This is due to the fact that many cells are only transiently hypoxic during this period. Continuous recordings from spatially fixed oxygen probes have also directly demonstrated temporal fluctuations in oxygenation (Lanzen et al., 2006). The results from these studies indicate that a substantial proportion of tumour cells experience transient periods of hypoxia lasting less than 1 hour.

The potentially rapid changes in oxygenation associated with perfusion-limited hypoxia present an additional problem associated with attempts to measure oxygenation in patient tumours. Such measurements are typically made only once, and it is unclear how representative they are of the actual oxygenation during treatment.

Heterogeneity amongst patients

Although there is large intratumour spatial and temporal heterogeneity, the variability in oxygenation between different tumours is even greater. Tumours with similar clinical characteristics can display very different patterns and overall levels of hypoxia at any given time. Figure 16.6 illustrates this fact using data obtained from a group of cervical tumours whose oxygenation status was determined using an oxygen electrode (Nordsmark et al., 2006). In these cases, the hypoxic fraction within a tumour was defined as the percentage of oxygen readings which were less than 5 mmHg. Defined in this way, the hypoxic fraction of individual tumours ranged from 0 to 100 per cent across 105 cervical cancers. About half of the tumours had hypoxic fractions above 50 per cent.

The heterogeneity in oxygenation among different patients is one of the features of tumour hypoxia that makes it so interesting to study. Because oxygenation differs markedly among patients, it can be used as a factor to categorize otherwise similarly presenting patients into different prognostic subgroups that may receive different treatment. Indeed, a recent multicentre meta-analysis identified the hypoxic fraction measured by oxygen electrodes as the most significant negative prognostic factor in radiotherapy-treated head and neck cancer (Fig. 16.7).

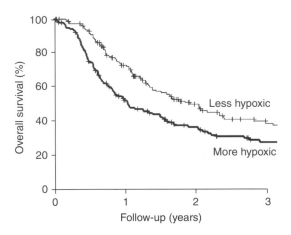

Figure 16.7 Overall survival rate for 397 patients with primary head and neck cancers. Measurements were performed with polarographic O_2-sensitive needle electrodes with multiple recordings along ±5 tracks for each patient. Thin and bold lines represent patients with less or more hypoxic tumours, respectively. More hypoxia was defined as a patient having more than 19 per cent of measurements yielding less than 2.5 mmHg O_2. From Nordsmark et al. (2005), with permission.

16.3 HYPOXIA AND ITS ASSOCIATION WITH THE MALIGNANT PHENOTYPE

The long-standing interest in tumour hypoxia within the radiation oncology community stems primarily from its association with radioresistance (see Chapter 15) and this aspect certainly remains an important contributor to patient response in the clinic (Tatum et al., 2006). However, clinical studies also support a role for hypoxia that is unrelated to treatment sensitivity. For example, in a study of uterine cervix cancers treated with surgery alone, patients with more hypoxic tumours had poorer disease-free and overall survival and more frequent parametrial spread as well as lymph–vascular space involvement (Fig. 16.8). This study, albeit small, indicated that hypoxic tumours are somehow biologically different from well-oxygenated tumours. Similarly, several clinical studies have demonstrated that hypoxia is a strong predictor for the presence of distant metastasis (e.g. Brizel et al., 1996).

Although a correlation between hypoxia and tumour progression, infiltration and metastasis has been established, these correlative studies cannot address whether this is a cause-and-effect relationship. In other words, is the increased malignancy a result of tumour hypoxia or is tumour hypoxia a

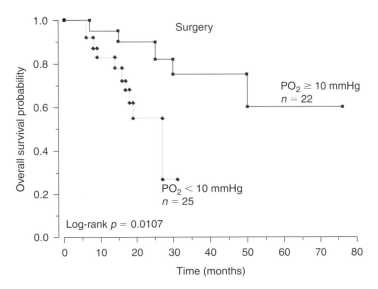

Figure 16.8 Overall survival probability for 47 patients with uterine cervix cancer treated with primary surgery. Measurements were performed with polarographic O_2-sensitive needle electrodes with multiple recordings along two tracks for each patient. Full or broken lines represent patients with median partial pressure of oxygen (PO_2) higher or lower than 10 mmHg respectively. From Hoeckel et al. (1996), with permission.

consequence of a more malignant tumour? This is not an easy question to answer and there is evidence supporting both of these possibilities.

16.4 HYPOXIA AND TUMOUR MALIGNANCY

Data from the laboratory and experimental tumour models indicate that hypoxia influences malignancy through at least three distinct mechanisms. The first is through the activation of physiological responses that facilitate adaptation to low oxygen, for example by increasing the rates of anaerobic glycolysis and angiogenesis. The second occurs by providing an adverse environment that allows the selection and outgrowth of cells that have increased tolerance to hypoxia and possibly other forms of stress. Finally, hypoxia has been shown to alter DNA repair capacity and to promote genomic instability in ways that can accelerate tumourigenesis.

Hypoxia-driven adaptation

During evolution, organisms have developed a number of different pathways whose function is to allow adaptation to low oxygen availability (Harris, 2002). Adaptation occurs at the cellular, tissue and whole-animal level. For example, hypoxia associated with high altitude causes increased production of erythropoietin (EPO), which stimulates uptake of oxygen by promoting the differentiation of red blood cells and synthesis of the oxygen carrier haemoglobin as well as endothelial cell proliferation. Similarly, during heavy exercise, oxygen consumption may exceed supply in muscle and cause hypoxia. The muscle cells respond to hypoxia by increasing their capacity to carry out anaerobic metabolism in order to produce sufficient ATP. The byproduct of anaerobic metabolism is lactate which causes pain in the muscles, a signal that exercise should be reduced. Hypoxia is also a powerful regulator of angiogenesis in both tumours and normal tissues. In fact, cellular responses to hypoxia play a fundamental role in controlling normal development of our vascular system.

Increased red blood cell and haemoglobin production, anaerobic metabolism and angiogenesis are adaptive processes that act to improve cellular oxygen supply and maintain energy homeostasis. Cancer cells use these same physiological response pathways to support the growth and spread of tumours. They switch to glycolysis for energy production and stimulate angiogenesis to improve oxygenation. In many cases, cancer cells have even undergone genetic alterations that allow them to hijack physiological responses to hypoxia, and they exhibit high rates of anaerobic metabolism and angiogenesis even during well-oxygenated conditions. This can occur through mutations in genes that regulate the hypoxic molecular response pathways to render them constitutively 'on' even during aerobic conditions. As noted above, however, tumour hypoxia persists despite high tumour vascularization, owing to poor organization and functionality of these vessels.

Hypoxia-driven selection of malignant cells

Despite adaptation, oxygen deficiency ultimately becomes toxic and results in cell death if it is severe and long-lasting. In a normal organism, this toxicity is often dealt with in a controlled manner by the induction of a highly regulated death process termed apoptosis. In this regard, the adverse clinical effect of tumour hypoxia may seem surprising, since one might expect hypoxia itself to be toxic to the tumour cells. Unfortunately, tumour cells are generally tolerant to hypoxia. This is partly because they often have mutations in genes that regulate apoptosis. In fact, hypoxia itself can evoke selection pressure against apoptosis-susceptible cells and thereby also promote the overall malignant potential of the tumour.

This principle of hypoxia-mediated selection has been elegantly illustrated in an experiment where rare cells that lack the tumour suppressor gene p53 (p53 knockout cells) are mixed with identical cells where p53 is functional and then exposed to periods of hypoxia (Graeber *et al.*, 1996). p53 is required for the induction of apoptosis in response to many stimuli, including hypoxia, and the knockout cells are therefore resistant to apoptosis. In the mixing experiment, the cells with functional p53 die during oxygen

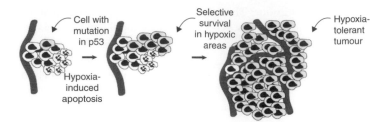

Figure 16.9 Selection of apoptosis-resistant cells in a hypoxic microenvironment. Early in tumour genesis, apoptosis-susceptible cells die rapidly if they experience hypoxia. In the genetically unstable tumour, a clonal mutation in an apoptosis gene (e.g. p53) arises that makes a cell resistant to hypoxia-induced death. Owing to its extended lifespan, this clone expands relative to the wild-type cells and eventually its progeny dominate the tumour mass.

deficiency, while the p53 knockout cells survive. The p53 knockout cells thus rapidly outgrow their counterparts and eventually dominate the cell population (Fig. 16.9). One can easily envisage this selection process occurring in a genetically unstable tumour. Single cells with random mutations that cause tolerance to hypoxia will have a growth advantage and expand relative to the other cells. Thus, hypoxia can act as a strong selective force during tumour development.

The selection of cells with increased hypoxia tolerance can occur through a number of different ways affecting various molecular pathways. Importantly, the genetic alterations selected for by hypoxia may also render the cells resistant to other forms of stress. Consequently a high level of tumour hypoxia may indicate that the tumour cells not only have a unique ability to survive against hypoxic exposure, but also an increased ability to survive during radiotherapy or other forms of cancer treatment. In other words, hypoxia can co-select highly resistant or highly malignant cells.

Hypoxia and genetic instability

Tumour progression is linked to the acquisition of a series of genetic changes and development of cancer is often accelerated by genetic instability (Bristow and Hill, 2008). Increased genetic instability can occur through mutations in genes that are responsible for the correct repair of damaged DNA, but may also occur during conditions of cell stress including hypoxia. Reporter gene and genomic minisatellite assays have shown that cells have increased mutation frequency and genetic instability when grown in the microenvironment of tumours compared with growth *in vitro*. Hypoxia and reoxygenation also causes aberrant DNA synthesis, leading to over-replication and gene amplification, which are other frequent alterations observed in cancer cells. Cycling oxygenation has particularly been linked to DNA damage through the production of reactive oxygen species (ROS) upon reoxygenation. This is accompanied by reduced expression of DNA repair genes under subsequent hypoxic conditions and functional decreases in the nucleotide excision repair (NER), mismatch repair (MMR) and homologous recombination (HR) pathways.

16.5 HYPOXIA RESPONSE PATHWAYS

Since hypoxia response pathways contribute to both hypoxia tolerance and overall malignancy, there is great interest in understanding these responses at the molecular level. Ultimately, this knowledge should lead to the development of hypoxia-specific biomarkers and new molecular targeting agents that can be tested in the clinic. Many of the biological changes that occur during hypoxia result from changes in gene expression, a process that is affected at many different levels, including chromatin remodelling, transcription, mRNA modification, mRNA translation and protein modifications. Although there are examples where hypoxia can affect gene expression at all of these levels, two in particular have emerged as important regulators of the biological changes

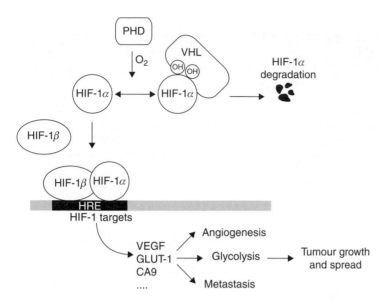

Figure 16.10 The regulation of hypoxia-inducible factor-1 (HIF-1). During normoxia, HIF-1α is hydroxylated by the PHD enzymes. This makes it a substrate for VHL–mediated proteasomal degradation. In the absence of oxygen, HIF-1α is stabilized and can dimerize with its partner HIF-1β to form the transcription factor HIF-1. This factor binds hypoxia–responsive elements (HRE) in the promoter of its target genes, resulting in increased transcription. These target genes regulate angiogenesis, metabolism and metastasis.

caused by hypoxia. These are changes in transcription and changes in mRNA translation.

16.6 HYPOXIA-INDUCIBLE FACTOR (HIF): THE MASTER TRANSCRIPTIONAL REGULATOR OF HYPOXIC RESPONSES

Many of the known changes in biology that occur during hypoxia in humans and other organisms are controlled by the activation of the HIF family of transcription factors (Semenza, 2007b). This is summarized in Fig. 16.10. The most widely expressed family member is HIF-1, although HIF-2 also functions in various cell types. Both HIF-1 and HIF-2 have similar functions and they regulate the transcriptional induction of more than 100 different known genes during hypoxia. These HIF targets regulate several important processes including erythropoiesis, metabolism, angiogenesis, invasion, proliferation and cell survival.

The HIF transcription factors consist of a constitutively expressed HIF-1β subunit, and an oxygen-sensitive HIF-1α or HIF-2α subunit. When oxygen is present, HIF-1α and HIF-2α are synthesized normally, but are unstable and degraded with a half-life of only about 5 min. Their degradation occurs because during aerobic conditions two proline amino acids are hydroxylated by enzymes known as the HIF PHDs (prolyl

hydroxylases) that use molecular oxygen as a cofactor. When they are hydroxylated, HIF-1α and HIF-2α are recognized by the von Hippel–Lindau (VHL) protein and targeted for ubiquitination and degradation. Under hypoxic conditions, HIF-1α and HIF-2α cannot be hydroxylated and thus are not recognized by VHL. This leads to their stabilization, allowing them to bind the HIF-1β subunit and activate gene transcription. Interestingly, the PHDs are themselves HIF transcriptional targets, thus establishing a negative feedback loop following the activation of HIF.

HIF activity as a hypoxia biomarker

The reduction in oxygen concentration required to stabilize and activate HIF is much less than that necessary to induce radioresistance. The dependency of HIF on oxygen concentration is determined by the enzymes that hydroxylate HIF-1α and HIF-2α. The HIF PHDs have a comparatively high K_m for oxygen. Thus, HIF becomes active when oxygen concentrations drop to only 1 or 2 per cent oxygen – a level that would cause virtually no increase in radioresistance. Consequently, the fraction of cells expressing HIF or HIF-dependent genes in a tumour can be significantly greater than the fraction of radiation-resistant cells. This is an important consideration in clinical studies that

SCCNij 51　　　　　　　　　　　　SCCNij 58

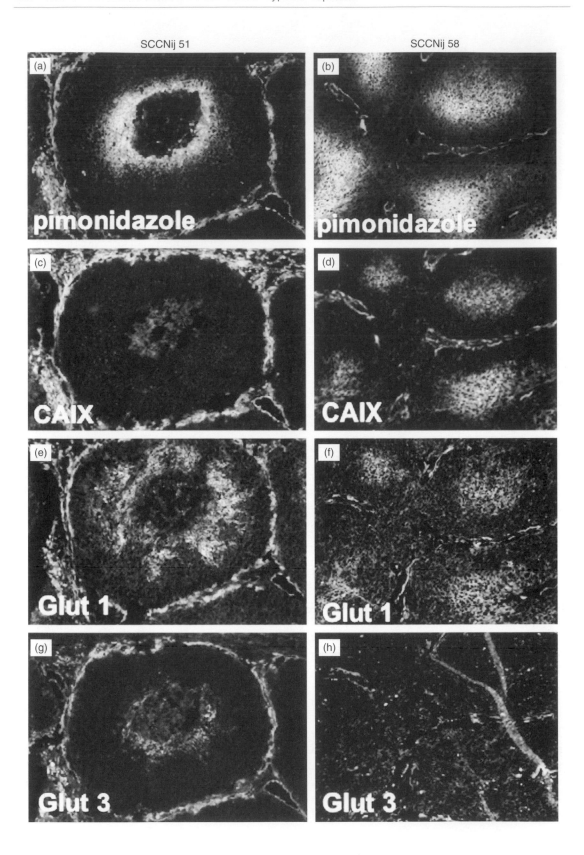

have investigated so-called 'endogenous' hypoxia markers. Several HIF target genes, including carbonic anhydrase 9 (*CA9*), glucose transporter 1 or 3 (*GLUT-1*, *GLUT-3*) and vascular endothelial growth factor (VEGF) have been used in studies to assess hypoxia. These markers are assessing HIF activity and thus reflect the type of hypoxia necessary to activate it. One should not expect that this will necessarily also reflect the radiobiological hypoxic fraction or the hypoxic fraction measured through other methods (Fig 16.11).

Although HIF is controlled primarily through oxygen, several common genetic alterations in cancer result in hypoxia-independent regulation of HIF-1α. *VHL* is a classic tumour suppressor gene, and its loss prevents degradation of HIF-1α and HIF-2α. Consequently, VHL-deficient tumours show constitutive HIF activity, and greatly enhanced angiogenesis. Oncogenic activation of the PI3-kinase and Ras pathways has also been reported to influence HIF-1α protein levels. This regulation also needs to be taken into account when using HIF targets as biomarkers of hypoxia. In some cases, HIF activation may occur in ways that are largely independent of hypoxia.

HIF as a target for therapy?

The activation of HIF and its target genes may be highly clinically relevant despite not always reflecting tumour hypoxia. The malignant cancer phenotype is highly linked to processes such as angiogenesis, metastasis and glycolysis which can all be stimulated by activation of HIF. Genetic alterations that cause constitutive activation of the HIF pathway can therefore be envisaged to both promote and reflect malignancy. On the basis of this, there is great interest in evaluating HIF and its transcriptional targets as prognostic factors, even in the absence of a direct correlation with hypoxia (Semenza, 2007a). Furthermore, the central role that HIF plays in regulating gene expression has caused widespread interest in its potential as a molecular target in cancer therapy. HIF-mediated gene expression presumably helps cells to survive better during low oxygen availability, so disrupting this signalling in tumours is expected to promote hypoxia-induced death. In this way, targeting HIF in cancer therapy can be seen as an attractive approach to complement radiotherapy, which kills well-oxygenated cells. The current efforts to target HIF have been spurred on by a detailed understanding of how HIF is regulated at the molecular level. This knowledge provides a basis for the targeting approach and makes the rational design of specific small-molecule inhibitors feasible. Experiments *in vitro* and *in vivo* have also provided some proof-of-principle supporting this approach. These studies have shown that cells which have been genetically engineered to lack functional HIF-1 die more rapidly from hypoxic stress and form fewer and slower growing tumours in animal models. A somewhat improved response to radiation has also been achieved experimentally when HIF has been targeted in established tumours using genetic approaches. It remains to be seen whether these encouraging results can be repeated and further improved with drugs that can be administered in the clinic.

16.7 HYPOXIA AND PROTEIN SYNTHESIS

Although HIF-mediated changes in transcription are important, they do not explain all of the biological changes that occur during hypoxia. On a genome-wide scale, a comparable number of genes are influenced through changes in their rate of protein synthesis. In light of the often acute and transient nature of hypoxic stress, it is not surprising that cells utilize fast-responding and reversible mechanisms such as those regulating protein synthesis (Wouters *et al.*, 2005). Protein synthesis

Figure 16.11 Different expression of hypoxia markers in two human squamous cell carcinoma xenograft models (SCCNij51 and SCCNij58). The images show the differences in localization of the exogenous marker pimonidazole (a and b) compared with three endogenous hypoxic markers: CAIX (c, d), GLUT-1 (e, f) and GLUT-3 (g, h) (all in green), relative to the vasculature (in red). From Rademakers *et al.* (2008), with permission from Elsevier. See colour plate section for full colour images.

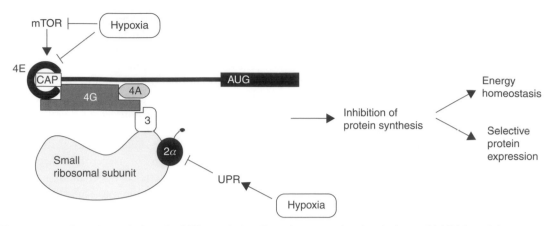

Figure 16.12 Hypoxic regulation of mRNA translation. Hypoxia causes phosphorylation and inhibition of the eukaryotic initiation factor 2 subunit α (eIF2α), preventing it from recruiting aminoacylated tRNA to the ribosome. Hypoxia also inhibits the interaction between eIF4E and eIF4G at the mRNA 5' cap structure, thereby preventing ribosome recruitment to the mRNA. This occurs through both mTOR-dependent and –independent mechanisms.

rates drop significantly during hypoxia because of a reduction in the rate at which mRNA transcripts are translated into protein. Protein synthesis is one of the most energy-consuming processes in the cell. Inhibition of protein synthesis in response to hypoxia has therefore been regarded as a means to conserve energy and maintain homeostasis.

The pathways that affect overall levels of protein synthesis during hypoxia (discussed below) also differentially influence specific genes through two different mechanisms. First, because proteins have different half-lives, inhibition of protein synthesis causes a selective enrichment of stable over labile proteins. This can alter cellular behaviour because several processes, including apoptosis, are regulated by the balance of proteins with different stability. Second, although overall levels of protein synthesis are reduced during hypoxia, this is a stringently regulated process that affects the production of individual proteins to a highly varying degree. The rate of synthesis of a particular gene product is determined by elements in the untranslated regions (UTRs) of its mRNA. These regions do not affect the composition of the protein, but instead function to regulate the stability and translation of the mRNA transcript. The mRNAs of some proteins contain elements in their UTRs that render them less affected by

hypoxia, and synthesis of some transcripts is even stimulated under hypoxic conditions. It is now recognized that regulation of mRNA translation has an important impact on the cellular proteome during hypoxia, especially at early times when it dominates the slower transcriptional responses.

mTOR and regulation of translation initiation

One of the ways that hypoxia affects protein synthesis is through inhibition of the mammalian target of rapamycin (mTOR) kinase signalling pathway (Koumenis and Wouters, 2006) as summarized in Fig. 16.12. This occurs in response to long-lasting moderate hypoxia (around 0.5 per cent O_2). Signalling through the mTOR pathway stimulates translation by increasing the availability of a rate-limiting eukaryotic mRNA translation initiation factors (eIF) called eIF4E. During hypoxic conditions, eIF4E becomes inactivated leading to reduced rates of protein synthesis. Because of its ability to control protein synthesis, mTOR is recognized as an important regulator of overall cellular metabolism and many different receptor signalling pathways influence cell growth and proliferation by this process. Consequently, mTOR is sensitive not only to oxygen but also to changes in energy levels and nutrient supply. Interestingly, many of the signalling pathways that converge on mTOR are frequently altered in cancer and lead to activation of mTOR and high rates of protein synthesis and proliferation as part of the oncogenic process. Possible tumour-specific regulation (or dysregulation) of the mTOR pathway has led to considerable interest in targeting this protein, and inhibitors such as rapamycin are currently in clinical trials in combination with other modalities including radiotherapy.

Endoplasmic reticulum stress and the unfolded protein response

Under more severe hypoxic conditions (less than about 0.02 per cent oxygen) hypoxia causes a rapid and more severe inhibition of protein synthesis (Wouters *et al.*, 2005). This effect results from the phosphorylation and inactivation of a subunit (α) of another important translation initiation factor, eIF2 (Fig. 16.2). The function of eIF2 is to recruit the first amino acid (methionine) to the mRNA transcript during the initiation of protein synthesis. Phosphorylation of eIF2α during hypoxia is carried out by activation of an endoplasmic reticulum (ER) transmembrane kinase called PERK. This kinase senses ER stress as part of a larger process called the unfolded protein response (UPR). During the UPR, PERK and two other proteins known as IRE-1 and ATF6 are activated as a consequence of the accumulation of unfolded or misfolded proteins within the ER. Together, these proteins function to prevent further ER stress both by inhibiting new protein synthesis and by increasing the folding capacity of the ER. Both PERK and IRE-1 are activated during hypoxia, suggesting that hypoxia may cause ER stress through protein misfolding and/or aggregation. It is believed that activation of the UPR during hypoxia protects cells against ER stress. Indeed, similar to HIF-1, genetically modified cells that lack proper ER stress responses mediated by either PERK or IRE-1 are sensitive to hypoxia and form slower growing tumours. Therefore, PERK and IRE-1 might also be future targets for oxygen-directed molecular cancer therapy.

Key points

1. Tumour oxygenation is heterogeneous with respect to severity, time and space.
2. Most tumours have some hypoxic cells.
3. High levels of hypoxia are associated with poor treatment outcome.
4. Hypoxia can select for outgrowth of cells with mutations.
5. Cellular responses to hypoxia influence malignancy.

■ BIBLIOGRAPHY

Bennewith KL, Durand RE (2004). Quantifying transient hypoxia in human tumor xenografts by flow cytometry. *Cancer Res* **64**: 6183–9.

Bristow RG, Hill RP (2008). Hypoxia and metabolism. Hypoxia, DNA repair and genetic instability. *Nat Rev Cancer* **8**: 180–92.

Brizel DM, Scully SP, Harrelson JM *et al.* (1996). Tumor oxygenation predicts for the likelihood of distant metastases in human soft tissue sarcoma. *Cancer Res* **56**: 941–3.

Graeber TG, Osmanian C, Jacks T *et al.* (1996). Hypoxia-mediated selection of cells with diminished apoptotic potential in solid tumours. *Nature* **379**: 88–91.

Harris AL (2002). Hypoxia – a key regulatory factor in tumour growth. *Nat Rev Cancer* **2**: 38–47.

Hoeckel M, Schlenger K, Aral B, Mitze M, Schaffer U, Vaupel P (1996). Association between tumor hypoxia and malignant progression in advanced cancer of the uterine cervix. *Cancer Res* **56**: 4509–15.

Konerding MA, Malkusch W, Klapthor B *et al.* (1999). Evidence for characteristic vascular patterns in solid tumours: quantitative studies using corrosion casts. *Br J Cancer* **80**: 724–32.

Koumenis C, Wouters BG (2006). 'Translating' tumor hypoxia: unfolded protein response (UPR)-dependent and UPR-independent pathways. *Mol Cancer Res* **4**: 423–36.

Lanzen J, Braun RD, Klitzman B, Brizel D, Secomb TW, Dewhirst MW (2006). Direct demonstration of instabilities in oxygen concentrations within the extravascular compartment of an experimental tumor. *Cancer Res* **66**: 2219–23.

Ljungkvist AS, Bussink J, Kaanders JH, van der Kogel AJ (2007). Dynamics of tumour hypoxia measured with bioreductive hypoxic cell markers. *Radiat Res* **167**: 127–45.

Magagnin MG, Koritzinsky M, Wouters BG (2006). Patterns of tumor oxygenation and their influence on the cellular hypoxic response and hypoxia-directed therapies. *Drug Resist Updat* **9**: 185–97.

Nordsmark M, Bentzen SM, Rudat V *et al.* (2005). Prognostic value of tumor oxygenation in 397 head and neck tumors after primary radiation therapy. An international multicenter study. *Radiother Oncol* **77**: 18–24.

Nordsmark M, Loncaster J, Aquino-Parsons C *et al.* (2006). The prognostic value of pimonidazole and tumour pO2 in human cervix carcinomas after radiation therapy: a prospective international multi-center study. *Radiother Oncol* **80**: 123–31.

Rademakers SE, Span PN, Kaanders JHAM, Sweep FCGJ, van der Kogel AJ, Bussink J (2008). Molecular aspects of tumour hypoxia. *Mol Oncol* **2**: 41–53.

Semenza GL (2007a). Evaluation of HIF-1 inhibitors as anticancer agents. *Drug Discov Today* **12**: 853–9.

Semenza GL (2007b). Hypoxia-inducible factor 1 (HIF-1) pathway. *Sci STKE* **407**: cm8.

Tatum JL, Kelloff GJ, Gillies RJ *et al.* (2006). Hypoxia: importance in tumor biology, noninvasive measurement by imaging, and value of its measurement in the management of cancer therapy. *Int J Radiat Biol* **82**: 699–757.

Thomlinson RH, Gray LH (1955). The histological structure of some human lung cancers and the possible implications for radiotherapy. *Br J Cancer* **9**: 539–49.

van Laarhoven HW, Bussink J, Lok J, Punt CJ, Heerschap A, van der Kogel AJ (2004). Effects of nicotinamide and carbogen in different murine colon carcinomas: immunohistochemical analysis of vascular architecture and microenvironmental parameters. *Int J Radiat Oncol Biol Phys* **60**: 310–21.

Vaupel P, Schlenger K, Knoop C, Hoeckel M (1991). Oxygenation of human tumors: evaluation of tissue oxygen distribution in breast cancers by computerized O_2 tension measurements. *Cancer Res* **51**: 3316–22.

Wouters BG, van den Beucken T, Magagnin MG, Koritzinsky M, Fels D, Koumenis C (2005). Control of the hypoxic response through regulation of mRNA translation. *Semin Cell Dev Biol* **16**: 487–501.

■ FURTHER READING

Fang JS, Gillies RD, Gatenby RA (2008). Adaptation to hypoxia and acidosis in carcinogenesis and tumor progression. *Semin Cancer Biol* **18**: 330–7.

Vaupel P (2008). Hypoxia and aggressive tumor phenotype: implications for therapy and prognosis. *Oncologist* **13**(Suppl 3): 21–6.

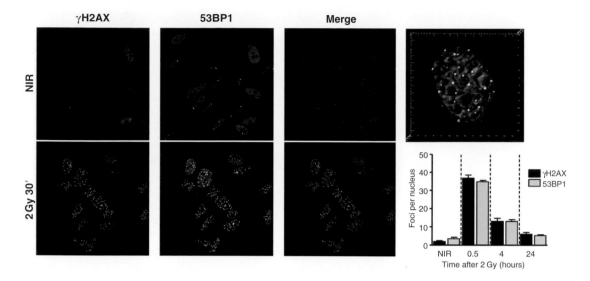

Figure 2.4 Examples of ionizing radiation-induced nuclear foci. Unirradiated and irradiated (2 Gy) cells have been fixed and stained with antibodies that recognize γH2AX and 53BP1, two proteins that interact at sites of DNA damage to form foci after induction of DNA double-strand breaks. These foci form rapidly and then resolve, consistent with the kinetics of DNA double-strand break rejoining. Photographs courtesy of Farid Jallai and Rob Bristow, Princess Margaret Hospital.

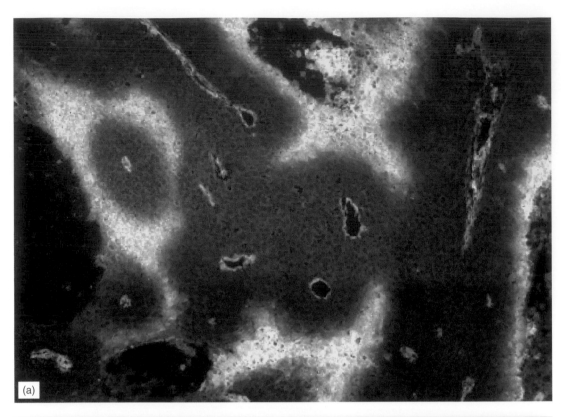

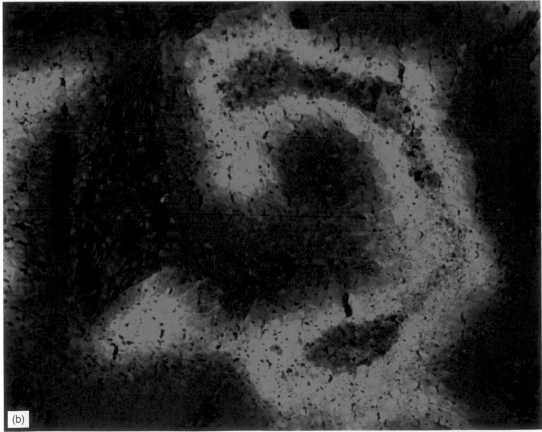

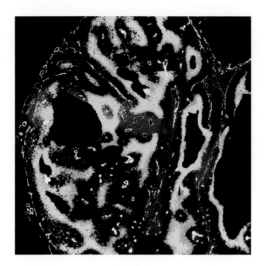

Figure 16.4 Composite binary image of a larger tumour area of the same tumour shown in Fig. 16.1a.

Figure 16.2 (a) Multimarker grey-scale image of human mucoepidermoid carcinoma MEC82 grown as xenograft, with vasculature (white), Hoechst 33342 (blue) staining nuclei of cells adjacent to perfused vessel, first hypoxia marker (pimonidazole, green), and second hypoxia marker (CCI-103F, red). Spatial co-localization of both markers (red and green) appears as yellow. At an injection interval of 2 hours, most of the hypoxic cells were labelled by both the first and second hypoxia markers. Acute (or transient) hypoxia is illustrated as an area that was not hypoxic at the time of the injection of the first marker but had become hypoxic at the time of the second hypoxia marker injection (red only). From Ljungkvist *et al.* (2007). (b) Grayscale image of C38 murine colon carcinoma, showing vessels (red) and hypoxia stained by pimonidazole (green). From van Laarhoven *et al.* (2004).

SCCNij 51 SCCNij 58

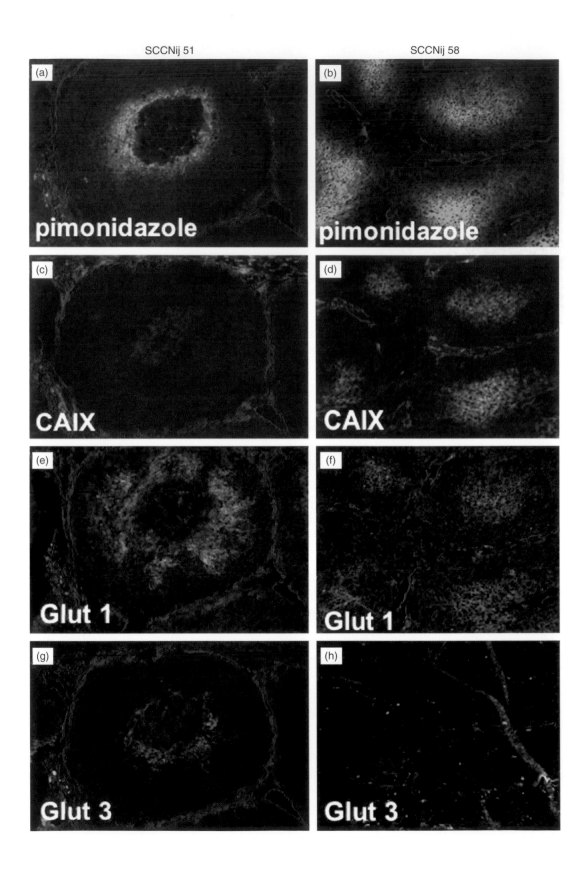

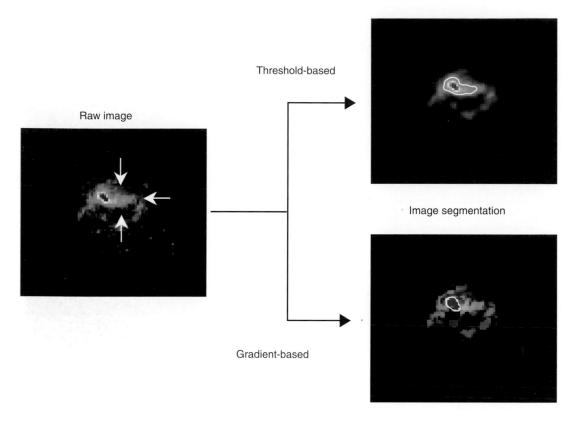

Raw image

Threshold-based

Image segmentation

Gradient-based

Figure 20.3 Comparison between a threshold-based and a gradient-based method for the automatic segmentation of a head and neck tumour during radiotherapy. The image is intrinsically noisier because of peritumoural radiation-induced mucositis. The gradient-based method led to a more specific tumour segmentation.

Figure 16.11 Different expression of hypoxia markers in two human squamous cell carcinoma xenograft models (SCCNij51 and SCCNij58). The images show the differences in localization of the exogenous marker pimonidazole (a and b) compared with three endogenous hypoxic markers: CAIX (c, d), GLUT-1 (e, f) and GLUT-3 (g, h) (all in green), relative to the vasculature (in red). From Rademakers *et al.* (2008 in press).

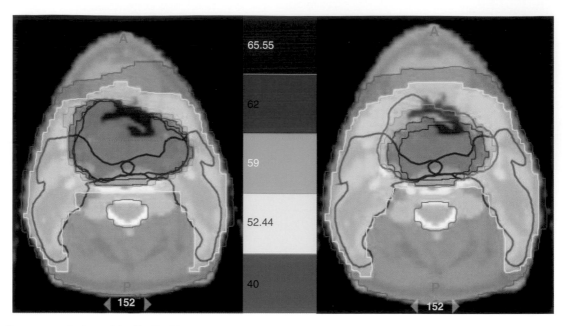

Figure 20.4 Patient with a T4–N0–M0 squamous cell carcinoma of the hypopharynx. The patient was treated using a simultaneous integrated boost approach delivering a dose of 55.5 Gy (30 fractions of 1.85 Gy) to the prophylactic planning target volume (PTV; delineated in dark blue) and a dose of 69 Gy (30 fractions of 2.3 Gy) to the therapeutic PTV (delineated in dark green). Comparison between a pretreatment computed tomography (CT)-based plan (left) and adaptive fluorodeoxyglucose positron emission tomography (FDG-PET)-based plan (right). On both plans, only the CT-based PTVs are depicted. A FDG-PET examination was performed before treatment and at 16 Gy, 24 Gy, 34 Gy and 44 Gy. The dose distribution was adapted to the progressive reduction of the FDG-PET gross tumour volume (GTV).

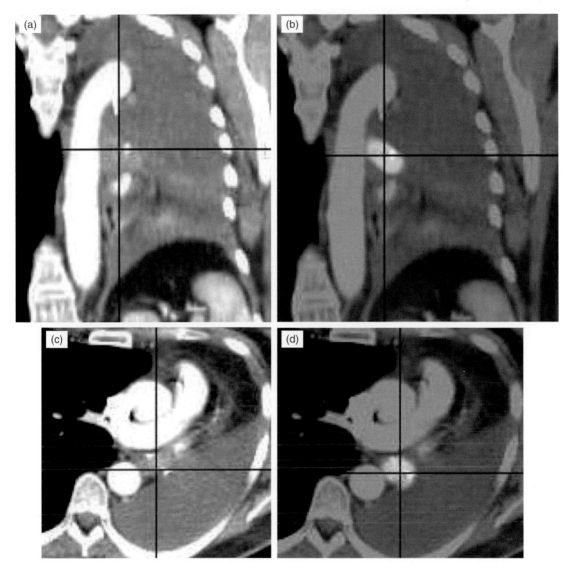

Figure 20.5 This example illustrates the role of fluorodeoxyglucose positron emission tomography (FDG-PET) for delineating the volume of a lung cancer. The images represent saggital (a) and axial (c) slices of a patient with a lung cancer located in the left hilar region, with retro-obstructive atelectasis of the entire left lung, associated with a major pleural effusion. The metabolic information provided by FDG-PET (b, d) shows that the tumour tissue is strictly located to the hilum. The delineation of the tumour margins is easier and more accurate with the help of FDG-PET, allowing for a significant modification of the target volume.

Therapeutic approaches to tumour hypoxia

MICHAEL R. HORSMAN AND ALBERT J. VAN DER KOGEL

17.1 INTRODUCTION

The radiobiological problem presented by hypoxia in tumours has been set out in the previous chapters; the present chapter describes a number of therapeutic approaches that have been designed to overcome this source of resistance. These primarily include decreasing hypoxia by increasing oxygen availability, chemically or physically radiosensitizing the hypoxic cells or preferentially killing this resistant cell population. Since inadequacy of the abnormal vascular supply to tumours is one reason why hypoxia develops, more recent attempts to improve tumour radiation response have involved specifically targeting the tumour blood supply.

17.2 RAISING THE OXYGEN CONTENT OF INSPIRED GAS

One of the earliest clinical attempts to eliminate hypoxia involved patients breathing high oxygen-content gas under hyperbaric conditions (Churchill-Davidson, 1968). An increase in barometric pressure of the gas breathed by the patient

during radiotherapy is termed 'hyperbaric oxygen (HBO) therapy' with pressures up to around 3 atmospheres having been used. Most trials were small in size and suffered from the use of unconventional fractionation schedules but the results demonstrated that HBO therapy was superior to radiotherapy given in air, especially when a few large fractions were applied (Overgaard, 1989). This was clearly seen in the largest of the multi-centre clinical trials of HBO, by the British Medical Research Council, in which the results from both advanced head and neck cancer and uterine cervix cancer showed a significant benefit in local tumour control and subsequent survival (Fig. 17.1). Benefit was not observed in bladder cancer; neither were these results confirmed by a number of smaller studies (Dische, 1985; Overgaard, 1989). In hindsight, the use of HBO therapy was discontinued somewhat prematurely. This was partly because of the introduction of chemical radiosensitizers and because of problems with patient compliance. It has been claimed that hyperbaric treatment caused significant suffering, but the discomfort associated with such a treatment must be considered minor compared

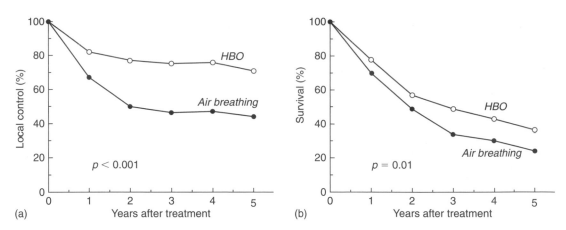

Figure 17.1 Results from the Medical Research Council hyperbaric oxygen (HBO) trial showing (a) actuarial local tumour control and (b) survival in patients with stage III carcinoma of the cervix randomized to receive either HBO (open symbols, 119 patients) or air breathing (closed symbols, 124 patients) in conjunction with conventional radiotherapy. Modified from Watson *et al.* (1978), with permission.

with the sometimes life-threatening complications associated with chemotherapy that is used with a less restrictive indication.

High-oxygen gas breathing, either as 100 per cent oxygen or carbogen (95 per cent oxygen + 5 per cent carbon dioxide) under normobaric conditions has also been used clinically to radiosensitize tumours, but failed to show significant therapeutic gain (Horsman *et al.*, 2007). One reason for this may have been the failure to achieve the optimum pre-irradiation gas breathing time (PIBT); a number of experimental studies have shown this to be critical for the enhancement of radiation damage and that results can vary from tumour to tumour. The failure of this approach may also have been related to the fact that normobaric oxygen would only be expected to deal with diffusion-limited chronic hypoxia and not with perfusion-limited acute hypoxia. Both the PIBT and the acute hypoxia phenomenon have been taken into account in the current ARCON clinical trials (see Section 17.5).

17.3 HYPOXIC CELL RADIOSENSITIZERS

The concept of chemical radiosensitization of hypoxic cells was introduced by Adams and Cooke (1969) when they showed that certain compounds were able to mimic oxygen and thus enhance radiation damage. They also demonstrated that the efficiency of sensitization was directly related to the electron affinity of the compounds. It was postulated that such agents would diffuse out of the tumour blood supply and, unlike oxygen, which is rapidly metabolized by tumour cells, they would be able to diffuse further, reach the more distant hypoxic cells, and thus sensitize them. Since these drugs mimic the sensitizing effect of oxygen they would not be expected to increase the radiation response of well-oxygenated cells in surrounding normal tissues; radiation tolerance should therefore not be compromised.

The first electron-affinic compounds to show radiosensitization were the nitrobenzenes. These were followed by the nitrofurans and finally nitroimidazoles, the most potent of which was found to be the 2-nitroimidazole, misonidazole. Its *in vitro* activity is illustrated in Fig. 17.2. Note that, in these experiments, misonidazole is radiation dose-modifying: the survival curves have the same extrapolation number (i.e. 4 in this case). The radiation response of hypoxic cells can thus be enhanced substantially by irradiating the cells in the presence of misonidazole; in fact, at a drug concentration of 10 mM the radiosensitivity of hypoxic cells approaches that of aerated cells.

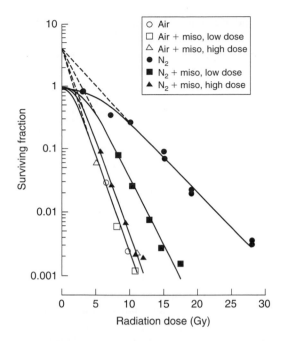

Figure 17.2 Survival curves for aerated and hypoxic Chinese hamster cells irradiated in the presence or absence of misonidazole. Low dose, 1 mM; high dose, 10 mM. From Adams (1977), with permission.

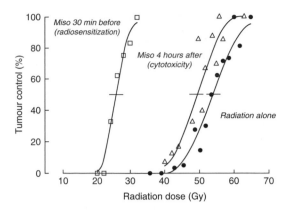

Figure 17.3 Local tumour control in C3H mouse mammary carcinomas measured 120 days after tumour irradiation. Mice were given misonidazole (1 g/kg, i.p.) either 30 min before or 4 hours after irradiation. The TCD_{50} (50 per cent tumour control probability) dose was reduced from 54 Gy in control animals to 26 Gy in the misonidazole-pretreated mice, equivalent to an enhancement ratio (SER) of 2.1. Misonidazole given 4 hours after irradiation gave a TCD_{50} of 49 Gy, an SER of 1.1.

The response of the aerated cells is unaffected, as expected for an oxygen-mimetic agent.

Radiosensitizers such as misonidazole also enhance radiation damage in experimental tumours *in vivo*, as shown in Fig. 17.3. The magnitude of the sensitizing effect is usually expressed by the sensitizer enhancement ratio (SER):

$$SER = \frac{\text{Radiation dose without sensitizer}}{\text{Radiation dose with sensitizer}}$$

for the same biological effect.

Large enhancement ratios (>2.0) have been found in a variety of animal tumours when the sensitizer was administered prior to single-dose irradiation. When misonidazole was combined with fractionated radiation, the SER values were lower. This probably results from reoxygenation between radiation fractions reducing the therapeutic impact of hypoxia. Also shown in Fig. 17.3 is the effect of giving misonidazole after irradiation, where a small but significant enhancement was seen. This obviously cannot be caused by hypoxic cell radiosensitization, but probably

results from the well-demonstrated observation that misonidazole is directly toxic to hypoxic cells – the level of cell killing increasing considerably with the duration of exposure to the sensitizer.

The first clinical studies of radiosensitizers were with metronidazole in brain tumours and together with encouraging laboratory studies of misonidazole they were followed by a boom in the late 1970s of trials exploring the potential of this latter agent as a radiosensitizer (Dische, 1985; Overgaard, 1989). However, most of the trials with misonidazole were unable to demonstrate a significant improvement in radiation response, although benefit was seen in some trials in certain subgroups of treated patients. This was certainly true for the Danish head and neck cancer trial (DAHANCA 2), which found a highly significant improvement in pharynx tumours but not in the prognostically better glottic carcinomas (Overgaard *et al.*, 1989). The generally disappointing clinical results with misonidazole may partly be because it was evaluated in unpromising tumour sites and with too few patients. However, the most likely explanation is the fact that the misonidazole doses

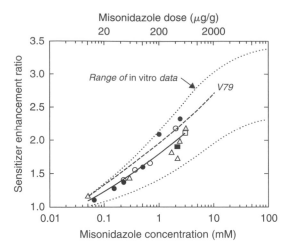

Figure 17.4 Sensitizer enhancement ratios determined *in vivo* using large, single radiation doses as a function of misonidazole dose (upper scale). The symbols indicate different tumour types. The solid line shows the best fit to the *in vivo* results. The dotted lines enclose the range of *in vitro* data (lower scale); data on V79 cells indicated by the dashed line. From Brown (1989), with permission.

were too low, being limited by the risk of neurotoxicity. Figure 17.4 summarizes data in mice for the dependence of sensitization on misonidazole concentration, in comparison with *in vitro* results. Although the SER for misonidazole increases with drug dose, the maximum tolerated misonidazole dose that can be given with standard clinical fractionated radiotherapy is around $0.5\,g/m^2$, which results in a tumour concentration of about $15\,\mu g/g$, and it is clear from the laboratory animal data that such a dose could only be expected to yield a small sensitizer enhancement ratio.

The difficulty in achieving sufficiently large clinical doses of misonidazole has led to a search for better radiosensitizing drugs (Coleman, 1988; Overgaard, 1994). Of the many compounds synthesized and tested, two of the most promising were etanidazole and pimonidazole (Overgaard, 1994). Etanidazole was selected as being superior to misonidazole for two reasons. First, although it has a sensitizing efficiency equivalent to that of misonidazole, it does have a shorter half-life *in vivo*, which should lead to reduced toxicity.

Second, it also has a reduced lipophilicity (a lower octanol/water partition coefficient) and is therefore less readily taken up in neural tissue, leading to less neurotoxicity. Etanidazole was tested in two large head and neck cancer trials, one in the USA and the other in Europe. In neither case was there a significant therapeutic benefit although in a later subgroup analysis a positive benefit was reported (Overgaard, 1998). Pimonidazole contains a side-chain with a weakly basic piperidine group. This compound is more electron-affinic than misonidazole and thus is more effective as a radiosensitizer; it is also uncharged at acid pH, thus promoting its accumulation in ischaemic regions of tumours. A pimonidazole trial was started in uterine cervix, but was stopped when it became evident that those patients who received pimonidazole showed a poorer response.

In Denmark, an alternative strategy was used and this involved searching for a less toxic drug and thus nimorazole was chosen. Although its sensitizing ability was less than could theoretically be achieved by misonidazole, nimorazole was far less toxic and thus could be given in much higher doses. At a clinically relevant dose the SER was approximately 1.3. Furthermore, the drug could be given in association with a conventional radiation therapy schedule and was therefore amenable to clinical use. When given to patients with supraglottic and pharyngeal carcinomas (DAHANCA 5), a highly significant benefit in terms of improved loco-regional tumour control and disease-free survival was obtained (Overgaard *et al.*, 1998). These results are shown in Fig. 17.5 and are consistent with the earlier DAHANCA 2 study for misonidazole. As a consequence, nimorazole has now become part of the standard treatment schedule for head and neck tumours in Denmark.

Additional studies are ongoing in an attempt to find other drugs that have low systemic toxicity but superior radiosensitization. In that context, two drugs are now in clinical testing. These are the nitroimidazole doranidazole, in which promising preliminary results were obtained in a phase III study with intraoperative radiotherapy in advanced pancreatic cancer, and the nitrotriazole derivative Sanazol, which in an International Atomic Energy Agency multicentre randomized trial (Dobrowsky *et al.*, 2007) in cervical cancer

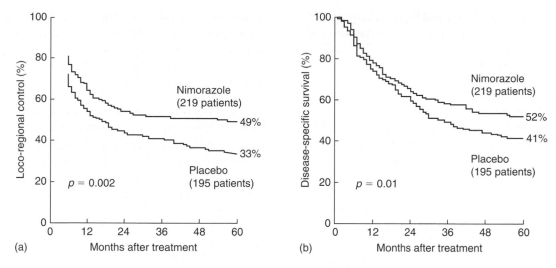

Figure 17.5 Results from the DAHANCA 5 study showing (a) actuarial estimated loco-regional tumour control and (b) disease-specific survival rate in patients randomized to receive nimorazole or placebo in conjunction with conventional radiotherapy for carcinoma of the pharynx and supraglottic larynx. From Overgaard *et al.* (1998), with permission.

was found to significantly increase local control and survival following radical radiotherapy.

17.4 MODIFICATION BASED ON HAEMOGLOBIN

It is well established that haemoglobin concentration is an important prognostic factor for the response to radiotherapy in certain tumour types, especially squamous cell carcinomas (Overgaard, 1989; Grau and Overgaard, 1997; Horsman *et al.*, 2007). Generally, patients with low haemoglobin levels have a reduced local-regional tumour control and survival probability (see Figure 15.8). While several mechanisms can be proposed to explain this relationship, tumour hypoxia is clearly one of the major factors.

Although there is no clear relationship between the 'steady-state' haemoglobin concentration and the extent of tumour hypoxia, both experimental and clinical studies have indicated that a rapid, albeit transient, increase of the haemoglobin concentration by transfusion can result in an increase in tumour oxygenation (Hirst, 1986). Furthermore, studies have shown that the amount of oxygen delivered to tumours by the blood is especially

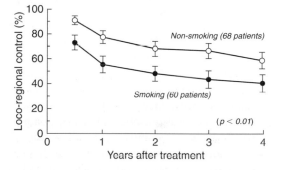

Figure 17.6 Influence of smoking during treatment on the outcome of radiotherapy in patients with advanced head and neck carcinoma. The local control probability was significantly poorer in patients who continued to smoke during radiotherapy, probably owing to reduced oxygen delivery to the tumour. Results from a prospective study in patients treated with curative radiotherapy alone; modified from Grau and Overgaard (1997).

important for a curative result. This is clearly illustrated in Fig. 17.6, in which patients with head and neck cancer who smoked were found to have a significantly lower loco-regional control than those who did not. Smoking can lead to a loss of more than 30 per cent of the oxygen-unloading capacity of the blood and this would be expected to significantly reduce tumour oxygenation and subsequently decrease tumour control (Grau and Overgaard, 1997).

The importance of haemoglobin has led to two randomized trials of the effect of transfusion in patients with low haemoglobin values (Overgaard et al., 1998; Fyles et al., 2000). Despite an initial positive report from the Canadian trial in uterine cervix carcinoma, both studies concluded that the use of such transfusions did not significantly improve treatment outcome. In the DAHANCA 5 study, transfusion was given several days prior to radiotherapy and adaptation may have occurred. Using preclinical data, Hirst (1986) hypothesized that any increase in tumour hypoxic fraction induced by anaemia will be only transient, with tumours adapting to the lowered oxygen delivery. Transfusing anaemic animals decreased tumour hypoxia, but this effect also was only transient and the tumours were able to adapt to the increased oxygen level. This suggests that when correcting for anaemia it may not necessarily be the final haemoglobin concentration itself which is important. Rather, an increasing haemoglobin concentration occurring at the time when the tumours are regressing during radiotherapy may be more likely to result in an increased oxygen supply to tumours and a subsequent improvement in response to radiotherapy.

Although a well-documented causal relationship between haemoglobin concentration, tumour oxygenation and response to radiotherapy has not been shown, it is nevertheless likely that such a relationship does exist and there is thus a rationale for investigating the possibility of improving the outcome of radiotherapy in relevant tumour sites in patients with low haemoglobin concentration given curative radiotherapy. The use of erythropoietin (EPO) is another approach for increasing haemoglobin levels and, unlike transfusion, such an increase would result in a gradual increase of oxygen supply over time. Several studies demonstrated that EPO was capable of producing such a gradual increase in haemoglobin concentration in patients with head and neck cancer (Henke et al., 1999) and several multicentre phase III studies were initiated to evaluate the importance of EPO in radiotherapy. However, a number of clinical studies, including two involving radiation therapy,

have shown that patients treated with EPO had a poorer outcome than the non-EPO treated control arms (Henke et al., 2003; Machtay et al., 2007). This may be related to non-haemopoietic effects of EPO and although this clearly raises concerns about the use of such agents to improve radiation therapy through a manipulation of haemoglobin levels, it does not make the concept of having a high haemoglobin concentration during radiation therapy an irrelevant issue.

17.5 OVERCOMING ACUTE HYPOXIA IN TUMOURS

Although the potential benefits of hypoxic cell modification in radiotherapy have been clearly demonstrated in a meta-analysis (see Section 17.7), the overall results of this approach are generally disappointing. One possible explanation for this may be the fact that most of the procedures used clinically operate against diffusion-limited chronic hypoxia, and they have little or no influence on perfusion-limited acute hypoxia (see Chapter 16). Experimental studies have demonstrated that nicotinamide, a vitamin B_3 analogue, can enhance radiation damage in a variety of murine tumours using both single-dose and fractionated schedules (Horsman, 1995). Typical results are illustrated in Fig. 17.7. This enhancement of radiation damage depends on tumour type, drug dose and the time of irradiation after drug administration, although it does appear to be independent of the route of administration. Nicotinamide can enhance radiation damage in normal tissues but generally these effects are less than are seen in tumours.

The mechanism of action of nicotinamide seems primarily that it prevents the transient fluctuations in tumour blood flow that lead to the development of acute hypoxia (Horsman et al., 1990). This finding led to the suggestion that the optimal approach would be to combine nicotinamide with treatments that specifically target chronic hypoxia. Benefit has been seen when nicotinamide was combined with hyperthermia, perfluorochemical emulsions, pentoxifylline and high oxygen-content gas breathing (Horsman, 1995). The combination of two potentially successful strategies, *Accelerated Radiotherapy to* overcome tumour cell proliferation with *Carb*Ogen and *N*icotinamide (ARCON) has been studied in various tumour sites, but most extensively in head and neck carcinoma (Kaanders *et al.*, 2002). A phase II clinical trial in 215 patients has shown very promising results in cancer of the larynx and oropharynx (Fig. 17.8). Two large multicentre phase III trials in bladder cancer (UK) and laryngeal cancer (The Netherlands) have recently been completed, and results should be available in 2010.

17.6 HYPOXIC CELL CYTOTOXINS: BIOREDUCTIVE DRUGS

Radioresistant hypoxic cells can also be eliminated by selectively killing them. This can be achieved with bioreductive drugs (McKeown *et al.*, 2007). These are compounds that undergo intracellular reduc-

tion to form active cytotoxic species, primarily under low oxygen tensions. The development of such agents arose following the discovery that electron-affinic radiosensitizers not only sensitize hypoxic cells to radiation but also are preferentially toxic to them (see Section 17.3). These drugs can be divided into three major groups, as illustrated in Fig. 17.9: quinones (e.g. mitomycin-C), nitroimidazoles (e.g. RSU-1069) and N-oxides (e.g. tirapazamine).

Mitomycin-C (MMC) is probably the prototype bioreductive drug. It has been used clinically for many years as a chemo-radiosensitizer, long before it was realized that it had preferential effects against hypoxic cells. It is activated by bioreduction to form products that crosslink DNA and therefore produce cell killing. Several randomized clinical trials in patients with squamous cell carcinoma of the head and neck have now been undertaken, specifically using MMC to counteract the effects of hypoxia.

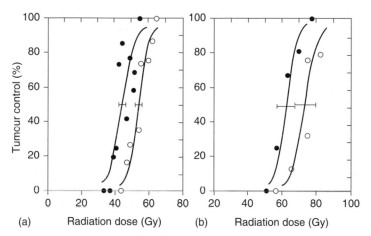

(a) Radiation dose (Gy) (b) Radiation dose (Gy)

Figure 17.7 Effect of an intraperitoneal injection of nicotinamide (500–1000 mg/kg) prior to local tumour irradiation on the level of tumour control measured as a function of the total radiation dose given either as (a) a single treatment to C3H mammary carcinomas or (b) in a fractionated schedule to the carcinoma NT. Results are for radiation alone (open symbols) or nicotinamide and radiation (closed symbols). Redrawn from Horsman *et al.* (2007), with permission from Elsevier.

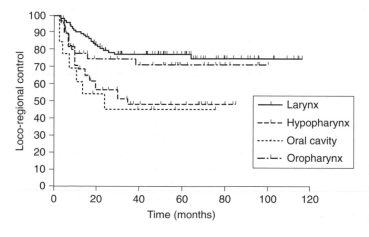

Time (months)

Legend:
— Larynx
— ⌐ — Hypopharynx
······ Oral cavity
— · ⌐ · Oropharynx

Figure 17.8 Results from a phase II trial of ARCON (see text) in 215 patients with head and neck cancer. Modified from Hoogsteen *et al.* (2006), with permission.

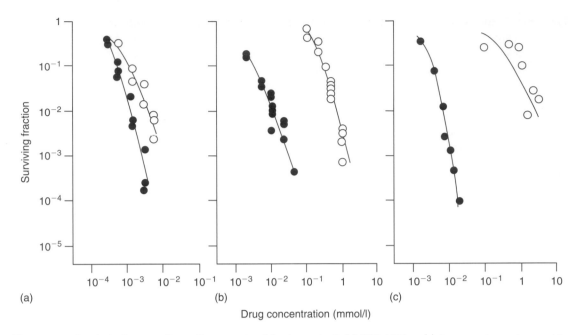

Figure 17.9 Survival of mammalian cells exposed to (a) mitomycin-C, (b) RSU-1069 or (c) tirapazamine under aerobic (open symbols) or hypoxic (closed symbols) conditions. Redrawn from Horsman *et al.* (2007), with permission from Elsevier.

Initial studies reported an improvement in local tumour control and/or survival, without any enhancement of radiation reactions in normal tissues. However, this has not been confirmed by more recent studies, perhaps not surprising when one considers that MMC actually has a very small differential killing effect between aerobic and hypoxic cells (Fig. 17.9). Also, in the clinical trials MMC was administered only once or twice during the entire course of radiotherapy, so its ability to preferentially kill hypoxic cells and thus enhance radiation therapy must have been limited. Attempts to find more efficient quinones have been undertaken and to that end porfiromycin and EO9 have been developed. While EO9 has gone through only preliminary phase I/II testing, porfiromycin was included in a prospective randomized trial in combination with radiation therapy in head and neck cancer, but was found to be no better than MMC.

The finding that misonidazole was preferentially toxic towards hypoxic cells led to numerous efforts to find other nitroimidazoles that were better. To that end RSU-1069 was developed. This compound has the classic 2-nitroimidazole radiosensitizing properties, but also an aziridine ring at the terminal end of the chain, which gave the molecule

substantial potency as a hypoxic cell cytotoxin, both *in vitro* and *in vivo*. In large-animal studies it was found to cause gastrointestinal toxicity and a less toxic prodrug was therefore developed (RB-6145) which is reduced *in vivo* to RSU-1069. Although this drug was found to have potent anti-tumour activity in experimental systems, further animal studies revealed that this drug induced blindness; this is perhaps not surprising when one realizes that the retina is hypoxic. Further development of this drug was then halted. However, other nitro-containing compounds including NLCQ-1, CB1954, SN23862 and PR-104 are currently under development.

Perhaps the most promising group of bioreductive drugs are the organic nitroxides, of which the benzotriazene di-*N*-oxide tirapazamine is the lead compound. The parent moiety shows limited toxicity towards aerobic cells, but after reduction under hypoxic conditions a product is formed that has been shown to be highly toxic and can substantially enhance radiation damage to tumours *in vivo*. Most clinical studies have involved combining tirapazamine with chemotherapy, although there have been a few trials with radiation ± chemotherapy. The results from the phase II trials generally showed promise, but in the few randomized trials

Table 17.1 Meta-analysis of randomized clinical trials of radiotherapy (RT) with a hypoxic-cell modifier

	Number of trials	Number of patients	RT + modifier (%)	RT alone (%)	Odds ratio (95% CL)
A. Summary of randomized trials					
Endpoint					
Loco-regional control	65	8652	52	45	1.29 (1.19–1.41)
Survival	77	10037	35	31	1.19 (1.09–1.29)
Distant metastases	21	4138	20	21	0.93 (0.80–1.07)
RT complications	26	3918	18	17	1.09 (0.93–1.29)
B. Loco-regional tumour control as a function of type of hypoxic modification					
Hypoxic modifier					
HBO/oxygen*	24	2667	59	49	1.47 (1.26–1.71)
Hypoxic sensitizer*	41	5974	48	42	1.24 (1.12–1.38)
Transfusion	1	135	84	69	2.27 (1.00–5.20)
C. Loco-regional tumour control as a function of tumour type and location					
Tumour site					
Head and neck	27	4250	46	39	1.35 (1.20–1.53)
Bladder	12	707	50	45	1.24 (0.93–1.67)
Uterine cervix	18	2877	65	58	1.31 (1.13–1.52)
Lung (NSCLC)	8	624	37	33	1.19 (0.85–1.65)
Oesophagus	2	192	30	26	1.25 (0.66–2.34)
All (group C) trials	65	8652	52	45	1.29 (1.19–1.41)

*Including one trial with hyperbaric oxygen (HBO) + misonidazole (124 patients).

CL, confidence limits; NSCLC, non-small cell lung carcinoma.

that have been completed the results have been somewhat disappointing. However, it has now been suggested that a benefit of tirapazamine might be achieved if one could select patients with hypoxic tumours by PET-imaging prior to treatment. Other *N*-oxides are currently under development, including chlorambucil *N*-oxide and AQ4N (banoxantrone), the latter being combined with radiation in a number of phase II trials.

17.7 META-ANALYSIS OF CONTROLLED CLINICAL TRIALS OF MODIFIED TUMOUR HYPOXIA

The clinical role of hypoxia is one of the most thoroughly addressed issues in radiotherapy and has been under investigation for many years. Of the numerous clinical trials that have been conducted during the last three decades, most have been inconclusive and this has raised serious concerns about

the real importance of hypoxia. This was addressed in a meta-analysis of all randomized clinical trials in which some form of hypoxic modification was performed in solid tumours undergoing radiotherapy with curative intent. The survey of published and unpublished data identified more than 11000 patients treated in 91 randomized clinical trials. The median number of patients per trial was 76 (range 14–626) and the trials involved HBO (31 trials), hypoxic cell radiosensitizers (53 trials), HBO and radiosensitizer (one trial), oxygen or carbogen breathing (five trials) and blood transfusion (one trial). Tumour sites were bladder (18 trials), uterine cervix (20 trials), central nervous system (CNS; 13 trials), head and neck (29 trials), lung (10 trials), oesophagus (two trials) and mixed site (one trial). These trials were analysed with regard to local tumour control (65 trials), survival (77 trials), distant metastases (21 trials) and complications resulting from radiotherapy (26 trials). The overall results are given in Table 17.1. The most relevant endpoint

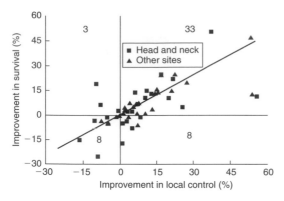

Figure 17.10 Results from 52 randomized trials of radiotherapy with/without hypoxic modification in which both local tumour control and survival data were obtained. A positive improvement in either survival or local control indicates that the hypoxic-modified arms were better than those of the controls. A strong correlation between both endpoints is indicated ($r = 0.69$; slope $= 0.81$). The figure shows that patients with head and neck carcinoma seem to have the most impressive benefit.

was considered to be local tumour control in view of the local nature of the radiation treatment, and this showed a significant improvement. This improvement persisted when the trials were evaluated separately for radiosensitizer or HBO treatment. When analysed according to site, significant improvements were found only for uterine cervix and head and neck. Overall survival was also significantly improved, again dominated by the head and neck patients, but no difference was found for distant metastases or radiation complications. The trials did use different fractionation schedules, including some large doses per fraction, but even for head and neck trials using conventional fractionation, the effect of hypoxic modification was still maintained with an odds ratio of 1.25 (range 1.08–1.45). Figure 17.10 shows the relationship between improvement in local control and subsequent improvement in survival. The trials shown in Fig. 17.10 are all of epithelial carcinomas, but patients with head and neck tumours generally achieved the greatest improvement in both local control and subsequent survival.

From this meta-analysis it appears that radiobiological hypoxic radioresistance may be marginal

in most adenocarcinomas. Future efforts should therefore be focused on squamous cell carcinoma, especially of the head and neck, at least when radiotherapy is given in conventional treatment schedules. The variation in the results among the trials certainly points towards a considerable heterogeneity among tumours with the same localization and histology. Thus, the need to predict the presence of hypoxia and especially the capacity for reoxygenation appears to be a key issue in order to optimize future clinical applications. The observations that polarographic oxygen electrode measurements were highly predictive for the outcome of radiotherapy in head and neck and cervix (see Chapter 16) indicates that a better selection of patients may be possible. The significant improvement obtained by manipulation of the hypoxic status of squamous tumours of the head and neck, and to a lesser extent cervix, indicates that the underlying biological rationale is probably sound, at least in these tumour sites. It would be logical, therefore, to direct future clinical studies of the hypoxic problem at these tumour types and sites.

17.8 VASCULAR TARGETING THERAPIES

The vascular supply to tumours is one of the major factors responsible for the development of hypoxia. The tumour vasculature develops from normal-tissue vessels by the process of 'angiogenesis'. This is an essential aspect of tumour growth, but this tumour neo-vasculature is primitive and chaotic in nature; it is often unable to meet the oxygen demands of rapidly expanding tumour regions, thus allowing hypoxia to develop (see Fig. 16.1). The importance of the tumour neo-vasculature in determining growth and the environmental conditions within a tumour makes it an attractive target for therapy and two approaches are currently in vogue (Horsman and Siemann, 2006). The first and most popular is the use of drugs to prevent angiogenesis from occurring, while the second involves the use of therapies that can specifically damage the already established vasculature. Examples of both angiogenesis inhibiting agents (AIAs) and vascular disrupting agents (VDAs) are given in Table 17.2.

Table 17.2 Strategies targeting the tumour vasculature

Approaches	Agents
Angiogenesis inhibitors	
Angiogenesis activator inhibitors	Anti-vascular endothelial growth factor (VEGF) antibodies (Avastin/ Bevacizumab, DC101), VEGF-trap
Receptor tyrosine kinase inhibitors	SU5416, SU6668, SU11248, SU11657, ZD6474, PTK787/ZK22854, IMC-1C11, c-Kit/Flt-3
Proteolysis inhibitors	Marimastat, Neovastat, AG-3340, Bay-12-9566, BMS-275291
Endothelial cell function inhibitors	Angiostatin, endostatin, TNP-470, thalidomide, ABT-510, thrombospondin, anginex, arginine deiminase
Integrin activity inhibitors	Vitaxin, cilengitide
Vascular disrupting agents	
Tubulin binding agents	Colchicine, combretastatin A-4 disodium phosphate (CA4DP), OXi4503, ZD6126, AVE8062, NPI2358, MN-029
Non-tubulin effectors	Tumour necrosis factor, flavone acetic acid (FAA), 5,6-dimethylxanthenone-4-acetic acid (DMXAA), 2-methoxyestradiol, arsenic trioxide, interleukins

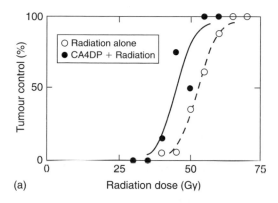 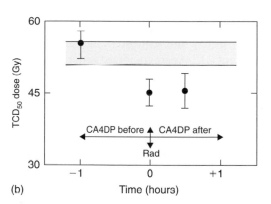

(a)   (b)

Figure 17.11 (a) Local tumour control in C3H mammary carcinomas measured 90 days after local tumour irradiation with single radiation doses either given alone (open symbols) or followed by a single intraperitoneal injection with CA4DP (250 mg/kg) 30 min later (closed symbols). (b) The TCD_{50} doses (radiation dose producing tumour control in 50 per cent of mice) with 95 per cent confidence intervals obtained from full radiation dose response curves for radiation alone (shaded area) or radiation with CA4DP given at various times before or after irradiating (closed symbols).

Although both types of vascular targeting agents have anti-tumour activity when used alone, significant improvements in tumour response have been observed when they are combined with radiation. With AIAs, the consensus opinion is that this improvement is the consequence of normalization of the tumour vasculature resulting in a decrease in tumour hypoxia. While there are certainly preclinical studies showing an improved tumour oxygenation status with AIA treatment, there are just as many studies showing no change and even a decrease in tumour oxygenation. These findings not only make it unclear as to the role of hypoxia in influencing the combination of AIAs with radiation, they also suggest that timing and sequencing of the two modalities may be critical for an optimal benefit.

The ability of VDAs to enhance radiation response is shown in Fig. 17.11. In these experiments tumour-bearing mice were injected with CA4DP, the lead VDA currently in clinical testing, shortly before or after locally irradiating the tumours. Although the drug alone had no effect on tumour control, it significantly enhanced the response to radiation when given after irradiating. Vascular disrupting agents damage tumour blood vessels leading to a reduced blood flow to the affected tumour region. This gives rise to local hypoxia and ischaemia, and ultimately cell death. Since hypoxic cells are already under stress as a result of oxygen and nutrient deprivation it is likely that these cells will be the first to die after this additional insult from vascular shut-down, and it is probably this effect that explains the enhancement of the radiation response. Additional studies suggest that these effects are tumour-specific. Figure 17.11 also shows that when VDAs are given prior to irradiating, no enhancement is seen, suggesting that although CA4DP kills some cells as a result of the vascular occlusion, there are other cells that become hypoxic yet survive and are a source of radiation resistance. This again raises the issue of timing and sequence, which is especially important if VDAs are combined with radiation in a fractionated schedule. However, when appropriate schedules designed to minimize the hypoxia-inducing effect of VDAs are used, a significant enhanced response has been observed with a fractionated radiation schedule. As a result, the combination of VDAs with radiation is currently under clinical evaluation.

Key points

1. Hypoxic cell radioresistance is a significant cause of failure in the local control of tumours, especially squamous cell carcinomas of the head and neck and cervix.
2. Clinical attempts to overcome hypoxic cell radioresistance using high oxygen-content gas breathing, chemical radiosensitizers or blood transfusions have shown mixed results. Meta-analysis of randomized trials does, however, demonstrate a significant benefit.

3. Since these treatments are designed to negate the effects of chronic hypoxia, additional benefit may be obtained by including a modifier of acute hypoxia such as nicotinamide in the treatment protocol.
4. Hypoxic cell cytotoxins (e.g. bioreductive drugs) also show promise as clinically relevant methods for eliminating radioresistance.
5. Since one of the major factors responsible for hypoxia is the inadequate vascular supply of tumours, preclinical studies are now suggesting that drugs which specifically target tumour blood vessels may provide a new approach to overcoming the hypoxia problem.

■ BIBLIOGRAPHY

Adams GE (1977). Hypoxic cell sensitizers for radiotherapy. In: Becker FF (ed.) *Cancer: a comprehensive treatise*, Vol. 6. New York: Plenum Press, 181–223.

Adams GE, Cooke MS (1969). Electron–affinic sensitization. I. A structural basis for chemical radiosensitizers in bacteria. *Int J Radiat Biol* **15**: 457–71.

Brown JM (1989). Keynote address: hypoxic cell radiosensitizers: where next? *Int J Radiat Oncol Biol Phys* **16**: 987–93.

Churchill-Davidson I (1968). The oxygen effect in radiotherapy: historical review. *Front Radiat Ther Oncol* **1**: 1–15.

Coleman CN (1988). Hypoxia in tumors: a paradigm for the approach to biochemical and physiologic heterogeneity. *J Natl Cancer Inst* **80**: 310–7.

Dische S (1985). Chemical sensitizers for hypoxic cells: a decade of experience in clinical radiotherapy. *Radiother Oncol* **3**: 97–115.

Dobrowsky W, Huigol NG, Jayatilake RS *et al.* (2007). AK-2123 (sanazol) as a radiation sensitizer in the treatment of stage III cervical cancer: results of an IAEA multicentre randomized trial. *Radiother Oncol* **82**: 24–9.

Fyles AW, Milosevic M, Pintilie M, Syed A, Hill RP (2000). Anemia, hypoxia and transfusion in patients with cervix cancer: a review. *Radiother Oncol* **57**: 13–9.

Grau C, Overgaard J (1997). Significance of hemoglobin concentration for treatment outcome. In: Molls M, Vaupel P (eds) *Medical radiology: blood perfusion and microenvironment of human tumours.* Heidelberg: Springer-Verlag, 101–12.

Henke M, Guttenberger R, Barke A, Pajonk F, Potter R, Frommhold H (1999). Erythropoietin for patients undergoing radiotherapy: a pilot study. *Radiother Oncol* **50**: 185–90.

Henke M, Laszig R, Rube C *et al.* (2003). Erythropoietin to treat head and neck cancer patients with anaemia undergoing radiotherapy: randomized, double-blind, placebo-controlled trial. *Lancet* **362**: 1255–60.

Hirst DG (1986). Anemia: a problem or an opportunity in radiotherapy? *Int J Radiat Oncol Biol Phys* **12**: 2009–17.

Hoogsteen IJ, Pop LA, Marres HA *et al.* (2006). Oxygen-modifying treatment with ARCON reduces the prognostic significance of hemoglobin in squamous cell carcinoma of the head and neck. *Int J Radiat Oncol Biol Phys* **64**: 83–9.

Horsman MR (1995). Nicotinamide and other benzamide analogs as agents for overcoming hypoxic cell radiation resistance in tumours. A review. *Acta Oncol* **34**: 571–87.

Horsman MR, Siemann DW (2006). Pathophysiologic effects of vascular-targeting agents and the implications for combination with conventional therapies. *Cancer Res* **66**: 11520–39.

Horsman MR, Chaplin DJ, Overgaard J (1990). Combination of nicotinamide and hyperthermia to eliminate radioresistant chronically and acutely hypoxic tumor cells. *Cancer Res* **50**: 7430–6.

Horsman MR, Lindegaard JC, Grau C, Nordsmark M, Overgaard J (2007). Dose–response modifiers in radiation therapy. In: Gunderson LL, Tepper JE (eds) *Clinical radiation oncology,* 2nd edn. Philadelphia: Churchill Livingstone, 59–73.

Kaanders JH, Bussink J, van der Kogel AJ (2002). ARCON: a novel biology-based approach in radiotherapy. *Lancet Oncol* **3**: 728–37.

Machtay M, Pajak TF, Suntharalingam M *et al.* (2007). Radiotherapy with or without erythropoietin for anemic patients with head and neck cancer: a randomized trial of the Radiation Therapy Oncology Group (RTOG 99–03). *Int J Radiat Oncol Biol Phys* **69**: 1008–17.

McKeown SR, Cowen RL, Williams KJ (2007). Bioreductive drugs: from concept to clinic. *Clin Oncol* **19**: 427–42.

Overgaard J (1989). Sensitization of hypoxic tumour cells – clinical experience. *Int J Radiat Biol* **56**: 801–11.

Overgaard J (1994). Clinical evaluation of nitroimidazoles as modifiers of hypoxia in solid tumors. *Oncol Res* **6**: 509–18.

Overgaard J (1998). Letter to the editor: Reply to Ben-Josef. *Radiother Oncol* **48**: 345–6.

Overgaard J, Hansen HS, Andersen AP *et al.* (1989). Misonidazole combined with split-course radiotherapy in the treatment of invasive carcinoma of larynx and pharynx: report from the DAHANCA 2 study. *Int J Radiat Oncol Biol Phys* **16**: 1065–8.

Overgaard J, Hansen HS, Overgaard M *et al.* (1998). A randomized double-blind phase III study of nimorazole as a hypoxic radiosensitizer of primary radiotherapy in supraglottic larynx and pharynx carcinoma. Results of the Danish Head and Neck Cancer Study (DAHANCA) Protocol 5–85. *Radiother Oncol* **46**: 135–46.

Watson ER, Halnan KE, Dische S *et al.* (1978). Hyperbaric oxygen and radiotherapy: a Medical Research Council trial in carcinoma of the cervix. *Br J Radiol* **51**: 879–87.

■ FURTHER READING

Brown JM, Giaccia AJ (1998). The unique physiology of solid tumors: opportunities (and problems) for cancer therapy. *Cancer Res* **58**: 1408–16.

Moeller BJ, Richardson RA, Dewhirst MW (2007). Hypoxia and radiotherapy: opportunities for improved outcomes in cancer treatment. *Cancer Metastasis Rev* **26**: 241–8.

Overgaard J (2007). Hypoxic radiosensitization: adored and ignored. *J Clin Oncol* **25**: 4066–74.

Combined radiotherapy and chemotherapy

VINCENT GRÉGOIRE AND MICHAEL BAUMANN

18.1 INTRODUCTION: CLINICAL OVERVIEW OF COMBINED RADIOTHERAPY AND CHEMOTHERAPY

In solid adult tumours, owing to its limited biological efficacy, chemotherapy is very seldom used as a sole curative treatment modality. It is, however, used more and more in combination with curative treatments such as surgery and radiotherapy, at least for locally advanced diseases. Chemotherapy can be delivered before a local treatment in an induction or neo-adjuvant setting, it can be delivered during a local treatment (i.e. during the course of radiotherapy) in a concomitant setting, and it can be delivered after a local treatment in an adjuvant setting. The rationale for these various schedules of administration will be discussed in Section 18.2. Table 18.1 summarizes the evidence-based data supporting the combined use of chemotherapy and radiotherapy in the most common adult tumours.

In brain glioblastoma, a recent EORTC–NCIC (European Organisation for Research and Treatment of Cancer–National Cancer Institute of Canada) study demonstrated that the concomitant and adjuvant use of temozolomide to standard brain radiotherapy (60 Gy in 6 weeks) was associated with a significant improvement in overall survival increasing from 10.4 per cent (radiotherapy alone arm) to 26.5 per cent following radiotherapy plus temozolomide (Stupp et al., 2005). Only minimal additional toxicity was observed in the combined modality group. The benefit of temozolomide was particularly striking in patients expressing a silencing of the MGMT (O-6-methyl-guanine DNA methyltransferase) DNA-repair gene by promoter methylation (Hegi et al., 2005).

In head and neck squamous cell carcinoma (SCC), meta-analyses have been conducted to ascertain the benefit and optimal scheduling of chemotherapy administration in relation to primary radiotherapy (Pignon et al., 2000; Budach et al., 2006). A significant benefit in survival was observed only when chemotherapy was associated concomitantly with radiotherapy. The benefit was higher in patients receiving platinum-based chemotherapy. The use of induction chemotherapy in patients with laryngeal or hypopharyngeal

Table 18.1 Evidence-based data supporting combined chemotherapy and radiotherapy

Disease site	Induction	Concomitant	Adjuvant	References
Brain glioblastoma	–	+ (level 2)	+ (level 2)	Stupp *et al.* (2005)
Head and neck SCC	± (level 1)	+++ (level 1)	– (level 2)	Budach *et al.* (2006), Pignon *et al.* (2000), Forastière *et al.* (2003), Cooper *et al.* (2004), Bernier *et al.* (2004)
Non-small cell lung cancer	+ (level 1)	+++ (level 1)	–	Rowell and O'Rourke (2004)
Small cell lung cancer	+++ (level 1)	+++ (level 1)	+++ (level 1)	Pignon *et al.* (1992)
Cancer of uterine cervix	± (level 1)	+++ (level 1)	–	Green *et al.* (2001, 2005), NACCCMA (2004)
Oesophageal carcinoma	–	+++ (level 1)	–	Wong & Malthaner (2006)
Rectal carcinoma	–	+++ (level 2)	–	Bosset *et al.* (2005a, b), Wolmark *et al.* (2000)
Anal carcinoma	–	+++ (level 2)	–	Bartelink *et al.* (1997)

Level of evidence: Level 1, multiple randomized studies/meta-analysis; Level 2, one or two randomized studies, requiring further confirmation.

SCC, squamous cell carcinoma.

SCC did not translate into a benefit, but was instead associated with a lower laryngectomy-free survival compared with concomitant chemoradiotherapy (Forastière *et al.*, 2003). In patients with a high risk of loco-regional recurrence after primary surgery (R1 or R2 resection, extracapsular tumour extension), postoperative concomitant chemoradiotherapy with 3-weekly cisplatin ($100 \, mg/m^2$) was also associated with a significant benefit in survival (Bernier *et al.*, 2004; Cooper *et al.*, 2004).

A meta-analysis has been conducted to determine the effectiveness and toxicity of concomitant chemoradiotherapy regimens compared with radiotherapy alone for non-small cell lung carcinoma (Rowell and O'Rourke, 2004). Fourteen randomized studies including 2393 patients were reviewed. At 2 years following treatment, there was a significant reduction in the death rate (relative risk of 0.93, $p = 0.01$) and a significant improvement in loco-regional progression-free survival (relative risk of 0.84, $p = 0.03$) and in progression-free survival at any site (relative risk of 0.90, $p = 0.005$) in favour of the combined treatment. In comparison with sequential chemotherapy and radiotherapy, concomitant treatment was associated with a 14 per cent reduction in the risk of death. The incidence of oesophagitis, neutropenia and anaemia were, however, significantly increased with concomitant chemoradiotherapy.

In limited stage small cell lung cancer, meta-analysis has also demonstrated the benefit of combining chemotherapy with thoracic radiotherapy, indicating an improved absolute overall survival of 5.4 ± 1.4 per cent at 3 years (Pignon *et al.*, 1992). Data are, however, conflicting regarding the optimal combination and timing between chemotherapy and radiotherapy and further clinical research is needed to resolve this issue (Pijls-Johannesma *et al.*, 2005).

In cancer of the uterine cervix, several meta-analyses have been performed to evaluate the benefit of combining radiotherapy with chemotherapy. A recent review including 24 trials totalling 4921 patients (from which data were available for 61–75 per cent of patients) has shown that concomitant chemoradiotherapy improved absolute survival by 10 per cent (95 per cent confidence interval 8–16 per cent) over radiotherapy alone (Green *et al.*,

2005). Cisplatin was the most commonly used chemotherapy. The benefit was observed for both loco-regional control (odds ratio of 0.61, $p < 0.0001$) and distant recurrence (odds ratio of 0.57, $p < 0.0001$) (Green et al., 2001). However, this improvement was associated with an increased risk of haematological and gastrointestinal early toxicities. A similar analysis was performed to evaluate the benefit of induction chemotherapy (NACCCMA Collaboration, 2004). The results are much more heterogeneous and no definite conclusion can be drawn. There was a trend towards improved survival for regimens with cisplatin dose intensities greater than 25mg/m^2 per week or cycle lengths shorter than 14 days. Conversely, in all other settings, a detrimental effect of induction chemotherapy on survival was found.

In localized oesophageal carcinoma, a meta-analysis of 19 randomized trials comparing radiotherapy and concomitant chemotherapy with radiotherapy alone has shown an absolute survival benefit of 9 per cent (95 per cent confidence interval 5–12 per cent) and 4 per cent (95 per cent confidence interval 3–6 per cent) at 1 year and 2 years, respectively (Wong and Malthaner, 2006). However, this benefit was associated with a significant increase in severe and life-threatening toxicities.

For patients with Dukes' stages B and C carcinoma of the rectum, a randomized study conducted by the NSABP (National Surgical Adjuvant Breast and Bowel Project) demonstrated that postoperative concomitant chemoradiotherapy reduced the incidence of loco-regional relapse compared with postoperative chemotherapy alone (13 per cent versus 8 per cent at 5 years, $p = 0.02$) (Wolmark et al., 2000). However, postoperative chemoradiotherapy did not have any influence on disease-free survival or overall survival. A recent EORTC randomized study demonstrated that the concomitant use of preoperative concomitant chemotherapy and radiotherapy was biologically more active than radiotherapy alone (Bosset et al., 2005a). Concomitant chemoradiotherapy was associated with a significant reduction in loco-regional relapse compared with radiotherapy alone, but did not have any effect on overall survival (Bosset et al., 2005b).

In patients with locally advanced squamous cell carcinoma of the anal canal, concomitant 5-fluorouracil, mitomycin and radiotherapy (45 Gy plus a boost of 15–20 Gy) resulted in an 18 per cent increase in 5-year loco-regional control and a 32 per cent increase in colostomy-free survival in comparison with radiotherapy alone (Bartelink et al., 1997). No significant difference in early and late side-effects was observed between the two arms.

In summary, the combined use of chemotherapy with radiotherapy has typically translated into a significant benefit in overall survival in sites where radiotherapy plays a substantial role. This benefit is mainly a consequence of an improvement in loco-regional control rather than a decrease in the risk of distant metastasis. In all the reported studies, the therapeutic ratio (defined as the advantage in efficacy over the disadvantage in toxicity) was, however, less clearly assessed and/or reported. In general, an increase in early toxicity was observed in all the trials. For late toxicity, systematic reporting of data is lacking, but the few available reports also indicate an increase in late radiation effects.

Even if the benefits of combined modality chemoradiotherapy appear irrefutable, the reported clinical trials generally do not allow any information to be derived on the actual underlying mechanisms of interaction between chemotherapeutic drugs and ionizing radiation. Have the benefits and side-effects resulted from a simple additivity of two effective therapeutic interventions, or from a more complex molecular interplay between the two modalities? If the latter is the case, was the combination of treatments appropriately designed based on the known mechanisms of interaction and the biodistribution and pharmacokinetics of the drugs?

18.2 INTERACTION BETWEEN CHEMOTHERAPY AND RADIOTHERAPY

Spatial cooperation

Spatial cooperation is the term used to describe the use of radiotherapy and chemotherapy to target disease in different anatomical sites. The commonest situation is where radiation is used to treat the primary tumour and chemotherapy is added to deal with systemic spread. There is an analogous situation in leukaemia where chemotherapy is the main treatment and radiotherapy is used to deal with disease in a 'seclusion site' such as the brain. Another example is the treatment of breast cancer where surgery and postoperative radiotherapy deal with the loco-regional disease and adjuvant chemotherapy deals with the micrometastatic disease.

If spatial cooperation is effective, this should result in a reduction of distant failures after the combined therapy. The successful exploitation of spatial cooperation depends critically on the effectiveness of the chemotherapy used. In the common solid tumours, chemotherapy seldom achieves a surviving fraction lower than 10^{-6}. Even small metastatic deposits of $< 0.1\,g$ may contain $10^7–10^8$ tumour cells and, if the majority of these are also clonogenic, standard chemotherapy may fail to control even a small amount of disseminated disease. For spatial cooperation to succeed more widely, we need more effective drugs or methods of specifically targeting existing drugs to the tumour cells, thus allowing dose escalation.

If the rationale underlying spatial cooperation between radiotherapy and chemotherapy is indeed to target different anatomical sites, the optimal way of combining these modalities is sequentially in order to avoid the likely increase in side-effects if given concomitantly.

Independent cell kill and 'shared' toxicity

This term describes the simple concept that if two effective therapeutic modalities can both be given at full dose then, even in the absence of interactive processes, the tumour response (total cell kill) should be greater than that achieved with either agent alone. To exploit this mechanism, the radiotherapy and chemotherapy should have non-overlapping toxicities and the chemotherapy should not enhance normal-tissue damage within the radiation field. Such a situation may be obtained by temporal separation of the two modalities but, even if this can be achieved without a negative influence on tumour control, the patient will probably have to tolerate a wider range

of toxic reactions. This needs to be taken into account when assessing the overall benefit. If independent cell killing can be successfully exploited, it could potentially lead to both improved local control and reduced distant failure, without any interactions between the modalities.

The treatment of early-stage Hodgkin's disease is a good illustration of this concept. Both radiation (mantle field irradiation, 40 Gy) and chemotherapy (including alkylating agents) are highly effective in providing long-term cure for these patients (Table 18.2). However, the use of both modalities is associated with a relatively high incidence of late complications (e.g. mainly induction of secondary solid tumours and cardiopathy for radiotherapy, and induction of lymphoma and leukaemia for chemotherapy). Hence, modern treatment of early-stage Hodgkin's disease combines different chemotherapy regimens (fewer courses and different drugs) with radiotherapy delivered on the involved fields only and to a lower dose. Long-term efficacy is similar. Data are not yet mature enough to inform conclusively about any reduced incidence of late toxicity, but it is expected to be 'shared' between the two modalities.

When independent cell kill is the mechanism of interaction between radiotherapy and chemotherapy, obviously the optimal way of combining these modalities is sequentially to avoid the likely increase in side-effects when given concomitantly.

Cellular and molecular interaction

This term describes the situation in which radiation and chemotherapy interact with each other at the cellular or molecular level such that the net effect is greater than the simple addition of the individual effects of the two modalities. As illustrated in Fig. 18.1, this interaction is likely to translate into a modification of the shape of the cell survival curves, i.e. a steeper slope of the tangent to the initial part of the curve (increase in the α parameter of the linear-quadratic model) for the combined treatment. A classical way of expressing the benefit of a combined treatment is through the use of a dose-modifying factor (DMF), which is defined as the ratio of isoeffective radiation doses in the absence and presence of the radiosensitizer.

Table 18.2 Comparative efficacy and toxicity between several treatment options for early-stage Hodgkin's disease

	Radiotherapy: extended field, 40Gy	Chemotherapy (MOPP–ABVD)	Chemotherapy–radiotherapy: involved field, <40Gy
10-year overall survival	80–90%	80–90%	≈ 90%
Complications (RR):			
Leukaemia induction	11.0	70.0	Not known yet
Lymphoma induction	21.0	22.0	Not known yet
Solid tumour induction	2.8	1.1	Not known yet
Cardiopathy	2.2–3.1	≈ 1.0	Not known yet

RR, relative risk.

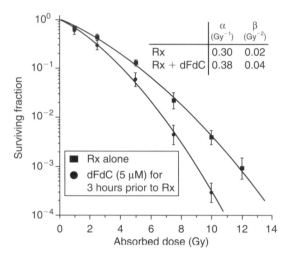

Figure 18.1 Head and neck SQD-9 cell-survival curves with or without preincubation with gemcitabine (dFdC) at a dose of 5 μM for 3 hours. In the presence of the drug, the initial slope of the cell survival curve is steeper, reflecting an interaction with ionizing radiation.

The concept of DMFs can be used in describing tumour effect or normal tissue toxicity.

A good clinical illustration of this type of interaction between chemotherapy and radiotherapy is in the treatment of locally advanced head and neck squamous cell carcinoma, in the meta-analysis of over 10 000 individual patients (Pignon *et al.*, 2000). Patients were categorized according to whether chemotherapy had been given before (induction chemotherapy), during (concomitant chemotherapy) or after radiotherapy (adjuvant chemotherapy). A significant absolute 5-year benefit of 8 per cent was found only when concomitant chemotherapy was given. For induction or adjuvant chemotherapy, the 5-year survival was improved

by only 1 per cent and 2 per cent, respectively. This example illustrates that the two modalities needed to be given within a narrow time-frame of opportunity to translate into a clinical benefit. This mechanism of interaction is likely to play a substantial role in achieving a benefit of combined chemoradiotherapy in the majority of solid tumours in adults.

18.3 MOLECULAR MECHANISMS OF INTERACTION BETWEEN CHEMOTHERAPY AND RADIOTHERAPY

Enhanced DNA/chromosome damage and repair

Little is known about the capacity of chemotherapeutic agents to increase the efficiency with which ionizing radiation induces DNA damage. Compounds such as iododeoxyuridine (IdUrd) and bromodeoxyuridine (BrdUrd) when incorporated into DNA have been shown to enhance radiation-induced DNA damage, likely through the production of reactive uracilyl radicals and halide ions, which in turn induce DNA single-strand-breaks (SSBs) in the neighbouring DNA (Iliakis *et al.*, 1991). However, several commonly used chemotherapy agents have been shown to inhibit the repair of radiation damage (i.e. DNA and/or chromosome damage). Examples are nucleoside analogues, cisplatin, bleomycin, doxorubicin and hydroxyurea. Some of these drugs inhibit the repair processes by interfering with the enzymatic machinery involved in the restoration of the DNA/ chromosome integrity. Fludarabine, for example, is a nucleoside analogue, which is incorporated

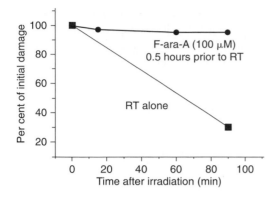

Figure 18.2 Inhibition of repair of chromosome breaks by the nucleoside analogue F-ara-A. Human lymphocytes were irradiated with a single X-ray dose of 2 Gy and incubated at 37°C in the presence or absence of F-ara-A. At 90 min post-irradiation, 70 per cent of the chromosome breaks have repaired in the control sample; in the sample incubated with F-ara-A, only 5 per cent of breaks have repaired. RT, radiotherapy.

into DNA and blocks DNA primase, DNA polymerase α and ε and DNA ligase, and which has been shown to inhibit the repair of chromosome break repair (Fig. 18.2) (Gregoire *et al.*, 1999).

Some of these drugs, like radiation, can directly produce DNA damage which manifests as DNA breaks, adducts and intercalation. For cisplatin, there is also an increase in the number of radiation-induced strand breaks. This might occur by conversion of radiation-induced SSBs to double strand breaks (DSBs) during the repair of DNA–platinum adducts. Inhibition of repair, or the conversion of SSBs to DSBs, has the effect of increasing the slope of the radiation survival curve and leads to an enhanced response (Fig. 18.1). Enhancement, which occurs as a result of repair inhibition, will be more pronounced in fractionated schedules than for single doses. A major problem with DNA repair inhibition as an exploitable mechanism for obtaining a therapeutic gain is the lack of evidence for a selective anti-tumour effect. For this strategy to be effective, some sort of tumour drug targeting may be required.

Cell-cycle synchronization

The vast majority of chemotherapeutic agents are inhibitors of cell division and are thus mainly active on proliferating cells. Agents such as gemcitabine, fludarabine, methotrexate and 5-fluorouracil inhibit various enzymes involved in DNA synthesis and repair in S-phase cells; agents such as etoposide, doxorubicin, alkylating agents and platinum compounds induce DNA strand breaks and DNA strand crosslinks in any phase of the cell cycle, but will only become potentially lethal in replicating cells; agents such as taxol, taxotere and *Vinca* alkaloids inhibit mitotic spindle formation and thus are mainly active during mitosis.

As a consequence of this cell-cycle phase selective cytotoxicity of chemotherapeutic agents, the remaining surviving cells will be synchronized. If radiation could be delivered when these synchronized cells have reached a more radiosensitive phase of the cell cycle (e.g. G2 mitosis), a tremendous potentiation of the radiation effect could be observed. Such a mechanism of interaction between drugs and ionizing radiation has often been reported in preclinical experimental models (Gregoire *et al.*, 1994). However, in clinics, because of the difficulty in assessing the appropriate timing between drug injection and radiotherapy delivery, it is unlikely that cell synchronization can be successfully exploited. Furthermore, considering that radiotherapy is typically delivered on a fractionated basis, it is also likely that this effect would be lost after a few fractions.

Enhanced apoptosis

Apoptosis (or interphase cell death) is a common mechanism of cell death induced by chemotherapeutic agents (Kaufmann and Earnshaw, 2000). These drugs can trigger one or more of the pathways leading to apoptosis. For the anti-metabolites, DNA incorporation is a necessary event to ensure a robust apoptotic response, hence the specific sensitivity of S-phase cells to these agents. Within this framework, it has been hypothesized that combining these drugs with ionizing radiation, which is very effective in inducing DNA SSBs or DSBs in every phase of the cell cycle, could facilitate their DNA incorporation and thus trigger an enhanced apoptotic reaction. This hypothesis was investigated in tumour models *in vivo*, using single doses of X-rays combined with gemcitabine (Milas *et al.*, 1999). An increased apoptotic response was indeed observed when the two modalities were combined, but comprehensive analysis of the data did not demonstrate any synergistic enhancement, only an additive effect.

Re-oxygenation

As discussed in Chapters 15 and 16, hypoxia, a common feature of the majority of human solid tumours, is associated with a poorer response to radiotherapy. One reason for this is that the functionally insufficient tumour vascular network does not permit an adequate diffusion of oxygen throughout the whole tumour mass. It has therefore been proposed that chemotherapy, by inducing some degree of tumour shrinkage, might facilitate a more even diffusion of oxygen and increase overall tumour oxygenation, which in turn would increase

tumour radiosensitivity. In the murine mammary carcinoma MCA-4, it was indeed shown that intratumoural PO_2 increased progressively in the few hours following taxol administration, from 6.2 mmHg in untreated tumours to 10.0 mmHg in treated tumours (Milas *et al.*, 1995). This progressive tumour reoxygenation was associated with a significant parallel increase in the tumour radioresponse compared with control animals that did not receive taxol. This mechanism, which likely could play a role with any chemotherapeutic drug, has, however, never been tested with other agents.

Inhibition of cell proliferation

Table 18.3 summarizes information from preclinical experiments on the mechanisms of interaction

Table 18.3 Summary of the preclinical data regarding the mechanisms of interaction between ionizing radiation and chemotherapeutic agents

	DNA damage Induction	Repair	Chromosome aberration	Cell cycle	Apoptosis	Re-oxygenation
Antimetabolites						
5-Fluorouracil	−	±	−	+	?	?
Methotrexate	?	?	?	?	?	?
Hydroxyurea	?	±	+	+	?	?
Gemcitabine	−	−	+	+	−	?
Fludarabine	−	−	+	+	−	?
Plant derivatives						
Vinca alkaloids	?	−	?	+	?	?
Etoposide	?	+?	−	+	+	?
Camptothecin	?	?	−	±	±	?
Taxanes	?	−	+	+	+	+
Antibiotics						
Doxorubicin	−	±	±	+	?	?
Mitomycin-C	?	?	−	?	?	?
Bleomycin	?	−	±	+	?	?
Actinomycin-D	?	+?	?	?	−	−
Alkylating agents						
Cisplatin	+?	+	?	−	?	?
BCNU	?	+	−	?	?	?
Cyclophosphamide	?	?	−	?	?	?

−, Not demonstrated; +, demonstrated; ±, conflicting data; ?, unknown.

BCNU, β-chloro-nitrosourea.

between chemotherapeutic agents and ionizing radiation. For the majority of these agents, the exact cellular and molecular mechanisms of interaction are not precisely known. Nevertheless, these agents are routinely used in the clinic and have been shown to be effective in combination with radiotherapy. Furthermore, even for those agents for which mechanisms of interaction with radiation have been elucidated in experimental models, it is unlikely that the clinical regimen has been designed to benefit fully from these interactions. Indeed, in the clinical setting, logistical considerations may come into play to explain ways in which drugs and radiotherapy are combined, and such considerations may not be entirely compatible with a full exploitation of the molecular and cellular interactions between drugs and ionizing radiation.

It is therefore reasonable to propose that a prominent mechanism of interaction between drugs and radiotherapy would be a simple inhibition of the cellular proliferation that takes place during the radiation interfraction interval. Such a mechanism is illustrated in Fig. 18.3 (Gregoire *et al.*, 1999). This interaction would be much less sensitive to the exact timing between drug and radiation dose delivery, provided that the drug is delivered at some point during the radiotherapy schedule. This being the case, it would be best to administer the drug towards the end of the radiation treatment course, when tumour cell repopulation had been triggered (see Chapter 10, Section 10.4). This was the rationale of a phase II trial conducted on head and neck squamous cell carcinoma, where two courses of cisplatin/5FU were given over the last 2 weeks of radiotherapy as a so-called 'chemoboost' (Corry *et al.*, 2000). Results were encouraging but have not yet been tested in a randomized phase III trial.

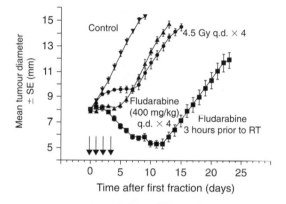

Figure 18.3 Regrowth delay experiment in a mouse sarcoma (SA-NH). Tumours (8 mm diameter) were treated with four daily i.p. administrations of fludarabine (arrows), irradiated with four daily fractions of 4.5 Gy, or given four daily doses of fludarabine 3 hours prior to four daily fractions of 4.5 Gy. Control mice were injected with saline. Each datum point represents the mean of nine or ten mice. When treated with radiation alone, tumours kept growing and only a 5.3 ± 0.5 (SEM) day regrowth delay was seen compared with control animals. During fludarabine treatment alone, tumour proliferation was inhibited, but tumours started growing again as soon as drug administration stopped; overall, a regrowth delay of 5.5 ± 0.7 (SEM) days was seen. When both modalities were combined, a decrease in tumour size was observed during treatment and the regrowth delay of 14.3 ± 0.9 (SEM) days was greater than the additive effect of the two modalities alone.

18.4 TOXICITY RESULTING FROM CONCOMITANT USE OF CHEMOTHERAPY AND RADIOTHERAPY

Early toxicity

As discussed in Chapter 13, early toxicity after radiotherapy (e.g. oral mucositis, skin reaction, oesophagitis, proctitis and bone marrow depletion) typically results from an imbalance between physiological loss of mature cells and renewal from the stem cells or the precursor cells. As mentioned above, all chemotherapeutic agents are active on proliferative cells, and thus on their own also produce an imbalance between precursors and mature cells. It is thus anticipated that concomitant association between drugs and radiation will result in an increased early toxicity. Table 18.4 summarizes experimental data on early toxicity observed during concomitant association between drug and radiation. It shows that, for all classes of drugs, an increase in radiation-induced

Table 18.4 Summary of the preclinical data regarding the toxicity of concomitant chemoradiation

	Early effects	Late effects
Antimetabolites		
5-Fluorouracil	+ (GI, skin)	?
Methotrexate	+ (GI)	?
Hydroxyurea	+ (GI)	?
Gemcitabine	+ (GI)	± (lung)
Fludarabine	+ (GI)	± (CNS)
Plant derivatives		
Vinca alkaloids	− (GI, BM)	?
Etoposide	?	?
Taxanes	+ (GI)	?
Antibiotics		
Doxorubicin	+ (GI, skin)	+ (heart, lung)
Mitomycin-C	+ (GI, BM)	+ (lung)
Bleomycin	+ (GI, skin)	+ (skin, lung)
Actinomycin-D	+ (GI, BM, skin)	+ (lung)
Alkylating agents		
Cisplatin	+ (GI)	+ (kidney)
BCNU	+ (GI)	+ (lung)
Cyclophosphamide	+ (GI, skin)	+ (lung, bladder, CNS)

BCNU, β-chloro-nitrosourea; BM, bone marrow; CNS, central nervous system; GI, gastrointestinal.
−, Not demonstrated; +, demonstrated; ±, conflicting data; ?, unknown.

early toxicity has been reported. These findings are in agreement with the clinical trials that compared radiotherapy alone with concomitant chemoradiation, which indicated a significant increase in early toxicity in the combined modality arm.

There is a considerable body of experimental data which demonstrates that normal-tissue damage after combined modality treatment is strongly influenced by the sequence and timing of the modalities. Many commonly used drugs cause a substantial increase in normal-tissue radiation injury when the modalities are given in close sequence but not when they are separated in time (Fig. 18.4) (Gregoire *et al.*, 1997). However, this finding conflicts with the requirement to use concomitant chemoradiation (thus with a narrow window of association) for improving loco-regional tumour control. Thus, unless pharmacokinetic

studies show a different pattern of drug biodistribution between tumour cells and normal cells, it is likely that the optimal sequence of drug administration for tumour radiosensitization is the one that will also produce the greatest increase in early radiation toxicity.

Late toxicity

In contrast to early radiation effects, which typically occur during treatment and in rapidly renewing tissues, late effects can affect all types of tissues after a latent period, which typically is expressed in months to years. Late damage also tends more to be irreversible and a radiation dose-dependency has been well documented in a large number of tissues. The pathophysiology of late radiation effects is discussed at length in

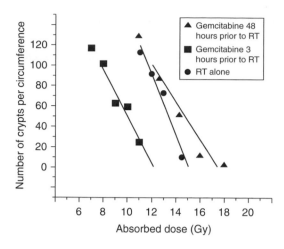

Figure 18.4 Radioenhancement of early jejunal damage after single-dose irradiation in mice. Mice were total body irradiated with single doses of 250 kV X-rays with or without prior administration (at 3 or 48 hours) of a single dose (150 mg/kg) of gemcitabine. The crypt cell regeneration assay was used. When injected 3 hours prior to irradiation, gemcitabine induced a marked radiosensitization (dose-modifying factor, DMF = 1.3). When injected 24 hours prior to irradiation a small radioprotection was observed (DMF = 0.9).

Chapter 13. Although it may involve various cell types, any therapeutic intervention that may affect the repair of radiation (DNA) damage in the tumour is likely to also increase late normal-tissue radiation damage (Table 18.4). Furthermore, the risk of late effects after combined chemoradiotherapy can be further increased when the drugs have a specific toxicity for tissues within the irradiated volume, such as bleomycin for lung toxicity, doxorubicin for cardiac toxicity and cisplatin for renal toxicity. In the clinical setting, the design of protocols and the choice of the various drugs to combine with radiotherapy needs to integrate this knowledge. For example, bleomycin should be avoided together with radiotherapy for tumours of the mediastinum. For postoperative irradiation of the left breast or chest wall in women receiving doxorubicin, adequate planning should be made to avoid irradiation of the myocardium.

18.5 THE THERAPEUTIC RATIO

The therapeutic ratio (TR), or therapeutic gain, is the relative expected benefit of a combined modality treatment, integrating both the tumour and the normal-tissue effects. It is defined as the ratio of DMFs for tumour over normal tissues. A therapeutic ratio above unity indicates that, overall, the combined modality treatment is relatively more effective for tumour control than for normal tissue toxicity; conversely, a therapeutic ratio below unity indicates that the combined treatment is relatively more toxic than beneficial. The therapeutic ratio needs to be determined for both early and late normal-tissue toxicity. Table 18.5 presents an example of a concomitant association of cisplatin and 5-fluorouracil with radiotherapy for the treatment of locally advanced SCC of the cervix (Morris *et al.*, 1999). It shows that, when early toxicity is taken into account, the therapeutic ratio is far below unity. However, although very distressful, early side-effects are usually manageable with extensive supportive care during treatment, and in this clinical example they fully resolved within a few weeks after the end of treatment. When late effects are considered, the therapeutic ratio is well above unity, illustrating the potential net benefit of the combined treatment strategy in this particular clinical setting.

When designing a new clinical trial or a new clinical strategy with concomitant chemotherapy and radiotherapy, one may need to slightly decrease the dose intensity of the standard treatment (i.e. radiotherapy) to obtain a therapeutic ratio above unity, but still have a beneficial effect at the tumour level. This was done in a trial comparing radiotherapy alone (70 Gy in 7 weeks) for locally advanced head and neck squamous cell carcinoma, with intercalated chemotherapy–radiotherapy (three cycles of 20 Gy in 2 weeks plus 1 week of cisplatin/5FU) (Merlano *et al.*, 1992). At 3 years, the overall survival was increased from 23 per cent to 41 per cent without any increase in early toxicity.

The choice between an 'equal toxicity' design or an 'equal dose' design must therefore be considered on a site-by-site basis depending on the objective of the trial or clinical strategy.

Table 18.5 Comparison of efficacy and side-effects after concomitant chemoradiotherapy for locally advanced squamous cell carcinoma of the cervix

	Radiotherapy alone[1] (%)	Chemoradiotherapy[2] (%)	Therapeutic ratio
Recurrence rate at 5 years	35	19	–
Early effects (grades 3–5)	5	45	0.2
Early effects (excluding haematological toxicity) (grades 3–5)	2	10	0.4
Late effects (grades 3–5)	11	12	1.7

[1]External pelvic radiotherapy up to 45 Gy in 4.5 weeks followed by a brachytherapy implant with a total dose equal to or greater than 85 Gy; $n = 193$.

[2]Cisplatin (75 mg/m^2, day 1) + 5-fluorouracil (1g/m^2 per day, days 1–4) $\times$ 3, every 3 weeks; $n = 195$.

Key points

1. Proper design combined drug and radiotherapy treatment depends on the objective desired. Sequential association (neo-adjuvant or adjuvant) is preferred when target cell populations are different and/or when the objective is to optimize the dose intensity of chemotherapy and radiotherapy in both chemosensitive and radiosensitive disease. Concomitant association is preferred when cellular or molecular interactions are used to improve loco-regional control of the disease.

2. Although several mechanisms of interaction between drugs and radiation have been identified (modulation of DNA and chromosome damage and repair, cell-cycle synchronization, enhanced induction of apoptosis, re-oxygenation), in a clinical setting it is most likely that a key benefit is the inhibition of tumour cell proliferation by drugs during the radiation interfraction interval.

3. Concomitant administration of chemotherapy and radiation gives increased early normal tissue toxicity due to inhibition of stem cell or precursor cell proliferation. Late normal-tissue damage is likely to be enhanced through inhibition of DNA repair, and by a specific mechanism of drug toxicity in sensitive tissues (e.g. doxorubicin in the heart, bleomycin in the lung).

4. The therapeutic ratio (TR) expresses the relative benefit of a combined modality treatment, integrating both the tumour and the normal-tissue effects. For 'equal dose' trials, TR is typically below unity for early toxicity and above unity for late radiation damage.

5. Several randomized trials with concomitant chemoradiotherapy have been conducted in brain, head and neck, lung, oesophagus, cervix and colorectal cancers. A significant increase in loco-regional control has been found in some disease sites (e.g. brain, head and neck, cervix) with a consequent improvement in patient survival.

■ BIBLIOGRAPHY

Bartelink H, Roelofsen F, Eschwege F *et al.* (1997). Concomitant radiotherapy and chemotherapy is superior to radiotherapy alone in the treatment of locally advanced anal cancer: results of a phase III randomized trial of the European Organization for Research and Treatment of Cancer Radiotherapy and Gastrointestinal Cooperative Groups. *J Clin Oncol* **15**: 2040–9.

Bernier J, Domenge C, Ozsahin M *et al.* (2004). Postoperative irradiation with or without concomitant chemotherapy for locally advanced head and neck cancer. *N Engl J Med* **350**: 1945–52.

Bosset JF, Calais G, Mineur L *et al.* (2005a). Enhanced tumoricidal effect of chemotherapy with preoperative radiotherapy for rectal cancer: preliminary results – EORTC 22921. *J Clin Oncol* **23**: 5620–7.

Bosset JF, Calais G, Mineur L *et al.* (2005b). Preoperative radiation (Preop RT) in rectal cancer: effect and timing of additional chemotherapy (CT) 5-year results of the EORTC 22921 trial. *J Clin Oncol (Meeting Abstracts)* **23**(Suppl. 16S): 3505.

Budach W, Hehr T, Budach V, Belka C, Dietz K (2006). A meta-analysis of hyperfractionated and accelerated radiotherapy and combined chemotherapy and radiotherapy regimens in unresected locally advanced squamous cell carcinoma of the head and neck. *BMC Cancer* **6**: 28.

Cooper JS, Pajak TF, Forastiere AA *et al.* (2004). Postoperative concurrent radiotherapy and chemotherapy for high-risk squamous-cell carcinoma of the head and neck. *N Engl J Med* **350**: 1937–44.

Corry J, Rischin D, Smith JG *et al.* (2000). Radiation with concurrent late chemotherapy intensification ('chemoboost') for locally advanced head and neck cancer. *Radiother Oncol* **54**: 123–7.

Forastière AA, Goepfert H, Maor M *et al.* (2003). Concurrent chemotherapy and radiotherapy for organ preservation in advanced laryngeal cancer. *N Engl J Med* **349**: 2091–8.

Green JA, Kirwan JM, Tierney JF *et al.* (2001). Survival and recurrence after concomitant chemotherapy and radiotherapy for cancer of the uterine cervix: a systematic review and meta-analysis. *Lancet* **358**: 781–6.

Green J, Kirwan J, Tierney J *et al.* (2005). Concomitant chemotherapy and radiation therapy for cancer of the uterine cervix. *Cochrane Database Syst Rev* CD002225.

Gregoire V, Van NT, Stephens LC *et al.* (1994). The role of fludarabine-induced apoptosis and cell cycle synchronization in enhanced murine tumor radiation response *in vivo*. *Cancer Res* **54**: 6201–9.

Gregoire V, Beauduin M, Rosier JF *et al.* (1997). Kinetics of mouse jejunum radiosensitization by 2′,2′-difluorodeoxycytidine (gemcitabine) and its relationship with pharmacodynamics of DNA synthesis inhibition and cell cycle redistribution in crypt cells. *Br J Cancer* **76**: 1315–21.

Gregoire V, Hittelman WN, Rosier JF, Milas L (1999). Chemoradiotherapy: radiosensitizing nucleoside analogues (review). *Oncol Rep* **6**: 949–57.

Hegi ME, Diserens AC, Gorlia T *et al.* (2005). MGMT gene silencing and benefit from temozolomide in glioblastoma. *N Engl J Med* **352**: 997–1003.

Iliakis G, Pantelias G, Kurtzman S (1991). Mechanism of radiosensitization by halogenated pyrimidines: effect of BrdU on cell killing and interphase chromosome breakage in radiation-sensitive cells. *Radiat Res* **125**: 56–64.

Kaufmann SH, Earnshaw WC (2000). Induction of apoptosis by cancer chemotherapy. *Exp Cell Res* **256**: 42–9.

Merlano M, Vitale V, Rosso R *et al.* (1992). Treatment of advanced squamous-cell carcinoma of the head and neck with alternating chemotherapy and radiotherapy. *N Engl J Med* **327**: 1115–21.

Milas L, Hunter N, Mason KA, Milross C, Peters LJ (1995). Tumor reoxygenation as a mechanism of taxol-induced enhancement of tumor radioresponse. *Acta Oncol* **34**: 409–12.

Milas L, Fujii T, Hunter N *et al.* (1999). Enhancement of tumor radioresponse *in vivo* by gemcitabine. *Cancer Res* **59**: 107–14.

Morris M, Eifel PJ, Lu J *et al.* (1999). Pelvic radiation with concurrent chemotherapy compared with pelvic and para-aortic radiation for high-risk cervical cancer. *N Engl J Med* **340**: 1137–43.

NACCCMA (Neoadjuvant Chemotherapy for Cervical Cancer Meta-Analysis) Collaboration (2004). Neoadjuvant chemotherapy for locally advanced cervix cancer. *Cochrane Database Syst Rev* CD001774.

Pignon JP, Arriagada R, Ihde DC *et al.* (1992). A meta-analysis of thoracic radiotherapy for small-cell lung cancer. *N Engl J Med* **327**: 1618–24.

Pignon JP, Bourhis J, Domenge C, Designe L (2000). Chemotherapy added to locoregional treatment for head and neck squamous-cell carcinoma: three meta-analyses of updated individual data. MACH-NC Collaborative Group. Meta-Analysis of Chemotherapy on Head and Neck Cancer. *Lancet* **355**: 949–55.

Pijls-Johannesma MC, De Ruysscher D, Lambin P, Rutten I, Vansteenkiste JF (2005). Early versus late chest radiotherapy for limited stage small cell lung cancer. *Cochrane Database Syst Rev* CD004700.

Rowell NP, O'Rourke NP (2004). Concurrent chemoradiotherapy in non-small cell lung cancer. *Cochrane Database Syst Rev* CD002140.

Stupp R, Mason WP, van den Bent MJ *et al.* (2005). Radiotherapy plus concomitant and adjuvant temozolomide for glioblastoma. *N Engl J Med* **352**: 987–96.

Wolmark N, Wieand HS, Hyams DM *et al.* (2000). Randomized trial of postoperative adjuvant chemotherapy with or without radiotherapy for carcinoma of the rectum: National Surgical Adjuvant Breast and Bowel Project Protocol R–02. *J Natl Cancer Inst* **92**: 388–96.

Wong R, Malthaner R (2006). Combined chemotherapy and radiotherapy (without surgery) compared with radiotherapy alone in localized carcinoma of the esophagus. *Cochrane Database Syst Rev* CD002092.

■ FURTHER READING

Browman GP, Hodson DI, Mackenzie RJ, Bestic N, Zuraw L (2001). Choosing a concomitant chemotherapy and radiotherapy regimen for squamous cell head and neck cancer: a systematic review of the published literature with subgroup analysis. *Head Neck* **23**: 579–89.

Steel GG (1988). The search for therapeutic gain in the combination of radiotherapy and chemotherapy. *Radiother Oncol* **11**: 31–53.

Steel GG, Peckham MJ (1979). Exploitable mechanisms in combined radiotherapy–chemotherapy: the concept of additivity. *Int J Radiat Oncol Biol Phys* **5**: 85–91.

Wouters A, Pauwels B, Lardon F, Vermorken JB (2007). Review: implications of in vitro research on the effect of radiotherapy and chemotherapy under hypoxic conditions. *Oncologist* **12**: 690–712.

Retreatment tolerance of normal tissues

WOLFGANG DÖRR AND FIONA A. STEWART

19.1 INTRODUCTION

Improvements in cancer therapy, particularly advances in medical radiation physics and radiation biology, have resulted in prolonged survival times and increased survival rates for a variety of malignancies over the past two decades. Surviving cancer patients are, however, at an increased risk of developing secondary neoplasms (see Chapter 25). The most important reason for this is that patients cured of one cancer still retain more risk (e.g. molecular predisposition) to develop a (second) tumour than any other person of similar age, gender, lifestyle, etc., who had not previously experienced the disease. Second, the aetiological factors associated with the first tumour, such as smoking for lung and head and neck tumours, or alcohol consumption for tumours of the head and neck or the oesophagus, or exposure to other carcinogens, can continue and hence promote the manifestation of a second malignancy. Of $>30\,000$ irradiated patients with a primary head and neck tumour, more than 20 per cent developed a second neoplasm (Hashibe *et al.*, 2005), out of which >80 per cent were found in the head and neck region, the oesophagus and the lung. Third, the therapy itself, radiation exposure as well as chemotherapy, is associated with an increased risk for second tumours. This is of particular importance for children and younger adults; childhood cancer survivors are at an up to 19-fold increased risk for developing another malignancy (Dickerman, 2007).

Such second primary tumours are observed within, or, more frequently, close to the initial high-dose treatment volume (Dörr and Herrmann, 2002). Moreover, recurrent tumours can develop within or close to the original gross tumour volume. Both second primary tumours and recurrences must be treated adequately, which frequently involves radiotherapy. Decisions regarding safe retreatment are very complex; for example, surgical options are frequently compromised by local responses (e.g. fibrosis) to the first treatment. Hence, for the development of curative or even palliative re-irradiation strategies, a number of parameters must be considered:

- initial radiotherapy: dose (EQD_2 – see below), volume, relationship to the required re-irradiation fields
- additional treatments for the first tumour (e.g. chemotherapy, 'biologicals')
- time interval between therapy courses
- organs and tissues involved
- alternative treatment options.

Obviously, if the radiation tolerance within a given volume of an organ has already been exceeded during the first treatment and function is lost (or loss is to be expected), then no further treatment can be administered to this volume regardless of the first dose. Therefore, this chapter focuses on scenarios where the initial radiation treatment was in the range of subtolerance doses, with the induction of only subclinical or minimal damage, and with possible long-term recovery or potential residual damage after longer periods. Based on the risk factors mentioned above, the potential tissue-specific morbidity caused by the second treatment, and its impact on the patient's quality of life, must be weighed against the expected benefits in terms of tumour response and survival.

This chapter summarizes the main findings from experimental and clinical studies on the re-irradiation tolerance of various normal tissues. Only clinical studies that provide information on one specific side-effect are included in the organ-specific sections. More general descriptions for entire tumour entities are reviewed in the section on clinical studies.

In order to compare data from studies with different fractionation regimes, we have recalculated the doses administered in these studies to obtain the equivalent dose in 2-Gy fractions (EQD_2) using the linear-quadratic (LQ) approach with α/β values of 10 Gy for early reactions and 3 Gy for late reactions (see Chapters 8 and 9). Tolerance doses (i.e. threshold doses above which defined grades of toxicity are observed) are referred to as the EQD_{2tol}. The intensity of both the initial treatment and the retreatment can be specified as a percentage of EQD_{2tol}.

19.2 EARLY TISSUE REACTIONS

Early tissue reactions are usually found in proliferating, turnover tissues (see Chapter 13, Section 13.2). Based on surviving stem cells within the irradiated volume or area, or on stem cells migrating into the irradiated tissue from non-irradiated sites, regeneration and restitution of tissue architecture and cellularity occurs, which should result in complete or partial restoration of the radiation tolerance.

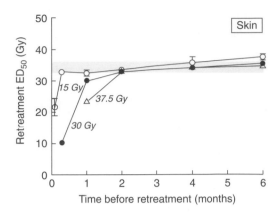

Figure 19.1 Retreatment tolerance of mouse skin at different times after initial treatments with 15–37.5 Gy. The vertical scale gives the retreatment dose required for a specified level of skin damage (ED_{50} for desquamation). The shaded area shows the range of ED_{50} doses for the same level of skin damage for previously untreated mice. Adapted from Terry et al. (1989), with permission.

Epidermis

Reports on the re-irradiation tolerance for early, epidermal skin reactions in rodents are consistent in demonstrating very good recovery from the initial damage with restoration of the radiation tolerance (Fig. 19.1). Recovery is faster after lower initial doses and is inversely proportional to the extent of (stem) cell kill (see Chapter 13, Fig. 13.3). After single radiation doses that induce clinical desquamation of the epidermis, complete restitution of the initial tolerance has been observed after 2 months (Terry et al., 1989). In another study with fractionated irradiation, high initial doses, causing severe acute damage, resulted in some residual damage even after 6 months, with the consequence of reduced tolerance (c. 80 per cent EQD_{2tol} after 10×5 Gy pretreatment), as demonstrated by increased early responses, particularly to high retreatment doses (Brown and Probert, 1975).

Oral and oesophageal mucosa

No preclinical animal data are available on re-irradiation effects in oral and oesophageal

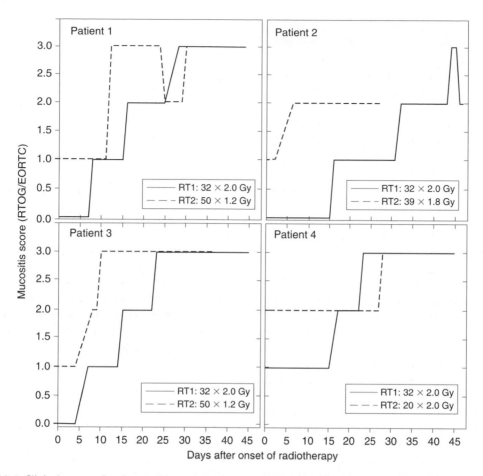

Figure 19.2 Clinical scores of oral mucositis according to Radiation Therapy Oncology Group (RTOG)/European Organisation for Research and Treatment of Cancer (EORTC) for four patients during their first course of radiotherapy (solid lines) and during re-irradiation (dashed lines). Dörr *et al.*, unpublished data.

mucosa. However, oral mucositis has been quantified after repeated radiotherapy courses with treatment breaks. If these breaks are in the range of 2 weeks, then mucositis developed with an identical time-course and severity after each of three treatment cycles (van der Schueren *et al.*, 1990). If the breaks are shorter, around 10 days, then the severity of oral mucositis can even be lower after a second cycle (Maciejewski *et al.*, 1991), as repopulation is still maximally active and can effectively counteract the cell kill right from the onset of re-irradiation.

However, early reactions after short treatment breaks do not necessarily reflect the responses to re-irradiation. Patients subject to re-irradiation in the head and neck region after longer intervals of

2–3 years may present with mucosal erythema (mucositis grade 1 according to RTOG/EORTC), or even focal lesions, even before the start of the second radiotherapy. More severe reactions (confluent: grade 3) are frequently observed earlier after re-irradiation than in the first radiation series (Fig. 19.2). This indicates mucosal atrophy, resulting in increased vulnerability and a reduction in the time required for cell depletion (see Chapter 13, Section 13.2).

Bone marrow

The potential and extent of long-term recovery in bone marrow is clearly dependent on the toxicity

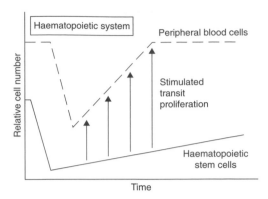

Figure 19.3 Changes in peripheral blood cell counts (dashed line) versus number of haematopoietic stem cell numbers in bone marrow (solid line). Earlier recovery of the peripheral cell number is based on stimulated transitproliferation, and does not reflect recovery of the stem cell population (i.e. restoration of radiation tolerance).

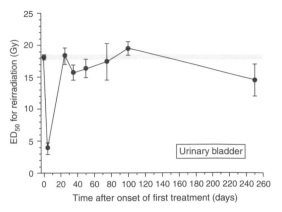

Figure 19.4 Retreatment tolerance of mouse urinary bladder (early damage) at different times after irradiation with 5×5.3 Gy over 1 week. The ordinate indicates the retreatment ED_{50} required for a 50 per cent reduction in bladder storage capacity (at 1–3 weeks after re-irradiation). The shaded area shows the ED_{50} for the effect in previously untreated mice. From Satthoff and Dörr, unpublished data.

of the initial treatment. At high doses, in the range used for total body irradiation as a conditioning regimen for bone marrow/stem cell/progenitor cell transplantation, the stem cell pool is irreversibly damaged and no recovery is possible without an external supply of stem cells. At more moderate doses, the first response of the bone marrow is the stimulation of transit divisions (see Chapter 13, Section 13.2), resulting in an increased output of differentiated cells per stem cell division. This counteracts cell depletion in the peripheral blood at early time-points (Fig. 19.3), but regeneration at the stem cell level may take much longer (Hendry and Yang, 1995). The toxicity of the initial treatment must therefore be considered carefully for re-irradiation, independently of blood cell counts that may be critically misleading.

Restitution of stromal elements, which closely interact with the stem–progenitor cell system in the bone marrow, may take even longer than for the haematopoietic system itself. At higher doses, no regeneration occurs and the marrow is irreversibly converted into fatty tissue. Thus in mice, irradiation with 6.5 Gy resulted in persistent damage in the stromal and the progenitor compartment after 1 year; the effect was even more pronounced when the initial exposure was fractionated over 15 days. It has also been demonstrated in

mice and dogs that this residual injury is more pronounced in neonates and younger animals than in adults (Hendry and Yang, 1995).

Urinary bladder

The early response of the urinary bladder, presenting as a reduction in storage capacity, is independent of urothelial cell depletion, which would not be expected during or shortly after radiotherapy, based on long turnover times of several months in this tissue (see Chapter 13). Re-irradiation tolerance of the urinary bladder with regard to early reactions, assessed as a > 50 per cent reduction in compliance capacity during the first 4 weeks after treatment, has been studied in mice. After an initial treatment with 5×5.3 Gy (inducing reduced compliance in *c.* 30 per cent of the animals), the original tolerance was restored between 25 days and 50 days (Fig. 19.4). Longer intervals were required after higher initial doses. At late time-points, reduced tolerance was found because of an overlap between the acute response to the re-irradiation and the onset of late damage from the first treatment.

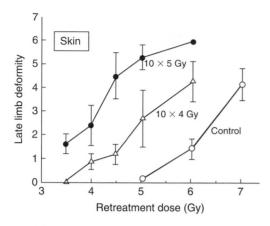

Figure 19.5 Retreatment tolerance for late hind-limb deformity in mice, as measured by fibrosis. Re-irradiation was with 10 fractions at the dose per fraction indicated on the abscissa, administered at 6 months after an initial treatment with 10 × 4 Gy or 10 × 5 Gy, or without previous irradiation. Redrawn from Brown and Probert (1975), with permission.

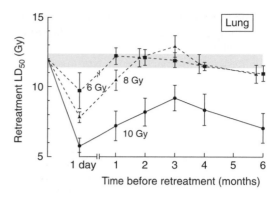

Figure 19.6 Retreatment tolerance of the mouse lung. The ordinate indicates LD_{50} values caused by pneumonitis for retreatment at the indicated times after priming treatment with 6, 8 or 10 Gy. The shaded area shows the LD_{50} value for previously untreated animals. Adapted from Terry *et al.* (1988), with permission.

19.3 LATE EFFECTS

Skin

Using hind-limb deformation as an endpoint for late subcutaneous fibrosis (Brown and Probert, 1975), there is a clear reduction in tolerance for re-irradiation after 6 months (Fig. 19.5). The effect of re-irradiation was much more pronounced after more aggressive initial radiation protocols (10 × 5 Gy vs 10 × 4 Gy). Also, this effect was markedly more prominent than for early skin reactions in the same animals (cf. epidermis in Section 19.2). Further studies similarly suggest a significantly poorer retreatment tolerance than for early reactions. In general, a reduction to 50–70 per cent of the $EQD2_{tol}$ is found after re-irradiation. However, there are contradictory studies, where very good retreatment tolerance has been demonstrated for late deformity endpoints (e.g. in pig skin; Simmonds *et al.*, 1989). In the mouse study, the reduced re-irradiation tolerance for late damage may have been influenced by the severity of early epidermal reactions in the first treatment, based on the development of consequential changes (see Chapter 13).

Lung

The response of the lung to irradiation occurs in two waves: pneumonitis as a delayed early effect, followed by late fibrosis. These effects, however, are not independent (see Chapter 13), indicating a strong consequential component. Moreover, the pathogenic processes appear to be connected, with continuous (subclinical) changes from the time of the initial radiation exposure.

In a mouse study using death from pneumonitis to evaluate lung re-irradiation tolerance (Terry *et al.*, 1988), there was complete recovery from an initial dose of 6–8 Gy (approximately 30–50 per cent of a full tolerance dose). The time to restitution was, depending on the initial dose, in the range of 1–2 months (Fig. 19.6). After higher initial doses (≥70 per cent of the initial tolerance), re-irradiation tolerance increased from 1 day to 3 months, at which time tolerance was approximately 75 per cent of tolerance in previously untreated mice. Yet, at 6 months a decline in retreatment tolerance was then observed. No later time-points were studied, and hence it is unclear whether this trend continued or also occurred after lower initial doses. The basis for the later decreased tolerance may be the development of (subclinical) fibrosis.

The remarkably good re-irradiation tolerance of the lung demonstrated in experimental studies only applies for the pneumonitis phase. It is likely that retreatment tolerance for late lung fibrosis may be poorer, although no conclusive evidence is available.

Kidney

The kidneys are among the most radiosensitive of organs, although the latent period before expression of clinically manifest radiation effects may be very long, particularly after low doses. Progressive, dose-dependent development of functional damage, without apparent recovery, has been clearly demonstrated in rodents (Stewart *et al.*, 1989, 1994). This is consistent with clinical observations of slowly progressive renal damage, which develops many years after irradiation. Based on the known dose-dependence of renal radiation injury, large initial doses ($\geqslant 14\,\text{Gy}$) result in complete loss of function and hence re-irradiation cannot cause any further damage.

After subtolerance doses, the absence of any clinically measurable renal dysfunction at the time of retreatment certainly cannot be interpreted as a sign that the tissue has regained full tolerance, because of progression of the subclinical effects. Experimental studies demonstrate that doses of radiation too low to produce overt renal damage nevertheless significantly reduce the tolerance to retreatment (Stewart *et al.*, 1989); none of these studies has demonstrated any long-term functional recovery of the kidney. After an initial dose of only 6 Gy (25 per cent of the $\text{EQD}_{2\text{tol}}$) the tolerance for retreatment actually decreases with time between 2 weeks and 26 weeks (Fig. 19.7). This is consistent with continuous progression of occult damage in the interval between treatments and implies that re-irradiation of the kidneys after any previous irradiation should be approached with extreme caution, if preservation of function is required.

Urinary bladder

Studies on the re-irradiation tolerance of mouse bladder have also not demonstrated any recovery

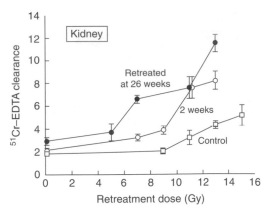

Figure 19.7 Dose–response curves for renal damage in mice at 35 weeks after re-irradiation. Retreatment was administered either 2 weeks (open circles) or 26 weeks (closed circles) after the initial treatment with 6 Gy. The response of age-matched control animals without previous irradiation (open squares) is also shown. Renal damage was worse for retreatment with the longer 26-week interval than for a shorter interval, indicating progression of subthreshold damage rather than recovery. From Stewart *et al.* (1989), with permission.

from late functional damage (as measured by increased urination frequency or reduced bladder compliance) for retreatment intervals of 12 or 40 weeks compared with short (1 day) intervals (Fig. 19.8). The latent period before expression of permanent functional damage was also much shorter in animals that were re-irradiated than in those after a single course of treatment, even after low, subtolerance initial doses (Stewart *et al.*, 1990; Dörr and Satthoff, unpublished data).

Spinal cord

Spinal cord has been studied most extensively with regard to retreatment, in various rodent species and in non-human primates. Moreover, clinical data are available. There is evidence for substantial long-term recovery, indicating that retreatment is feasible.

Analyses of data obtained on re-irradiation of rodent spinal cord, using paralysis as an endpoint, are illustrated in Fig. 19.9. In juvenile animals,

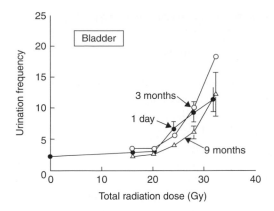

Figure 19.8 Dose–response curves for late urinary bladder damage in mice after irradiation with two doses separated by 1 day (closed circles), 3 months (open circles) or 9 months (open triangles). The total dose for a given effect did not increase with increasing time from first treatment. From Stewart *et al.* (1990), with permission.

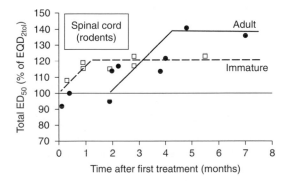

Figure 19.9 Long-term recovery after irradiation of rodent cervical cord. The total cumulative isoeffective dose (for 50 per cent paresis) is expressed as a percentage of EQD_{2tol} (equivalent tolerance dose at 2 Gy) and as a function of the interval between initial and re-irradiation dose. Data are for 3-week-old (open circles) and adult (closed circles) rats. Data from Ruifrok *et al.* (1992), White and Hornsey (1980), van der Kogel *et al.* (1982), with permission.

long-term recovery started early and maximum retreatment tolerance was observed after 1–2 months; the maximum total dose (initial plus re-irradiation) was 120 per cent of the tolerance for previously untreated animals (Ruifrok *et al.*, 1992). The higher the initial dose was, the lower

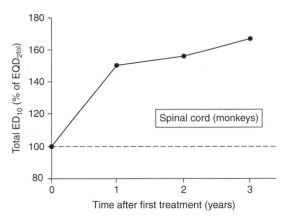

Figure 19.10 Total tolerance (initial plus retreatment) of monkey spinal cord. Retreatment was performed after 1–3 years after an initial dose of 44 Gy (i.e. 60 per cent of tolerance dose at 2 Gy, EQD_{2tol}). All treatments were given with 2.2 Gy per fraction. Data from Ang *et al.* (2001), with permission.

was the tolerance to re-irradiation. In adult animals, restitution started with a delay of several months and reached a maximum of *c.* 140 per cent of the original tolerance after 5–6 months (White and Hornsey, 1980; van der Kogel *et al.*, 1982). These data were confirmed in an extensive study in rats for different levels of initial damage (Wong and Hao, 1997).

An extensive re-irradiation study was performed in non-human primates (Ang *et al.*, 1993, 2001). In these experiments, an 8-cm length of the cervical cord was initially irradiated with 20 fractions of 2.2 Gy, which is equivalent to about 60 per cent of the ED_{50} for a 50 per cent incidence of paralysis (76 Gy in 2.2-Gy fractions). After 1, 2 or 3 years the non-symptomatic monkeys were re-irradiated with graded doses in fractions of 2.2 Gy. Only a few animals developed paralysis with the retreatment doses administered; therefore, the data must be compared at a 10 per cent incidence level of paralysis rather than at 50 per cent. The re-irradiation ED_{10} increased from 55 Gy after 1 year, to 59 Gy after 2 years to 66 Gy after 3 years. The total EQD_{2tol} for initial and retreatment doses amounted to 150 per cent, 156 per cent and 167 per cent for retreatment after 1, 2, or 3 years, respectively (Fig. 19.10). Hence, despite a different time-course in rodents and primates, the extent of long-term recovery in spinal cord, using paralysis as an end-point, is similar, and may be adopted for re-irradiation of patients.

Some clinical analyses of radiation myelopathy after re-irradiation of spinal cord are available. Nieder *et al.* (2006) summarized data from a total of 78 patients re-irradiated to the spinal cord with various regimens. Their conclusion was that, if the interval between the two radiotherapy courses was longer than 6 months, and the EQD_2 in each course was $\leqslant$ 48 Gy, the risk for myelopathy was small after a total EQD_2 of 68 Gy. In a smaller series, no myelopathies were seen after a cumulative EQD_{2tol} of 125 per cent to 172 per cent, with intervals between the series of 4 months to 13 years.

For calculation of the re-irradiation tolerance for spinal cord, the initial tolerance must be defined. Both human and primate data (Baumann *et al.*, 1994) demonstrate that, at an EQD_2 of 55 Gy, the incidence of myelopathy is clearly <3 per cent. At a dose of 60 Gy, the incidence of myelopathy is about 5 per cent for doses per fraction < 2.5 Gy and for one fraction per day. This level of risk may be acceptable in a re-irradiation situation, which is frequently the last curative option for the patient. Assuming, for example, that a patient received an initial dose to the spinal cord of $EQD_2 = 40$ Gy, this leaves a 20-Gy tolerance from the first irradiation. Restitution of 40 per cent of the initial dose amounts to $EQD_2 = 16$ Gy; hence re-irradiation with a dose of 36 Gy can probably be administered to the spinal cord in 2-Gy fractions. However, the dose to the spinal cord is usually less than the dose to the PTV, which must be included in the calculation of the initial dose. Moreover, the pronounced fractionation effect of the spinal cord can be exploited by administering hyperfractionated re-irradiation. Based on these considerations, re-irradiation with a curative intent is often possible.

In an analysis of clinical cases of myelopathy (Wong *et al.*, 1994), the mean latent time before clinical symptoms became manifest after a single course of radiotherapy ($EQD_2 = 60.5$ Gy) was 18.5 months ($n = 24$). After re-irradiation to a total dose of $EQD_2 = 74$ Gy ($n = 11$), myelopathies were observed after a significantly shorter mean latent time of 11.4 months. These data are in line with results from the preclinical studies.

Summary of experimental data

Figure 19.11 summarizes results from experimental studies for re-irradiation tolerance in tissues where recovery following a range of initial treatments has been evaluated. Both the initial and the retreatment radiation exposures are shown as a percentage of the tolerance dose for a defined level of damage, calculated in terms of EQD_{2tol} using the appropriate α/β ratio for each tissue. The dashed lines indicate the relationship that would be expected if no long-term reconstitution of tolerance would occur. Data points for retreatment above the dashed line (in skin, lung and cord) indicate some long-term recovery in the tissue. Where the data points fall below the dashed line (kidney), this indicates a progressive reduction of tissue tolerance with time after the initial irradiation rather than recovery. The general conclusion is that, on the basis of studies in experimental animals, several normal tissues are able to tolerate considerable retreatment with radiation. The phenomenon is not, however, universal.

19.4 CLINICAL STUDIES

In some clinical studies, overall incidences of side-effects (without specification of the complications) after primary or re-irradiation are compared; these studies will be reviewed here. However, the vast majority of the increasing number of clinical reports on re-irradiation do not include data from simultaneous control groups with primary irradiation of the same site, and hence do not provide quantitative information. It must also be emphasized that most of the clinical studies have enrolled patients over long periods, and therefore provide only limited information because of changes, for example, in irradiation techniques and side-effect scoring. Moreover, many studies include highly variable radiotherapy (and chemotherapy) protocols and curative as well as palliative treatment intent.

Head and neck

Kasperts *et al.* (2005) reviewed 27 retreatment studies of head and neck cancer, where the second

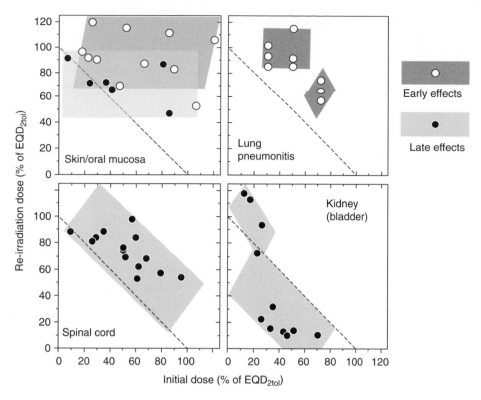

Figure 19.11 Summary of retreatment tolerance from experimental studies reported in the literature. Both the initial and retreatment doses have been calculated as a percentage of equivalent tolerance dose at 2 Gy (EQD_{2tol}). The dashed line indicates the residual tissue tolerance if no long-term restitution occurred. Data points above the dashed line (in skin, lung and cord) indicate some long-term recovery, while data below this line (kidney, bladder) point towards a progressive reduction of tissue tolerance with time after the initial irradiation.

irradiation was performed as teletherapy or brachytherapy, in combination with chemotherapy or after surgery. Major late complications were fibrosis, mucosal ulceration/necrosis, and osteoradionecrosis. Despite the toxicity, they recommended high-dose re-irradiation. Similar side-effects were reported by De Crevoisier *et al.* (1998) in a series of 169 patients re-irradiated to cumulative doses of 120 Gy (re-irradiation 60–65 Gy). After initial irradiation with 68 Gy, plus 67 Gy in the second series, Salama *et al.* (2006) found grade 4–5 late reactions (osteoradionecrosis, carotid haemorrhage, myelopathy and neuropathy) in a total of 18 per cent of the patients, with > 16 per cent fatalities. Lee *et al.* (2007) re-irradiated 105 patients with head and neck tumours with 59.4 Gy after initial doses of 62 Gy. Severe early and late complications were found in 23 per cent and

15 per cent of the patients; the latter comprised mainly temporal lobe necrosis, hearing loss, dysphagia and trismus. Lee *et al.* (2000) compared late complications (excluding xerostomia) in more than 3600 patients given a single course of radiotherapy and 487 patients given a second course of radiotherapy for nasopharyngeal carcinoma. The observed incidence of normal tissue injury was clearly lower than expected in the retreatment series, indicating partial long-term recovery of the head and neck tissues, particularly with intervals ⩾2 years.

General conclusions from these and other studies in head and neck tumours are that good local control rates of over 30 per cent can be achieved with total retreatment doses of at least 50–60 Gy, but that lower doses are ineffective. Serious complications in up to 60 per cent of long-term survivors are generally associated with higher total cumulative doses and short intervals before retreatment.

Breast

Re-irradiation for breast cancer, as partial breast irradiation, can be delivered either as conformal external-beam irradiation (e.g. with electrons) or as interstitial brachytherapy, with an acceptable incidence of side-effects, but less acceptable results with regard to cosmesis. After chest wall re-irradiation, severe grade 4 reactions are observed in ≤10 per cent of the patients (Harms *et al.*, 2004).

Lung

In recurrent lung cancer, re-irradiation with doses of 10–70 Gy (median 50 Gy, 1.8–3.0 Gy per fraction) after initial treatment with 30–80 Gy (median 60 Gy, 1.5–2.0 Gy per fraction) was studied in 34 patients (Okamoto *et al.*, 2002). No radiation myelopathy was observed; major toxicities were symptomatic pneumonitis (56 per cent) and oesophagitis (18 per cent). Palliative retreatment was associated with lower levels of oesophagitis than the initial treatment and no increase in pneumonitis. The retreatment doses are, of course, much lower than the initial doses and most patients will succumb to their disease before late damage (i.e. lung fibrosis) has time to be expressed.

Rectum

Re-irradiation for rectal cancer was carried out with doses of 15–49.2 Gy plus fluorouracil (5FU)-based chemotherapy after a median interval of 19 months (Mohiuddin *et al.*, 2002). Cumulative doses were 70.6–108.0 Gy. Early toxicity comprised ≥ grade 3 diarrhoea, mucositis and skin desquamation, requiring treatment breaks or cessation (15 per cent); late sequelae were fistula (4 per cent) and colo-anal strictures (2 per cent). All toxicities were independent of radiation dose. Valentini *et al.* (2006) studied retreatment (hyperfractionation, chemotherapy) after initial doses of

≤55 Gy (median interval 27 months). Re-irradiation doses were 30 Gy plus a boost of 10.8 Gy with 2 × 1.2 Gy per day. Late toxicities were skin fibrosis and urinary complications requiring nephrostomy at an acceptable incidence.

Cervix uteri

Early experience of retreatment for recurrent cervical cancer was not encouraging. Local control and survival rates were generally poor (10–20 per cent long-term survival) and complication rates were high (30–50 per cent). Several more recent studies, in which patients were carefully selected on the basis of volume and location of the cancer, have demonstrated much better results, particularly for retreatment using brachytherapy. In these studies, long-term survivals of 60 per cent with a severe complication rate below 15 per cent could be achieved after full-dose retreatment. Favourable conditions were small tumour volume, second primary malignancies and retreatment with brachytherapy; unfavourable conditions were recurrent cancer, large tumour volume and retreatment with external-beam therapy. Re-irradiation, mainly by brachytherapy, of vaginal recurrences of carcinomas of the cervix has been tried with 20–40 Gy in three to five fractions in 3–4 weeks (Xiang *et al.*, 1998). Side-effects were severe, with rectal changes (14 per cent), haematuria (12 per cent) and fistula (12 per cent).

Summary of clinical data

These clinical data clearly indicate that re-irradiation is an option for patients with recurrent or second tumours. However, the risk of normal-tissue damage and impact on the quality of life, as well as possible alternative therapeutic approaches, must be taken into account. If a second course of radiotherapy has to be administered, this should be done with maximum care. Optimum conformation of the planning target volume is required. For radiobiological reasons, in order to reduce the risk of late effects, hyperfractionation protocols should be considered, at least for curative treatments.

Key points

1. If the tolerance within a given tissue volume has already been exceeded during the first treatment, and loss of function is present or expected soon, then re-irradiation is not possible without loss of function.

2. For early effects, restitution of the original tolerance may be complete after low to moderate doses, and after tissue-specific and dose-dependent time intervals. At high doses, residual damage may remain for longer intervals, particularly at the stem cell level, which is not necessarily reflected by the number of differentiated cells in the functional tissue compartments (e.g. blood cell counts for bone marrow).

3. For some late-responding tissues, partial (central nervous system, lung) or complete (skin) restoration of tolerance is observed after low and moderate initial doses (< 60 per cent of the initial tolerance). For example, spinal cord can safely be re-irradiated to a total of 140 per cent of the initial EQD_{2tol}.

4. In some late responding tissues (kidney, urinary bladder), progression of damage at a subclinical level must be expected, thus precluding re-irradiation without exceeding tolerance.

5. Alternative treatment options must be considered before re-irradiation.

6. If (curative) re-irradiation is to be administered, optimum treatment planning (dose conformation) and a proper choice of fractionation protocol (hyperfractionation) are required.

■ BIBLIOGRAPHY

Ang KK, Price RE, Stephens LC *et al.* (1993). The tolerance of primate spinal cord to re-irradiation. *Int J Radiat Oncol Biol Phys* **25**: 459–64.

Ang KK, Jiang GL, Feng Y, Stephens LC, Tucker SL, Price RE (2001). Extent and kinetics of recovery of occult spinal cord injury. *Int J Radiat Oncol Biol Phys* **50**: 1013–20.

Baumann M, Budach V, Appold S (1994). Radiation tolerance of the human spinal cord. *Strahlenther Onkol* **170**: 131–9.

Brown JM, Probert JC (1975). Early and late radiation changes following a second course of irradiation. *Radiology* **115**: 711–6.

De Crevoisier R, Bourhis J, Domenge C *et al.* (1998). Full-dose re-irradiation for unresectable head and neck carcinoma: experience at the Gustave-Roussy Institute in a series of 169 patients. *J Clin Oncol* **16**: 3556–62.

Dickerman JD (2007). The late effects of childhood cancer therapy. *Pediatrics* **119**: 554–68.

Dörr W, Herrmann T (2002). Second primary tumors after radiotherapy for malignancies. Treatment-related parameters. *Strahlenther Onkol* **178**: 357–62.

Harms W, Krempien R, Grehn C *et al.* (2004). Re-irradiation of chest wall local recurrences from breast cancer. *Zentralbl Gynakol* **126**: 19–23.

Hashibe M, Ritz B, Le AD, Li G, Sankaranarayanan R, Zhang ZF (2005). Radiotherapy for oral cancer as a risk factor for second primary cancers. *Cancer Lett* **220**: 185–95.

Hendry JH, Yang F (1995). Response of bone marrow to low LET irradiation. In: Hendry JH, Lord BI (eds) *Radiation toxicology: bone marrow and leukaemia*. London: Taylor & Francis, 91–116.

Kasperts N, Slotman B, Leemans CR, Langendijk JA (2005). A review on re-irradiation for recurrent and second primary head and neck cancer. *Oral Oncol* **41**: 225–43.

Lee AW, Foo W, Law SC *et al.* (2000). Total biological effect on late reactive tissues following re-irradiation for recurrent nasopharyngeal carcinoma. *Int J Radiat Oncol Biol Phys* **46**: 865–72.

Lee N, Chan K, Bekelman JE *et al.* (2007). Salvage re-irradiation for recurrent head and neck cancer. *Int J Radiat Oncol Biol Phys* **68**: 731–40.

Maciejewski B, Zajusz A, Pilecki B *et al.* (1991). Acute mucositis in the stimulated oral mucosa of patients during radiotherapy for head and neck cancer. *Radiother Oncol* **22**: 7–11.

Mohiuddin M, Marks G, Marks J (2002). Long-term results of re-irradiation for patients with recurrent rectal carcinoma. *Cancer* **95**: 1144–50.

Nieder C, Grosu AL, Andratschke NH, Molls M (2006). Update of human spinal cord re-irradiation tolerance based on additional data from 38 patients. *Int J Radiat Oncol Biol Phys* **66**: 1446–9.

Okamoto Y, Murakami M, Yoden E *et al.* (2002). Re-irradiation for locally recurrent lung cancer previously treated with radiation therapy. *Int J Radiat Oncol Biol Phys* **52**: 390–6.

Ruifrok AC, Kleiboer BJ, van der Kogel AJ (1992). Re-irradiation tolerance of the immature rat spinal cord. *Radiother Oncol* **23**: 249–56.

Salama JK, Vokes EE, Chmura SJ *et al.* (2006). Long-term outcome of concurrent chemotherapy and re-irradiation for recurrent and second primary head-and-neck squamous cell carcinoma. *Int J Radiat Oncol Biol Phys* **64**: 382–91.

Simmonds RH, Hopewell JW, Robbins ME (1989). Residual radiation-induced injury in dermal tissue: implications for retreatment. *Br J Radiol* **62**: 915–20.

Stewart FA, Luts A, Lebesque JV (1989). The lack of long-term recovery and re-irradiation tolerance in the mouse kidney. *Int J Radiat Biol* **56**: 449–62.

Stewart FA, Oussoren Y, Luts A (1990). Long-term recovery and re-irradiation tolerance of mouse bladder. *Int J Radiat Oncol Biol Phys* **18**: 1399–406.

Stewart FA, Oussoren Y, van Tinteren H, Bentzen SM (1994). Loss of re-irradiation tolerance in the kidney with increasing time after single or fractionated partial tolerance doses. *Int J Radiat Biol* **66**: 169–79.

Terry NH, Tucker SL, Travis EL (1988). Residual radiation damage in murine lung assessed by pneumonitis. *Int J Radiat Oncol Biol Phys* **14**: 929–38.

Terry NH, Tucker SL, Travis EL (1989). Time course of loss of residual radiation damage in murine skin assessed by retreatment. *Int J Radiat Biol* **55**: 271–83.

Valentini V, Morganti AG, Gambacorta MA *et al.* (2006). Preoperative hyperfractionated chemoradiation for locally recurrent rectal cancer in patients previously irradiated to the pelvis: a multicentric phase II study. *Int J Radiat Oncol Biol Phys* **64**: 1129–39.

van der Kogel AJ, Sissingh HA, Zoetelief J (1982). Effect of X-rays and neutrons on repair and regeneration in the rat spinal cord. *Int J Radiat Oncol Biol Phys* **8**: 2095–7.

van der Schueren E, van den Bogaert W, Vanuytsel L, van Limbergen E (1990). Radiotherapy by multiple fractions per day (MFD) in head and neck cancer: acute reactions of skin and mucosa. *Int J Radiat Oncol Biol Phys* **19**: 301–11.

White A, Hornsey S (1980). Time dependent repair of radiation damage in the rat spinal cord after X-rays and neutrons. *Eur J Cancer* **16**: 957–62.

Wong CS, Hao Y (1997). Long-term recovery kinetics of radiation damage in rat spinal cord. *Int J Radiat Oncol Biol Phys* **37**: 171–9.

Wong CS, van Dyk J, Milosevic M, Laperriere NJ (1994). Radiation myelopathy following single courses of radiotherapy and retreatment. *Int J Radiat Oncol Biol Phys* **30**: 575–81.

Xiang EW, Shu-mo C, Ya-qin D, Ke W (1998). Treatment of late recurrent vaginal malignancy after initial radiotherapy for carcinoma of the cervix: an analysis of 73 cases. *Gynecol Oncol* **69**: 125–9.

■ FURTHER READING

Morris DE (2000). Clinical experience with retreatment for palliation. *Semin Radiat Oncol* **10**: 210–21.

Nieder C, Milas L, Ang KK (2000). Tissue tolerance to re-irradiation. *Semin Radiat Oncol* **10**: 200–9.

Stewart FA (1999). Re-treatment after full-course radiotherapy: is it a viable option? *Acta Oncol* **38**: 855–62.

Stewart FA, van der Kogel AJ (1994). Retreatment tolerance of normal tissues. *Semin Radiat Oncol* **4**: 103–11.

Molecular image-guided radiotherapy with positron emission tomography

VINCENT GRÉGOIRE, KARIN HAUSTERMANS AND JOHN LEE

20.1 INTRODUCTION: MOLECULAR IMAGING AND ITS POTENTIAL USE IN MODERN RADIOTHERAPY

Molecular imaging, also referred to as biological imaging or functional imaging, is the use of non-invasive imaging techniques that enable the visualization of various biological pathways and physiological characteristics of tumours and/or normal tissues. In short, it mainly refers (but not only) to positron emission tomography (PET) and functional magnetic resonance imaging (fMRI). In clinical oncology, molecular imaging offers a unique opportunity to allow an earlier diagnosis and staging of the disease, to contribute to the selection and delineation of the optimal target volumes for radiotherapy and, to a lesser extent, for surgery, to evaluate the response early in the treatment or after its completion, and to help in the early detection of recurrence (Fig. 20.1). From the viewpoint of experimental oncology, molecular imaging may also facilitate and speed up the process of drug development by allowing faster and cheaper pharmacokinetic and biodistribution studies.

For target volume selection and delineation, anatomic imaging modalities such as computed tomography (CT), and to a lesser extent magnetic resonance imaging (MRI), remain the most widely used modalities. Over the last few years, however, the use of molecular imaging and in particular the use of positron-labelled fluorodcoxyglucosc (FDG-PET) has become increasingly widespread. Provided that appropriate tracers are used, molecular imaging with PET enables the visualization of the various molecular pathways in tumours, including metabolism, proliferation, oxygen delivery and consumption, and receptor or gene expression, all of which may be important in the response to ionizing radiation.

The goal of radiotherapy treatment planning is to select and delineate target volumes (and organs at risk) based on all the available diagnostic information and on the knowledge of the physiology of the disease (i.e. the probability of local and nodal infiltration). This is done in part by using various imaging modalities, which depict more or less accurately the true tumour extent. The difficulty with using imaging modalities is that none of them has a sensitivity (no false negatives) or a

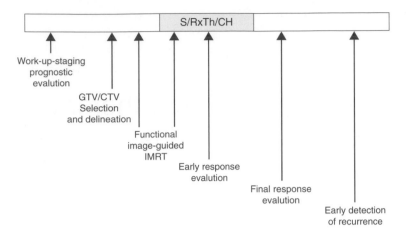

Figure 20.1 Relative timescale illustrating the various opportunities for the use of biological imaging in oncology. S/Rx Th/Ch, surgery and/or radiotherapy and/or chemotherapy.

specificity (no false positives) of 100 per cent. Thus, false negatives and false positives for depicting neoplastic processes occur.

How the sensitivity and specificity of a particular imaging modality influences the radiotherapy planning process depends on the underlying objective of the treatment. If, for a particular disease, the objective is to avoid missing tumour at any cost, a highly sensitive approach needs to be selected. This will give a lower specificity, resulting in inclusion of non-neoplastic tissue into the target volume. However, this approach reduces the likelihood that neoplastic cells are missed. If, on the other hand, the aim is to avoid including non-neoplastic cells into the target volume to protect normal tissue, a highly specific approach needs to be selected. However, this reduces the sensitivity of the approach and increases the risk of missing tumour cells. Therefore, the additional use of PET in treatment planning, and of FDG-PET in particular, has assumed increasing importance to the point where many radiation oncologists now believe that target volume selection and delineation cannot be adequately performed without the use of PET.

When incorporating PET into treatment planning, its sensitivity and specificity should be compared with CT and with pathological verification of tumour extent from surgical sampling, if available. The potential impact of PET on treatment planning needs to be determined. For example, if an additional lymph node is visualized with a new imaging modality known to be more specific than

the standard modality, it might be legitimate to increase the target volume(s) beyond what would have been given using a standard procedure; conversely, if fewer nodes are visualized with a new imaging modality known to be more sensitive than the standard modality, it might be legitimate to decrease the target volume(s) below what would have been given using a standard procedure.

Table 20.1 summarizes data on the specificity and sensitivity of FDG-PET and CT (or MRI) for lymph node staging in lung cancer, head and neck cancer, cervical cancer, oesophageal cancer and colorectal cancer, comparing with surgical lymph node sampling as the gold standard. In head and neck tumours, CT and FDG-PET performed with a comparable diagnostic accuracy. A potentially interesting use of FDG-PET is in the staging of node-negative patients (as assessed by other imaging modalities) where the issue could be to avoid treating the neck nodes if an FDG-PET examination also turns out to be negative. However, in the node-negative neck, the sensitivity of FDG-PET, compared with the examination of the pathology specimen after a neck node dissection, is only around 70 per cent (Stuckensen *et al.*, 2000). This is not surprising in light of the fact that in node-negative patients who underwent a prophylactic neck node dissection, microscopic nodal infiltration could nevertheless be observed in up to 30 per cent of cases (Shah, 1990). Thus the rather low signal-to-background ratio of FDG and the limited spatial resolution of the cameras currently

Table 20.1 Comparison between computed tomography (CT) (or magnetic resonance imaging, MRI) and fluorodeoxyglucose positron emission tomography (FDG-PET) for nodal staging

Site	Sensitivity (%)		Specificity (%)		Reference
	CT	FDG–PET	CT	FDG–PET	
Head and neck cancer	36–86	50–96	56–100	88–100	Menda and Graham (2005)
Non-small cell lung cancer	45	80–90	85	85–100	Birim *et al.* (2005)
Cervix carcinoma	57–73[1]	75–91	83–100[1]	92–100	Rose *et al.* (1999), Sugawara *et al.* (1999), Reinhardt *et al.* (2001)
Oesophageal cancer	11–87	30–78	28–99	86–98	van Westreenen *et al.* (2004)
Colorectal carcinoma	29	29	96	85	Abdel-Nabi *et al.* (1998)

[1]CT or MRI.

preclude the detection of microscopic disease with PET and, therefore, compared with anatomic imaging modalities such as CT and MRI, it is unlikely that FDG-PET will be of any value in selecting nodal target volumes in the neck.

Conversely, when evaluating the added value of FDG-PET in non-small cell lung cancer (NSCLC), the opposite is true. The sensitivity for staging of lymph nodes in lung cancer is significantly higher for FDG-PET than for CT. This implies that a negative PET scan could result in substantially reduced target volumes and permit focusing on the primary tumour.

In esophageal cancer, the sensitivity of FDG-PET is similar to that of CT. Conversely, FDG-PET is very specific for the staging of lymph nodes outside of the mediastinum (e.g. supra-clavicular or coeliac lymph nodes). If such lymph nodes are detected with FDG-PET, it is legitimate to enlarge the selection (thus the delineation) of the target volume (Vrieze *et al.*, 2004).

In para-aortic lymph nodes of patients with cervix carcinoma, although based on a limited number of patients, FDG-PET is also reported to be much more specific than CT or MRI, thus supporting the inclusion of these nodes in case of positive PET findings. It has also been shown that FDG-PET positive findings in the para-aortic region were a predictor of overall survival after treatment with radiotherapy and chemotherapy (Grigsby *et al.*, 2001).

In colorectal carcinoma, FGD-PET was slightly more specific than CT for the detection of lymph node infiltration (Table 20.1), but owing to the quasi-systematic use of preoperative chemoradiotherapy on the whole pelvis, the value of this finding is unclear. However, it might be useful to support a change in the therapeutic management in cases of a positive lymph node outside of the pelvic cavity.

The data in Table 20.1 were obtained with PET cameras, whereas centres are increasingly being equipped with dual PET/CT systems. Few systematic comparisons between the diagnostic accuracy of standalone PET and integrated PET/CT have been performed. Overall, diagnostic accuracy might be improved by the use of dual PET/CT cameras (Bar-Shalom *et al.*, 2003; Antoch *et al.*, 2004). It is, however, interesting to note that, although logistically more demanding, the performance of the side-by-side PET and CT comparison was almost as good as the dual cameras (Antoch *et al.*, 2004). Whatever the improved diagnostic accuracy of combined PET and CT examinations, the results of more extensive comparisons between PET/CT and PET alone have to be awaited before definitive conclusions can be drawn.

20.2 IMAGE ACQUISITION AND RECONSTRUCTION WITH PET

In oncology, PET has been used routinely as a diagnostic tool for detection of lesions. By contrast, volume delineation on PET images appears as a relatively recent trend in radiotherapy. In comparison with simple diagnosis, volume delineation requires greater care in acquisition, reconstruction and processing of PET images, in order to minimize the uncertainty on tumour boundaries and achieve reasonable volume accuracy.

First, it is useful to recall some inherent limitations of PET (Tarantola *et al.*, 2003). For many physical reasons (e.g. optimal size of detector chosen for efficiency reasons, positron energy, etc.) whose discussion is beyond the scope of this chapter, the resolution of PET images is lower than images from CT or MR: typical PET cameras have about four times lower resolution than modern CT scans, which explains the blurry aspect of PET images. Also, because PET is an emission modality, its images suffer from a high noise level. The injected dose of the tracer must be limited for obvious radioprotective reasons. Moreover, many positron disintegrations occur outside the field of view of the PET camera where they do not contribute to the image but can add additional noise (scattered events). Both the low resolution and the high noise level must be taken into account when selecting suitable acquisition protocols and reconstruction procedures. In summary, the best sensitivity is achieved with three-dimensional (3D) acquisition; this also allows a good trade-off between tracer-injected dose, acquisition duration and patient comfort. Regarding reconstruction protocols, iterative algorithms such as Ordered Subsets Expectation Maximization (OSEM) is preferred, especially for accurate volumetric assessment. This reconstruction method is, however, quite slow and may not be suitable for routine diagnostic PET acquisition.

After the images have been reconstructed, further enhancements can be achieved by filtering and deblurring. Filtering aims at further reducing the noise to enhance the gradient between the background activity and the signal of interest. When image quality is essential, as it is for automatic segmentation, an anisotropic diffusion filter or bilateral filter is preferred to the typical Gaussian filter (Nagayoshi *et al.*, 2005). A typical example of what image filtering does is shown in Fig. 20.2. Image deblurring aims at restoring sharp edges between voxels of low activity and those of high activity. Such methods require an accurate knowledge of the resolution characteristics of the PET camera. In addition, because of the longer computation time required by those techniques, small objects (with a size approximating the resolution of the camera) cannot be correctly segmented.

20.3 PET IMAGE SEGMENTATION

The accurate determination of the volume and shape of the tumour from PET images remains a challenge and an incompletely resolved issue. Although most of the reports on the segmentation of PET images have dealt with non-small cell lung cancer, various methods have been already tested to determine the outline of FDG-positive tissue in patients with head and neck squamous carcinoma (HNSSC) (Erdi *et al.*, 1997).

The easiest and simplest method consists of visual interpretation of the PET images and definition of the tumour contours by an experienced nuclear medicine physician or a radiation oncologist (Ciernik *et al.*, 2003). However, this method appears highly debatable. First, the threshold level of the PET image, which depends on the display windowing, strongly influences the visual assessment of the tumour boundaries. Moreover, the visual delineation of objects is a subjective approach that will necessarily lead to substantial intra- and interobserver variability.

Within this framework, the development of objective and reproducible methods for segmenting PET images has become crucial. The simplest method relies on the choice of a fixed threshold of activity (i.e. a given percentage of the maximal activity within the tumour, for distinguishing between malignant and surrounding normal tissues). Using a fixed threshold of 50 per cent of the maximal activity to automatically segment a primary tumour of the head and neck region, tumour volumes delineated from PET images with FDG were larger than those delineated with CT in 25 per cent of the cases (Paulino *et al.*, 2005). However, results from this study have to be viewed with caution since the relevance of an arbitrary fixed threshold appears questionable. Indeed, it has been shown that the threshold required to match macroscopic laryngectomy specimens used as a 'gold standard' varied from one specimen to another between 36 per cent and

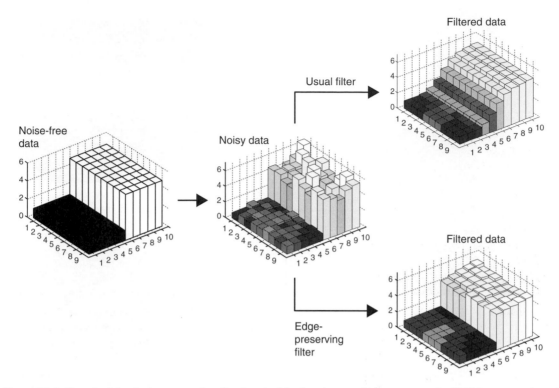

Figure 20.2 The principle of edge-preserving filtering. An 'ideal' positron emission tomography (PET) image consists of two regions, one with a low activity and another with a higher activity (on left). The activity is depicted with bars of varying height. 'Real' PET scanners do not yield noise-free images, and a simulation of a noisy 'real' image is depicted in the centre. From there, two different filters have been used. The top right image is obtained with a usual Gaussian filter, whereas the bottom right image results from the application of an edge-preserving filter. This 'real' image is much closer to the 'ideal' image.

73 per cent of the maximal activity (Gregoire *et al.*, 2005). Reinforced by the absence of validation studies, these data clearly illustrate that methods based on fixed thresholds are not adequate for accurately segmenting tumours from PET images.

The use of an adaptive threshold is an elegant option that could eliminate the drawbacks of methods described above. Adaptive thresholding relies on a model that determines the appropriate threshold of activity according to the signal-to-background ratio. This method has been shown to be accurate for segmenting PET images in a series of pharyngo-laryngeal tumours (Daisne *et al.*, 2004). Although validated as a reliable segmentation method, it nevertheless presents some drawbacks. For example, it is unclear whether the method is valid across different centres as it depends on so many centre-dependent parameters such as the

camera and its point spread function (PSF), and the reconstruction and filtering method. Also, this method is not ideal for images with low signal to background ratios, such as encountered in peritumoural inflammation induced by radiotherapy or in undifferentiated tumours.

Gradient-based segmentation methods, which are used for CT, cannot be directly employed for PET because of its poor resolution. However, image restoration tools, such as edge-preserving filters and deblurring algorithms (see Section 20.2), partly overcome the problems of blur and noise and may enable gradient-based segmentation techniques to be adopted. Preliminary experiments have shown encouraging results with segmentation of phantom objects and head and neck tumours based on the combination of watershed transform and hierarchical cluster analyses

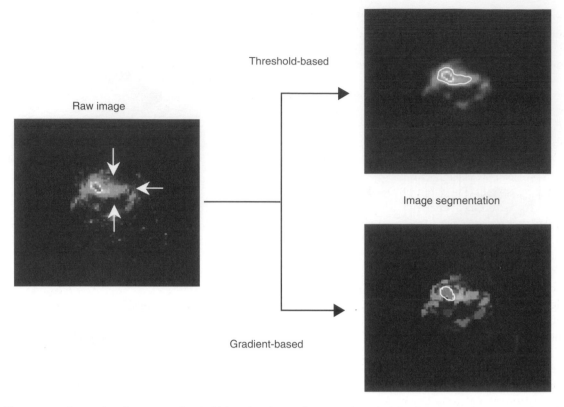

Figure 20.3 Comparison between a threshold-based and a gradient-based method for the automatic segmentation of a head and neck tumour during radiotherapy. The image is intrinsically noisier because of peritumoural radiation-induced mucositis. The gradient-based method led to a more specific tumour segmentation. See colour plate section for full colour image.

(Geets *et al.*, 2007a). The main advantage of this approach is that it is purely data-driven; no underlying model or calibration curve is necessary, except the knowledge of the scanner PSF. Consequently, both the applicability of the method and its spread could be increased since it could still yield a reasonable segmentation in difficult cases (e.g. an image with low signal-to-background ratio), where threshold-based methods usually fail. A typical example is the use of FDG-PET during radiotherapy (Fig. 20.3). The combination of radio-induced mucositis, which increases the background signal, together with the reduction in tumour uptake secondary to the treatment response, leads to a drastic decrease in signal-to-background ratio. In this context, resolving the residual tumour from the surrounding inflammatory area requires powerful segmentation methods

that are able to detect gradient-intensity crests of low magnitude and/or delayed imaging acquisition.

20.4 USING PET IMAGES FOR TREATMENT PLANNING

Brain tumours

Unlike other tissues, the brain almost exclusively metabolizes glucose to meet its energy demands. Consequently, the accumulation of FDG in normal brain tissue is very high and this limits the use of FDG-PET for brain tumour imaging. Thus, compared with MRI, FDG-PET provides additional information for radiotherapy planning only in a minority of cases. This is because of the small difference in contrast between viable tumour and normal white matter even for many high-grade tumours. Because uptake of ^{11}C-labelled methionine ([^{11}C]-MET) in normal brain parenchyma is low, MET-PET is superior to FDG-PET in the assessment of tumour dimensions. The most important radiolabelled amino acid tracers used for brain imaging are ^{11}C-labelled MET, [132]I-labelled α-methyl-tyrosine (IMT) and ^{18}F-labelled O-(2) fluoroethyl-L-tyrosine (FET). The short half-life of [^{11}C]-MET limits its clinical usefulness to centres with on-site cyclotrons. However, FET is an attractive alternative, as it was shown that MET-PET and FET-PET were equal in their ability to diagnose vital glioma tumour tissue (Weber et al., 2000).

The uptake of MET is correlated to prognosis and higher MET uptake has been seen in grade III or IV gliomas, compared with low-grade gliomas. Moreover, oligodendrogliomas tend to show a higher uptake of MET than astrocytomas, which is probably linked to oligodendroglial cellular differentiation (Herholz et al., 1998). However, a number of studies have provided controversial findings on the accuracy of tracer uptake in determining tumour grade (e.g. Schmidt et al., 2001).

There are only limited data available on the usefulness of MET-PET in radiotherapy treatment planning. Several studies have shown that the margins of tumours, as assessed by PET with amino acid tracers, are frequently wider than those assessed by MRI or CT (Jacobs et al., 2002). MET-PET detects solid parts of brain tumours as well as the infiltration area with high sensitivity (87 per cent) and specificity (87 per cent) and this phenomenon can be even more pronounced in low-grade tumours and diffuse gliomatosis because of their lack of contrast enhancement on MRI (Kracht et al., 2004). Sensitivity and specificity of MET-PET in differentiating between non-tumour tissue and low-grade gliomas was 76 per cent and 87 per cent, respectively (Herholz et al., 1998). In 14 patients of whom 13 had low-grade astrocytomas, MET-PET was helpful in delineating the gross tumour volume (GTV) in 27 per cent, whereas PET findings either correlated with MRI (46 per cent) or were less distinctive in 27 per cent (Nuutinen et al., 2000). In meningiomas, difficulties in tumour delineation may occur as these tumours frequently infiltrate and because contrast enhancement in the normal tissues may be comparable to that of the tumour. Meningioma borders

can be more accurately defined on the basis of MET-PET/CT (Grosu et al., 2003; Sweeney et al., 2003). In conclusion, MET-PET can be helpful in delineating brain tumours for radiotherapy planning but more studies, especially with the alternative FET, tracer are needed to recommend its use in daily radiation treatment planning (Grosu et al., 2005).

Head and neck squamous cell carcinoma

As discussed above, the value of FDG-PET for the selection of target volumes in the head and neck area has yet to be demonstrated. Indeed, its sensitivity and specificity for the assessment of head and neck node infiltration does not differ significantly from that of CT or MRI (Table 20.1). However a study in 20 patients with mostly locally advanced disease demonstrated an increase in sensitivity with the use of a hybrid PET/CT compared with CT alone and showed that PET/CT-based radiation treatment would have significantly changed the dose distribution (Schwartz et al., 2005). These findings need to be confirmed prospectively in larger study populations before it can be implemented into routine use.

In contrast, FDG-PET has been shown to be of value for the delineation of the primary tumour GTV by comparing 3D registration of CT, MRI and FDG-PET images of oropharyngeal, hypopharyngeal and laryngeal squamous cell carcinomas (Daisne et al., 2004). In a subset of laryngeal tumours, the imaging modalities were also registered with the actual surgical specimen taken as a 'gold standard'. It was found that MRI did not provide any added value to CT, either in terms of volumetric GTV assessment or in terms of reduced interobserver variability (Geets et al., 2005). In contrast, FDG-PET demonstrated higher accuracy in delineating GTV with a statistically significant reduction in the target volumes. All three imaging modalities, however, failed to visualize the extent of superficial tumour, illustrating their limitations in spatial resolution. Interestingly, the differences observed between CT and FDG-PET for the GTV delineation translated into significant differences in clinical target volume (CTV) and planning target volume (PTV) delineation. When comparative

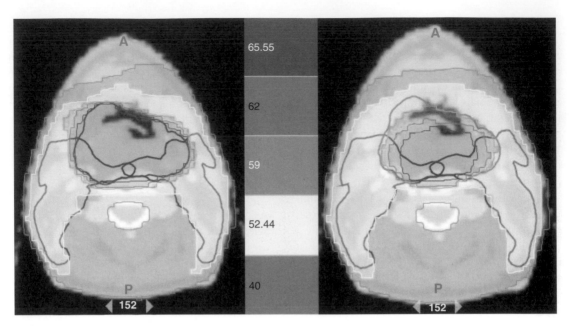

Figure 20.4 Patient with a T4–N0–M0 squamous cell carcinoma of the hypopharynx. The patient was treated using a simultaneous integrated boost approach delivering a dose of 55.5 Gy (30 fractions of 1.85 Gy) to the prophylactic planning target volume (PTV; delineated in dark blue) and a dose of 69 Gy (30 fractions of 2.3 Gy) to the therapeutic PTV (delineated in dark green). Comparison between a pretreatment computed tomography (CT)-based plan (left) and adaptive fluorodeoxyglucose positron emission tomography (FDG-PET)-based plan (right). On both plans, only the CT-based PTVs are depicted. A FDG-PET examination was performed before treatment and at 16 Gy, 24 Gy, 34 Gy and 44 Gy. The dose distribution was adapted to the progressive reduction of the FDG-PET gross tumour volume (GTV). See colour plate section for full colour image.

3D-conformal radiotherapy (CRT) plans were made, FDG-PET-based plans were more conformal than the CT-based plans and reductions in the isodose volumes with subsequent reductions in the dose to the surrounding normal tissues were observed in the PET-based plans (Geets *et al.*, 2006). This could have important consequences as it paves the way for possible dose escalation to the target volumes; in a proof-of-concept study on 15 patients with head and neck tumours, it was shown that an increase in dose per fraction (to 2.5 Gy and 3 Gy per fraction) could be safely delivered to the FDG-PET-based PTV during part of the treatment (Vanderstraeten *et al.*, 2006).

During a course of fractionated radiotherapy, it is anticipated that both anatomical and functional tumour changes will occur. Re-assessment of the tumour during radiotherapy with subsequent adaptation of the plan might thus allow a much tighter dose distribution to the target volumes

with consequent decrease of the total irradiated volume. In the hypopharynx, it has been shown (Geets *et al.*, 2007b) that the GTV progressively decreases during radiotherapy and that adaptive treatment could lead to a significant reduction in the high-dose volume in some cases (Fig. 20.4).

Non-small cell lung cancer (NSCLC)

Fluorodeoxyglucose-PET has a higher sensitivity/specificity for nodal staging than CT and might thus alter the GTV either by detecting unnoticed metastatic lymph nodes or by down-staging a CT false-positive mediastinal nodal station. Because of the particularly high sensitivity, the second situation is more frequent (Table 20.1). In a series of 44 patients, it was shown that FDG-PET altered the stage of the disease in 11 patients (25 per cent) by down-staging 10 of these patients

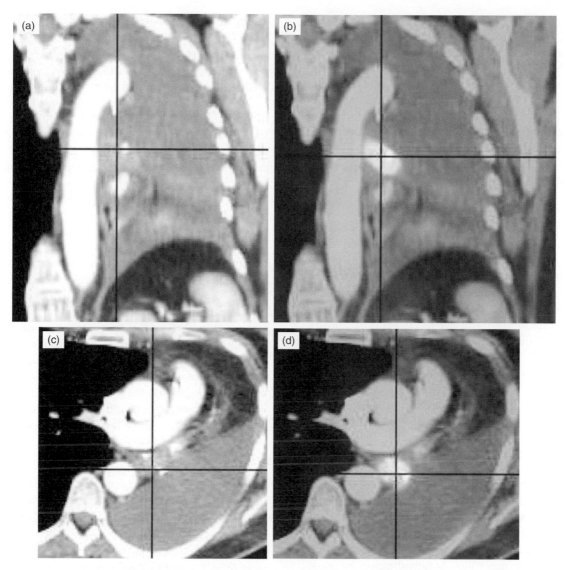

Figure 20.5 This example illustrates the role of fluorodeoxyglucose positron emission tomography (FDG-PET) for delineating the volume of a lung cancer. The images represent saggital (a) and axial (c) slices of a patient with a lung cancer located in the left hilar region, with retro-obstructive atelectasis of the entire left lung, associated with a major pleural effusion. The metabolic information provided by FDG-PET (b, d) shows that the tumour tissue is strictly located to the hilum. The delineation of the tumour margins is easier and more accurate with the help of FDG-PET, allowing for a significant modification of the target volume. See colour plate section for full colour image.

(De Ruysscher *et al.*, 2005b). As a consequence, the GTV based on FDG-PET was, on average, smaller than the GTV defined on CT. In a simulation study, it has been shown that for the same expected toxicity to lungs, spinal cord and oesophagus, the dose to the tumour could be increased by 25 per cent, resulting in a potentially higher tumour control probability of 24 per cent for PET-CT planning compared with 6.3 per cent for CT alone (De Ruysscher *et al.*, 2005a). In addition to better detection of true positive lymph nodes, FDG-PET further alters the definition of GTV by discriminating tumour tissue from atelectasis or necrosis (Fig. 20.5). Other studies have reported that FDG-PET alters the GTV in 22–62 per cent of the patients (Bachaud *et al.*, 2005) and PET, especially PET-CT, imaging has been shown to significantly reduce the inter-observer variability, as well as the intraobserver variability (Ashamalla *et al.*, 2005; Fox *et al.*, 2005). In a modelling study, it was reported in 21 patients with N2–N3 NSCLC that the use of PET-CT for radiotherapy planning resulted in a lower radiation exposure of the oesophagus and the lungs, allowing a significant dose escalation to the tumour (van der Wel *et al.*, 2005).

To date, only a few studies have prospectively included PET with FDG in radiotherapy planning and actually addressed its impact on local tumour control and survival. Selective mediastinal node irradiation based on PET with FDG has yielded a low rate of isolated nodal failure, suggesting that reducing the target volume does not result in worse local control (De Ruysscher *et al.*, 2005b).

Some issues related to the use of PET in lung cancer radiotherapy remain unresolved. First, tumour delineation/contouring by PET is still unsatisfactory, as discussed in Section 20.3. The appropriate activity threshold to be used to automatically delineate the tumour contours varies with the size of the tumour and the tumour-to-background ratio (Yaremko *et al.*, 2005). It has been suggested that the area of lower uptake (which has been named the 'anatomic biologic halo') immediately surrounding the most metabolic part of the tumour be included in the GTV defined from PET (Ashamalla *et al.*, 2005). Including this 'halo' resulted in a better dose coverage of the PTVs. Standardization is needed, since the use of different delineation techniques for FDG leads to different GTVs (Nestle *et al.*, 2005).

The second methodological issue, of particular importance in lung cancer radiation therapy, is tumour motion during PET imaging and radiotherapy. The PET images are usually acquired during free breathing. Usual emission scan duration for PET is 5–10 min per bed position for conventional PET. For PET/CT, the short CT scan is used for attenuation correction. To increase the accuracy of tumour volume delineation, respiratory gating techniques should be implemented (Boucher *et al.*, 2004).

Esophageal tumour

As already discussed, FDG-PET is particularly specific for lymph node detection outside of the mediastinum, which might help to optimize the radiation target volume (Table 20.1). In an analysis of the additional value of FDG-PET for optimization of the CTV in 30 patients with advanced oesophageal cancer (Vrieze *et al.*, 2004), discordances between conventional staging modalities, including CT and oesophageal endoscopic ultrasound (EUS), for the detection of lymph node involvement were found in 14 out of 30 patients (47 per cent). In eight patients, the involved lymph nodes were detected only on CT/EUS, which would have led to a decrease in the CTV in three of them if PET alone had been used. In contrast, PET with FDG was the only detector of lymph node involvement in six patients, resulting in a possible larger CTV in three of these patients (10 per cent). The authors concluded that the high specificity of FDG-PET for lymph node detection justifies its use for treatment volume adaptation in case of positive findings, while the low sensitivity of FDG-PET (i.e. false-negative lymph nodes) would give an erroneous reduction of the CTV. Whether the role of FDG-PET in esophageal treatment planning will lead to a therapeutic gain without increasing the toxicity remains unanswered.

Another study evaluated the impact of CT and FDG-PET in conformal radiotherapy in 34 patients with oesophageal carcinoma referred for radical chemo-radiation (Moureau-Zabotto *et al.*, 2005). After manual delineation of the GTV on both modalities, CT and PET were co-registered. Image fusion (GTV-PET was used as overlay to GTV-CT) resulted in a reduction of the GTV in 12 patients (25 per cent) and an increase in seven patients (21 per cent). Modification of the GTV affected the PTV in 18 patients and affected the percentage of lung volume receiving more than 20 Gy in 25 patients (74 per cent), with a dose reduction in 12 patients and a dose increase in 13 patients. A similar study was performed with an integrated PET/CT scanner (Leong *et al.*, 2004). Here, the GTV was enlarged in 9 out of 10 (90 per cent) patients by a median volume of 22 per cent (range 3–100 per cent) when PET with FDG information was added to the CT-based GTV. In three patients, the

PET-avid disease was also excluded from the PTV defined on CT, which would have resulted in a geographical miss. In 16 patients confirming the possible role of FDG-PET/CT in radiotherapy treatment planning for oesophageal cancer (Howard *et al.*, 2004), CT-derived GTVs were compared with GTVs contoured on PET/CT images by means of a conformality index (CI). The mean CI was 0.46, suggesting a significant lack of overlap between the GTVs in a large proportion of patients. The use of PET/CT in treatment planning for patients with oesophageal cancer is now being evaluated in a prospective trial. Another preliminary finding on incorporating EUS and PET scanning in the treatment planning process of 25 patients with oesophageal carcinoma showed that the measured tumour length was significantly longer on CT than on PET with FDG (Konski *et al.*, 2005). The authors concluded that PET could be of additional help in the treatment planning. Although EUS measurements of the tumour length were as accurate as PET measurements, the results of EUS are difficult to translate into the planning process. A major drawback of this study was the lack of comparison with pathology findings after surgery.

Rectal cancer

The usefulness of FDG-PET for the initial staging of colorectal cancer has been investigated. Preoperative PET may be useful for the diagnosis of the primary tumour, but it is of limited value for detecting metastasis to the regional lymph nodes (Table 20.1). The potential use of PET/CT in radiotherapy planning for rectal cancer has been addressed in only one study (Ciernik *et al.*, 2005) which evaluated the accuracy of target volume definition with FDG-PET in 11 patients using an integrated PET/CT system. They found that the PET-defined GTV did not correlate well with the pathologic tumour volume. However, this study should be interpreted with caution, as there are several methodological weaknesses. First, pretreatment PET/CT was compared with pathological specimens obtained after preoperative chemoradiotherapy. Second, a fixed threshold was used and a so-called 'standardized region-growing

algorithm' to segment the target volumes. This procedure omits the selection and delineation of the CTV, which contains all pelvic regions that are at risk for subclinical disease in rectal cancer, including the internal iliac lymph node regions (Roels *et al.*, 2006).

Although FDG-PET has a high sensitivity for colorectal cancer, there are some limitations in specificity, mainly owing to FDG uptake by macrophages. This limitation becomes important when assessing tumour volume during treatment or when assessing response to chemoradiation, as radiation induces mucositis of the rectal wall surrounding the tumour. In this regard, efforts are being made to develop new ^{18}F-labelled tracers that might be more tumour specific.

Even if PET can provide additional functional information, its usefulness in the treatment of rectal cancer patients is still questionable and needs to be evaluated in prospective trials using a strict methodology. Its benefit might be of little interest in preoperative 3D-CRT, as the total mesorectum included in the CTV will be surgically removed anyway. However, it may become more important when 'dose painting' to relevant biological regions is achieved with simultaneous integrated boost techniques. Whether this in turn can improve patient outcome in terms of local control and/or sphincter preservation has to be tested in future trials. Moreover, there remain problems that require specific attention, such as image co-registration and variations in patient setup, in organ motion (e.g. bowel movements) and in organ shape (e.g. bladder filling). The use of an integrated PET/CT is the modality of choice when it comes to more accurate registration in this site. However, there are still small variations possible because of the elastic properties of the rectal wall resulting in distortions of the rectum (and tumour) during the time of acquisition. Displacements of the rectal wall/tumour could also induce geographical misses when dose escalation to small volumes is planned.

Cervix cancer

As already mentioned in Section 20.1 (Table 20.1), FDG-PET appears to be of particular value in detecting para-aortic lymph node involvement.

Based on these findings, a proof-of-concept study has been reported on four patients in whom FDG-PET was used to guide intensity-modulated radiation therapy (IMRT) treatments by altering the GTV selection with inclusion of para-aortic lymph nodes (Mutic *et al.*, 2003). Fluorodeoxyglucose-PET has also been used to delineate the GTV (fixed threshold of 40 per cent of the maximum activity) in 24 patients treated by brachytherapy and external 3D-CRT (Lin *et al.*, 2005). This preliminary study has indicated the benefit of FDG-PET in improving the coverage of large tumours. However, confirmatory studies on larger series of patients are needed before it is possible to ascertain the exact role of FDG-PET for volume delineation of cervix tumours.

20.5 THERAGNOSTIC IMAGING FOR RADIATION ONCOLOGY

Recent developments in molecular imaging have created opportunities to probe the heterogeneity of the tumour biology. In addition to FDG, which is likely to be a surrogate of tumour burden and hence of clonogen density, tracers of hypoxia, such as fluoromisonidazole (F-Miso), 3,3,3-trifluoro-propylamine (EF3), fluoro-erythronitroimidazole (FETNIM) or copper-diacetyl-*bis*N4-methylthiosemicarbazone (Cu-ATSM), of proliferation such as 5-bromo-2'-fluoro-2'-deoxyuridine (BFU) or 3'-deoxy-3'-fluorothymidine (FLT), and of receptor expression such as epithelial growth factor receptor (EGFR), have been developed.

Among the PET tracers for hypoxia, F-Miso is the most widely reported but no studies have yet used the tracer to actually define a sub-GTV, which would benefit from a higher radiation dose. There are still several questions that remain open regarding the use of these hypoxia tracers for treatment planning purpose. For example, it is still unclear whether all the tracers are imaging similar biological characteristics, and thus could be interchangeable. In a recent study comparing F-Miso and EF3 in mouse tumour models, it has been shown that these two tracers might not have the same specificity for cellular hypoxia, and thus may not identify identical hypoxic fractions within a GTV (Mahy *et al.*, 2008).

Fluorothymidine (FLT) is a tracer which images DNA synthesis and cellular proliferation by entering the salvage pathway of DNA synthesis. It is thus not incorporated into DNA as the native nucleotides. Amino acids, like FLT, are of interest because they do not seem to accumulate in inflammatory processes and could therefore provide a more specific tumour label (Been *et al.*, 2004). Comparison between FLT and FDG-PET imaging in colorectal cancer has demonstrated lower standardized uptake value (SUV) values for FLT compared with FDG. No correlation was found between the uptake of both tracers, confirming that FLT and FDG detect distinct processes. It has been found that FLT is a valuable tracer for improvement of the specificity for the detection of colorectal tumours. The lack of FLT uptake in inflammatory cells, which are present during and after radiotherapy and/or chemotherapy, makes FLT a promising agent to measure the response to anti-cancer therapy. Preclinical and clinical studies in colorectal cancer show a good correlation between FLT uptake and proliferation (Francis *et al.*, 2004). However, as FLT is not incorporated into DNA, results of clinical PET studies with FLT should be interpreted carefully, taking into account previous treatment and bearing in mind that FLT uptake observed *in vivo* might result from various mechanisms with possibly divergent influences.

Although limitations certainly exist regarding the use of these various tracers, their integration into the treatment planning process could give a clearer view of the biological pathways involved in radiation response, and hence could be used to 'paint' or 'sculpt' the dose in various subvolumes using IMRT. Along this line of investigation, 'dummy run' studies have been reported with FDG and Cu-ATSM (Chao *et al.*, 2001; De Ruysscher *et al.*, 2005a). Although these studies demonstrate the feasibility of the concept of dose-painting, no clinical validation has been undertaken.

In all the studies on target volume definition to date, it has been assumed that, even when defined with regard to specific biological pathways, GTVs were homogeneous and did not vary during the course of a radiation treatment. Hence, a radiation dose homogeneously distributed in space and time is delivered (i.e. a so-called four-dimensional homogeneous dose distribution. This is likely to be an oversimplification of the biological reality, as tumours are known to be heterogeneous with respect to pathways of importance for radiation response, and are also known to progressively shrink, at least some of them, during treatment.

Bentzen (2005) has proposed the term 'theragnostic' to describe the use of molecular imaging to assist in prescribing the distribution of radiation dose in four dimensions (i.e. the three spatial dimensions plus time). This is undoubtedly a challenging research topic, which could potentially revolutionize the process of radiotherapy planning and delivery. However, several issues need to be resolved. From a planning point of view, the challenge will be to establish the correspondence between a PET signal intensity (or a PET image segmentation) and a prescribed dose, thus evolving the concept of dose-painting into dose-painting by number (Alber *et al.*, 2003). We will also need to develop the tools to register in space and time the various images and the dose distributions acquired throughout the therapy. To this end, non-rigid registration techniques will be required as tumour and/or normal-tissue shrinkage is expected during the course of a radiotherapy treatment. From a biological viewpoint, the challenge will be to relate a change in tracer uptake to a change in the underlying biology, thus requiring a comprehensive biological validation of the concept of dose-painting or dose-painting by number in experimental models. However, although much research still needs to be done, it is likely that during the next 10 years these concepts and procedures will be increasingly incorporated into clinical radiotherapy.

types. Given the considerable range of PET accuracies across different tumour types, its role will not be identical in the different tumour locations.
3. In using PET for volume segmentation, image acquisition, reconstruction and analysis need new standards favouring image quality over reconstruction speed.
4. Observer-independent segmentation of PET images is required for automatic delineation of the GTV. Gradient-based methods appear more robust than threshold-based methods, especially in difficult cases (low uptake and/or peritumoural inflammation) encountered during radiotherapy treatment.
5. The use of molecular imaging for treatment planning is under validation in various disease sites. It has shown encouraging results in head and neck and lung tumours.
6. 'Theragnostic' has been proposed to describe the use of molecular imaging to assist in prescribing the distribution of radiation dose in four dimensions – the three spatial dimensions plus time. It is a challenging concept at the frontier between radiation oncology, radiation biology and radiation physics that still requires thorough testing.
7. Before proper validation of the use of various PET tracers has been performed, and all methodological aspects have been fully optimized, it is reasonable to say that the use of PET for treatment planning purposes should not be used on a routine basis, but should remain in the clinical research arena.

Key points

1. Molecular imaging is the use of non-invasive imaging techniques (e.g. PET, fMRI) that enable the visualization of various biological pathways and physiological characteristics of tumours and normal tissues.
2. FDG-PET may be of benefit for the selection of target volumes depending on its sensitivity and specificity for various tumour

■ BIBLIOGRAPHY

Abdel-Nabi H, Doerr RJ, Lamonica DM *et al.* (1998). Staging of primary colorectal carcinomas with fluorine-18 fluorodeoxyglucose whole-body PET: correlation with histopathologic and CT findings. *Radiology* **206**: 755–60.

Alber M, Paulsen F, Eschmann SM, Machulla HJ (2003). On biologically conformal boost dose optimization. *Phys Med Biol* **48**: N31–5.

Antoch G, Saoudi N, Kuehl H *et al.* (2004). Accuracy of whole-body dual-modality fluorine-18-2-fluoro-2-deoxy-D-glucose positron emission tomography and computed tomography (FDG-PET/CT) for tumor staging in solid tumors: comparison with CT and PET. *J Clin Oncol* **22**: 4357–68.

Ashamalla H, Rafla S, Parikh K *et al.* (2005). The contribution of integrated PET/CT to the evolving definition of treatment volumes in radiation treatment planning in lung cancer. *Int J Radiat Oncol Biol Phys* **63**: 1016–23.

Bachaud JM, Marre D, Dygai I *et al.* (2005). [The impact of ^{18}F-fluorodeoxyglucose positron emission tomography on the 3D conformal radiotherapy planning in patients with non-small cell lung cancer]. *Cancer Radiother* **9**: 602–9.

Bar-Shalom R, Yefremov N, Guralnik L *et al.* (2003). Clinical performance of PET/CT in evaluation of cancer: additional value for diagnostic imaging and patient management. *J Nucl Med* **44**: 1200–9.

Been LB, Suurmeijer AJ, Cobben DC, Jager PL, Hoekstra HJ, Elsinga PH (2004). [^{18}F]FLT-PET in oncology: current status and opportunities. *Eur J Nucl Med Mol Imaging* **31**: 1659–72.

Bentzen SM (2005). Theragnostic imaging for radiation oncology: dose-painting by numbers. *Lancet Oncol* **6**: 112–7.

Birim O, Kappetein AP, Stijnen T, Bogers AJ (2005). Meta-analysis of positron emission tomographic and computed tomographic imaging in detecting mediastinal lymph node metastases in nonsmall cell lung cancer. *Ann Thorac Surg* **79**: 375–82.

Boucher L, Rodrigue S, Lecomte R, Benard F (2004). Respiratory gating for 3-dimensional PET of the thorax: feasibility and initial results. *J Nucl Med* **45**: 214–9.

Chao KS, Bosch WR, Mutic S *et al.* (2001). A novel approach to overcome hypoxic tumor resistance: Cu-ATSM-guided intensity-modulated radiation therapy. *Int J Radiat Oncol Biol Phys* **49**: 1171–82.

Ciernik IF, Dizendorf E, Baumert BG *et al.* (2003). Radiation treatment planning with an integrated positron emission and computer tomography (PET/CT): a feasibility study. *Int J Radiat Oncol Biol Phys* **57**: 853–63.

Ciernik IF, Huser M, Burger C, Davis JB, Szekely G (2005). Automated functional image-guided radiation treatment planning for rectal cancer. *Int J Radiat Oncol Biol Phys* **62**: 893–900.

Daisne JF, Duprez T, Weynand B *et al.* (2004). Tumor volume in pharyngolaryngeal squamous cell carcinoma: comparison at CT, MR imaging, and FDG PET and validation with surgical specimen. *Radiology* **233**: 93–100.

De Ruysscher D, Wanders S, Minken A *et al.* (2005a). Effects of radiotherapy planning with a dedicated combined PET-CT-simulator of patients with non-small cell lung cancer on dose limiting normal tissues and radiation dose-escalation: a planning study. *Radiother Oncol* **77**: 5–10.

De Ruysscher D, Wanders S, van Haren E *et al.* (2005b). Selective mediastinal node irradiation based on FDG-PET scan data in patients with non-small-cell lung cancer: a prospective clinical study. *Int J Radiat Oncol Biol Phys* **62**: 988–94.

Erdi YE, Mawlawi O, Larson SM *et al.* (1997). Segmentation of lung lesion volume by adaptive positron emission tomography image thresholding. *Cancer* **80**: 2505–9.

Fox JL, Rengan R, O'Meara W *et al.* (2005). Does registration of PET and planning CT images decrease interobserver and intraobserver variation in delineating tumor volumes for non-small-cell lung cancer? *Int J Radiat Oncol Biol Phys* **62**: 70–5.

Francis DL, Visvikis D, Costa DC *et al.* (2004). Assessment of recurrent colorectal cancer following 5-fluorouracil chemotherapy using both ^{18}FDG and ^{18}FLT PET. *Eur J Nucl Med Mol Imaging* **31**: 928.

Geets X, Daisne JF, Arcangeli S *et al.* (2005). Inter-observer variability in the delineation of pharyngo-laryngeal tumor, parotid glands and cervical spinal cord: comparison between CT-scan and MRI. *Radiother Oncol* **77**: 25–31.

Geets X, Daisne JF, Tomsej M, Duprez T, Lonneux M, Gregoire V (2006). Impact of the type of imaging modality on target volumes delineation and dose distribution in pharyngo-laryngeal squamous cell carcinoma: comparison between pre- and per-treatment studies. *Radiother Oncol* **78**: 291–7.

Geets X, Lee JA, Bol A, Lonneux M, Gregoire V (2007a). A gradient-based method for segmenting FDG-PET images: methodology and validation. *Eur J Nucl Med Mol Imaging* **34**: 1427–38.

Geets X, Tomsej M, Lee JA (2007b). Adaptive biological image-guided IMRT with anatomic and functional imaging in pharyngo-laryngeal tumors: impact on target volume delineation and dose distribution using helical tomotherapy. *Radiother Oncol* **85**: 105–15.

Gregoire V, Daisne JF, Geets X (2005). Comparison of CT- and FDG-PET-defined GT. *Int J Radiat Oncol Biol Phys* **63**: 308–9.

Grigsby PW, Siegel BA, Dehdashti F (2001). Lymph node staging by positron emission tomography in patients with carcinoma of the cervix. *J Clin Oncol* **19**: 3745–9.

Grosu AL, Lachner R, Wiedenmann N et al. (2003). Validation of a method for automatic image fusion (BrainLAB System) of CT data and ^{11}C-methionine-PET data for stereotactic radiotherapy using a LINAC: first clinical experience. *Int J Radiat Oncol Biol Phys* **56**: 1450–63.

Grosu AL, Piert M, Weber WA et al. (2005). Positron emission tomography for radiation treatment planning. *Strahlenther Onkol* **181**: 483–99.

Herholz K, Holzer T, Bauer B et al. (1998). ^{11}C-methionine PET for differential diagnosis of low-grade gliomas. *Neurology* **50**: 1316–22.

Howard A, Mehta MP, Ritter MA et al. (2004). The value of PET/CT in gross tumor volume delineation in lung and esophagus cancer. *Int J Radiat Oncol Biol Phys* **60**(Suppl. 1): S536–7.

Jacobs AH, Winkler A, Dittmar C et al. (2002). Molecular and functional imaging technology for the development of efficient treatment strategies for gliomas. *Technol Cancer Res Treat* **1**: 187–204.

Konski A, Doss M, Milestone B, Haluszka O, Hanlon A, Freedman G, Adler L (2005). The integration of 18-fluoro-deoxy-glucose positron emission tomography and endoscopic ultrasound in the treatment-planning process for esophageal carcinoma. *Int J Radiat Oncol Biol Phys* **61**: 1123–8.

Kracht LW, Miletic H, Busch S et al. (2004). Delineation of brain tumor extent with ^{11}C]L-methionine positron emission tomography: local comparison with stereotactic histopathology. *Clin Cancer Res* **10**: 7163–70.

Leong T, Everitt C, Yuen K et al. (2004). A prospective study to evaluate the impact of coregistered PET/CT images on radiotherapy treatment planning for esophageal cancer. *Int J Radiat Oncol Biol Phys* **60**(Suppl. 1): S139–40.

Lin LL, Mutic S, Malyapa RS et al. (2005). Sequential FDG-PET brachytherapy treatment planning in carcinoma of the cervix. *Int J Radiat Oncol Biol Phys* **63**: 1494–501.

Mahy P, de Bast M, de Groot T et al. (2008). Comparative pharmacokinetics, biodistribution, metabolism and hypoxia-dependent uptake of [18F]-EF3 and [18F]-MISO in rodent tumors model. *Radiother Oncol* (in press).

Menda Y, Graham MM (2005). Update on ^{18}F-fluorodeoxyglucose/positron emission tomography and positron emission tomography/computed tomography imaging of squamous head and neck cancers. *Semin Nucl Med* **35**: 214–9.

Moureau-Zabotto L, Touboul E, Lerouge D et al. (2005). Impact of CT and ^{18}F-deoxyglucose positron emission tomography image fusion for conformal radiotherapy in esophageal carcinoma. *Int J Radiat Oncol Biol Phys* **63**: 340–5.

Mutic S, Malyapa RS, Grigsby PW et al. (2003). PET-guided IMRT for cervical carcinoma with positive para-aortic lymph nodes: a dose-escalation treatment planning study. *Int J Radiat Oncol Biol Phys* **55**: 28–35.

Nagayoshi M, Murase K, Fujino K et al. (2005). Usefulness of noise adaptive non-linear Gaussian filter in FDG-PET study. *Ann Nucl Med* **19**: 469–77.

Nestle U, Kremp S, Schaefer-Schuler A et al. (2005). Comparison of different methods for delineation of ^{18}F-FDG PET-positive tissue for target volume definition in radiotherapy of patients with non-small cell lung cancer. *J Nucl Med* **46**: 1342–8.

Nuutinen J, Sonninen P, Lehikoinen P et al. (2000). Radiotherapy treatment planning and long-term follow-up with [(11)C]methionine PET in patients with low-grade astrocytoma. *Int J Radiat Oncol Biol Phys* **48**: 43–52.

Paulino AC, Koshy M, Howell R, Schuster D, Davis LW (2005). Comparison of CT- and FDG-PET-defined gross tumor volume in intensity-modulated radiotherapy for head-and-neck cancer. *Int J Radiat Oncol Biol Phys* **61**: 1385–92.

Reinhardt MJ, Ehritt-Braun C, Vogelgesang D et al. (2001). Metastatic lymph nodes in patients with cervical cancer: detection with MR imaging and FDG PET. *Radiology* **218**: 776–82.

Roels S, Duthoy W, Haustermans K et al. (2006). Definition and delineation of the clinical target volume for rectal cancer. *Int J Radiat Oncol Biol Phys* **65**: 1129–42.

Rose PG, Adler LP, Rodriguez M, Faulhaber PF, Abdul-Karim FW, Miraldi F (1999). Positron emission tomography for evaluating para-aortic nodal metastasis in locally advanced cervical cancer before surgical staging: a surgicopathologic study. *J Clin Oncol* **17**: 41–5.

Schmidt D, Gottwald U, Langen KJ *et al.* (2001). 3-[^{123}I]Iodo-alpha-methyl-L-tyrosine uptake in cerebral gliomas: relationship to histological grading and prognosis. *Eur J Nucl Med* **28**: 855–61.

Schwartz DL, Ford EC, Rajendran J *et al.* (2005). FDG-PET/CT-guided intensity modulated head and neck radiotherapy: a pilot investigation. *Head Neck* **27**: 478–87.

Shah JP (1990). Patterns of cervical lymph node metastasis from squamous carcinomas of the upper aerodigestive tract. *Am J Surg* **160**: 405–9.

Stuckensen T, Kovacs AF, Adams S, Baum RP (2000). Staging of the neck in patients with oral cavity squamous cell carcinomas: a prospective comparison of PET, ultrasound, CT and MRI. *J Craniomaxillofac Surg* **28**: 319–24.

Sugawara Y, Eisbruch A, Kosuda S, Recker BE, Kison PV, Wahl RL (1999). Evaluation of FDG PET in patients with cervical cancer. *J Nucl Med* **40**: 1125–31.

Sweeney RA, Bale RJ, Moncayo R *et al.* (2003). Multimodality cranial image fusion using external markers applied via a vacuum mouthpiece and a case report. *Strahlenther Onkol* **179**: 254–60.

Tarantola G, Zito F, Gerundini P (2003). PET instrumentation and reconstruction algorithms in whole-body applications. *J Nucl Med* **44**: 756–69.

Vanderstraeten B, Duthoy W, De Gersem W, De Neve W, Thierens H (2006). [^{18}F]fluoro-deoxy-glucose positron emission tomography ([^{18}F]FDG-PET) voxel intensity-based intensity-modulated radiation therapy (IMRT) for head and neck cancer. *Radiother Oncol* **79**: 249–58.

van der Wel A, Nijsten S, Hochstenbag M *et al.* (2005). Increased therapeutic ratio by ^{18}FDG-PET CT planning in patients with clinical CT stage N2-N3M0 non-small-cell lung cancer: a modeling study. *Int J Radiat Oncol Biol Phys* **61**: 649–55.

van Westreenen HL, Westerterp M, Bossuyt PM *et al.* (2004). Systematic review of the staging performance of ^{18}F-fluorodeoxyglucose positron emission tomography in esophageal cancer. *J Clin Oncol* **22**: 3805–12.

Vrieze O, Haustermans K, De Wever W *et al.* (2004). Is there a role for FGD-PET in radiotherapy planning in esophageal carcinoma? *Radiother Oncol* **73**: 269–75.

Weber WA, Wester HJ, Grosu AL *et al.* (2000). *O*-(2-[^{18}F]fluoroethyl)-L-tyrosine and L-[methyl-^{11}C]methionine uptake in brain tumours: initial results of a comparative study. *Eur J Nucl Med* **27**: 542–9.

Yaremko B, Riauka T, Robinson D, Murray B, McEwan A, Roa W (2005). Threshold modification for tumour imaging in non-small-cell lung cancer using positron emission tomography. *Nucl Med Commun* **26**: 433–40.

■ FURTHER READING

Apisarnthanarax S, Chao KS (2005). Current imaging paradigms in radiation oncology. *Radiat Res* **163**: 1–25.

Bradbury M, Hricak H (2005). Molecular MR imaging in oncology. *Magn Reson Imaging Clin N Am* **13**: 225–40.

Chapman JD, Schneider RF, Urbain JL, Hanks GE (2001). Single-photon emission computed tomography and positron-emission tomography assays for tissue oxygenation. *Semin Radiat Oncol* **11**: 47–57.

Rohren EM, Turkington TG, Coleman RE (2004). Clinical applications of PET in oncology. *Radiology* **231**: 305–32.

van de Wiele C, Lahorte C, Oyen W *et al.* (2003). Nuclear medicine imaging to predict response to radiotherapy: a review. *Int J Radiat Oncol Biol Phys* **55**: 5–15.

Molecular-targeted agents for enhancing tumour response

MICHAEL BAUMANN AND VINCENT GRÉGOIRE

21.1 INTRODUCTION

Combined radiochemotherapy is now firmly established in clinical practice for a wide spectrum of tumours. Randomized trials have shown that, in many cases, this strategy may lead to better local control and survival than radiotherapy alone. The radiobiological basis for radiochemotherapy and its current results are reviewed in Chapter 18. In this present chapter we emphasize that, despite their proven benefit, currently available chemotherapeutic drugs are far from being perfect for combining with radiotherapy (Krause *et al.*, 2006). Tumour cell kill by chemotherapy at clinically achievable doses is minor compared with that caused by radiation. Only in a relatively small proportion of patients is chemotherapy sufficiently effective to destroy subclinical metastatic deposits. Normal tissue toxicity is frequently increased after combined radiochemotherapy, which may limit doses of drugs or radiation. For these reasons it is obvious that more effective and less toxic substances are needed to further improve the results of systemic therapies combined with radiation.

Substantial research is ongoing in the design of so-called targeted anti-cancer drugs. These drugs, also called molecular-targeted drugs, more or less specifically interfere with those molecular pathways which keep cells alive, and which allow cells to communicate with their environment and with other cells, or which govern the response of cells against stressors, including radiation. Important examples of such molecular processes are outlined in Chapter 23. Recent advances in the field of biotechnology and cell biology have made it possible to unravel the details of this molecular signalling, and new pathways of molecular crosstalk are being detected at a rapid pace. As many of these pathways may be specifically inhibited or modified, the number of novel biology-driven drugs whose potential for radiotherapy warrants evaluation is increasing rapidly.

Rationale for combining molecular-targeted drugs with radiotherapy

Several reasons make the combination of molecular-targeted agents with irradiation a promising

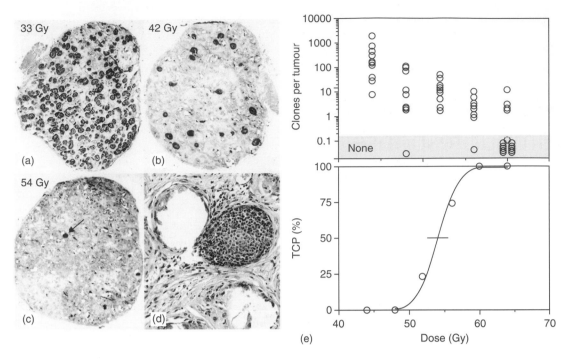

Figure 21.1 Pattern of clonal regeneration of stem cells in the AT17 mouse mammary carcinoma after irradiation with single doses of (a) 33 Gy, (b) 42 Gy and (c) 54 Gy under clamp hypoxic conditions. With increasing irradiation dose, the number of colonies per section decreases, after 54 Gy only one surviving colony was found (arrow, close-up shown in d). (e, upper) The number of surviving stem cells for individual AT17 tumours measured at day 19 after single dose irradiation under clamp hypoxia; (e, lower) local tumour control (symbols) at 18-month follow-up and the calculated tumour control probabilities (TCP, line) for AT17 tumours irradiated with the same single doses under clamp hypoxia. The increase in local tumour control corresponds closely to the proportion of tumours without surviving stem cells. From Krause *et al.* (2006), with permission.

avenue for preclinical and clinical cancer research (Krause *et al.*, 2006):

- The radiobiological basis of the response of tumours and normal tissues has been extensively studied and can in many cases be described not only qualitatively but also quantitatively (see Chapter 5).
- The molecular mechanisms underlying the radiobiology are being increasingly well understood and may be specifically targeted (see Chapters 2, 3 and 23).
- Molecular targets are often differentially expressed in tumours and normal tissues, offering a possible therapeutic gain (see Chapter 22).
- Molecular-targeted agents are in themselves not curative in solid tumours, whereas radiotherapy

is highly efficient in eradicating cancer stem cells. As discussed in Chapter 5, it can be estimated from Poisson statistics that on average only 0.1–2.3 cancer stem cells per tumour survive at local tumour control probabilities between 10 per cent and 90 per cent (i.e. in the 'curative' dose range). This means that recurrences after high-dose radiotherapy may be caused by only one or few cancer stem cells. This is illustrated in Fig. 21.1, where histological sections of irradiated AT17 mouse mammary carcinomas are compared with the dose–response curve for local control in the same tumour model. A unique feature of the AT17 tumour is that regrowth of surviving cancer stem cells after irradiation can be directly visualized and measured as colony formation *in vivo* (Kummermehr and Trott, 1997; Krause *et al.*, 2006). Figure 21.1a–c shows that, with increasing dose, the number of colonies per section decreases, and that after 54 Gy a single surviving colony was found (close up shown in Fig. 21.1d). Figure 21.1e shows the number of surviving clonogenic cells per tumour for groups of tumours treated with increasing doses. The number of colonies per tumour decreases and the proportion of tumours without any surviving cancer stem cell increases with increasing radiation dose. The histological data correspond well with the observed rate of permanent local tumour control after irradiation in the same tumour model. Those tumours that are not completely sterilized after irradiation with doses in the curative range (in this experiment >50 Gy) typically contain only one to a maximum of 100 surviving cancer stem cells. Thus, even if a novel molecular-targeted agent has the potential to kill only a few cancer stem cells, or if it interferes in mechanisms of radioresistance of tumours, its combination with radiotherapy may still lead to an improvement in local tumour control.

Research strategies to evaluate targeted drugs for radiotherapy

The large number of potential cellular target molecules and the rapid emergence of new drugs to interact with these targets requires a rational, radiobiology-driven approach for target selection. Attractive targets for drugs to be used specifically within the context of radiotherapy would be (over)expressed in a high proportion of tumours frequently treated by radiation, would not be expressed by normal tissues surrounding the tumour, would be linked to poor loco-regional tumour control after radiotherapy alone and would ideally be associated with known radiobiological mechanisms of tumour radioresistance (Krause *et al.*, 2006). Identification of such targets requires specific research on preclinical model tumours and on tumour material of patients treated by radiotherapy. The biological data obtained from the tumours should be compared with high-quality clinical outcome data which incorporate comprehensive information on dose, fractionation and known prognostic factors. Appropriate multivariate methods should be applied, not only in determining prognostic factors but also in assessing the results of biomarker studies. A good example of rational target identification in the context of radiotherapy is the epidermal growth factor receptor (EGFR), which will be discussed below.

In developing new molecular-targeted agents for use with radiation, the initial evaluation is typically performed on cells in culture. Endpoints include inhibition of cell proliferation, and colony formation after irradiation with and without drug. However, it should be kept in mind that effects *in vitro* do not necessarily translate into the same effect *in vivo*. Typical problems are that higher drug concentrations can be achieved *in vitro* than *in vivo*, that the expression of target molecules may be different *in vitro* and *in vivo*, that cell culture conditions may significantly influence cell survival, and that many microenvironmental factors that are present in tumours (e.g. hypoxia, low pH, cell–cell interactions) are usually not reflected in cell culture (reviewed in Krause *et al.*, 2006). However, because of the high number of potential targets, there is currently no practical alternative to initially screening molecular-targeted drugs combined with radiation using *in vitro* models. Experiments on cells in culture are also very important for unravelling the mechanisms of action of effects observed in animals or in clinical studies.

The final step in the preclinical investigation of new targeted drugs for radiotherapy should include experiments on tumour models *in vivo*. The design and experimental endpoints of such studies are discussed in Chapter 7. For the discussion here, it is important to discriminate volume-dependent endpoints such as tumour regression or tumour growth delay from local tumour control. Those cells which may form a recurrence after therapy (i.e. cancer stem cells) constitute only a small proportion of all cancer cells, whereas the bulk of tumour cells are non-tumourigenic (Hill and Milas, 1989; Clarke *et al.*, 2006). Thus, changes in tumour volume after therapy are governed by the changes in the mass of tumour cells, that is, primarily by the non-stem cells. In contrast, local tumour control is dependent on the

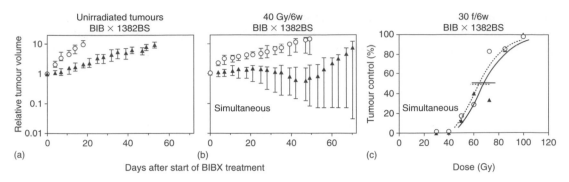

Figure 21.2 Effect of epithelial growth factor receptor (EGFR) tyrosine kinase inhibitors (TKIs) on the tumour volume of unirradiated (a) and irradiated (b) FaDu HNSCC xenografts (40 Gy, 30 fractions, 6 weeks) and on local tumour control after 30 fractions within 6 weeks (c). Open symbols, control tumours; closed symbols, tumours treated with the TKI simultaneously with irradiation. Error bars show 95% CI. Adapted from Baumann and Krause (2004), with permission.

complete inactivation of the subpopulation of cancer stem cells (Baumann *et al.*, 2008). The majority of current preclinical studies in cancer research use volume-dependent endpoints. This carries a substantial risk that new treatments may be optimized for their effect on the bulk of non-stem cancer cells, with no improvement in the curative potential. That there exist such different effects of molecular-targeted agents when combined with radiation on non-stem cells and cancer stem cells is supported by several recent studies that have shown a dissociation of tumour volume-dependent endpoints and tumour control (reviewed in Krause *et al.*, 2006; Baumann *et al.*, 2008). An example is shown in Fig. 21.2, in which inhibition of the epithelial growth factor receptor (EGFR) led to pronounced regression and growth delay of the tumour without improving local tumour control. Overall, these experiments support the principle that radiotherapy-specific preclinical research strategies need to be applied to test the efficacy of molecular-targeted drugs combined with radiation, and that cancer stem cell-specific endpoints such as local tumour control should be used whenever possible (see Chapter 7).

Some specific aspects need also to be mentioned with regard to testing molecular-targeted drugs for radiotherapy in clinical trials (Baumann, 2006). First, preclinical data should be available from combining the drug with radiation, and there should be a valid radiobiological rationale to combine exactly the selected drug in the selected tumour entity. As outlined above, preclinical data

on tumour volume-dependent endpoints might not be sufficient, as these do not always reflect survival of cancer stem cells which determine the outcome of curative radiotherapy. Furthermore, biomarkers which are established for use of the drug alone or combined with chemotherapy do not necessarily also work for the combination with radiation. Therefore, extensive biological co-investigations should be part of all clinical trials on combined modality treatments to establish radiotherapy-specific prognostic and predictive tests (see below). Lastly, the effects of molecular-targeted drugs on cancer stem cells are weak compared with the effects of radiation where clear and often very steep dose–response relationships exist for tumours as well as for normal tissues. If the (biologically effective) radiation dose and the dose distribution is not standardized and of high quality, an effect of a new drug may be easily missed or normal tissue reactions might be increased.

Unfortunately this preclinical and clinical research strategy has so far not been fully established in research laboratories and industry, leading to inadequate access to new drugs with specific activity when combined with radiotherapy (Baumann, 2006). Today's laboratory mass screening of candidate anti-cancer drugs is usually done in the absence of radiotherapy. Thus, candidate compounds that are not effective alone, but could be promising for radiosensitizing tumour cells, will not be selected. Furthermore, preclinical studies usually apply new compounds as monotherapy or in combination with chemotherapeutic agents, but not combined with radiotherapy. New drugs that are eventually included in clinical trials are usually tested in combination with radiotherapy only after they have shown promise alone or in combination with chemotherapy. Again, this selection could miss important opportunities (Baumann, 2006).

Targeted drugs and distant metastases

A 'perfect' targeted drug for radiotherapy may have no impact on the survival of cancer cells when given without irradiation, but effectively decreases mechanisms of radiation resistance, thereby improving local tumour control. However, subclinical distant metastases might be already present outside the irradiated volume. The drug, because of its ineffectiveness without irradiation, will not eradicate these subclinical metastases, and the patient may succumb from distant metastases despite the fact that the primary tumour is controlled. This is a fundamental difference between a (pure) targeted radiation modifier and chemotherapeutic drugs that may kill tumour cells by themselves and, thus, when combined with radiotherapy, may help to eradicate both the primary tumour and distant metastases. Therefore, most researchers aim to develop targeted drugs that also have efficacy against cancer cells by themselves and which can eradicate subclinical metastases. Alternatively, pure radiation modifiers may be combined with radiation plus chemotherapy. In such trimodality treatments, systemic chemotherapy (potentially enhanced by the targeted drug) would be directed against the metastatic deposits, whereas radiotherapy, enhanced in its effect by the targeted drug and possibly by the chemotherapeutic agent, would eradicate the primary tumour. It should be noted that such novel strategies would not necessarily have to utilize concurrent radiochemotherapy which for most cancers is today's standard of care.

21.2 EGFR INHIBITORS

Preclinical data in model tumours

In murine tumour models, a significant correlation between EGFR expression and radiation dose needed to achieve 50 per cent local tumour control (TCD_{50}) after single-dose exposure was demonstrated (Akimoto et al., 1999). These results may be explained by a higher number, an increased cellular radioresistance or greater hypoxia of cancer stem cells in EGFR-overexpressing tumours. A correlation has also been observed between accelerated repopulation of cancer stem cells and the expression kinetics of EGFR in one of several human squamous cell carcinoma models, suggesting that the EGFR might also be involved in specific radiobiological mechanisms of resistance in fractionated radiotherapy (Petersen et al., 2003; Eicheler et al., 2005; Baumann et al., 2007). It is important to note that not only EGFR expression but also the ligand-independent activation of the receptor by radiation may be involved in radioresistance (Schmidt-Ullrich et al., 1999).

A promising approach therefore is to combine radiotherapy with drugs that target the EGFR. Such drugs can be either monoclonal antibodies against the EGFR or small molecules that specifically inhibit phosphorylation of the EGFR (tyrosine kinase inhibitors, TKIs). Figure 21.3 shows the downstream molecular pathways that may be altered by these two approaches. For a large number of tumour cell lines in vitro it has been demonstrated that EGFR inhibition with or without irradiation results in reduced cell proliferation. For some but not all of these cell lines, a radiosensitizing effect could also be shown, which, at least in part, seems to be related to inhibition of repair of DNA damage (reviewed in Baumann et al., 2007). Also, for many tumour models in vivo, prolonged growth delay was demonstrated for different EGFR inhibitors combined with radiotherapy (reviewed in Baumann and Krause, 2004). Experiments demonstrated improved local tumour control when the monoclonal anti-EGFR antibody C225 was given with single dose or fractionated irradiation (Nasu et al., 2001; Krause et al., 2005b; Milas et al., 2007).

Several radiobiological mechanisms may explain the observed effects: direct inactivation of cancer stem cells by the drug, cellular radiosensitization, reduced repopulation and improved reoxygenation are all possible (Krause et al., 2005a; Baumann et al., 2007). It is interesting to note that, to date, improved local tumour control

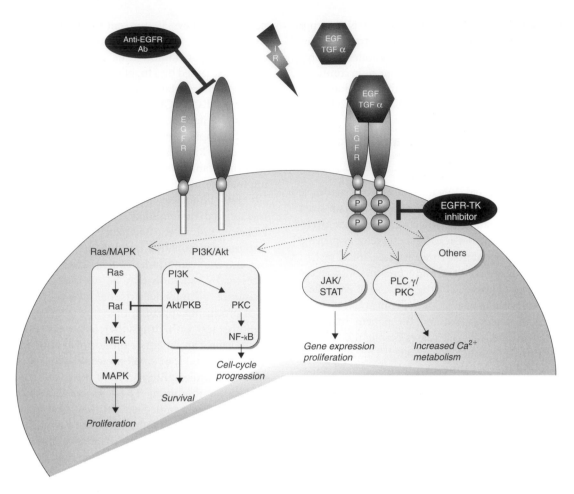

Figure 21.3 Schematic illustration of epithelial growth factor receptor (EGFR)-mediated signal transduction. Activation of the EGFR by its ligands or by irradiation results in a homodimerization of two EGFRs or a heterodimerization with another member of the EGFR family, followed by internalization and autophosphorylation of the intracellular tyrosine kinase (TK) domain. Different cascades can be activated, leading to proliferation, enhanced cell survival and cell-cycle progression. The EGFR can be inhibited by monoclonal antibodies (mAbs), which block extracellular dimerization and lead to internalization of the EGFR–mAb complex, degradation and down-modulation of the EGFR. The TK inhibitors pass the cellular membrane and block phosphorylation of the tyrosine kinase. From Baumann and Krause (2004), with permission.

in preclinical studies has been shown only for anti-EGFR antibodies but not for EGFR TKIs, even when tested in exactly the same tumour models. This suggests that immune-response reactions might be important. It also should be noted that there is considerable heterogeneity in the efficacy of EGFR inhibitors between different tumour models and between different drugs, thus calling for better understanding of the mechanisms

of action and for predictive tests within the context of radiotherapy.

Clinical data

HEAD AND NECK CANCER

The greatest clinical experience so far has been reported for head and neck cancer. The EGFR is

Table 21.1 Comparison between radiotherapy alone and radiotherapy plus cetuximab in patients with locally advanced head and neck squamous cell carcinoma

	Radiotherapy alone (%) ($n = 213$)	Radiotherapy + cetuximab (%) ($n = 211$)	p
Anti-tumour efficacy			
3-year loco-regional control	34	47	<0.01
3-year progression-free survival	31	42	0.04
3-year overall survival	45	55	0.05
Adverse effects (grades 3–5)			
Mucositis	52	56	0.44
Dysphagia	30	26	0.45
Radiation dermatitis	18	23	0.27
Acneiform rash	1	17	<0.001

Data from Bonner et al. (2006).

highly expressed in head and neck squamous cell carcinoma and, in a retrospective Radiation Therapy Oncology Group (RTOG) study on patients with locally advanced tumours treated by radiotherapy alone, EGFR expression has been shown to be an independent prognostic factor for both overall survival and disease-free survival (Ang et al., 2002); patients whose tumours overexpressed the EGFR did significantly worse than patients who did not. These clinical observations on the negative impact of EGFR expression on the outcome of radiotherapy support the concept that EGFR inhibition might counteract mechanisms of intrinsic radioresistance. It was also shown in retrospective analyses from the DAHANCA (Danish Head and Neck Cancer) and the CHART (continuous *h*yperfractionated *a*ccelerated *r*adio*t*herapy) trials that only patients with high EGFR expression benefited from accelerated radiotherapy (Bentzen et al., 2005; Eriksen et al., 2005). In line with preclinical results discussed above, these data suggest that the EGFR may be involved in accelerated repopulation of cancer stem cells.

Cetuximab (C225 or Erbitux) is, at the time of writing, the leading monoclonal antibody against EGFR that has been tested clinically. A phase I study in patients with advanced head and neck squamous cell carcinoma has evaluated the safety profile of this antibody in association with radiotherapy alone, and has recommended the use of a loading dose of 400–500 mg/m^2 followed by weekly injection at a dose of 250 mg/m^2 (Robert et al., 2001). Based on these data, a randomized phase III trial comparing radiotherapy alone with the same radiotherapy with a loading dose (400 mg/m^2) followed by weekly doses (250 mg/m^2) of C225 was undertaken in patients with stage III or IV squamous cell carcinoma (SCC) of the oropharynx, hypopharynx and larynx (Bonner et al., 2006). Patients were stratified according to the radiotherapy regimen (70 Gy in 35 fractions in 7 weeks or 72.0–76.8 Gy in 60–64 fractions in 7 weeks, or 72.0 Gy in 42 fractions over 6 weeks), the performance status, the nodal involvement (N0 versus N+) and the T-stage (T1–T3 versus T4). A total of 424 patients were randomized. With a median follow-up of 54 months, patients treated with the combined treatment did significantly better than patients treated by radiotherapy alone in term of loco-regional control, progression-free survival and overall survival (Table 21.1). The rate of distant metastasis was not different between the two arms and, although some differences were observed when subgroup analysis was performed, the study was not powered to detect any significant difference between them. An interesting observation of this trial was that, with the exception of acneiform rash, no difference was observed between the two groups regarding toxicity and, in particular, radiation-induced acute side-effects (Table 21.1). Also, for palliative treatment of head and neck squamous cell carcinoma (HNSCC), addition of cetuximab to cisplatin has been shown, in a phase III trial, to be superior to cisplatin alone (Burtness *et al.*, 2005).

Other monoclonal antibodies directed against the EGFR have been developed and are being tested in various clinical phases. H-R3 is a humanized antibody that has been tested in a phase I trial in combination with radiotherapy in patients with locally advanced disease (Crombet *et al.*, 2004). A phase II trial is ongoing in HNSCC. The safety profile of Zalutumumab (HuMax-EGFr), a fully humanized monoclonal antibody, has been evaluated in patients with metastatic or recurrent HNSCC (Bastholt *et al.*, 2005). This antibody is undergoing testing in concomitant association with radiotherapy for locally advanced HNSCC. Panitumumab (ABX-EGF) and matuzumab (EMD 72000) are also fully humanized antibodies against EGFR (Foon *et al.*, 2004; Kim, 2004) and have been tested in various human tumours, but no study so far has been reported on combination with radiation.

For EGFR TKIs, so far, no phase III trial has been reported in HNSCC. A phase II trial on ZD1839 (gefitinib, Iressa) in patients with metastatic or recurrent HNSCC reported a response rate of 11 per cent and a disease control rate of 53 per cent for daily doses of 500 mg (Cohen *et al.*, 2003). For daily doses of 250 mg, the response rate was much lower (Cohen *et al.*, 2005). Interestingly, in both studies, a correlation was reported between the incidence of skin rash and the tumour response. No study has yet been reported on Iressa combined with radiotherapy or radiochemotherapy. A randomized phase II trial is currently ongoing in previously untreated patients with locally advanced HNSCC treated with concomitant radiochemotherapy. In a phase II trial, a modest response rate of 4 per cent was also reported with erlotinib (Tarceva) used in monotherapy in heavily pretreated patients with recurrent or metastatic disease (Soulieres *et al.*, 2004). No data on concomitant use of Tarceva with radiotherapy has been reported.

OTHER TUMOUR SITES

At the time of writing, no phase III trials have been reported on the combination of radiotherapy with anti-EGFR antibodies in sites other than HNSCC. Cetuximab and panitumumab have been shown in phase III trials to be effective in palliative treatment of chemotherapy-refractory colorectal cancer. It is interesting to note that cetuximab, when given simultaneously with neoadjuvant radiochemotherapy in patients with rectal carcinoma, showed inferior complete pathological response rates compared with historical data on radiochemotherapy alone in two different phase II studies (Machiels *et al.*, 2007; Rodel *et al.*, 2008).

With EGFR TKIs, one phase III trial has been reported on the combination with radiotherapy in patients with non-small cell lung cancer (NSCLC). Administration of gefitinib after the end of radiochemotherapy was compared with radiochemotherapy alone; the trial was stopped early because survival was significantly better after radiochemotherapy alone (Kelly *et al.*, 2007). Without radiotherapy, EGFR TKIs have been tested in several phase III trials in NSCLC and in one trial on pancreatic cancer (reviewed in Krause and Baumann, 2008). In NSCLC the results were only positive when the TKIs were given alone, whereas no improvement in tumour response or survival were observed when the TKIs were combined with chemotherapy. This contrasts with pancreatic cancer, in which addition of erlotinib to gemcitabine improved survival.

Overall, the data reported so far indicate that addition of targeted drugs to established anti-cancer treatments will not always improve the results, even if the drug when given alone is effective. This calls for careful preclinical and clinical research into exactly the setting intended for use before introduction of novel drugs into multi-modality treatments.

21.3 ANTI-ANGIOGENIC DRUGS

Very early tumour foci can be fed by diffusion alone; however, at a diameter larger than 1–2 mm, tumours need perfused blood vessels for further growth. For this neo-angiogenesis, the vascular endothelial growth factor (VEGF) plays an important role. A potential advantage of targeting VEGF signalling is that there is almost no physiological neo-angiogenesis in adults, thus making this target tumour-specific. The VEGF receptor (VEGFR) is expressed preferentially on endothelial cells and its activation is known to induce endothelial cell proliferation, migration and survival. High levels of VEGF are associated with poor prognoses in patients. In preclinical experiments, VEGFR inhibitors have been shown to radiosensitize endothelial cells and to inhibit the proliferation and survival of endothelial cells and, secondarily, of tumour cells. Application of an anti-VEGFR antibody in combination with short-term fractionated irradiation led to improved local control in two different tumour models *in vivo* (Kozin *et al.*, 2001). With a VEGFR thymidine kinase inhibitor, prolonged tumour growth delay could be shown after combination with fractionated irradiation in different tumour models; however, this effect did not translate into improved local tumour control (Zips *et al.*, 2003, 2005). Interpreting these data, potential radiobiological effects on tumour hypoxia need to be considered. In theory, anti-angiogenic drugs could increase hypoxia by reduction of the vessel density. However, improvement of tumour cell oxygenation by reduction of the interstitial fluid pressure and oxygen consumption and by normalization of the chaotic tumour vasculature is also possible (Jain, 2005). Preclinical data on the impact of transient normalization of the tumour vasculature for tumour response after irradiation are contradictory.

Anti-angiogenic substances are also being tested clinically in combination with radiotherapy. A randomized trial has been performed in stage III NSCLC in which induction chemotherapy was followed by concomitant radiochemotherapy. The patients were randomized to receive AE-941 (Neovastat), a shark cartilage extract with anti-angiogenic properties, or placebo at the start of induction chemotherapy and continuing after radiochemotherapy as maintenance therapy. This trial was closed early because of insufficient accrual after 384 patients and showed no effect on overall survival (Lu *et al.*, 2007). Early clinical experience is also available for the monoclonal anti-VEGF antibody bevacizumab (Avastin) in rectal cancer. A proof of concept study was performed with bevacizumab and radiotherapy in six patients with locally advanced adenocarcinoma of the rectum (Willett *et al.*, 2004). Patients received

bevacizumab 2 weeks before neoadjuvant fluorouracil (5FU)-based radiochemotherapy. Twelve days after the first infusion of bevacizumab, overall improvement in the efficiency of blood vessels was observed, as measured by various endpoints such as blood flow, blood volume, microvascular density and fluorodeoxyglucose (FDG) uptake, and this supports the concept of transient normalization of tumour perfusion with anti-angiogenic drugs, allowing a more effective delivery of oxygen and chemotherapeutic agents (Jain, 2005). Early tumour response rates after bevacizumab combined with radiochemotherapy are encouraging in phase I clinical trials. However, some in-field intestinal toxicity has occurred, underlining the need for further investigations to clarify the therapeutic potential of bevacizumab to improve the results of radiochemotherapy in gastrointestinal cancer (Willett *et al.*, 2005; Crane *et al.*, 2006).

21.4 INHIBITORS OF THE PHOSPHOINOSITIDE-3-KINASE (PI3K)/PROTEIN KINASE B (AKT) PATHWAY

Signal transduction of PI3K/AKT is an important downstream pathway of the receptor tyrosine kinases. Its activation results in increased cell survival and contributes to radioresistance. The mammalian target of rapamycin (mTOR) is a key signal transduction molecule of the PI3K/AKT pathway and constitutive mTOR activation contributes to radioresistance. However, using clonogenic endpoints *in vitro*, mTOR inhibition by rapamycin could not be shown to radiosensitize U87 glioma cells. When given combined with irradiation ($4 \times 4\,Gy$ over 18 days) in the same tumour model, tumour growth delay was significantly prolonged compared with irradiation alone (Eshleman *et al.*, 2002) and a significant effect on growth delay of U87 tumours could be shown in another *in vivo* experiment in the same tumour model. However, using a fractionated irradiation schedule with daily irradiation over 5 days and daily application of rapamycin, neither tumour growth delay nor local tumour control (TCD_{50}) were influenced by addition of the drug (Weppler *et al.*, 2007). At the time of writing, rapamycin derivatives are in clinical phase I–III trials in combination with radiotherapy in different tumour entities.

21.5 INHIBITORS OF THE RAS PATHWAY

Ras is a downstream molecule of several growth factor receptors, among others the EGFR. Its signal transduction leads to proliferation of tumour cells. Many human tumours overexpress activated H- or K-Ras isoforms, which may increase tumour radioresistance by promoting aberrant survival signals. Inhibition of the enzyme farnesyl transferase prevents Ras activation (reviewed in Chinnaiyan *et al.*, 2006). Farnesyl transferase inhibitors (FTIs) have been shown to radiosensitize tumour cells *in vitro* and to reduce tumour growth when combined with single-dose irradiation *in vivo*. Using an *ex-vivo* clonogenic assay, reduced survival of clonogenic tumour cells has been demonstrated after single-dose irradiation combined with a FTI in two different tumour models. This effect was considerably higher in *H-RAS* mutated than *H-RAS* wildtype tumour cells (Cohen-Jonathan *et al.*, 2000; Delmas *et al.*, 2002). Studies with tumour-control endpoints have not yet been performed. In clinical phase I trials, FTI combined with radiotherapy in NSCLC, HNSCC and pancreatic cancer has shown acceptable toxicity (Hahn *et al.*, 2002; Martin *et al.*, 2004).

21.6 HISTONE DEACETYLASE INHIBITORS

The main mechanisms underlying the effects of histone deacetylase (HDAC) inhibitors are physical modifications of the chromatin structure and hyper-acetylation of histone proteins, which leads to relaxation of the chromatin and possibly to radiosensitization of tumour cells. Indeed, HDAC inhibitors such as valproic acid have been shown in preclinical experiments to radiosensitize tumour cells *in vitro* and to inhibit tumour growth when combined with single-dose irradiation *in vivo* (reviewed in Chinnaiyan *et al.*, 2006). At the time of writing there are no data from studies using local tumour control endpoints. Valproic acid is currently being tested in combination with radiochemotherapy in phase II clinical trials in glioblastoma.

21.7 CYCLOOXYGENASE-2 INHIBITORS

Cyclooxygenase-2 (COX-2), an enzyme involved in prostaglandin synthesis, is overexpressed in a variety of human cancers and has been associated with poor prognosis after radiotherapy. Selective COX-2 inhibitors have been shown to increase the radiosensitivity of human glioma and lung cancer cells *in vitro*. In human tumour xenografts, COX-2 inhibitors have prolonged tumour growth delay and improved local tumour control after irradiation (Liao *et al.*, 2007). Early clinical trials combining COX-2 inhibitors with radiotherapy have not shown unexpected toxicity (Ganswindt *et al.*, 2006). However, because of cardiovascular problems observed in patients receiving long-term treatment with COX-2 inhibitors for inflammation and pain, several clinical trials were terminated and not reported. However, in light of the promising preclinical data, short-term use of COX-2 inhibitors combined with radiotherapy still appears to be a highly attractive avenue for further research.

21.8 OTHER TARGETED DRUGS

The combination of radiation with a variety of other targeted drugs, including tumour necrosis factor-related apoptosis-inducing ligand (TRAIL), DNA repair inhibitors, broad-spectrum tyrosine kinase inhibitors and inhibitors of cell adhesion molecules, have shown promising effects when combined with radiation *in vitro* or *in vivo*. Clinical data are not yet available.

21.9 CONCLUSIONS

Tumour response and duration of patient survival after treatment with molecular-targeted agents in combination with radiotherapy varies considerably between different classes of drugs, different substances within one class of drugs and different combination schedules, but also between individual patients. To date, this heterogeneity has been best studied for the combination of radiotherapy with EGFR inhibitors. To rationally prescribe the many emerging molecular-targeted drugs within the context of radiotherapy, development and introduction of biomarkers is of high importance. Owing to specific interactions of molecular-targeted drugs with the biological effects of irradiation, biomarkers are expected to differ for radiation oncology compared with application of the drugs alone or within chemotherapy treatment schedules and therefore need to be established and tested separately. An example of this principle are the activating *K-RAS* mutations that have been shown to be negatively correlated with the effect of EGFR TKIs given alone or combined with chemotherapy in NSCLC, whereas preclinical data show radiosensitizing effects for EGFR TKIs. There are still more open than answered questions in the field of biomarkers for combined radiotherapy and molecular-targeted agents (Krause and Baumann, 2008). Further research into the mechanisms of action of these novel combined approaches will eventually contribute to the development of valid biomarkers, enabling clinicians to take full advantage of the potential of molecular-targeted drugs for improving radiotherapy.

Key points

1. Molecular-targeted drugs specifically modify intracellular or intercellular signal transduction and may thereby radiosensitize tumours.
2. Molecular targets are often differentially expressed in tumours and normal tissues, offering the possibility of a therapeutic gain.
3. Radiotherapy offers a particularly promising scenario for utilizing targeted anti-cancer agents. These drugs by themselves kill only a few cancer stem cells and are not curative in solid tumours, whereas radiotherapy is highly efficient in eradicating cancer stem cells. When combined with radiation, the additional cell kill by the drug may enhance the curative potential of radiotherapy.
4. Identification and testing of molecular-targeted drugs for radiotherapy requires a radiotherapy-specific research strategy. The addition of targeted drugs to radiation may promote tumour regression and prolong tumour growth delay without improving local tumour control. As tumour control reflects the survival of cancer stem cells, this endpoint should be used whenever possible.
5. Considerable inter-tumoural and inter-substance heterogeneity exists for the efficacy of targeting the same pathway. This calls for better understanding of the mechanisms of action of molecular-targeted drugs in combination with radiation, and for the development of predictive assays.

■ BIBLIOGRAPHY

Akimoto T, Hunter NR, Buchmiller L, Mason K, Ang KK, Milas L (1999). Inverse relationship between epidermal growth factor receptor expression and radiocurability of murine carcinomas. *Clin Cancer Res* **5**: 2884–90.

Ang K, Berkey BA, Tu X *et al.* (2002). Impact of epidermal growth factor receptor expression on survival and pattern of relapse in patients with advanced head and neck carcinoma. *Cancer Res* **62**: 7350–6.

Bastholt L, Specht L, Jensen K *et al.* (2005). A novel fully human monoclonal antibody against epidermal growth factor receptor (EGFR). First clinical and FDG-PET imaging results from a phase I/II trial conducted by the Danish Head and Neck Cancer Study Group (DAHANCA) in patients with squamous cell carcinoma of the head and neck (SCCHN). *J Clin Oncol* **23**: 507S.

Baumann M (2006). Keynote comment: Radiotherapy in the age of molecular oncology. *Lancet Oncol* **7**: 786–7.

Baumann M, Krause M (2004). Targeting the epidermal growth factor receptor in radiotherapy: radiobiological mechanisms, preclinical and clinical results. *Radiother Oncol* **72**: 257–66.

Baumann M, Krause M, Dikomey E *et al.* (2007). EGFR-targeted anti-cancer drugs in radiotherapy: preclinical evaluation of mechanisms. *Radiother Oncol* **83**: 238–48.

Baumann M, Krause M, Hill R (2008). Exploring the role of cancer stem cells in radioresistance. *Nat Rev Cancer* **8**: 545–54.

Bentzen SM, Atasoy BM, Daley FM *et al.* (2005). Epidermal growth factor receptor expression in pretreatment biopsies from head and neck squamous cell carcinoma as a predictive factor for a benefit from accelerated radiation therapy in a randomized controlled trial. *J Clin Oncol* **23**: 5560–7.

Bonner JA, Harari PM, Giralt J *et al.* (2006). Radiotherapy plus cetuximab for squamous-cell carcinoma of the head and neck. *N Engl J Med* **354**: 567–78.

Burtness B, Goldwasser MA, Flood W, Mattar B, Forastiere AA (2005). Phase III randomized trial of cisplatin plus placebo compared with cisplatin plus cetuximab in metastatic/recurrent head and neck cancer: an Eastern Cooperative Oncology Group study. *J Clin Oncol* **23**: 8646–54.

Chinnaiyan P, Allen GW, Harari PM (2006). Radiation and new molecular agents, part II: targeting HDAC, HSP90, IGF-1R, PI3K, and Ras. *Semin Radiat Oncol* **16**: 59–64.

Clarke MF, Dick JE, Dirks PB *et al.* (2006). Cancer stem cells – perspectives on current status and future directions: AACR Workshop on Cancer Stem Cells. *Cancer Res* **66**: 9339–44.

Cohen EE, Rosen F, Stadler WM *et al.* (2003). Phase II trial of ZD1839 in recurrent or metastatic squamous cell carcinoma of the head and neck. *J Clin Oncol* **21**: 1980–7.

Cohen EE, Kane MA, List MA *et al.* (2005). Phase II trial of gefitinib 250 mg daily in patients with recurrent and/or metastatic squamous cell carcinoma of the head and neck. *Clin Cancer Res* **11**: 8418–24.

Cohen-Jonathan E, Muschel RJ, Gillies McKenna W *et al.* (2000). Farnesyltransferase inhibitors potentiate the antitumor effect of radiation on a human tumor xenograft expressing activated HRAS. *Radiat Res* **154**: 125–32.

Crane CH, Ellis LM, Abbruzzese JL *et al.* (2006). Phase I trial evaluating the safety of bevacizumab with concurrent radiotherapy and capecitabine in locally advanced pancreatic cancer. *J Clin Oncol* **24**: 1145–51.

Crombet T, Osorio M, Cruz T *et al.* (2004). Use of the humanized anti-epidermal growth factor receptor monoclonal antibody h-R3 in combination with radiotherapy in the treatment of locally advanced head and neck cancer patients. *J Clin Oncol* **22**: 1646–54.

Delmas C, Heliez C, Cohen-Jonathan E *et al.* (2002). Farnesyltransferase inhibitor, R115777, reverses the resistance of human glioma cell lines to ionizing radiation. *Int J Cancer* **100**: 43–8.

Eicheler W, Krause M, Hessel F, Zips D, Baumann M (2005). Kinetics of EGFR expression during fractionated irradiation varies between different human squamous cell carcinoma lines in nude mice. *Radiother Oncol* **76**: 151–6.

Eriksen JG, Steiniche T, Overgaard J (2005). The influence of epidermal growth factor receptor and tumor differentiation on the response to accelerated radiotherapy of squamous cell carcinomas of the head and neck in the randomized DAHANCA 6 and 7 study. *Radiother Oncol* **74**: 93–100.

Eshleman JS, Carlson BL, Mladek AC, Kastner BD, Shide KL, Sarkaria JN (2002). Inhibition of the mammalian target of rapamycin sensitizes U87 xenografts to fractionated radiation therapy. *Cancer Res* **62**: 7291–7.

Foon KA, Yang XD, Weiner LM *et al.* (2004). Preclinical and clinical evaluations of ABX-EGF, a fully human anti-epidermal growth factor receptor antibody. *Int J Radiat Oncol Biol Phys* **58**: 984–90.

Ganswindt U, Budach W, Jendrossek V, Becker G, Bamberg M, Belka C (2006). Combination of celecoxib with percutaneous radiotherapy in patients with localised prostate cancer – a phase I study. *Radiat Oncol* **1**: 9.

Hahn SM, Bernhard EJ, Regine W *et al.* (2002). A phase I trial of the farnesyltransferase inhibitor L-778,123 and radiotherapy for locally advanced lung and head and neck cancer. *Clin Cancer Res* **8**: 1065–72.

Hill RP, Milas L (1989). The proportion of stem cells in murine tumors. *Int J Radiat Oncol Biol Phys* **16**: 513–8.

Jain RK (2005). Normalization of tumor vasculature: an emerging concept in antiangiogenic therapy. *Science* **307**: 58–62.

Kelly K, Chansky K, Gaspar LE *et al.* (2007). Updated analysis of SWOG 0023: a randomized phase III trial of gefitinib versus placebo maintenance after definitive chemoradiation followed by docetaxel in patients with locally advanced stage III non-small cell lung cancer. *J Clin Oncol* **25**: 18S, abstract 7513.

Kim T (2004). Technology evaluation: Matuzumab, Merck KGaA. *Curr Opin Mol Ther* **6**: 96–103.

Kozin SV, Boucher Y, Hicklin DJ, Bohlen P, Jain RK, Suit HD (2001). Vascular endothelial growth factor receptor-2-blocking antibody potentiates radiation-induced long-term control of human tumor xenografts. *Cancer Res* **61**: 39–44.

Krause M, Baumann M (2008). Clinical biomarkers of kinase activity: examples from EGFR inhibition trials. *Cancer Metastasis Rev* **27**: 387–402.

Krause M, Ostermann G, Petersen C *et al.* (2005a). Decreased repopulation as well as increased reoxygenation contribute to the improvement in local control after targeting of the EGFR by C225 during fractionated irradiation. *Radiother Oncol* **76**: 162–7.

Krause M, Schutze C, Petersen C *et al.* (2005b). Different classes of EGFR inhibitors may have different potential to improve local tumour control after fractionated irradiation: a study on C225 in FaDu hSCC. *Radiother Oncol* **74**: 109–15.

Krause M, Zips D, Thames HD, Kummermehr J, Baumann M (2006). Preclinical evaluation of molecular-targeted anticancer agents for radiotherapy. *Radiother Oncol* **80**: 112–22.

Kummermehr J, Trott KR (1997). Tumour stem cells. In: Potten CS (ed.) *Stem cells.* London: Academic Press, 363–400.

Liao Z, Mason KA, Milas L (2007). Cyclo-oxygenase-2 and its inhibition in cancer: is there a role? *Drugs* **67**: 821–45.

Lu C, Lee JJ, Komaki R *et al.* (2007). A phase III study of AE-941 with induction chemotherapy (IC) and concomitant chemoradiotherapy (CRT) for stage III non-small cell lung cancer (NSCLC) (NCI T99-0046, RTOG 02-70, MDA 99-303). *J Clin Oncol* **25**: 18S, abstract 7527.

Machiels JP, Sempoux C, Scalliet P *et al.* (2007). Phase I/II study of preoperative cetuximab, capecitabine, and external beam radiotherapy in patients with rectal cancer. *Ann Oncol* **18**: 738–44.

Martin NE, Brunner TB, Kiel KD *et al.* (2004). A phase I trial of the dual farnesyltransferase and geranylgeranyltransferase inhibitor L-778,123 and radiotherapy for locally advanced pancreatic cancer. *Clin Cancer Res* **10**: 5447–54.

Milas L, Fang FM, Mason KA, Valdecanas D, Hunter N, Koto M, Ang KK (2007). Importance of maintenance therapy in C225-induced enhancement of tumor control by fractionated radiation. *Int J Radiat Oncol Biol Phys* **67**: 568–72.

Nasu S, Ang KK, Fan Z, Milas L (2001). C225 antiepidermal growth factor receptor antibody enhances tumor radiocurability. *Int J Radiat Oncol Biol Phys* **51**: 474–7.

Petersen C, Eicheler W, Frömmel A, Krause M, Balschukat S, Zips D, Baumann M (2003). Proliferation and micromilieu during fractionated irradiation of human FaDu squamous cell carcinoma in nude mice. *Int J Radiat Biol* **79**: 469–77.

Robert F, Ezekiel MP, Spencer SA *et al.* (2001). Phase I study of anti-epidermal growth factor receptor antibody cetuximab in combination with radiation therapy in patients with advanced head and neck cancer. *J Clin Oncol* **19**: 3234–43.

Rodel C, Arnold D, Hipp M *et al.* (2008). Phase I-II trial of cetuximab, capecitabine, oxaliplatin, and radiotherapy as preoperative treatment in rectal cancer. *Int J Radiat Oncol Biol Phys* **70**: 1081–6.

Schmidt-Ullrich RK, Contessa JN, Dent P *et al.* (1999). Molecular mechanisms of radiation-induced accelerated repopulation. *Radiat Oncol Investig* **7**: 321–30.

Soulieres D, Senzer NN, Vokes EE, Hidalgo M, Agarwala SS, Siu LL (2004). Multicenter phase II study of erlotinib, an oral epidermal growth factor receptor tyrosine kinase inhibitor, in patients with recurrent or metastatic squamous cell cancer of the head and neck. *J Clin Oncol* **22**: 77–85.

Weppler SA, Krause M, Zyromska A, Lambin P, Baumann M, Wouters BG (2007). Response of U87 glioma xenografts treated with concurrent rapamycin and fractionated radiotherapy: possible role for thrombosis. *Radiother Oncol* **82**: 96–104.

Willett CG, Boucher Y, di Tomaso E *et al.* (2004). Direct evidence that the VEGF-specific antibody bevacizumab has antivascular effects in human rectal cancer. *Nat Med* **10**: 145–7.

Willett CG, Boucher Y, Duda DG *et al.* (2005). Surrogate markers for antiangiogenic therapy and dose-limiting toxicities for bevacizumab with radiation and chemotherapy: continued experience of a phase I trial in rectal cancer patients. *J Clin Oncol* **23**: 8136–9.

Zips D, Krause M, Hessel F *et al.* (2003). Experimental study on different combination schedules of VEGF-receptor inhibitor PTK787/ZK222584 and fractionated irradiation. *Anticancer Res* **23**: 3869–76.

Zips D, Hessel F, Krause M (2005). Impact of adjuvant inhibition of vascular endothelial growth factor receptor tyrosine kinases on tumor growth delay and local tumor control after fractionated irradiation in human squamous cell carcinomas in nude mice. *Int J Radiat Oncol Biol Phys* **61**: 908–14.

■ FURTHER READING

Cengel KA, McKenna WG (2005). Molecular targets for altering radiosensitivity: lessons from Ras as a pre-clinical and clinical model. *Crit Rev Oncol Hematol* **55**: 103–16.

Colevas AD, Brown JM, Hahn S, Mitchell J, Camphausen K, Coleman CN (2003). Development of investigational radiation modifiers. *J Natl Cancer Inst* **95**: 646–51.

Dent P, Yacoub A, Contessa J *et al.* (2003). Stress and radiation-induced activation of multiple intracellular signaling pathways. *Radiat Res* **159**: 283–300.

Tofilon PJ, Saxman S, Coleman CN (2003). Molecular targets for radiation therapy: bringing preclinical data into clinical trials. *Clin Cancer Res* **9**: 3518–20.

Biological response modifiers: normal tissues

WOLFGANG DÖRR

22.1 INTRODUCTION

Modulation of radiation effects in normal tissues is closely related to the pathogenetic cascade of changes which eventually results in the loss of tissue function (see Chapter 13). The sequences of early changes at the subcellular, cellular and tissue level, and their consequences, are illustrated in Fig. 22.1. Options for interventions are given at any of the pathogenetic steps, from the very early induction of free radicals to the delayed proliferative changes in early-reacting tissues or even the late fibrotic remodelling in late-responding organs. This chapter will summarize the principles that can be applied to modulate radiation effects in normal tissues in general, and present selected investigations as examples to illustrate the efficacy of the different strategies. It must be emphasized, however, that at the time of writing the vast majority of approaches to modifying normal tissue side-effects are still experimental and remain to be validated in clinical studies.

This chapter does not focus on modification of normal-tissue effects by radiotherapy treatment planning (i.e. dose fractionation or modification of overall treatment time; see Chapters 8, 9 and 11), or by a reduction in the exposed volume (see Chapter 14). Moreover, only those strategies for biological response modification are reviewed which have already been tested in preclinical investigations in experimental animals or in first clinical trials; *in vitro* studies in cell or tissue culture systems, without confirmation of applicability to the *in vivo* situation, are not included here. Also, the symptomatic management of already clinically manifest normal-tissue reactions is excluded as this is dealt with in guidelines and textbooks for supportive care in radiation oncology.

One major prerequisite for the reasonable clinical application of normal-tissue response modifiers is the association with a therapeutic gain. This can be achieved either by selectivity for normal tissues and hence exclusion of similar effects

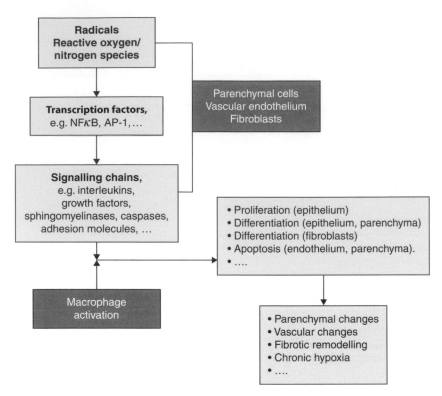

Figure 22.1 The 'molecular' pathogenetic cascade of normal-tissue effects. Radiation primarily induces free radicals, which then generate reactive oxygen and other reactive molecular species. Indirectly, this results in the activation of nuclear transcription factors, which consequently leads to modulation of various signalling chains. The orchestrated response of all tissue components, plus the contribution of macrophages, results in various changes at the cellular and tissue level.

in tumours, or by a relatively greater effect on normal tissues compared with tumours.

Terminology

According to the conclusions of a National Cancer Institute (NCI) workshop on normal tissue protection (Stone *et al.*, 2004), interventions in the development of radiation effects should be termed as:

- *prophylaxis, protection* – if applied pre-exposure
- *mitigation* – if applied during or shortly after exposure, before clinically manifest symptoms occur (i.e. during the latent time)
- *treatment, management or therapy* – in the symptomatic phase.

This obviously applies to short-term exposure (e.g. during radiation accidents) but must be modified for radiotherapy, which is given over a course of several weeks (Fig. 22.2). In radiotherapy, prophylactic approaches must comprise not only interventions before exposure, but also until the threshold dose is reached for a specific side-effect (see Chapter 13). However, it must be emphasized that some signalling cascades are activated by the first radiation dose(s) of radiotherapy (Fig. 22.1). These become clinically relevant only if the tissue-specific tolerance doses are exceeded, or in a case of retreatment (see Chapter 19). Hence there is an overlap between prophylaxis, defined clinically, and mitigation, in terms of interaction with early processes at a molecular level. Prevention is a term frequently used to describe interventions that are applied before the

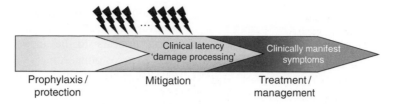

Figure 22.2 A terminology for intervention strategies in normal-tissue radiation effects. Based on the terminology developed for accidental radiation exposure (Stone *et al.*, 2004), in radiotherapy prophylaxis or protection is defined as any measure applied before the threshold dose for the specific side-effect is reached. Subsequently, but before the manifestation of clinical symptoms, mitigation strategies are used. Afterwards, in the symptomatic phase, treatment or management of side-effects is required.

onset of clinical symptoms, and hence refers to prophylaxis as well as mitigation.

Study protocols and endpoints

Most of the (*in vivo*) studies on biological response modification in normal tissues have been performed with single-dose irradiation. Aside from radiological accidents or attacks, there are only a few situations where this is relevant for radiation oncology. These include stereotactic radiotherapy, intraoperative irradiation, brachytherapy with few high-dose fractions, and perhaps treatments given over short periods, such as total-body irradiation as a conditioning treatment for stem/progenitor cell transplantation.

For application to standard external-beam radiotherapy, protection and mitigation strategies must be tested using experimental fractionation protocols as close to the clinical situation as possible (i.e. comprising daily fractionation with doses in the clinical range, administered over several weeks). The latter is required, for example, in order to test for potential interactions, beneficial or counterproductive, with repopulation processes in both tumours and normal tissues (see Chapters 10 and 11).

Modification approaches must be investigated for endpoints that are clinically relevant. For example, studies into modulation of skin or mucosal erythema are appropriate only if the associated pain reaction is concomitantly assessed, and may be entirely irrelevant for the epithelial, ulcerative response. The same applies for the relevance of endpoints used in studies of late effects.

22.2 MODIFICATION OF NORMAL-TISSUE OXYGEN LEVELS

The oxygen partial pressure in normal tissues, with few exceptions (e.g. cartilage), is normally above the range where the oxygen effect is important (see Chapter 15). Therefore, any reduction in oxygen levels (i.e. by induction of hypoxia) could be expected to reduce radiosensitivity. This has been demonstrated experimentally for total body hypoxia as well as for local hypoxia.

Systemic hypoxia

A systemic reduction of oxygen partial pressure can be achieved by breathing air with a reduced oxygen concentration. The protection factor is defined as the dose required for a specific effect with reduced oxygen compared with the dose giving the same effect with normal oxygen breathing. In single-dose studies, protection factors in the range of 1.2–1.4 have been observed. An increase in the binding of oxygen to haemoglobin, for example by the drug BW12C, developed as an agent for the treatment of sickle cell anaemia, results in reduced availability of oxygen in normal tissues, with protection factors between 1.0 and 1.3.

Yet, in radiotherapy the induction of systemic hypoxia must also be expected to be associated with an increase in the fraction of hypoxic cells within the tumour, and hence an increase in tumour radioresistance (see Chapter 15). Therefore, this strategy is inherently precluded for the amelioration of radiotherapy complications.

Local hypoxia

Local hypoxia in skin, by a pressure-induced reduction of blood flow, was one of the first instances where the radiobiological oxygen effect was described (see Chapter 15). Alternatively, in radiotherapy for head and neck tumours, 'cryotherapy' (i.e. oral cooling) may be applied (Stokman *et al.*, 2006) and patients are asked to chew ice chips before irradiation, in order to reduce the blood flow in the oral mucosa via vasoconstriction. Experimental studies have also demonstrated mucoprotective effects of local administration of vasoconstricting drugs in rectum and skin. If such approaches are considered, however, care must be taken to ensure that the target response, particularly of superficial tumours, is not affected.

22.3 RADICAL SCAVENGING AND CELLULAR DETOXIFICATION

The induction of free radicals is one of the earliest intracellular events after radiation exposure (Fig. 22.1). Administration of radical scavenging agents or, alternatively, the stimulation of endogenous detoxification mechanisms, has therefore been proposed to reduce the subsequent damage of biomolecules and consequently cellular and tissue radiation effects. The administration of antioxidants in combination with radiotherapy remains controversial. However, recent reviews conclude that antioxidants do not counteract the effectiveness of cytotoxic therapies. Clinical studies are available for the use of α-tocopherol (vitamin E), other vitamins, β-carotene, melatonin, retinol palmitate and others, and, with few exceptions, a beneficial effect of these drugs has been concluded (Moss, 2007; Simone *et al.*, 2007a,b). The most prominent example of all the drugs proposed for radical scavenging is WR2271 (amifostine). Intracellular detoxification strategies also include superoxide dismutase (SOD) and glutathione peroxidase stimulation via selenium.

Amifostine (WR2721, Ethyol)

Amifostine is an organic thiophosphate compound that has been suggested for amelioration of

radiation effects in a variety of normal tissues (Kouvaris *et al.*, 2007). The most promising application appears to be in reducing radiation-induced xerostomia. A meta-analysis (Sasse *et al.*, 2006) suggested positive effects also for other tissues, but non-blinded studies were included in this review. With regard to radiation-induced early oral mucositis, the results for the efficacy of amifostine are conflicting (reviewed in Fleischer and Dörr, 2006), which may be partly attributed to differences in dosing and timing of the drug in different studies. A recent phase III study even reported a marginally significant increase in severe mucositis in the amifostine arm (Buentzel *et al.*, 2006).

Intravenous administration of amifostine is associated with significant side-effects, such as nausea and hypotension, as well as skin reactions. Therefore, subcutaneous or topical applications have been suggested as alternative routes, and have been shown to be effective in experimental studies. In combination with clinically relevant, daily fractionation protocols (Fleischer and Dörr, 2006), amifostine was effective in reducing oral mucositis in a mouse model in the first treatment week only, but not in the second week of fractionation (Fig. 22.3). If radical scavenging were the only mechanism of action, similar effects in both treatment weeks would be expected, and therefore additional mechanisms must be postulated, such as a shortening of the latent time to the onset of repopulation processes (see Chapter 11).

The selectivity of amifostine for normal tissues is controversial, and tumour effects cannot be excluded (Andreassen *et al.*, 2003). Hence, further clinical trials are still required to determine the best application of this drug.

Superoxide dismutase

Radioprotective gene therapy with the transgene for manganese superoxide dismutase (SOD) has been administered to various organs, including lung, oesophagus, oral cavity, oropharynx, and urinary bladder. Application prior to (single-dose) irradiation has resulted in a significant reduction of tissue injury in several organ systems in rodent models (Greenberger and Epperly, 2007).

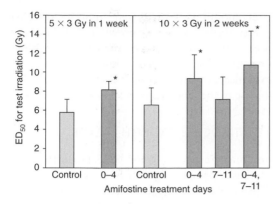

Figure 22.3 Modulation of oral mucositis in mice by amifostine, using radiation fractionation studies. Mouse tongue mucosa was irradiated with 5 × 3 Gy per week over 1 or 2 weeks, and each protocol was terminated by graded test doses to generate complete dose–effect curves. The ED_{50} for test irradiation (the dose at which an ulceration is expected in 50 per cent of the animals) therefore represents a read-out of the residual radiation tolerance of the tissue at the time of test irradiation. Amifostine administered in the first week of fractionation consistently resulted in a significant increase in mucosal tolerance (*, $p < 0.05$). In contrast, administration of amifostine in the second week of the 2-week fractionation protocol had no significant effect. Data from Fleischer and Dörr (2006).

Selenium

Selenium stimulates glutathione peroxidase, which is supposed to reduce the level of toxic oxygen compounds in irradiated cells. Only a few data are available on potential tumour effects of selenium which, however, do not suggest any detrimental effect (Dörr, 2006). After total-body irradiation of rats, a clear increase in animal survival was found after administration of sodium selenite. Protection of salivary glands by sodium selenite has also been found in preclinical studies in rats (Sagowski *et al.*, 2005).

In a study on the effects of selenium on oral mucositis (Gehrisch and Dörr, 2007), a significant effect was found for both systemic and local administration in combination with single-dose irradiation, with protection factors of 1.3–1.4. With 1 week of fractionation, a significant increase in isoeffective doses for oral mucositis (mouse) was observed for both routes of administration, equivalent to compensation of two or three dose fractions. With administration of selenium in the first week of a 2-week fractionation protocol, an effect similar to that seen for only 1 week of fractionation was observed. However, selenium given in week 2 alone, or in weeks 1 and 2 together, did not result in any significant change in isoeffective doses compared with irradiation alone, similar to the results with amifostine. If the effects of selenium were based only on increased radical scavenging by activation of glutathione peroxidase, then a similar effect of administration in either week would be expected. Therefore, as with amifostine, mechanisms independent of the antioxidative effects have been suggested, such as a shortening of the lag phase to effective repopulation. Currently, clinical data do not provide a basis for any recommendation either in favour of or against selenium supplementation in cancer patients.

22.4 GROWTH FACTORS

For modulation of radiotherapy complications by growth factors or cytokines, two aspects must be considered. First, exogenous growth factors may be applied in order to activate or stimulate tissue-specific endogenous signalling cascades. Second, growth factor signalling has been shown to change after radiation exposure or during fractionated radiotherapy; hence inhibition of upregulated signalling cascades may be applied either by antibodies against the growth factor or the respective receptors or by downstream interaction (e.g. by receptor tyrosine kinase inhibitors).

Exogenous growth factors

A variety of growth factors have been studied for their potential to modulate normal-tissue effects of radiotherapy. Most prominent examples are haematopoietic growth factors – granulocyte colony-stimulating factor (G-CSF) and granulocyte–macrophage colony-stimulating factor (GM-CSF) – to ameliorate radiation effects in the bone marrow, but also in other tissues, such as oral mucosa. Keratinocyte growth factor (KGF) has been demonstrated to effectively ameliorate the radiation response of oral and other mucosal membranes (Dörr, 2003).

With regard to late complications in the lung, conflicting data have emerged from various studies using fibroblast growth factor-2 (FGF-2). In the central nervous system and the kidney, insulin-like growth factor-1 (IGF-1) as an anti-apoptotic factor for oligodendrocytes and their progenitor cells, and platelet-derived growth factor (PDGF) as a survival factor of progenitor cells, have been suggested as strategies to prevent the development of radiation-induced necrosis.

Several interleukins, as well as angiogenic growth factors, such as FGF-1 and FGF-2 and vascular endothelial growth factor (VEGF) and others, have been proposed for the modification of gastrointestinal reactions to irradiation.

HAEMATOPOIETIC GROWTH FACTORS

Growth factors and their involvement in radiation pathogenesis and their potential to modulate radiation effects have been most extensively studied in the haematopoietic system. At all levels of the cellular differentiation sequence, the respective growth factors that trigger cells into the next step are known (Nieder et al., 2003). Stimulation of progenitor cells by G-CSF or GM-CSF has been demonstrated in numerous preclinical and clinical studies. The administration was initially established for the management of leukopenia in cancer patients (Ganser and Karthaus, 1996). Erythropoietin (EPO) was introduced for the treatment of cancer- or therapy-related anaemia (Bokemeyer et al., 2007). Other factors including c-mpl ligand (megakaryocyte growth and development factor, thrombopoietin) are under investigation.

Both GM-CSF and G-CSF have repeatedly been tested for their potential to ameliorate oral mucositis. Recent guidelines recommend not to apply GM-CSF mouthwashes for the prevention of oral mucositis in the transplant setting. In head and neck cancer patients undergoing radiotherapy, a placebo-controlled, randomized study has demonstrated no significant effect of systemic administration of GM-CSF on the severity or duration of oral mucositis (Ryu et al., 2007).

It should be noted that tumour-protective effects of haematopoietic growth factors have also been demonstrated experimentally for various tumour types and, as this cannot yet be excluded in clinical application, great caution is required in the use of these agents (Nieder et al., 2003).

KERATINOCYTE GROWTH FACTOR

Keratinocyte growth factor (KGF-1, palifermin) is synthesized predominantly by mesenchymal cells (fibroblasts). The target cells are the epithelial cells in a variety of tissues. The factor has been tested in preclinical models for its potential to ameliorate radiation effects in oral mucosa, skin, intestine, lung and urinary bladder. Positive effects have been found in all studies.

The most extensive studies have been carried out in mouse oral mucosa (Dörr, 2003). In single-dose studies, the dose-modification factors were between 1.7 and 2.3, depending on the KGF treatment protocol. In combination with single-dose irradiation, repeated KGF administration is required to achieve a significant effect. However, the treatment with KGF is effective even if given after irradiation, which offers some options for accidental radiation exposure. In contrast, KGF treatment during fractionated radiotherapy, given as only a single injection at the beginning of the weekend break, was as effective as repeated applications over the entire weekend. An increase in the effect was observed with up to four repeated treatments at consecutive weekends (Fig. 22.4), starting before the onset of radiotherapy (Dörr et al., 2005).

In a large, randomized, placebo-controlled, double-blinded phase III study in patients receiving total body irradiation and high-dose chemotherapy in preparation for peripheral blood progenitor cell transplantation, treatment with palifermin resulted in a highly significant reduction in the incidence and duration of oral mucositis (Spielberger et al., 2004). A phase III study in patients with radio(chemo)therapy for head and neck tumours has been undertaken.

The mechanisms through which KGF acts remain currently unclear. One component may be the stimulation of proliferation and the modification of differentiation (reduction of cell loss) in the epithelial tissues (Dörr, 2003). However, KGF

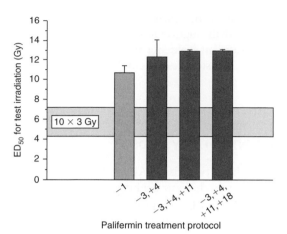

Figure 22.4 The effect of repeated applications of palifermin over subsequent weekends on the incidence of oral mucosal ulcerations in the mouse. Mouse tongue mucosa was irradiated with 10 × 3 Gy over 2 weeks. Palifermin was given before the onset of radiotherapy (day −1), or over 2, 3, or 4 subsequent weekends. Each protocol was terminated by graded test doses to generate complete dose–effect curves. The ED_{50} for test irradiation (the dose at which an ulceration is expected in 50 per cent of the animals) can be regarded as a measure of the mucosal tolerance at the time of test irradiation. Palifermin resulted in a highly significant increase in mucosal tolerance in all protocols tested. However, addition of a third palifermin injection on day +11 yielded only a minor increase in ED_{50} values, and a further injection on day +18 had no further effect. Data from Dörr *et al.* (2005).

has been demonstrated to also modulate the response of vascular endothelial cells and macrophages to irradiation, which appears to contribute to a complex mechanism of action.

Inhibition of growth factor signalling

Among the most prominent growth factor signalling cascades for which upregulation in early responding normal tissues after irradiation has been observed are the epidermal growth factor (EGF) pathway (upregulation of the receptor, EGFR) and the tumour necrosis factor-α (TNF-α) pathway (upregulation of the growth factor).

For late-responding tissues, a significant stimulation of transforming growth factor-β (TGF-β) has been reported. These processes might therefore be targeted in order to modify normal-tissue radiation effects.

EPIDERMAL GROWTH FACTOR SIGNALLING

The epidermal growth factor receptor is over-expressed in a variety of tumours and hence may represent one specific target for improving the tumour effects of radiotherapy (see Chapter 21). However in animal models, upregulation of EGFR expression in early-responding tissues by irradiation has also been shown. Therefore, targeting of EGFR may also modify normal-tissue effects of radiotherapy, in addition to the radiation-independent side-effects of some of the drugs used, such as skin changes. In mouse oral mucosa, EGFR inhibition by a specific tyrosine kinase inhibitor (BIBX1382BS) during fractionated irradiation did not have a significant effect (Fehrmann and Dörr, 2005). However, preliminary results (Dörr *et al.*, unpublished) using another tyrosine kinase inhibitor as well as an anti-EGFR antibody suggest that the normal-tissue effects may be drug-specific.

TUMOUR NECROSIS FACTOR-α SIGNALLING

Tumour necrosis factor-α is a growth factor with a profound role in inflammatory processes, and upregulation in normal tissues by irradiation has been demonstrated and is usually considered to promote the radiation response of these normal tissues. Therefore, inhibition of TNF-α signalling might be beneficial. Drugs directed against TNF-α signalling (e.g. infliximab) are already used clinically for treating Crohn's disease, rheumatoid arthritis and psoriasis. However, in mouse kidney, treatment with infliximab significantly exacerbated radiation nephropathy (Nieder *et al.*, 2007). This example clearly illustrates that the hypotheses underlying any strategy for intervention into the biological processes associated with the response of normal tissues to irradiation must be carefully tested in relevant preclinical models before clinical testing is undertaken.

TRANSFORMING GROWTH FACTOR-β SIGNALLING

Although the essential role of TGF-β for the development of radiation-induced fibrosis is well documented (see Chapter 13), approaches to inhibit TGF-β signalling have emerged only recently. One strategy is to inhibit the activation of TGF-β from its latent form, which, at least in the lung, is regulated by the integrin alpha(v)beta6. Treatment of irradiated mice with a monoclonal antibody against this integrin has prevented fibrosis (Puthawala *et al.*, 2008).

22.5 ANTI-INFLAMMATORY TREATMENTS

Glucocorticoids

Standard anti-inflammatory approaches with glucocorticoids are frequently applied as symptomatic, supportive treatment in order to manage oedema and pain associated with the inflammatory component of radiation-induced side-effects (e.g. in central nervous system, lung or skin). However, no conclusive results are available for this class of drugs for specific targeting of inflammatory processes in order to prevent radiotherapy side effects.

Non-steroidal anti-inflammatory drugs (NSAIDs)

As with corticoids, NSAIDs, particularly acetylic salicylic acid (ASA), are frequently used for the symptomatic management of inflammatory signs of (early) radiation side-effects. However, some preclinical studies have addressed the potential of ASA to specifically target the biological mechanisms of normal-tissue complications. In a first study in mouse kidney, ASA was administered as an antithrombotic agent (Verheij *et al.*, 1995). This treatment resulted in a significant prolongation of the latent time to development of renal failure. In a further study in mouse urinary bladder (Dörr *et al.*, 1998), where ASA was applied in order to reduce the increase in detrusor muscle

tone during the early-response phase, which is mediated through arachidonic acid metabolites, the treatment yielded a significant restoration of the bladder storage capacity.

Others

ESSENTIAL FATTY ACIDS

Essential fatty acids (EFAs) are known to interact with the arachidonic acid metabolism by shifting the endproducts into an anti-inflammatory direction. In pig skin, oral administration of EFAs resulted in a clear reduction in the severity of both early and late skin reactions (Hopewell *et al.*, 1994). Similarly, in mouse urinary bladder, EFA treatment has yielded a reduction in the incidence of late effects (Dörr *et al.*, unpublished).

INHIBITORS OF CYCLOOXYGENASE-2 (COX-2)

Similar to EGFR-inhibitors (see Section 22.4), COX-2-inhibitors have been proposed as drugs that specifically target the metabolism of tumours, where COX-2 is frequently upregulated. However, upregulation of COX-2 is also seen in normal tissues, particularly during the early response; the relevance of these changes is unknown. In studies on mouse tongue mucosa, a clear decrease in radiation effects has been seen when the COX-2 inhibitor celecoxib is administered during daily fractionated radiotherapy (Dörr *et al.*, unpublished).

22.6 MODULATION OF MACROPHAGE ACTIVITY

The relevance of macrophage responses to normal-tissue side-effects is controversial. For late effects, such as radiation pneumopathy, a contribution of alveolar macrophages to the orchestrated reaction of the tissue has been clearly demonstrated (see Chapter 13). Changes in macrophage activation have also been observed as early radiation side-effects. However, their relevance to the clinical manifestation of the actual side-effects remains obscure.

Selective modulation of macrophage activity has been tested in a rat model of radiation proctitis (Sassy *et al.*, 1991). Tetrachlorodecaoxide (TCDO, WF10) is a drug that activates macrophages, but then regulates their activity at an intermediate level. Treatment of rats at early time-points after irradiation resulted in a clear prolongation of the time to onset of late proctitis. Administration at later time-points also significantly reduced the severity of the response. For early radiation-induced oral mucositis in the mouse, local administration of TCDO appears to reduce the response to daily fractionated irradiation, while no effect is observed with single-dose irradiation (Schmidt and Dörr, unpublished). Similarly, the immunomodulator JBT3200, a bacterial wall component, seems to reduce the oral mucosal response during fractionated irradiation but is largely ineffective in combination with single-dose irradiation (Dörr *et al.*, unpublished).

22.7 STIMULATION OF PROLIFERATION IN EARLY-RESPONDING TISSUES

The severity of early radiation effects during fractionated irradiation is clearly related to the regeneration response of the tissue, shown by repopulation (see Chapter 11). Therefore, stimulation of cell production in epithelial tissues has been tested for its potential to reduce early complications of radiotherapy. In addition to the administration of growth factors (Section 22.4), removal of the superficial epithelia layers may increase the normal trigger for proliferation in the germinal compartment. In skin, this can be achieved by 'tape stripping' or hair plucking, which, however, has been tested only in combination with single-dose irradiation. In accordance with the more rapid turnover of the epidermis, epidermal reactions started earlier than in unstimulated skin.

Similar observations, with single-dose irradiation, have been made in mouse oral mucosa after ablation of the superficial keratin layers by applying mild silver nitrate solution as an astringent (Dörr and Kummermehr, 1992). However, when fractionated irradiation was applied, stimulated proliferation translated into an increased radiation tolerance, which was attributed to an earlier onset of repopulation processes. These data have been validated in a clinical study with accelerated radiotherapy for head and neck tumours, but, although the proliferative effect was demonstrated in mucosal biopsies, it could not be confirmed with conventional fractionation (Dörr *et al.*, 1995). It was concluded that, for effective stimulation of repopulation, an early switch from asymmetrical to symmetrical divisions (see Chapter 11) is required in addition to stimulated proliferation, which is achieved only during accelerated but not during conventional fractionation. Alternatively, low-level laser treatment can be successfully administered to oral mucosa in head and neck cancer patients to remove superficial material and the effectiveness of this approach has been demonstrated in two prospective clinical studies (Genot-Klastersky *et al.*, 2008).

22.8 STRATEGIES TO REDUCE CHRONIC OXIDATIVE STRESS

For late effects in normal tissues, a long-lasting perpetuation of the production of reactive oxygen and nitrogen species appears to play an essential role. Therefore, strategies have been developed to interrupt this chronic oxidative stress cascade and have been tested for fibrotic changes in skin, using a combination of pentoxifylline (PTX) and tocopherol (vitamin E) as anti-oxidative agents.

In breast cancer patients ($n = 24$) with manifest radiation skin fibrosis, a clear regression of the fibrotic lesions was observed at 6 months after treatment with PTX and tocopherol in a randomized, placebo-controlled trial (Delanian *et al.*, 2003). These results, however, could not be confirmed in a larger, double-blind placebo-controlled trial in breast cancer patients (Gothard *et al.*, 2004), or in a further trial in patients after pelvic radiotherapy (Gothard *et al.*, 2005).

22.9 INTERVENTION IN THE ANGIOTENSIN PATHWAY

The angiotensin system appears to be involved in the development of fibrosis, at least in the lung, presumably through interactions with TGF-β signalling. In the kidney, angiotensin converting enzyme (ACE)-induced hypertension also contributes to the development of the radiation response. Therefore, ACE inhibitors, such as captopril, and antagonists of the angiotensin II type 1 (AT1) and type 2 (AT2) receptor, have been tested for their potential to mitigate or treat late radiation effects, particularly in kidney and lung.

In a rat model of total-body irradiation and bone marrow transplantation, resulting in nephropathy, the drugs have been shown to effectively prevent kidney sequelae of irradiation (Moulder et al., 2007). All drugs also were effective in the treatment of kidney damage. Obviously, different modes of action are relevant at different periods (i.e. for mitigation and treatment). As a hypothesis, mitigation may be based on the suppression of the renin–angiotensin system, but treatment of established nephropathy is based on (additional) blood pressure control.

In two models of radiation injury of the lung (total-body irradiation, hemithorax irradiation), inhibition of ACE or AT1 receptors was found to be effective in the prevention of radiation pneumonitis and fibrosis (Molteni et al., 2000).

It should be noted that these studies were done with high single doses of radiation, given locally (lung) or as total-body irradiation in combination with chemotherapy, which may alter the pathobiology of the radiation effects. Therefore, validation of the results in studies with conventional fractionation protocols is desirable.

22.10 STEM CELL THERAPY

A novel, potentially selective approach for the amelioration of normal-tissue radiation effects is treatment with (adult) stem cells. This includes the administration of bone marrow (i.e. haematopoietic plus mesenchymal stem cells) or mesenchymal stem cells, or the mobilization of autologous stem cells by growth factors (e.g. G-CSF). These strategies have been tested in preclinical models of radiation injury in skin, salivary glands, intestine and oral mucosa.

Transplantation of bone marrow

Transplantation of (syngeneic) bone marrow has been studied for its potential to ameliorate oral mucositis in the mouse (Dörr et al., unpublished). Following single-dose irradiation, transplantation between days 0 and 10 did not result in any change in the mucosal response. In contrast, transplantation during daily fractionated irradiation resulted in a reduction in mucosal reactions, particularly if the stem cell treatment was administered at time-points later in the irradiation regimen.

Transplantation of mesenchymal stem cells

Systemically administered mesenchymal stem cells (MSCs) appear to home in specifically on (radiation) injured tissues. Systemic administration of human MSCs reduced the severity of the response and improved healing in human skin transplanted onto nude mice (Francois et al., 2007). Similarly, in the intestine, intravenous MSC transplantation accelerated crypt regeneration in a mouse model (Semont et al., 2006). In mouse oral mucosa, intravenous administration of MSCs at various time-points during daily fractionated irradiation has significantly reduced the incidence of confluent oral mucositis (Haagen and Dörr, unpublished data).

Mesenchymal stem cell therapy has also been applied successfully as part of the therapy of skin lesions in patients after radiation accidents (e.g. Lataillade et al., 2007).

Mobilization of bone marrow stem cells

Release of stem cells from the bone marrow can be stimulated by growth factors, such as G-CSF, and other drugs, such as inhibitors of the receptor for the stromal cell-derived factor 1 (SDF-1, CXCL12), which regulates the retention of the stem cells in the bone marrow. It must be noted that mobilization of stem cells by G-CSF (at least in the mouse) affects both haematopoietic and mesenchymal stem cells.

Treatment of mice with G-CSF induced the homing of bone marrow cells to irradiated sub-mandibular glands (Lombaert *et al.*, 2006), and was associated with increased gland weight, number of acinar cells, and salivary flow rates. In mouse oral mucosa (Dörr *et al.*, unpublished data), administration of G-CSF resulted in a clear reduction of radiation-induced mucositis after single-dose irradiation, particularly when the maximum number of stem cells in the circulation was induced at a time when the mucosal regeneration phase was about to start. Similarly, during daily fractionated irradiation, a maximum number of circulating stem cells was most effective at the time when radiation-induced repopulation processes (see Chapter 12) were effective (Fig. 22.5). In histological studies, only individual haematopoietic cells were found in the submucosal and mucosal tissues, without any indication of clonal expansion or transdifferentiation.

Administration of tissue-specific stem cells

Transplantation of bone marrow stem or progenitor cells is known to restore the bone marrow after myeloablative treatments. However, reliable methods to identify stem cells specific for other tissues and, more importantly, to stimulate these cells to proliferate *in vitro* are in only the early stages of development. These are prerequisites in order to achieve cell numbers sufficient for transplantation.

In a rat model, intraglandular transplantation of salivary gland-specific stem cells resulted in long-term restoration of salivary gland morphology and function (Lombaert *et al.*, 2008).

Mechanisms of action

In rat salivary glands, improved morphology and function are not associated with any transdifferentiation of bone marrow cells into salivary gland cells. Similarly, the reduction in oral mucosal reactions to single-dose or fractionated irradiation in mouse oral mucosa is not linked to any clonal expansion of either mesenchymal or haematopoietic cells or to transdifferentiation into an epithelial

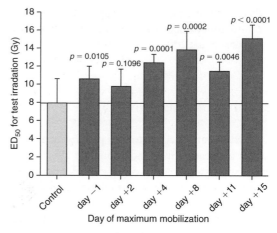

Figure 22.5 The effect of the mobilization of bone marrow stem cells on oral mucosal tolerance in mice. Daily fractionated irradiation was given with 5×3 Gy per week over 3 weeks, and the protocols were terminated by graded test doses in order to generate dose–effect curves, using the ED_{50} values as a measure of the residual tissue tolerance. Bone marrow stem cells were mobilized by two daily injections of granulocyte colony-stimulating factor (G-CSF) over 4 days. This protocol has been shown to result in a maximum number of circulating stem cells at day 10 after the first injection. This maximum mobilization effect was adjusted to various time-points during the fractionation protocol, shown on the abscissa. With the exception of day $+2$, all mobilization protocols yielded a significant reduction in the incidence of oral mucosal ulcerations. The effect was most pronounced at later time-points, when mucosal repopulation processes (see Chapter 11) were maximally stimulated. Data from Dörr *et al.* (unpublished).

cell type. For irradiated skin, the data are less consistent, with some indication of transdifferentiation processes. Two alternative mechanisms of action must hence be considered: (1) homing of stem cells into radiation-damaged sites and production of paracrine factors that locally stimulate tissue regeneration; or (2) release of such factors by stem cells, which are still in the circulation. Further research is required in order to identify the relevant modes of action and to design optimum stem cell treatment strategies.

In contrast to bone marrow stem cells, tissue-specific stem cells (including haematopoietic stem cells in the bone marrow) do appear to differentiate into functional cells (e.g. in salivary glands; Lombaert *et al.*, 2008).

22.11 CONCLUSIONS

A variety of approaches for the prophylaxis, mitigation or treatment of radiation side-effects have been suggested, based on the biology of the response of the tissues to irradiation. It must be emphasized that, at the time of writing, these interventions are predominantly experimental. A few cases of strategies that have already been translated into clinical studies have been described above.

Moreover, it must be noted that many experimental studies have been carried out only in combination with single-dose irradiation. This could reflect clinical scenarios of stereotactic irradiation, brachytherapy or myeloablative conditioning for stem cell transplantation. However, this clearly lacks relevance for fractionated radiotherapy given over several weeks where, for example, repopulation processes in early-responding tissues are a factor dominating the radiation tolerance of these tissues (see Chapter 11). Parallel studies with single and fractionated doses of radiation have clearly demonstrated that the results can be contradictory, such as for bone marrow transplantation in oral mucosa (see Section 22.10). During fractionated irradiation, intervention at intervals before the onset of repopulation can result in effects that are different from intervention at later times, as has been demonstrated for administration of amifostine or selenium to ameliorate oral mucositis (see Section 22.3).

Some approaches, such as stimulation of proliferation for a reduction of early epithelial radiation effects, or a reduction of the chronic oxidative stress response in irradiated tissues for the prophylaxis or treatment of late radiation sequelae in skin or lung, have been tested in clinical trials, but with conflicting results. A number of 'targeted' interventions (e.g. administration of growth factors or stem cell therapy) appear to act through several different mechanisms, which deserve further investigation.

In general, modification of normal-tissue responses to radiation exposure requires a thorough preclinical testing with appropriate *in vivo* (animal) models, analysing clinically relevant endpoints after irradiation with adequate (fractionation) protocols. The mechanisms of action of effective interventions must then be clarified in order to develop optimal clinical strategies.

In order to guarantee a clinical benefit, possible tumour effects of the normal tissue modification strategies must also be assessed. This must be done under the same premises with regard to suitability of the *in vivo* models, relevance of treatment protocols and endpoints. A therapeutic gain is achieved only if the target normal tissue demonstrates significantly greater radioprotection than any reduction in the radiation effect in the tumour being treated.

Key points

1. Strategies for modification of normal tissue responses to irradiation must be based on the underlying pathobiology.
2. Interventions in the processing of radiation damage can be directed against any step of the pathogenetic cascade from early production of free radicals to late tissue changes. The mechanisms of action underlying the protective effects must be clarified in order to design optimum clinical protocols.
3. Before clinical application, modification approaches must be thoroughly tested in animal models, with relevant irradiation protocols and endpoints. Results from single-dose and fractionation studies can be divergent.
4. Comparison with potential tumour effects is essential in order to achieve a therapeutic gain.
5. Most promising, with first clinical studies, are the interaction with growth factor signalling, the interruption of chronic oxidative stress cascades in late tissue reactions, and the treatment (mobilization and transplantation) with stem cells, both haematopoietic and mesenchymal.

■ BIBLIOGRAPHY

Andreassen CN, Grau C, Lindegaard JC (2003). Chemical radioprotection: a critical review of amifostine as a cytoprotector in radiotherapy. *Semin Radiat Oncol* **13**: 62–72.

Bokemeyer C, Aapro MS, Courdi A *et al.* (2007). EORTC guidelines for the use of erythropoietic proteins in anaemic patients with cancer: 2006 update. *Eur J Cancer* **43**: 258–70.

Buentzel J, Micke O, Adamietz IA, Monnier A, Glatzel M, de Vries A (2006). Intravenous amifostine during chemoradiotherapy for head-and-neck cancer: a randomized placebo-controlled phase III study. *Int J Radiat Oncol Biol Phys* **64**: 684–91.

Delanian S, Porcher R, Balla-Mekias S, Lefaix JL (2003). Randomized, placebo-controlled trial of combined pentoxifylline and tocopherol for regression of superficial radiation-induced fibrosis. *J Clin Oncol* **21**: 2545–50.

Dörr W (2003). Oral mucosa: response modification by keratinocyte growth factor. In: Nieder C, Milas L, Ang KK (eds) *Modification of radiation response: cytokines, growth factors and other biological targets*. Berlin: Springer-Verlag, 113–22.

Dörr W (2006). Effects of selenium on radiation responses of tumor cells and tissue. *Strahlenther Onkol* **182**: 693–5.

Dörr W, Kummermehr J (1992). Increased radiation tolerance of mouse tongue epithelium after local conditioning. *Int J Radiat Biol* **61**: 369–79.

Dörr W, Jacubek A, Kummermehr J, Herrmann T, Dolling-Jochem I, Eckelt U (1995). Effects of stimulated repopulation on oral mucositis during conventional radiotherapy. *Radiother Oncol* **37**: 100–7.

Dörr W, Eckhardt M, Ehme A, Koi S (1998). Pathogenesis of acute radiation effects in the urinary bladder. Experimental results. *Strahlenther Onkol* **174**(Suppl 3): 93–5.

Dörr W, Reichel S, Spekl K (2005). Effects of keratinocyte growth factor (palifermin) administration protocols on oral mucositis (mouse) induced by fractionated irradiation. *Radiother Oncol* **75**: 99–105.

Fehrmann A, Dörr W (2005). Effect of EGFR-inhibition on the radiation response of oral mucosa: experimental studies in mouse tongue epithelium. *Int J Radiat Biol* **81**: 437–43.

Fleischer G, Dörr W (2006). Amelioration of early radiation effects in oral mucosa (mouse) by intravenous or subcutaneous administration of amifostine. *Strahlenther Onkol* **182**: 567–75.

Francois S, Mouiseddine M, Mathieu N *et al.* (2007). Human mesenchymal stem cells favour healing of the cutaneous radiation syndrome in a xenogenic transplant model. *Ann Hematol* **86**: 1–8.

Ganser A, Karthaus M (1996). Clinical use of hematopoietic growth factors. *Curr Opin Oncol* **8**: 265–9.

Gehrisch A, Dörr W (2007). Effects of systemic or topical administration of sodium selenite on early radiation effects in mouse oral mucosa. *Strahlenther Onkol* **183**: 36–42.

Genot-Klastersky MT, Klastersky J, Awada F *et al.* (2008). The use of low-energy laser (LEL) for the prevention of chemotherapy- and/or radiotherapy-induced oral mucositis in cancer patients: results from two prospective studies. *Support Care Cancer* 2008; [epub ahead of print].

Gothard L, Cornes P, Earl J *et al.* (2004). Double-blind placebo-controlled randomised trial of vitamin E and pentoxifylline in patients with chronic arm lymphoedema and fibrosis after surgery and radiotherapy for breast cancer. *Radiother Oncol* **73**: 133–9.

Gothard L, Cornes P, Brooker S *et al.* (2005). Phase II study of vitamin E and pentoxifylline in patients with late side effects of pelvic radiotherapy. *Radiother Oncol* **75**: 334–41.

Greenberger JS, Epperly MW (2007). Review. Antioxidant gene therapeutic approaches to normal tissue radioprotection and tumor radiosensitization. *In Vivo* **21**: 141–6.

Hopewell JW, van den Aardweg GJ, Morris GM *et al.* (1994). Amelioration of both early and late radiation-induced damage to pig skin by essential fatty acids. *Int J Radiat Oncol Biol Phys* **30**: 1119–25.

Kouvaris JR, Kouloulias VE, Vlahos LJ (2007). Amifostine: the first selective-target and broad-spectrum radioprotector. *Oncologist* **12**: 738–47.

Lataillade JJ, Doucet C, Bey E *et al.* (2007). New approach to radiation burn treatment by dosimetry-guided surgery combined with autologous mesenchymal stem cell therapy. *Regen Med* **2**: 785–94.

Lombaert IM, Wierenga PK, Kok T, Kampinga HH, deHaan G, Coppes RP (2006). Mobilization of bone marrow stem cells by granulocyte colony-stimulating factor ameliorates radiation-induced damage to salivary glands. *Clin Cancer Res* **12**: 1804–12.

Lombaert IM, Brunsting JF, Wierenga PK *et al.* (2008). Rescue of salivary gland function after stem cell transplantation in irradiated glands. *PLoS ONE* **3**: e2063.

Molteni A, Moulder JE, Cohen EF *et al.* (2000). Control of radiation-induced pneumopathy and lung fibrosis by angiotensin-converting enzyme inhibitors and an angiotensin II type 1 receptor blocker. *Int J Radiat Biol* **76**: 523–32.

Moss RW (2007). Do antioxidants interfere with radiation therapy for cancer? *Integr Cancer Ther* **6**: 281–92.

Moulder JE, Fish BL, Cohen EP (2007). Treatment of radiation nephropathy with ACE inhibitors and AII type-1 and type-2 receptor antagonists. *Curr Pharm Des* **13**: 1317–25.

Nieder C, Jeremic B, Licht T, Zimmermann FB (2003). Hematopoietic tissue II: role of colony-stimulating factors. In: Nieder C, Milas L, Ang KK (eds) *Modification of radiation response: cytokines, growth factors and other biological targets*. Berlin: Springer-Verlag, 103–12.

Nieder C, Schnaiter A, Weber WA *et al.* (2007). Detrimental effects of an antibody directed against tumor necrosis factor alpha in experimental kidney irradiation. *Anticancer Res* **27**: 2353–7.

Puthawala K, Hadjiangelis N, Jacoby SC *et al.* (2008). Inhibition of integrin alpha(v)beta6, an activator of latent transforming growth factor-beta, prevents radiation-induced lung fibrosis. *Am J Respir Crit Care Med* **177**: 82–90.

Ryu JK, Swann S, LeVeque F *et al.* (2007). The impact of concurrent granulocyte macrophage-colony stimulating factor on radiation-induced mucositis in head and neck cancer patients: a double-blind placebo-controlled prospective phase III study by Radiation Therapy Oncology Group 9901. *Int J Radiat Oncol Biol Phys* **67**: 643–50.

Sagowski C, Wenzel S, Jenicke L, Metternich FU, Jaehne M (2005). Sodium selenite is a potent radioprotector of the salivary glands of the rat: acute effects on the morphology and parenchymal function during fractioned irradiation. *Eur Arch Otorhinolaryngol* **262**: 459–64.

Sasse AD, Clark LG, Sasse EC, Clark OA (2006). Amifostine reduces side effects and improves complete response rate during radiotherapy: results of a meta-analysis. *Int J Radiat Oncol Biol Phys* **64**: 784–91.

Sassy T, Breiter N, Trott KR (1991). Effects of tetrachlorodecaoxide (TCDO) in chronic radiation lesions of the rat colon. *Strahlenther Onkol* **167**: 191–6.

Semont A, Francois S, Mouiseddine M *et al.* (2006). Mesenchymal stem cells increase self-renewal of small intestinal epithelium and accelerate structural recovery after radiation injury. *Adv Exp Med Biol* **585**: 19–30.

Simone CB, Simone NL, Simone V, Simone CB (2007a). Antioxidants and other nutrients do not interfere with chemotherapy or radiation therapy and can increase kill and increase survival, Part 1. *Altern Ther Health Med* **13**: 22–8.

Simone CB, Simone NL, Simone V, Simone CB (2007b). Antioxidants and other nutrients do not interfere with chemotherapy or radiation therapy and can increase kill and increase survival, Part 2. *Altern Ther Health Med* **13**: 40–7.

Spielberger R, Stiff P, Bensinger W *et al.* (2004). Palifermin for oral mucositis after intensive therapy for hematologic cancers. *N Engl J Med* **351**: 2590–8.

Stokman MA, Spijkervet FK, Boezen HM, Schouten JP, Roodenburg JL, de Vries EG (2006). Preventive intervention possibilities in radiotherapy- and chemotherapy-induced oral mucositis: results of meta-analyses. *J Dent Res* **85**: 690–700.

Stone HB, Moulder JE, Coleman CN *et al.* (2004). Models for evaluating agents intended for the prophylaxis, mitigation and treatment of radiation injuries. Report of an NCI Workshop, December 3–4, 2003. *Radiat Res* **162**: 711–28.

Verheij M, Stewart FA, Oussoren Y, Weening JJ, Dewit L (1995). Amelioration of radiation nephropathy by acetylsalicylic acid. *Int J Radiat Biol* **67**: 587–96.

■ FURTHER READING

Bentzen SM (2006). Preventing or reducing late side effects of radiation therapy: radiobiology meets molecular pathology. *Nat Rev Cancer* **6**: 702–13.

Brizel DM (2007). Pharmacologic approaches to radiation protection. *J Clin Oncol* **25**: 4084–9.

Coleman CN, Stone HB, Moulder JE, Pellmar TC (2004). Medicine. Modulation of radiation injury. *Science* **304**: 693–4.

Delanian S, Lefaix JL (2007). Current management for late normal tissue injury: radiation-induced fibrosis and necrosis. *Semin Radiat Oncol* **17**: 99–107.

Greenberger JS (2008). Gene therapy approaches for stem cell protection. *Gene Ther* **15**: 100–8.

Moulder JE, Cohen EP (2007). Future strategies for mitigation and treatment of chronic radiation-induced normal tissue injury. *Semin Radiat Oncol* **17**: 141–8.

23

Molecular targeting and patient individualization

ADRIAN C. BEGG

23.1 INTRODUCTION

Radiotherapy is effective as a single modality. It is prescribed either alone or as an adjuvant therapy in more than half of all cancer patients. Improvements in radiotherapy have been considerable over the last two decades, in large measure owing to improvements in instrumentation, machine software and diagnostic techniques, enabling more accurate dose delivery to the tumour while minimizing the dose to surrounding healthy tissue. Despite these technical improvements, some patients still fail after radiotherapy and some still develop severe side-effects. Improvements are thus still needed. These improvements can, in principle, be achieved from the biological rather than the technical side.

One approach is to try and make tumour cells more sensitive to radiation. This can be done using drugs, usually small molecules, since these often have some pharmacological advantages, but also with antibodies to surface receptors linked to radioresistance pathways (e.g. epidermal growth factor receptor, EGFR). In addition, the expression of specific genes can be altered using short antisense RNA, short interference RNA (siRNA) or aptamers, all aimed at genes involved in radioresistance.

Some commonly used anti-cancer drugs are already known to radiosensitize cells, in addition to being cytotoxic. Cisplatin is a good example. However, future improvements must come from applying more tumour-specific drugs, and cisplatin and most other cytotoxic agents are not tumour specific, often causing serious side-effects in normal tissues. What is therefore needed is sufficient knowledge of the molecular biology of individual tumours, elucidating which pathways are deregulated. These pathways can then be attacked, providing a measure of tumour specificity. In the future, the combination of more accurate and complete molecular diagnostic methods, together with development of a wider range of radiosensitizing treatment options (drugs, antibodies or genetic manipulation, targeted to a range of pathways affecting the radiation response), will allow treatments tailored to the individual, maximizing tumour cell kill and minimizing normal-tissue damage.

This chapter describes which pathways can be targeted to increase cell killing by radiation. In addition, it will review current molecular diagnostic methods for finding the deregulated pathways in individual tumours, ultimately aiding the choice of tumour-specific treatments. It is important to keep in mind at the outset that making all cells more radiosensitive is relatively easy, while making tumour cells more radiosensitive than normal-tissue cells is considerably more difficult, but is the goal that must be achieved to improve cancer therapy.

23.2 MOLECULAR TARGETING

DNA repair

The ability to repair DNA damage is probably the most important determinant of resistance to ionizing radiation. The most important pathways are those for repairing base damages, single-strand breaks (SSBs) and double-strand breaks (DSBs); for details, see Chapter 2. They include base excision repair (BER), the related single-strand break repair pathway (SSBR), and two pathways for repairing double-strand breaks, namely homologous recombination (HR) and non-homologous end-joining (NHEJ). To a lesser extent, radiation also produces DNA–DNA and DNA–protein crosslinks, particularly under hypoxic irradiation conditions. Crosslink repair involves yet other genes. There are experimental data on cell lines showing that interfering in any of these pathways can make cells more sensitive to radiation, although interference with DSB repair usually produces the greatest increases in sensitivity.

DNA polymerase beta (polβ) is a central enzyme in both BER and SSBR. Cells deficient in polβ, or expressing a dominant negative construct to polβ, thereby inhibiting its function, have been shown to be more sensitive to ionizing radiation *in vitro* under certain conditions (Vermeulen *et al.*, 2007). In addition, cells deficient in XRCC1, a

central helper protein in BER and SSBR, have also been shown to be more radiosensitive than wild-type cells (Thompson *et al.*, 1990). A number of drugs have also been developed that are capable of inhibiting polβ. Some of these have been shown to modify the response of cells *in vitro* to alkylating agents and radiosensitizing thymidine analogues, which produce a type of damage repaired primarily by BER. At least one of these (methoxyamine) has also been tested in animal tumour models and shown to potentiate the action of alkylating agents, although it has not been tested with radiation (Liu and Gerson, 2004). Inhibitors also exist for APEX1, another central protein in BER, and can potentiate the response to some drugs (Luo and Kelley, 2004), although they have not been tested with radiation. Finally, small-molecule drugs have also been developed which inhibit poly-ADP-ribose polymerase 1 (PARP1), a critical break detector protein in SSBR. The PARP inhibitors and methoxyamine are the only drugs designed to target BER and SSBR which are now entering clinical trials.

Targeting double-strand break repair (DSBR) has received considerable attention, since this can substantially increase radiosensitivity, as shown from studies with knockout cells deficient in one of these essential genes. DNA-PKcs (DNA-dependent protein kinase) is a key enzyme in the major pathway of NHEJ. Several drugs have been developed against this enzyme and been shown to inhibit DNA repair and radiosensitize cells. These agents can also sensitize cells to DSB-inducing drugs such as etoposide (direct) and cisplatin (indirect). Tumour specificity is an issue here, since DNA-PKcs is also central to DNA repair in normal tissues. This is exemplified by severe combined immunodeficiency (SCID) mice, which are deficient in DNA-PKcs and which show hypersensitivity to radiation in all normal tissues examined.

MRN and ATM

Sensing DNA breaks and signalling their presence in order to halt the cell cycle and recruit repair proteins is an important aspect of the damage response after radiation. Inhibition of sensing and signalling can thus also lead to radiosensitization. The MRN complex of three proteins acting together, MRE11, RAD50 and NBS1, is central to damage detection and signalling (see Chapter 2), and knocking out one or more of these genes leads to a marked increase in radiosensitivity. One of their functions is to activate ATM (gene is mutated in ataxia telangiectasia), which is a crucial damage signalling molecule. Several natural compounds such as caffeine and newly developed more-specific drugs (Hickson *et al.*, 2004) can inhibit this enzyme. These drugs can abrogate the checkpoint response after irradiation, can reduce DNA repair and can lead to radiosensitization. Some of these drugs are undergoing clinical development. Tumour specificity is an issue here, since normal tissues also rely on MRN and ATM for an efficient damage response.

The PI3K/AKT pathway

One of the most important signal transduction pathways affecting the response to radiation is that involving phosphoinositide-3-kinase (PI3K) and protein kinase B (AKT) (see Chapter 21). Activation by phosphorylation of AKT, a key molecule in the pathway, is associated with resistance to radiation in both preclinical and clinical studies. Activation can be caused by overexpression of EGFR, deletion or mutation of the tumour suppressor PTEN, mutational activation of the RAS oncogene, and others (Valerie *et al.*, 2007). Many drugs have been developed that are targeted to different members of this pathway, and several of these drugs have been shown to radiosensitize cells. Some of these have already shown promise in clinical trials (see Chapter 21). Tumours often overexpress EGFR, or express oncogenic RAS or contain inactivating PTEN mutations, leading to a degree of tumour specificity for further attacks on this pathway.

Nuclear factor kappa B (NFκB)

NFκB is a transcription factor associated with a protective survival response after DNA damage. Radiation activates the NFκB pathway in a number of cell types, and inhibiting this activation by both genetic and chemical methods has been shown to lead to an increase in apoptosis. This

pathway has therefore also been proposed as a target for radiosensitizing tumour cells (Magne *et al.*, 2006). Some proteasome inhibitors (see below) also affect the NFκB pathway, and part of their effect may result from inhibition of NFκB. Inhibitors have also been developed to the upstream activator IKK, which increase the apoptotic response.

Proteasomes

Protein turnover, and its precise control, is essential for many cellular processes and for cell survival. The most common way the cell degrades proteins is to tag them with ubiquitin (requiring special enzymes) which then results in the protein being fed to a degradation organelle, the proteasome. This is a proteinase complex responsible for degrading most intracellular proteins, including those important for cell-cycle regulation and apoptosis. Several proteasome inhibitors have been found, including peptidyl aldehydes, lactacystin and a dipeptide boronic acid analogue (bortezomib). Proteasome inhibitors have been shown to induce apoptosis and to sensitize malignant cells in culture, and tumours *in vivo*, to radiation (Weber *et al.*, 2007) and to some chemotherapy agents. The exact mechanisms are unknown, although effects on the cell cycle, on the NFκB signalling pathway and on apoptosis probably play a role, since all these can under some circumstances affect radiosensitivity. It has also been reported that transformed (malignant) cells are more sensitive to such inhibitors than normal cells, implying a degree of tumour specificity. Why this should be so is not clear, although, if confirmed, it would make proteasome inhibitors promising agents for improving radiotherapy. At least one of these agents, bortezomib, is approved for clinical use.

Chromatin structure

Histone acetylation is another potential target for radiosensitization. Efficient DNA repair is usually associated with modifications of the chromatin structure in order to recruit repair proteins and facilitate their access to damage; these changes then have to be reversed on completion of repair. One important type of chromatin modification is the acetylation of histones, the proteins that form nucleosomes. Acetylation of histones removes a positive charge, reducing the affinity between histones and DNA and allowing easier access of transcription and other factors. The degree of histone acetylation is determined by competition between histone acetylases (HATs; putting on acetyl groups) and histone deacetylases (HDACs; taking them off). A number of HDAC inhibitors have been developed and found to have anti-tumour activity in preclinical cancer models. In addition, they can also significantly enhance tumour cell radiosensitivity (Cerna *et al.*, 2006). The mechanisms are not entirely understood, but presumably relate to the recruitment of repair factors and/or resetting the chromatin after repair. The HDAC inhibitors are undergoing clinical trials as single agents, and in combination with radiotherapy.

Checkpoints

Blocks at various stages of the cell cycle are a universal feature of the response of mammalian cells to irradiation (see Chapter 2). However, the link between the presence or length of these blocks and cell kill after irradiation is often weak. Thus for the G1/S and intra-S checkpoints, abrogation of the blocks can be achieved by genetic manipulation of one or more checkpoint genes without altering radiosensitivity. However, two distinct G2 checkpoints exist, one rapid and dose independent and the other slow and dose dependent (see Chapter 2), and the dose-dependent block appears to be associated with radiosensitivity (Xu *et al.*, 2002). Abrogation of this block increases radiosensitivity and it therefore represents a target for improving radiotherapy. In addition, abrogation of two or more blocks can be more effective than removing one block. Inhibition of the G2 checkpoint thus appears to more effectively sensitize cells to DNA damage if the cells also lack the G1 checkpoint, as in cells with mutant p53. This, in principle, provides some tumour specificity, since a large proportion of human cancers have p53 pathway mutations while the surrounding normal tissues will not. Drugs such as caffeine and pentoxyfylline can abrogate the G2 block and increase radiosensitivity. These drugs also inhibit

ATM, and so whether the effects seen are solely because of reducing damage-induced cell-cycle delays or effects on repair is not clear. At the time of writing, one drug, 7-hydroxystaurosporine (UCN-01), which also abrogates the G2 block and radiosensitizes cells, is undergoing clinical testing.

Apoptosis

Cells often die from apoptosis after irradiation or chemotherapy (although other forms of death can also dominate in solid tumours, see Chapter 3). It has therefore been proposed that increasing apoptosis would increase the effects of radiotherapy (Belka *et al.*, 2004). Several apoptosis inducers have shown synergy in combination with radiation in preclinical models, such as perifosine (an alkylphospholipid compound with structural similarity to phospholipids that are the main constituents of cellular membranes), TRAIL [tumour necrosis factor (TNF)-related apoptosis inducing ligand], gossypol (a natural compound from cotton seeds), and others. It has not been proven that the synergy seen between radiation and these compounds is caused by the increases observed in apoptosis, since apoptosis does not always correlate with clonogenic cell kill (cells not dying of apoptosis can die in other ways, see Chapter 3). There is also no obvious reason why this approach should be tumour specific other than the observation that tumours often arise by evading apoptosis (Hanahan and Weinberg, 2000), leading to the conjecture that restoring apoptosis sensitivity might restore treatment sensitivity.

Hypoxia

Targeting hypoxia to increase tumour radiosensitivity is an attractive approach since the occurrence of hypoxia is almost exclusively restricted to tumours. The aim here is to make only the hypoxic cells more radiosensitive, or to selectively kill hypoxic cells. Many preclinical and clinical studies have shown the feasibility and effectiveness of this approach. Chapters 16 and 17 discuss the biology of hypoxia and ways to combat it.

23.3 THE QUESTION OF TUMOUR SPECIFICITY

Most DNA repair pathways operate universally and equally well in normal tissues and tumours (Table 23.1a). There is no known consistent tumour specificity concerning expression or function of DNA repair genes, or ATM and other damage detectors, or for chromatin modifications associated with repair or for the NFκB pathway. A partial exception is the HR pathway for repairing DSBs. This operates only in proliferating cells (S/G2 phase), and is therefore proliferation specific. Tumours tend to exhibit higher proliferation rates than normal tissues, especially compared with late-reacting normal tissues after radiotherapy. This provides partial tumour specificity. Targeting homologous recombination may also reduce hypoxic radioresistance, thereby contributing to tumour specificity (Sprong et al., 2006). However, no drugs have yet been described that specifically inhibit HR proteins.

Proteasome inhibitors have been reported to work better on transformed cells, but it is not yet known how general this observation is.

The attraction of targeting DNA repair, including damage sensing and signalling, is that it is an excellent way of making cells more radiation sensitive (Choudhury et al., 2006). However, as stated above, in most cases it suffers from a lack of tumour specificity. There are two possible ways in which to increase tumour specificity. The first is to deliver the sensitizing drug or other sensitizing agent (e.g. siRNA, antibody) specifically to the tumour. This remains an elusive goal, and has yet to succeed sufficiently well to improve clinical cancer treatment using either cytotoxic agents alone or as radiosensitizers. Progress in this area would certainly help the application of the approaches discussed here.

The second approach is to attack tumours where they are already weakened (Table 23.1b). Since almost all malignant tumours are genetically

Table 23.1 DNA repair as a target for improving radiotherapy

	Pathway	Role	Tumour specificity	Reason
(a)	BER/SSBR	Base damage/SSBR	No	Important for repairing damage in normal tissue and tumour
	HR	DSB repair	Partial	Lower hypoxic radioresistance if mutated; proliferation dependent
	NHEJ	DSB repair	No	Important for repairing damage in normal tissue and tumour
	ATM	Sensing DSB	No	Important for repairing damage in normal tissue and tumour
	MRN	Sensing DSB	No	Important for repairing damage in normal tissue and tumour
	Pathway	Role	Mutations in cancer	Possible ways to exploit
(b)	BER/SSBR	Base damage/SSBR	Yes	Anti-HR drug (reduce backup repair pathway)
	HR	DSB repair	Yes	PARP inhibitor (anti-SSBR; reduce backup repair pathway)
	NHEJ	DSB repair	Yes	Anti-NHEJ drug (greater effect on tumour weakened by pathway mutation)
	ATM	Sensing DSB	Yes	Anti-ATM drug (greater effect on tumour weakened by pathway mutation)
	MRN	Sensing DSB	Yes	Anti-MRN drug (greater effect on tumour weakened by pathway mutation)

BER, base excision repair; SSBR, single-strand break repair; HR, homologous recombination; NHEJ, non-homologous end-joining; ATM, gene mutated in ataxia telangiectasia; MRN, MRN complex (MRE11, RAD50, NBS1); DSB, double-strand break; PARP: poly-ADP-ribose polymerase.

Table 23.2 Drugs for improving radiotherapy: tumour specificity of targets

	Tumour specificity	Remarks
Intrinsic radiosensitivity		
DNA repair	Partial	Only some pathways (e.g. HR); or if mutations in pathway (see Table 23.1)
Cell-cycle checkpoints	Partial	Only some checkpoints affect radiosensitivity (see Chapter 2); will also affect proliferating normal tissues
Cell death (e.g. pro-apoptotic)	Partial?	Tumours are less apoptosis prone?
Signal transduction (e.g. PI3K)	Partial	If overexpression of target, and/or activation of pathway
Hypoxia	Yes	Tumours are usually hypoxic, normal tissues rarely; acute and chronic hypoxia may require different approaches
Repopulation		
Anti-cell-cycle drugs	Partial	Tumours proliferate more rapidly than late-reacting normal tissues
Signal transduction (e.g. EGFR)	Partial	Tumours proliferate more rapidly than late-reacting normal tissues; if overexpression of target, and/or activation of pathway

EGFR, epidermal growth factor receptor; HR, homologous recombination.

unstable, mutations or deletions of many genes are often found in a tumour, which result in losses of gene or pathway function. This includes DNA repair genes. Therefore agents that reduce expression or inhibit function of a gene or pathway which is already compromised by genetic mutation in the tumour are likely to have more effect on such a tumour than on surrounding normal tissues with fully functional repair pathways. This idea remains speculative, and requires a detailed knowledge of deregulated pathways in individual tumours. An example from the chemotherapy world is the dramatically increased effect of PARP inhibitors in tumours with reduced homologous recombination, such as are found in *BRCA1/2* heterozygous individuals because BRCA genes are important for homologous recombination (Helleday *et al.*, 2007). Similar combinations with radiation are therefore being sought, but, without such tumour specificity, the therapeutic gain from using general radiosensitizers will remain limited.

Of the three main factors affecting the response to fractionated irradiation, hypoxia remains the most obvious tumour-specific target (Table 23.2), since tumours almost always contain hypoxic areas whereas normal tissues rarely do. Tumour proliferation, or repopulation, can be attacked with anti-proliferative drugs. These drugs will also adversely affect proliferating normal tissues leading to enhanced early reactions, but should have much less effect on the dose-limiting late-reacting normal tissues.

23.4 PATIENT INDIVIDUALIZATION

The goal of much current research is to develop rapid and robust methods enabling us to understand enough about each patient and their tumour to be able to choose the best treatment for that individual. At present, treatment choice is usually based on parameters such as tumour site, histological type, tumour stage and performance status. Within these broad categories, some tumours show less response to radiotherapy than others. If these tumours could be identified before treatment, alternative therapies might be selected that may give a better chance of cure than the standard therapy. This may involve one of the targeted therapies discussed above.

Individual patients also differ in their tolerance of radiation therapy. Among a group of patients given the same treatment protocol, some suffer more severe normal-tissue reactions than others. It is these severe reactors that limit the dose of radiation that can be prescribed to a group of patients. If severe reactors could be identified prior to therapy it might be possible to improve their management (e.g. by reducing their treatment dose, applying anti-fibrosis or anti-thrombotic therapies, etc.) as well as that of the rest of the patient group (e.g. by increasing their dose).

The following sections will deal with these two aspects of the individualization of radiation therapy: predicting tumour response and predicting normal-tissue response.

23.5 WHAT DETERMINES TUMOUR RESPONSE AFTER RADIOTHERAPY?

Determinants of tumour response to radiotherapy can be put into three broad categories: intrinsic radiosensitivity, proliferation rate and the extent of hypoxia. These are largely independent, such that a group of intrinsically radiosensitive tumours could have a range of proliferation rates and degrees of hypoxia; a group of tumours with high proliferation rates could have a range of radiosensitivities and degrees of hypoxia, etc. These three factors should thus be considered separately, and the goal is to measure them all to maximize the chance of accurately predicting response. In addition to these radiobiological parameters, other factors that can determine success or failure are tumour size at the time of treatment and the metastatic potential of the tumour. Large tumours are harder to control than small tumours simply because there are more cells to kill, which will require higher doses. This will be true even if intrinsic radiosensitivity, hypoxia and repopulation rates are equal at small and large tumour sizes. Tumour size should therefore be taken into account when assessing the performance of a predictive assay. Metastatic potential is clearly important for survival but should be considered separately from factors affecting local tumour control.

23.6 MEASURING SINGLE PARAMETERS

Intrinsic radiosensitivity

Malignant tumours are intrinsically genetically unstable, and there is ample evidence from cell lines, animal tumour models and in the clinic that this leads to a wide variation in intrinsic radiosensitivity, even between tumours of similar origin and histological type. Attempts have been made to assess the radiosensitivity of human tumours by explanting cells directly from biopsies, irradiating them in culture and measuring colony-forming ability, usually specifying surviving cell fraction after 2 Gy (SF2). Such studies have shown that tumour cell radiosensitivity is a significant and independent prognostic factor for radiotherapy outcome in carcinoma of both the cervix (West *et al.*, 1997) and head and neck (Bjork-Eriksson *et al.*, 2000). The disadvantages of the colony assay are its poor success rate for human tumours (<70 per cent) and the time needed to produce data (often up to 4 weeks). Subsequent studies have evaluated alternative assays that generate results in less than a week. Examples include chromosome damage, DNA damage, glutathione levels and apoptosis. However, comparing these assays with the 'gold standard' of clonogenic cell death in cell lines has shown variable results. Similarly, some clinical studies with such assays have shown correlations with radiotherapy outcome while others have not. It can be concluded that these functional, usually cell-based, assays have limited clinical utility as predictive assays but have been useful in confirming one mechanism underlying differences in response of tumours to radiotherapy.

Hypoxia

Tumour hypoxia is a key factor involved in determining not only resistance to treatment but also malignant progression. Evidence for an association between measurements of hypoxia in individual human tumours and response to radiation therapy has been summarized in Chapters 15–17.

Hypoxia has also been shown to be a negative prognostic factor after treatment with chemotherapy or surgery. The latter is consistent with data showing that hypoxia plays a key role in tumour progression by promoting both angiogenesis and metastasis (see Chapter 16).

One method to measure tumour hypoxia includes using thin polarographic glass electrodes (Eppendorf) which are inserted into tumours, producing several measurements along each track, thus providing multiple oxygen tension measurements per tumour. This direct method of measuring hypoxia has limitations in that it is only suitable for accessible tumours. Hypoxia-specific chemical probes such as pimonidazole (Raleigh et al., 2000) and EF5 (Evans et al., 2000) have been developed and are in clinical use. These and similar compounds are usually nitroimidazoles, which undergo bioreduction only under hypoxic conditions, followed by binding of reduced products onto macromolecules. Bound adducts can be detected with specific antibodies, allowing measurement by immunohistochemistry, immunofluorescence or flow cytometry. Some studies have shown a good correlation of pimonidazole binding with outcome after radiotherapy, as in head and neck cancer (Kaanders et al., 2002), while others have not, as in cervix cancer (Nordsmark et al., 2006).

The use of fluorinated derivatives of such bioreductive drugs also allows their detection by non-invasive positron emission tomography (PET) (Krause et al., 2006). This approach has the additional advantage of sampling the whole tumour and not just a small part of it. These drugs depend upon hypoxia for their reduction, although there are other factors that can influence their quantification and make them a less direct measure of hypoxia than is the case with electrodes. However, such agents are useful for quantifying hypoxia in human tumours, although they require administration of a drug. Other methods that are being evaluated to measure tumour hypoxia in the clinic include cross-sectional imaging using computed tomography (CT), magnetic resonance spectroscopic (MRS) imaging and magnetic resonance imaging (MRI) (Padhani et al., 2007).

Another possible surrogate marker of hypoxia is tumour vascularity, because of the known association between hypoxia and angiogenesis, and the fact that oxygen is delivered via a tumour blood supply that varies from ordered to chaotic. A variety of methods have been used to score vascularity, including intercapillary distance, vascular density, vascular 'hot-spots' and the proportion of tumour areas greater than a fixed distance from a vessel. Some of these methods have shown a positive correlation with outcome, while others have been negative (West et al., 2001a).

Repopulation

The importance of tumour proliferation is most clearly shown by the higher doses required to control a tumour when overall treatment time is increased (see Chapters 8 and 10). Further evidence comes from studies showing loss of local tumour control as a result of gaps in treatment, whether planned or unplanned. There is also increasing evidence from randomized trials that accelerated regimes can improve outcome (Chapter 10).

Methods for measuring tumour proliferation include counting the mitotic index (proportion of mitoses in tissue sections), determining the proportion of cells in the S phase of the cell cycle by DNA flow cytometry, measuring the tumour potential doubling time (T_{pot}) with thymidine analogues such as iododeoxyuridine (IdUrd) and bromodeoxyuridine (BrdUrd), and using antibodies to detect proliferation-associated proteins. A multicentre analysis of over 470 head and neck cancer patients treated with radiotherapy alone showed a lack of significance of T_{pot} as a predictor (Begg et al., 1999). A number of other studies have shown a significant although usually weak correlation between labelling index and radiotherapy outcome. Therefore pretreatment labelling index (LI) or T_{pot} measurements are apparently not sufficiently robust for determining tumour cell proliferation during radiotherapy. Proliferation, or repopulation, during fractionated radiotherapy is clearly an important factor determining outcome, but reliable ways to measure it are not yet available. A greater understanding at the cell and molecular levels is needed of why, in some tumours, radiation damage leads to an accelerated repopulation response, but in others it does not. This may be related to differences in the cytokine and growth-factor pathways.

23.7 MEASURING MULTIPLE PARAMETERS (GENOME WIDE)

The response of a tumour to radiotherapy is complex, determined broadly by the three factors mentioned above (intrinsic radiosensitivity, hypoxia and repopulation), each in turn controlled by many genes and pathways, some of which may be dysfunctional or overactive in a particular tumour. It is therefore unlikely that measuring a single factor, or expression of single genes, will provide a reliable predictor of how the tumour will respond to treatment. To maximize the chance of reliably predicting the success of a treatment in an individual, multiple factors, or multiple genes, need to be measured, both in the tumour and in the patient.

Methods for measuring genetic alterations on a genome-wide scale have made enormous progress in the last few years, including those for studying DNA changes, mRNA expression and protein expression. Application of these methods has already shown great promise for tumour diagnosis and prognosis, in addition to providing powerful new methods for fundamental studies of tumour (and other) biology. These genome-wide assays are now being applied to improve prediction in cancer treatments (see Fig. 23.1 for summary scheme).

The DNA level (comparative genomic hybridization, methylation)

Comparative genomic hybridization (CGH) allows tumour and normal-tissue DNA to be compared, producing a map of the loci in the chromosomes which are either deleted or amplified in the tumour (Pinkel and Albertson, 2005). This was originally achieved by hybridizing fluorescently labelled DNAs (e.g. tumour DNA green, normal DNA red) to metaphase spreads of normal cells. This technique has been superseded by hybridizing the labelled DNAs to a glass slide on which thousands of DNA probes, each representing a part of the genomic DNA, are spotted in an array (called array CGH, or aCGH). The advantage is reproducibility of the arrays, greater resolution because of the use of small DNA probes spaced closely on the array, and greater flexibility (widely spaced probes covering the whole genome, or closely spaced probes for part of a chromosome). Each of the observed genetic alterations covers megabases of DNA, but this is often sufficient to indicate genes of interest. Patterns of genomic changes have been correlated with outcome in several studies, although few after radiation (van den Broek *et al.*, 2007). Matching such genomic DNA changes with gene expression data (microarrays, see below) can help pinpoint relevant genomic regions and relevant genes (Adler *et al.*, 2006).

Methylation is a further factor at the DNA level which affects gene expression. Methylation of cytosines in promoter regions of genes can switch

LEVEL   PROCESS   ASSAY

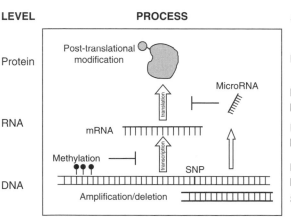

Proteomics

MicroRNA profiling

Expression profiling

Methylation profiling

SNP, CGH

Figure 23.1 Genetic screening methods. The genome can be screened at three levels (left) using different assays (right). The scheme (middle) shows the relationship between the biological processes. Combining results from more than one assay will give a better indication of the deregulation of important pathways, which could then be targets of therapy. CGH, comparative genomic hybridization; SNP, single nucleotide polymorphism.

them off by altering the binding of specific proteins (transcription factors) necessary to initiate transcription. A number of methods have been designed to measure methylation status, and although these are not quite yet genome wide, they are likely to become so in the near future. Methods are based on affinity purification of methylated DNA, or fractionation of (un)methylated DNA using methyl-sensitive restriction enzymes, or chemical modification of unmethylated cytosines; in each case, microarray detection can be used for monitoring many loci. Such measurements, representing the epigenetic status of the genome, are also likely to help monitor which pathways are deregulated in tumours.

The RNA level (microarrays)

Expression microarrays are small chips (often glass slides) containing many thousands of DNA sequences in spots, one DNA sequence per spot. The DNA can be cDNA (messenger RNA back-translated into more stable complementary DNA) but more usually oligomers (short DNA chains) representing the partial sequence of a gene. Messenger RNA, representing all expressed genes, is extracted from the tumour or other sample of interest, then fluorescently labelled and added to the chip, where each labelled RNA hybridizes only to the spot for that gene having the complementary DNA sequence. Genes which are highly expressed in the tumour then result in bright spots on the array, while lowly expressed genes show low signals. After hybridization, the array is scanned automatically and rapidly to measure the expression of all genes. Current arrays can hold almost all the genes in the human genome, estimated to be around 30 000.

Several studies have reported finding gene sets, or signatures, which predict the response to drugs or to radiation. In these studies, expression profiles of each sample are correlated with treatment sensitivity using specific statistical (bioinformatics) methods, such as supervised hierarchical clustering. Some of these studies have employed a range of cell lines with different treatment sensitivities, while others have studied a series of clinical tumours in which mRNA has been extracted

from pretreatment biopsies and the results correlated with subsequent treatment outcome. The technique thus shows promise as a predictor of outcome. However, at the present time, there are almost no examples of predictive signatures specific for a particular treatment such as radiation, although signatures have been found for combined radiation and drug treatments (Pramana *et al.*, 2007).

Before such expression signatures can be used in the clinic to select treatment options, they require rigorous testing and validation. Usually this first involves a single institute trial in which a signature is found on a group of patient samples and tested on a second independent group. This is usually done on frozen samples from patients for whom treatment outcome is already known. If sensitivity and specificity are high for distinguishing good and poor outcomes, the signature should then be tested prospectively on a larger group of patients, preferably in a multicentre trial. At the time of writing, only a few signatures, mainly for breast cancer, and mainly for predicting the probability of metastasis, are in the prospective stage (Bogaerts *et al.*, 2006). Most studies have been underpowered (low sample numbers) and/or have not included appropriate independent validation.

The statistical methods that are employed to extract a set of genes distinguishing good and bad response consider each gene independently, and are also independent of any biological knowledge. The hope is that the genes appearing in the signature are causal for the response, and that they, or their molecular pathways, also represent drug targets for intervention. In this way, not only can response be predicted, but appropriate treatments could be indicated. A second approach starts from the biology. A set of genes on known pathways relevant to the treatment can be tested, such as DNA repair genes, or hypoxia-inducible genes or proliferation genes. The rationale is that, while individual genes may not provide a strong enough predictor, several genes on the same pathway might do so. Such gene sets can be tested on clinical microarray data to see if they can split tumours into good and bad responders. This approach has shown good success with hypoxia (Chi *et al.*, 2006), a serum response signature (Chang *et al.*, 2005) and others. Signatures have also been derived from cell lines with different radiosensitivities, although such radiosensitivity signatures have not yet been adequately tested in clinical series.

The RNA level (microRNA)

MicroRNAs (miRNA) are small non-coding RNAs of 19–24 nucleotides that generally down-regulate gene expression by inhibiting protein translation. It is estimated that miRNAs affect expression of up to 30 per cent of the genes in the mammalian genome. They have been shown to play a role in development, differentiation and apoptosis, and to be involved in initiation and progression of human cancers. More recently, miRNA profiling has shown the potential to predict treatment outcome (Garzon et al., 2006). The use of miRNA profiling rather than, or together with, mRNA profiling and other genome-wide techniques holds promise for more accurate prediction in the future.

The protein level (proteomics)

Since proteins (rather than mRNA) carry out the actual cellular functions, expression profiling at the protein level should, in principle, be better than at the mRNA level. However, proteins are an order of magnitude more diverse in structure, making such profiling more difficult. Despite this, rapid progress is being made, including antibody chips and mass spectrometry in various forms (Domon and Aebersold, 2006). Proteomics using powerful mass spectrometry methods as clinical predictors has so far been restricted mainly to the study of serum proteins, and usually for early detection and treatment monitoring.

In addition, simple immunohistochemistry has been made more 'high throughput' by the use of tissue microarrays, in which hundreds of small paraffin-embedded tumour samples from different patients are placed on one microscope slide (Simon and Sauter, 2002). Staining with a particular antibody can then be done simultaneously for all tumours in a clinical series. Scoring and registration of the data can also be automated. This is far from genome wide, since candidate protein targets (and the antibodies which detect

them) must be chosen based on prior knowledge, and are usually restricted to up to 30 markers. However, this method is ideal for testing potential predictive markers in retrospective series.

23.8 PREDICTION OF NORMAL-TISSUE TOLERANCE

The existence of individuals with extreme sensitivity to ionizing radiation was first realized with the publication of a study showing the hypersensitivity of fibroblasts cultured from a patient with ataxia telangiectasia (Taylor et al., 1975). Then, in the 1980s, increasing evidence was found for a range of radiosensitivities within the population even without known genetic syndromes. Further evidence for differences in cellular radiosensitivity as a determinant of normal-tissue response to radiotherapy came from studies showing that inherent differences between individuals dominated normal-tissue reactions more than other contributing factors (Turesson et al., 1996). It was realized that the 5 per cent most sensitive individuals within a patient population limit the dose that can be safely applied in radiotherapy, but as it is not known beforehand who these sensitive patients are, radiation doses to most patients may be too low, jeopardizing the overall chance of cure.

In the 1990s, studies were carried out to test whether the in vitro radiosensitivity of normal cells could predict the severity of normal-tissue damage. In general, no correlations were seen with acute radiation effects. Several small studies showed correlations between fibroblast radiosensitivity and the severity of late effects (e.g. Johansen et al., 1994) but were not confirmed in subsequent larger studies (Russell et al., 1998; Peacock et al., 2000). There have been two large studies using peripheral blood lymphocytes and both showed that their radiosensitivity correlated with the severity of late effects (West et al., 2001b).

More rapid assays have also been evaluated, including the measurement of chromosome damage (Russell et al., 1995) and DNA damage (Kiltie et al., 1999). Although some significant correlations with late effects have been reported, other studies have shown no relationship. A general problem has been that experimental (assay) variability has been relatively large compared with inter-individual differences in radiosensitivity.

Although clonogenic cell survival is a crucial concept for local tumour control, it may be less significant for late normal-tissue damage. For example, the radiosensitivity of fibroblasts from a fibrosis-prone mouse strain was found to be identical to that from a fibrosis-resistant strain (Dileto and Travis, 1996). Therefore, other factors clearly influence the response of normal tissues to radiation. Cytokines are known to play an important role (Rodemann and Bamberg, 1995; Bentzen, 2006). For example, transforming growth factor-β (TGF-β) is a key cytokine in fibrosis development (see Chapter 13.3), influencing fibroblast proliferation and differentiation. This is a growing and important area of research, and increased understanding of the molecular pathogenesis of radiation

injury may lead to better predictions of the radiation response of normal tissues.

Genome-wide screens are beginning to be used for predicting adverse reactions to radiotherapy. Single nucleotide polymorphisms (SNPs) in candidate genes thought to influence normal-tissue radiation injury have shown some promising results (Chang-Claude *et al.*, 2005; Andreassen *et al.*, 2006). Expression profiling of patient lymphocytes irradiated *ex vivo* has also produced signatures correlating with the severity of normal-tissue injury (Svensson *et al.*, 2006). The results of all these studies need validating in larger independent patient series. The advantage of the SNP approach is that easily accessible lymphocytes are ideal for the measurements. In contrast, expression profiles in lymphocytes may not be a relevant surrogate for the target tissue (usually non-lymphoid) or

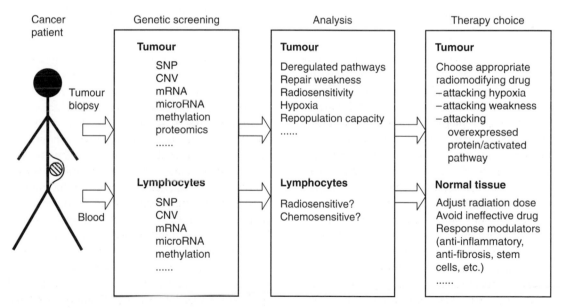

Figure 23.2 A schematic representation of how genetic screening can be combined with new molecular-targeted agents for individualizing therapy in the future. Samples are taken from both tumour and normal tissue and subjected to genome-wide screening methods. Analyses related to sensitivity, resistance and pathway deregulation will indicate where to attack each tumour, while protecting or sparing normal tissues. Examples: phosphoinositide-3-kinase (PI3K) pathway activation in the tumour together with high hypoxia would indicate attacking both these problems (e.g. anti-*AKT*/*EGFR*/*RAS* drug, plus hypoxic cytotoxin or hypoxic radiosensitizer). If normal-tissue screening indicated the patient is fibrosis-prone, anti-fibrosis therapies [related to the transforming growth factor-β (TGF-β) pathway] could be applied during follow-up. CNV, copy number variation; SNP, single nucleotide polymorphism.

response type, for example fibrosis or telangiectasia. In addition to SNPs, variations in DNA copy number and in DNA methylation patterns are now also being investigated and may further increase predictive power in the future.

23.9 HOW SHOULD CLINICIANS RESPOND TO PREDICTION RESULTS?

If and when reliable predictive assays are developed, their use will depend on the availability of alternative treatments. For example, patients with very hypoxic tumours could be assigned to treatments that include hypoxia-modifying or hypoxia-exploiting agents (e.g. ARCON, tirapazamine, etc; see Chapter 17). The type of hypoxia (chronic or acute) may also determine which modifying strategy to use. Tumours with fast repopulation potential would be candidates for accelerated fractionation, or radiotherapy combined with drugs designed to combat proliferation (e.g. EGFR inhibitors). In the short term, patients with radioresistant tumours may benefit from switching to an alternative therapeutic modality such as surgery or chemotherapy, combined chemoradiotherapy or the radiation dose to the tumour could be increased using some form of conformal radiotherapy where possible. In the long term, the goal is to be able to obtain a complete genetic picture of each tumour, thereby understanding why a tumour is radioresistant, allowing a rational choice of tumour-specific radiosensitizing drugs of the types described in the first section of this chapter. Rapid progress is being made in developing techniques for monitoring tumour genetics and this, coupled with the increasing pace of development of molecular-targeted drugs, should mean that more tumour-specific therapies with lower toxicity should emerge in the not too distant future. Finally, if reliable information were available for predicting the risk of severe normal-tissue effects, possible strategies would be to reduce the radiation dose for radiosensitive individuals, to offer a radioprotective agent (assuming the agent does not also protect tumours), or to use a post-radiotherapy strategy designed to reduce vascular and parenchymal consequences of irradiation, such as anti-TGF-β and anti-inflammatory approaches.

23.10 SUMMARY

Designing treatments which are tailored to the individual patient requires, first, extensive knowledge of the genetics of that individual and of their tumour. Second, the availability of a considerable array of agents that attack specific genes or pathways is essential. An agent (drug, antibody, peptide, siRNA, etc.) can then be chosen for that individual with the greatest chance of a therapeutic effect when combined with radiation (Fig. 23.2). With the rapid development of genome-wide screening approaches, providing massive new information on tumour genetics, there has been considerable progress in the area of outcome prediction. It is hoped and anticipated that this will soon lead to more rational therapies.

Key points

1. Impeding DNA repair pathways can significantly increase cellular radiosensitivity. However, there is no known consistent tumour specificity concerning expression or function of DNA repair genes, or ATM and other damage detectors, or for chromatin modifications associated with repair or for the NFκB pathway. Hypoxia is the most tumour-specific therapeutic target.

2. Intrinsic tumour cell radiosensitivity is a significant and independent prognostic factor for radiotherapy outcome in carcinomas both of the cervix and of the head and neck, but functional, usually cell-based, measurements have limited clinical utility as predictive assays.

3. Tumour hypoxia has been shown to be a negative prognostic factor after treatment with radiotherapy, chemotherapy or surgery and the predictive capability of several pathology-based and PET/CT/MRI markers is being evaluated clinically.

4. Tumour proliferation, or repopulation, during fractionated radiotherapy, is an important factor determining outcome, but no reliable ways to measure it are yet available.

5. Methods for studying DNA changes, mRNA expression and protein expression have already shown great promise in tumour diagnosis and prognosis. These genome-wide assays are now being applied to improve prediction in cancer treatments.

6. Reliable and rapid tests are not yet available for predicting the risk of severe normal-tissue effects.

■ BIBLIOGRAPHY

Adler AS, Lin M, Horlings H, Nuyten DS, van de Vijver MJ, Chang HY (2006). Genetic regulators of large-scale transcriptional signatures in cancer. *Nat Genet* **38**: 421–30.

Andreassen CN, Alsner J, Overgaard M, Sorensen FB, Overgaard J (2006). Risk of radiation-induced subcutaneous fibrosis in relation to single nucleotide polymorphisms in TGFB1, SOD2, XRCC1, XRCC3, APEX and ATM – a study based on DNA from formalin fixed paraffin embedded tissue samples. *Int J Radiat Biol* **82**: 577–86.

Begg AC, Haustermans K, Hart AA *et al.* (1999). The value of pretreatment cell kinetic parameters as predictors for radiotherapy outcome in head and neck cancer: a multicenter analysis. *Radiother Oncol* **50**: 13–23.

Belka C, Jendrossek V, Pruschy M, Vink S, Verheij M, Budach W (2004). Apoptosis-modulating agents in combination with radiotherapy-current status and outlook. *Int J Radiat Oncol Biol Phys* **58**: 542–54.

Bentzen SM (2006). Preventing or reducing late side effects of radiation therapy: radiobiology meets molecular pathology. *Nat Rev Cancer* **6**: 702–13.

Bjork-Eriksson T, West C, Karlsson E, Mercke C (2000). Tumor radiosensitivity (SF2) is a prognostic factor for local control in head and neck cancers. *Int J Radiat Oncol Biol Phys* **46**: 13–19.

Bogaerts J, Cardoso F, Buyse M *et al.* (2006). Gene signature evaluation as a prognostic tool: challenges in the design of the MINDACT trial. *Nat Clin Pract Oncol* **3**: 540–51.

Cerna D, Camphausen K, Tofilon PJ (2006). Histone deacetylation as a target for radiosensitization. *Curr Top Dev Biol* **73**: 173–204.

Chang HY, Nuyten DS, Sneddon JB *et al.* (2005). Robustness, scalability, and integration of a wound-response gene expression signature in predicting breast cancer survival. *Proc Natl Acad Sci USA* **102**: 3738–43.

Chang-Claude J, Popanda O, Tan XL *et al.* (2005). Association between polymorphisms in the DNA repair genes, XRCC1, APE1, and XPD and acute side effects of radiotherapy in breast cancer patients. *Clin Cancer Res* **11**: 4802–9.

Chi JT, Wang Z, Nuyten DS *et al.* (2006). Gene expression programs in response to hypoxia: cell type specificity and prognostic significance in human cancers. *PLoS Med* **3**: e47.

Choudhury A, Cuddihy A, Bristow RG (2006). Radiation and new molecular agents part I: targeting ATM-ATR checkpoints, DNA repair, and the proteasome. *Semin Radiat Oncol* **16**: 51–8.

Dileto CL, Travis EL (1996). Fibroblast radiosensitivity *in vitro* and lung fibrosis *in vivo*: comparison between a fibrosis-prone and fibrosis-resistant mouse strain. *Radiat Res* **146**: 61–7.

Domon B, Aebersold R (2006). Mass spectrometry and protein analysis. *Science* **312**: 212–17.

Evans SM, Hahn S, Pook DR *et al.* (2000). Detection of hypoxia in human squamous cell carcinoma by EF5 binding. *Cancer Res* **60**: 2018–24.

Garzon R, Fabbri M, Cimmino A, Calin GA, Croce CM (2006). MicroRNA expression and function in cancer. *Trends Mol Med* **12**: 580–7.

Hanahan D, Weinberg RA (2000). The hallmarks of cancer. *Cell* **100**: 57–70.

Helleday T, Lo J, van Gent DC, Engelward BP (2007). DNA double-strand break repair: from mechanistic understanding to cancer treatment. *DNA Repair (Amst)* **6**: 923–35.

Hickson I, Zhao Y, Richardson CJ *et al.* (2004). Identification and characterization of a novel and specific inhibitor of the ataxia-telangiectasia mutated kinase ATM. *Cancer Res* **64**: 9152–9.

Johansen J, Bentzen SM, Overgaard J, Overgaard M (1994). Evidence for a positive correlation between *in vitro* radiosensitivity of normal human skin fibroblasts and the occurrence of subcutaneous fibrosis after radiotherapy. *Int J Radiat Biol* **66**: 407–12.

Kaanders JH, Wijffels KI, Marres HA *et al.* (2002). Pimonidazole binding and tumor vascularity predict for treatment outcome in head and neck cancer. *Cancer Res* **62**: 7066–74.

Kiltie AE, Ryan AJ, Swindell R *et al.* (1999). A correlation between residual radiation-induced DNA double-strand breaks in cultured fibroblasts and late radiotherapy reactions in breast cancer patients. *Radiother Oncol* **51**: 55–65.

Krause BJ, Beck R, Souvatzoglou M, Piert M (2006). PET and PET/CT studies of tumor tissue oxygenation. *Q J Nucl Med Mol Imaging* **50**: 28–43.

Liu L, Gerson SL (2004). Therapeutic impact of methoxyamine: blocking repair of abasic sites in the base excision repair pathway. *Curr Opin Investig Drugs* **5**: 623–7.

Luo M, Kelley MR (2004). Inhibition of the human apurinic/apyrimidinic endonuclease (APE1) repair activity and sensitization of breast cancer cells to DNA alkylating agents with lucanthone. *Anticancer Res* **24**: 2127–34.

Magne N, Toillon RA, Bottero V *et al.* (2006). NF-kappaB modulation and ionizing radiation: mechanisms and future directions for cancer treatment. *Cancer Lett* **231**: 158–68.

Nordsmark M, Loncaster J, Aquino-Parsons C *et al.* (2006). The prognostic value of pimonidazole and tumour pO_2 in human cervix carcinomas after radiation therapy: a prospective international multi-center study. *Radiother Oncol* **80**: 123–31.

Padhani AR, Krohn KA, Lewis JS, Alber M (2007). Imaging oxygenation of human tumours. *Eur Radiol* **17**: 861–72.

Peacock J, Ashton A, Bliss J *et al.* (2000). Cellular radiosensitivity and complication risk after curative radiotherapy. *Radiother Oncol* **55**: 173–8.

Pinkel D, Albertson DG (2005). Array comparative genomic hybridization and its applications in cancer. *Nat Genet* **37**(Suppl): S11–7.

Pramana J, van den Brekel MW, van Velthuysen ML *et al.* (2007). Gene expression profiling to predict outcome after chemoradiation in head and neck cancer. *Int J Radiat Oncol Biol Phys* **69**: 1544–52.

Raleigh JA, Chou SC, Calkins-Adams DP, Ballenger CA, Novotny DB, Varia MA (2000). A clinical study of hypoxia and metallothionein protein expression in squamous cell carcinomas. *Clin Cancer Res* **6**: 855–62.

Rodemann HP, Bamberg M (1995). Cellular basis of radiation-induced fibrosis. *Radiother Oncol* **35**: 83–90.

Russell NS, Arlett CF, Bartelink H, Begg AC (1995). Use of fluorescence *in situ* hybridization to determine the relationship between chromosome aberrations and cell survival in eight human fibroblast strains. *Int J Radiat Biol* **68**: 185–96.

Russell NS, Grummels A, Hart AA *et al.* (1998). Low predictive value of intrinsic fibroblast radiosensitivity for fibrosis development following radiotherapy for breast cancer. *Int J Radiat Biol* **73**: 661–70.

Simon R, Sauter G (2002). Tissue microarrays for miniaturized high-throughput molecular profiling of tumors. *Exp Hematol* **30**: 1365–72.

Sprong D, Janssen HL, Vens C, Begg AC (2006). Resistance of hypoxic cells to ionizing radiation is influenced by homologous recombination status. *Int J Radiat Oncol Biol Phys* **64**: 562–72.

Svensson JP, Stalpers LJ, Esveldt-van Lange RE *et al.* (2006). Analysis of gene expression using gene sets discriminates cancer patients with and without late radiation toxicity. *PLoS Med* **3**: e422.

Taylor AM, Harnden DG, Arlett CF *et al.* (1975). Ataxia telangiectasia: a human mutation with abnormal radiation sensitivity. *Nature* **258**: 427–9.

Thompson LH, Brookman KW, Jones NJ, Allen SA, Carrano AV (1990). Molecular cloning of the human XRCC1 gene, which corrects defective DNA strand break repair and sister chromatid exchange. *Mol Cell Biol* **10**: 6160–71.

Turesson I, Nyman J, Holmberg E, Oden A (1996). Prognostic factors for acute and late skin reactions in radiotherapy patients. *Int J Radiat Oncol Biol Phys* **36**: 1065–75.

Valerie K, Yacoub A, Hagan MP *et al.* (2007). Radiation-induced cell signaling: inside-out and outside-in. *Mol Cancer Ther* **6**: 789–801.

van den Broek GB, Wreesmann VB, van den Brekel MW, Rasch CR, Balm AJ, Rao PH (2007). Genetic abnormalities associated with chemoradiation resistance of head and neck squamous cell carcinoma. *Clin Cancer Res* **13**: 4386–91.

Vermeulen C, Verwijs-Janssen M, Cramers P, Begg AC, Vens C (2007). Role for DNA polymerase beta in response to ionizing radiation. *DNA Repair (Amst)* **6**: 202–12.

Weber CN, Cerniglia GJ, Maity A, Gupta AK (2007). Bortezomib sensitizes human head and neck carcinoma cells SQ20B to radiation. *Cancer Biol Ther* **6**: 156–9.

West CM, Cooper RA, Loncaster JA, Wilks DP, Bromley M (2001a). Tumor vascularity: a histological measure of angiogenesis and hypoxia. *Cancer Res* **61**: 2907–10.

West CM, Davidson SE, Elyan SA *et al.* (2001b). Lymphocyte radiosensitivity is a significant prognostic factor for morbidity in carcinoma of the cervix. *Int J Radiat Oncol Biol Phys* **51**: 10–5.

West CM, Davidson SE, Roberts SA, Hunter RD (1997). The independence of intrinsic radiosensitivity as a prognostic factor for patient response to radiotherapy of carcinoma of the cervix. *Br J Cancer* **76**: 1184–90.

Xu B, Kim ST, Lim DS, Kastan MB (2002). Two molecularly distinct G(2)/M checkpoints are induced by ionizing irradiation. *Mol Cell Biol* **22**: 1049–59.

■ FURTHER READING

West CM, McKay MJ, Holscher T *et al.* (2005). Molecular markers predicting radiotherapy response: report and recommendations from an International Atomic Energy Agency technical meeting. *Int J Radiat Oncol Biol Phys* **62**: 1264–73.

Protons and other ions in radiotherapy

WOLFGANG DÖRR AND MICHAEL C. JOINER

24.1 INTRODUCTION

The physical characteristics of light and heavy ion radiation beams, as well as of neutrons, were introduced in Chapter 6. In this chapter, we will review the biological properties of ions (and neutrons) with relevance to radiotherapy, and summarize the recent experience and status of proton and heavy ion radiotherapy.

The major difference between radiotherapy with photons and ions is in the spatial distribution of physical dose. For photons, independent of energy, the maximum dose is deposited close to the entrance surface of the matter that is penetrated. In contrast, ions enter tissue with a low dose and the maximum dose deposition occurs within the so-called Bragg peak, at a depth depending on the beam energy. Behind this Bragg peak region, for protons no significant further dose is deposited, and in the case of heavy ions only a minor dose, owing to some nuclear fragments, is deposited.

A second advantage of ions over megavoltage X-rays is the steep dose gradient at the beam margins, with a reduction from 90 per cent to 10 per cent within few millimetres. This sharpness in the beam definition is even more pronounced for heavy ions than for protons, by a factor of approximately three. Moreover, in the case of heavy ions,

a small amount of positron emission (^{11}C, ^{15}O) is generated via nuclear reactions, and this can be exploited to visualize the dose distribution by positron emission tomography (PET).

24.2 BIOLOGICAL CHARACTERISTICS OF HIGH-LINEAR ENERGY TRANSFER (LET) BEAMS

Figure 24.1 illustrates that only minor changes occur in the total dose required for various biological effects (acutely responding tissues indicated with dashed lines and late-responding tissues with solid lines) with changes in dose per fraction for high-LET radiation (neutrons). Compared with low-LET radiation, particularly for late tissue endpoints, these changes are significantly less pronounced (Withers *et al.*, 1982). Figure 24.1 should be compared with Fig. 8.1, which shows these relationships for a similar range of tissues exposed to fractionated low-LET radiation. This comparison is illustrated schematically in Fig. 24.2 and the following conclusions can be drawn:

1 There is much less effect of dose fractionation (i.e. of dose per fraction) for high-LET radiation, either in acutely responding or in

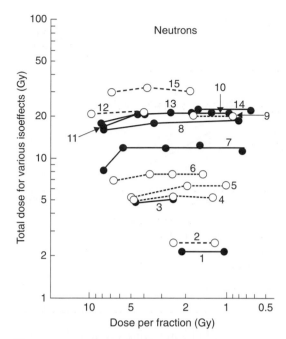

Figure 24.1 Summary of published data on isoeffect curves for neutrons as a function of dose per fraction in various tissues of mice and rats. Broken lines indicate data on acute-responding tissues; solid lines are for late-responding tissues. Compare with Fig. 8.1. Key: 1, thyroid function; 2, haemopoietic colonies; 3, vertebral growth; 4, spermatogenic colonies; 5, fibrosarcomas; 6, jejunum colonies; 7, lung LD_{50}; 8, lumbar nerve root function; 9 and 12, skin desquamation; 10, skin contraction; 11, skin late changes; 13, spinal cord; 14, oral mucosa necrosis; 15, skin necrosis. From Withers *et al.* (1982), with permission.

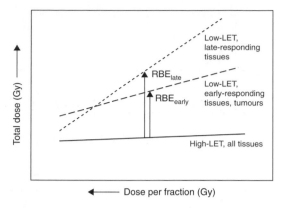

Figure 24.2 Illustration of the changes in isoeffective total doses with decreasing dose per fraction for acute- and late-responding tissues and tumours, for irradiation with high-linear energy transfer (LET) or low-LET radiation, respectively. The corresponding definition of relative biological effectiveness (RBE) values is indicated.

late-responding tissues (Fig. 24.1). Tissue responses to high-LET radiations (heavy ions, neutrons) therefore demonstrate substantially higher α/β ratios than low-LET (photon) beam responses, as is also the case for cell lines *in vitro* (see Fig. 6.2).

2. For photons, the total dose increases more steeply with decreasing dose per fraction for late-responding than for early-responding tissues, reflecting the smaller α/β ratios for late-responding tissues (see Chapters 8 and 9). The relative biological effectiveness (RBE) therefore rises rapidly with decreasing dose per fraction for late-responding tissues and more gradually for early-responding tissues.

3. The RBE values for late tissue responses are not intrinsically higher than for acute responses. However, because of their faster increase as dose is reduced, the RBE values for late tissue responses tend to be higher than for early tissue response at lower doses per fraction, especially at or below 2 Gy per (X-ray) fraction.

To further illustrate this last point, Fig. 24.3 demonstrates the rise in neutron RBE (compared with photons) with decreasing dose per fraction in epidermis, as an example of an early-responding tissue, and kidney (a late-responding tissue). In this example, the RBE for d(16)-Be neutrons in kidney was greater than in epidermis at an X-ray dose per fraction of 2 Gy, but lower for a more highly penetrating p(62)-Be neutron therapy beam. Therefore, compared with conventional photon therapy, late renal damage would be increased more substantially relative to early reactions (and perhaps relative to tumour response) by treating with a low-energy neutron beam, but late renal injury would actually be spared with the high-energy neutron radiation.

It must be emphasized that these relationships are clearly specific for the tissues and the high-LET beams studied. Similar relationships between other early- and late-responding tissues may not follow

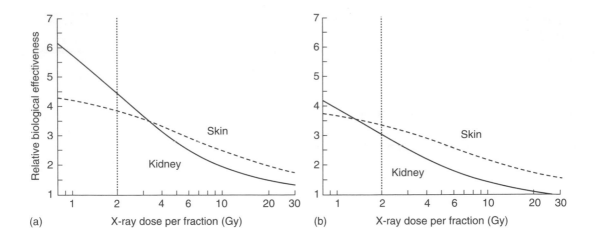

Figure 24.3 Comparison of relative biological effectiveness (RBE) values for mouse skin and kidney exposed to two different neutron beams: (a) d(16)-Be; (b) p(64)-Be. From Joiner (1988), with permission.

the same pattern and so must be evaluated individually in each case and for each treatment condition to determine whether high-LET radiation would result in a biological therapeutic gain. It is not true that late reactions are always worse after high-LET therapy for the same level of acute injury, but they may be in some cases unless the physical characteristics of a charged particle high-LET beam can be used to reduce the radiation dose to critical normal tissues. It should be noted that a d(16)-Be neutron beam has similar depth–dose characteristics to ortho-voltage X-rays, whereas a p(62)-Be neutron therapy beam can produce treatment plans comparable to a 4 MV X-ray beam.

Less comprehensive data are available on fractionation effects with heavy ion or proton beams. However, the loss of the fractionation dose-sparing effect, which has been described above for neutrons, is consistently less pronounced for heavy ions. However, protons must be considered – biologically, with regard to dose fractionation – as similar to photons. For both radiation qualities, heavy ions as well as protons, slight changes in RBE with dose per fraction cannot be excluded (Gerweck and Kozin, 1999). For these reasons, the number of fractions in ion radiotherapy protocols is currently close to that applied in photon therapy. For the biological reasons described above, higher doses per fraction and fewer fractions may

be possible, but supporting preclinical (*in vivo*) and clinical data are currently not available, and hence changes in fractionation protocols must be considered carefully.

24.3 DOSE SPECIFICATION AND ION RADIOTHERAPY PLANNING

For protons used in radiotherapy (in contrast to the extraterrestrial cosmic proton flux), a RBE factor of 1.1 is generally accepted and used routinely in clinical treatment planning programmes (Paganetti *et al.*, 2002). Most experimental studies on the biological effectiveness for various endpoints have yielded RBE values between 1.05 and 1.25 (Tepper *et al.*, 1977; Urano *et al.*, 1984; ICRP, 2003). However, there might be a higher RBE value for effects within the terminal few millimetres of the beam (Gerweck and Kozin, 1999).

For heavy ions, in the last *c.* 2 cm of the track, an increase in RBE is seen up to values of 2–4 (Kramer *et al.*, 2003). In the entrance channel, the biological effectiveness of heavy ions is considered only slightly higher than for protons. Complex mathematical/biophysical models are usually applied for heavy-ion treatment planning (Kramer and Scholz, 2000; Scholz *et al.*, 2006).

The dose in ion beam radiotherapy is described in gray equivalents (GyE) or cobalt gray equivalents (CGE). The GyE or CGE is equal to the measured physical dose in grays multiplied by the RBE factor. Note that the term 'equivalent dose' in sievert (Sv) is commonly used for radiation protection purposes, with a totally different meaning from that in the present context of therapy; these should not be confused (Wambersie *et al.*, 2006).

For radiotherapy applications, an ion beam must be extended in the lateral and longitudinal directions in order to adequately cover the clinical target volume. Depth variations can be achieved by passive absorbers (see Chapter 6, Section 6.6) or, in modern configurations, by active variation of the accelerator energy. Similarly, variations in width can be accomplished with passive devices such as scattering foils or with magnetic deflectors (pencil scanning beam). Use of beam scanning techniques will clearly result in a reduction of the normal tissue included in the high-dose volume. However, passive absorbers can increase the dose deposition outside the target volume (e.g. by neutrons that are generated at end energies $>10\,$MeV). Furthermore, proton and heavy ion beams are much more sensitive to tissue inhomogeneities than photons. Therefore, optimum conformation of the high-dose volume for minimization of normal-tissue exposure on one hand and best coverage of the planning target volume to avoid marginal recurrences on the other are highly demanding with regard to planning and technical execution of ion beam radiotherapy. Immobilization and image guidance are extremely important to limit set-up uncertainties to $<2\,$mm. In order to determine the necessary proton range, the density of tissue according to Hounsfield units obtained from planning computed tomography (CT) images is converted into stopping power of tissue.

The complexity of proton or heavy ion radiotherapy renders these treatments more expensive than photon radiation therapy. In a financial analysis (Goitein and Jermann, 2003), a ratio of 2.4 for cost per fraction of proton versus photon treatment was found. However, projected reductions in both construction and operational costs may reduce this ratio to 2 or even 1.5 (MacDonald *et al.*, 2006).

24.4 RADIOTHERAPY WITH PROTONS

More than 45 000 patients have so far been treated with proton therapy worldwide. The results of clinical studies with protons have recently been subject to comprehensive reviews (MacDonald *et al.*, 2006; Brada *et al.*, 2007; Lodge *et al.*, 2007; Olsen *et al.*, 2007), and will be briefly summarized here.

Most of the early treatments were performed at physics research facilities. Because of the limited time-slots for therapy, the vast majority of patients ($>20\,000$) have so far been treated for uveal melanoma, where the dose is delivered within a few days. Tumour control can be achieved in more than 95 per cent of the patients, with low rates of enucleation. Analysis of the available clinical data, however, has not provided unequivocal evidence that proton therapy is superior to photon irradiation in patients with ocular melanomas (Brada *et al.*, 2007).

Treatment of chordomas and chondrosarcomas at the base of the skull is clearly compromised by adjacent critical structures (brainstem, spinal cord, optic nerve and chiasm). The requirement of high doses in a precise location renders proton therapy attractive. In chondrosarcomas, 5-year local control rates can be as high as over 90 per cent, and are somewhat lower for chordomas, as well as for spinal and paraspinal tumours. The incidence of severe toxicities is clearly below 10 per cent. However, there are still insufficient clinical data available to formally compare toxicity after proton therapy and conventional treatment, for both chordoma and chondrosarcoma (Brada *et al.*, 2007).

Proton treatment of glioblastoma multiforme with 90 CGE in a combined proton–photon protocol resulted in a median survival time of 20 months, but the incidence of radionecrosis was high. Protons may also be used for single fraction radiosurgery, such as for vestibular schwannoma (Weber *et al.*, 2003) and other intracranial neoplasms.

At least 2000–3000 patients have received proton therapy for prostate cancer. The results with regard to tumour control have not been consistently better than with photons. However, fewer side-effects have been observed: standard photon techniques used over the last 30 years have resulted in severe side-effects in about 15 per cent of the patients; modern photon techniques are expected to reduce the incidence to 1–3 per cent, and proton treatment to ≤1 per cent (Cox, 2007). However, a comprehensive analysis (Lodge *et al.*, 2007) has shown an incidence of side-effects (≥grade 2) of 10–30 per cent for protons and 10–40 per cent for photons.

Other malignancies being tested with proton therapy are head and neck, breast, gastrointestinal and lung tumours (MacDonald *et al.*, 2006).

24.5 RADIOTHERAPY WITH HEAVY IONS

Heavy ion radiotherapy is more experimental than proton therapy, although some clinical data are available and have been reviewed (Schulz-Ertner *et al.*, 2003; Greco and Wolden, 2007; Lodge *et al.*, 2007). In a series of 67 patients treated with carbon ions for tumours of the base of skull (Schulz-Ertner *et al.*, 2003) with a median tumour dose of 60 GyE, actuarial 3-year local control rates were 100 per cent for chondrosarcomas and 81 per cent for chordomas, comparable to the results with protons. For squamous cell carcinomas, the results with carbon ion therapy seem also to be similar to protons or photons. For adenoid cystic carcinomas, higher local tumour control rates (>75 per cent) are found with carbon ions than with photons (<50 per cent) (Lodge *et al.*, 2007). For prostate tumours, 5-year local control rates of 95–100 per cent are reported, with ≥grade 2 genitourinary or gastrointestinal toxicity in 1–6 per cent of the patients.

Based on the biological properties of heavy ion beams (Section 24.2), with experimental evidence that higher doses per fraction are associated with a relatively more pronounced reduction in RBE (Fig. 24.2) for (late-responding) normal tissues compared with tumours (Denekamp *et al.*, 1997; Ando *et al.*, 2005), introduction of hypofractionated protocols has been suggested for clinical testing (Tsujii *et al.*, 2004; Schulz-Ertner and Tsujii, 2007).

24.6 SECOND CANCERS

Theoretically, radiotherapy with protons or other ions should, by a reduction of the integral dose outside the planning target volume, decline the risk of secondary tumours without compromising tumour control rates. Miralbell *et al.* (2002) compared the potential influence of proton dose distribution with that of conformal photon treatments or intensity-modulated radiotherapy (IMRT) for the risk of second malignancies. Protons (with or without intensity modulation) clearly decreased the estimated risk compared with photon planning (with or without intensity modulation). However, these expectations have not yet been validated in experimental or clinical studies. Moreover, the advantages of protons over photons may only apply if beam scanning is available, and not for passive modulation (Schneider *et al.*, 2002; Brenner and Hall, 2008), because of neutron generation (Section 24.3).

24.7 ION RADIOTHERAPY IN PAEDIATRIC ONCOLOGY

Radiotherapy in children must be considered more critical than in adult patients. Long-term growth deficiencies and developmental deficits must be expected. Moreover, children are at a higher risk for secondary tumours. In an analysis of children treated with radiation (Gold *et al.*, 2004), 8.3 per cent of patients developed a second cancer, mostly within the treatment field, with a median latency of 15.5 years. The cumulative risk of second cancer was 13 per cent at 30 years. Therefore, proton or heavy ion radiotherapy may be preferred for the treatment of childhood malignancies because of the reduction in normal-tissue exposure.

Clinical reports of paediatric ion beam radiotherapy so far include various central nervous system (CNS) tumours, retinoblastoma and medulloblastoma. For medulloblastoma, local control has been in the range of that anticipated with photons but morbidity was found to be low compared with historical results.

24.8 CONCLUSIONS AND FUTURE DIRECTIONS

The current evidence for the clinical efficacy of proton radiotherapy is predominantly based on non-randomized trials (Brada *et al.*, 2007; Lodge *et al.*, 2007; Olsen *et al.*, 2007). In the most common cancers, it seems unlikely that protons perform substantially better than optimized photon treatment; only a subgroup of patients with particular tumour localizations and configurations, or particular tumour biology (e.g. hypoxia) may benefit, which still must be proven in clinical trials. For ethical reasons some tumour sites (e.g. at the base of the skull), currently treated by ions at many centres, and where the dose distribution advantages are obvious, cannot be subject to randomized clinical trials. Furthermore, a reduction of rare and really late adverse effects (e.g. secondary malignancies and cardiac morbidity) is unlikely to be detected in sufficiently powered clinical investigations.

Based on prospective and retrospective studies, proton irradiation emerges as the treatment of choice for some ocular and skull base tumours. For prostate cancer, the results have been comparable to those from the best photon therapy series. However, heavy ion therapy is still in an experimental phase (Lodge *et al.*, 2007).

For the future, one interest is in combining protons with chemotherapy (Cox, 2007), as exposure of normal tissues that may develop combined side-effects can be reduced in proton radiotherapy. Also, the introduction of intensity-modulated proton therapy may be attractive because of its superior dose distributions compared with standard proton therapy (Miralbell *et al.*, 2002; MacDonald *et al.*, 2006).

Key points

1. Protons and other ions allow for dose deposition with steep dose gradients.
2. A minor fractionation effect is found for high-LET radiation (heavy ions, neutrons), while protons are comparable to photons.
3. The RBE of protons is 1.1. The RBE for heavy ions varies within the track, with low values within the entrance channel and high values of 2–4 at the Bragg peak.
4. The RBE for heavy ions and neutrons increases with decreasing dose per fraction, and is more pronounced for late radiation responses than for acute normal-tissue and tumour effects.
5. Doses for ion irradiation are specified in CGE or GyE, which is the absorbed dose multiplied by the RBE value.
6. Proton radiotherapy has been administered for various tumour entities/localizations which require precise, highly conformal dose deposition. The clinical application is mainly based on non-controlled trials. Heavy ion therapy is even more experimental.
7. The risk for second cancers is conceptually reduced with ion treatment compared with photons, as the integral normal-tissue dose is reduced, given that active beam shaping (pencil beam scanning) is used rather than passive devices. This concept, however, has not yet been validated in clinical studies.
8. Ion therapy may be preferred for some indications in paediatric oncology, because of the reduced risk for the induction of second neoplasms.

■ BIBLIOGRAPHY

Ando K, Koike S, Uzawa A *et al.* (2005). Biological gain of carbon-ion radiotherapy for the early response of tumor growth delay and against early response of skin reaction in mice. *J Radiat Res (Tokyo)* **46**: 51–7.

Brada M, Pijls-Johannesma M, De Ruysscher D (2007). Proton therapy in clinical practice: current clinical evidence. *J Clin Oncol* **25**: 965–70.

Brenner DJ, Hall EJ (2008). Secondary neutrons in clinical proton radiotherapy: a charged issue. *Radiother Oncol* **86**: 165–70.

Cox J (2007). Current and future status of proton-beam radiation therapy in radiation oncology. *Clin Adv Hematol Oncol* **5**: 303–5.

Denekamp J, Waites T, Fowler JF (1997). Predicting realistic RBE values for clinically relevant radiotherapy schedules. *Int J Radiat Biol* **71**: 681–94.

Gerweck LE, Kozin SV (1999). Relative biological effectiveness of proton beams in clinical therapy. *Radiother Oncol* **50**: 135–42.

Goitein M, Jermann M (2003). The relative costs of proton and X-ray radiation therapy. *Clin Oncol* **15**: S37–50.

Gold DG, Neglia JP, Potish RA, Dusenbery KE (2004). Second neoplasms following megavoltage radiation for pediatric tumors. *Cancer* **100**: 212–3.

Greco C, Wolden S (2007). Current status of radiotherapy with proton and light ion beams. *Cancer* **109**: 1227–38.

ICRP (2003). Relative biological effectiveness (RBE), quality factor (*Q*), and radiation weighting factor (w_R). ICRP Publication 92. *Ann ICRP* **33**: 1–117.

Joiner MC (1988). A comparison of the effects of p(62)-Be and d(16)-Be neutrons in the mouse kidney. *Radiother Oncol* **13**: 211–24.

Kramer M, Scholz M (2000). Treatment planning for heavy-ion radiotherapy: calculation and optimization of biologically effective dose. *Phys Med Biol* **45**: 3319–30.

Kramer M, Weyrather WK, Scholz M (2003). The increased biological effectiveness of heavy charged particles: from radiobiology to treatment planning. *Technol Cancer Res Treat* **2**: 427–36.

Lodge M, Pijls-Johannesma M, Stirk L, Munro AJ, De Ruysscher D, Jefferson T (2007). A systematic literature review of the clinical and cost-effectiveness of hadron therapy in cancer. *Radiother Oncol* **83**: 110–22.

MacDonald SM, DeLaney TF, Loeffler JS (2006). Proton beam radiation therapy. *Cancer Invest* **24**: 199–208.

Miralbell R, Lomax A, Cella L, Schneider U (2002). Potential reduction of the incidence of radiation-induced second cancers by using proton beams in the treatment of pediatric tumors. *Int J Radiat Oncol Biol Phys* **54**: 824–9.

Olsen DR, Bruland OS, Frykholm G, Norderhaug IN (2007). Proton therapy – a systematic review of clinical effectiveness. *Radiother Oncol* **83**: 123–32.

Paganetti H, Niemierko A, Ancukiewicz M *et al.* (2002). Relative biological effectiveness (RBE) values for proton beam therapy. *Int J Radiat Oncol Biol Phys* **53**: 407–21.

Schneider U, Agosteo S, Pedroni E, Besserer J (2002). Secondary neutron dose during proton therapy using spot scanning. *Int J Radiat Oncol Biol Phys* **53**: 244–51.

Scholz M, Matsufuji N, Kanai T (2006). Test of the local effect model using clinical data: tumour control probability for lung tumours after treatment with carbon ion beams. *Radiat Prot Dosimetry* **122**: 478–9.

Schulz-Ertner D, Tsujii H (2007). Particle radiation therapy using proton and heavier ion beams. *J Clin Oncol* **25**: 953–64.

Schulz-Ertner D, Nikoghosyan A, Thilmann C *et al.* (2003). Carbon ion radiotherapy for chordomas and low-grade chondrosarcomas of the skull base. Results in 67 patients. *Strahlenther Onkol* **179**: 598–605.

Tepper J, Verhey L, Goitein M, Suit HD (1977). In vivo determinations of RBE in a high energy modulated proton beam using normal tissue reactions and fractionated dose schedules. *Int J Radiat Oncol Biol Phys* **2**: 1115–22.

Tsujii H, Mizoe JE, Kamada T *et al.* (2004). Overview of clinical experiences on carbon ion radiotherapy at NIRS. *Radiother Oncol* **73**(Suppl 2): S41–9.

Urano M, Verhey LJ, Goitein M *et al.* (1984). Relative biological effectiveness of modulated proton beams in various murine tissues. *Int J Radiat Oncol Biol Phys* **10**: 509–14.

Wambersie A, Hendry JH, Andreo P *et al.* (2006). The RBE issues in ion-beam therapy: conclusions of a joint IAEA/ICRU working group regarding quantities and units. *Radiat Prot Dosimetry* **122**: 463–70.

Weber DC, Chan AW, Bussiere MR *et al.* (2003). Proton beam radiosurgery for vestibular schwannoma: tumor control and cranial nerve toxicity. *Neurosurgery* **53**: 577–86.

Withers HR, Thames HD, Peters LJ (1982). Biological bases for high RBE values for late effects of neutron irradiation. *Int J Radiat Oncol Biol Phys* **8**: 2071–6.

■ FURTHER READING

Brada M, Pijls-Johannesma M, De Ruysscher D (2007). Proton therapy in clinical practice: current clinical evidence. *J Clin Oncol* **25**: 965–70.

Brenner DJ, Hall EJ (2008). Secondary neutrons in clinical proton radiotherapy: a charged issue. *Radiother Oncol* **86**: 165–70.

Lodge M, Pijls-Johannesma M, Stirk L, Munro AJ, De Ruysscher D, Jefferson T (2007). A systematic literature review of the clinical and cost-effectiveness of hadron therapy in cancer. *Radiother Oncol* **83**: 110–22.

MacDonald SM, DeLaney TF, Loeffler JS (2006). Proton beam radiation therapy. *Cancer Invest* **24**: 199–208.

Olsen DR, Bruland OS, Frykholm G, Norderhaug IN (2007). Proton therapy – a systematic review of clinical effectiveness. *Radiother Oncol* **83**: 123–32.

Second cancers after radiotherapy

KLAUS RÜDIGER TROTT

25.1 INTRODUCTION

Age is the most important risk factor for developing cancer and for dying from cancer. The risk of developing cancer within the following year changes little between the end of childhood and the age of 40 years. In women the risk increases earlier than in men, yet in both sexes the most dramatic increase is after the age of 60 years, as demonstrated in Fig. 25.1. Table 25.1 shows the risk of developing cancer within 5 years after treatment (i.e. the commonly practised follow-up time after radiotherapy for patients treated at the age of 50, 55, 60, 65, 70 or 75 years), assuming that cancer rates follow those found in the general population, as shown in Fig. 25.1. Since there is no convincing evidence that the development of one cancer protects against the development of another, we may conclude that, during the typical follow-up period of a patient treated for cancer with curative intent, a relatively large proportion of patients will present with a second cancer. This frequency will vary between 1 per cent and more than 10 per cent, depending on age and sex. The results of epidemiological studies described below indicate that in cancer patients, after curative radiotherapy, the increased lifespan of cured

patients is by far the most important risk factor leading to second cancers. This risk, determined from cancer registry data which cover entire populations, may be further increased by individual

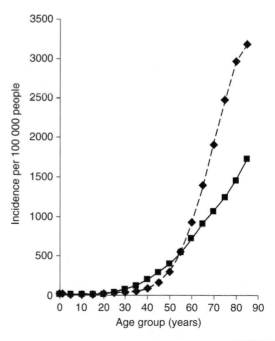

Figure 25.1 Average annual cancer incidence in the UK by gender and age attained. Diamonds, male; squares, female.

Table 25.1 The spontaneous cancer incidence risk within a follow-up period of 5 years, in patients treated at different ages

Age at treatment (years)	Cancer risk within the next 5 years (%)	
	Males	Females
50	1.5	2.0
55	2.5	2.7
60	5.0	3.6
65	7.0	4.6
70	10.0	5.4
75	12.5	6.3

Data from UK, England and Wales 1983–1987.

factors such as specific carcinogen exposure or by genetic predisposition.

It has been generally accepted that the majority of cancers are causally related to exposure of the individual to common carcinogens, the most important being dietary factors and smoking which, together, cause more than 50 per cent of all cancers (Doll and Peto, 1981). Most carcinogens are known to be related to more than one type of cancer. Smoking, for example, is causally related to cancer of the lung, the bladder and the head and neck. This means that a patient who has been cured of bladder cancer, for example, independent of the treatment modality, will have a greater risk than other members of the general population to develop, for example, lung cancer. The size of this increased individual risk is difficult to determine. However, in the quantification of treatment-related second cancer risks in epidemiological studies, methods have to be used which eliminate or reduce the potential bias related to specific carcinogen exposure. The best approaches are the determination of radiation dose dependence of risk or the comparison of different curative treatment modalities for the same type and stage of cancer.

The risk for the development of specific cancers is also influenced by genetic predisposition. The strength of this predisposition varies between gene mutations. Well-known examples of strong genetic predisposition are mutations of the *Rb* gene (predisposing for retinoblastoma and osteosarcoma) and of the *BRCA1* gene (predisposing for early

breast cancer and ovarian cancer). The fact that these, and probably most, predisposing cancer gene mutations are associated with more than one type of cancer also means that people cured of one of those cancers have a higher than average probability of developing the other cancers associated with the respective mutation. However, the impact of genetic predisposition on the risk of developing a second cancer after cure from the first cancer is difficult to assess at the present state of knowledge. The most obvious example is the high risk of children treated with radiotherapy for retinoblastoma to develop osteosarcomas in the irradiated volume.

Finally, some of the modalities used to treat cancer have proven to have carcinogenic potential. A large number of studies have been published exploring the impact of various chemotherapy and radiotherapy schedules as well as their combination on the incidence of second cancers. The most detailed and comprehensive analysis of studies carried out up to 2003 has been published by van Leeuwen and Travis (2005).

It is particularly in those cancer patients who were treated as children or young adults for cancers such as Hodgkin's and non-Hodgkin's lymphoma, testicular cancer and paediatric malignancies that it is becoming increasingly apparent that the most important cause of death in long-term survivors is second cancers causally related to the methods of treatment of the first cancer. Radiotherapy and chemotherapy are both implicated in the induction of those second malignancies. In general, chemotherapy is mostly related to the induction of leukaemia, in particular acute myeloid leukaemia (AML), most of which occur within 10 years after primary treatment. Radiotherapy is more related to the induction of solid cancers, the vast majority having longer latency with risk persisting for several decades or maybe even life-long. There are strong indications that radiotherapy also co-increases the risk of second leukaemia and that chemotherapeutic drugs also co-increase the risk of solid cancers after radiotherapy.

The risk of treatment-related second cancers is commonly determined by the comparison of the frequency of second cancers after different treatments such as surgery versus radiotherapy or with the general population. From this, a ratio of frequencies is calculated that indicates relative risk (RR) of cancers caused by a specific treatment. These RR values tend to vary greatly between different second cancers for the same primary cancer and, in many cases such as leukaemia after treatment of Hodgkin's lymphoma, may assume very high values. Although RR values form the basis of epidemiological and statistical analyses, they may be misleading in the evaluation of the clinical problem. Since many treatment-related cancers (particularly those with high RR values) are rare in the general population, a high RR may still translate into a low absolute risk. Therefore, absolute excess risk, which estimates the excess number of second malignancies per 10 000 patients per year, better reflects the second malignancy burden of treated patients than RR values (van Leeuwen and Travis, 2005).

25.2 ESTIMATING THE RISK OF RADIATION-INDUCED SECOND CANCERS AFTER CURATIVE RADIOTHERAPY OF CANCERS IN ADULT PATIENTS

Radiation is a well-established carcinogen. Therefore, it has to be assumed that successful curative radiotherapy of cancer may, in some cases, also cause a new, second cancer in addition to age-related cancer risks. In radiation protection, estimation of radiation-induced cancer follows a method which has been developed by the International Commission on Radiological Protection (ICRP) for preventive purposes in radiation worker populations. It is largely based on data derived from epidemiological studies in populations exposed to whole-body low-dose irradiation, in particular the lifespan study of the Japanese atomic bomb survivors. The method of risk estimation involves three steps of calculation:

1. Calculate the mean organ dose for the different organs at risk such as lung, stomach, colon, bone marrow and others.
2. Multiply the mean organ dose by the relevant organ weighting factor which ranges from 0.01 for skin to 0.12 for the four organs listed above.

3. Add up the weighted mean organ doses for all organs at risk. This weighted total body dose is called 'effective dose'. This effective dose is then multiplied by the appropriate risk factor that varies between 4 and 10 per cent per Gy, depending on age and exposure rate, to calculate the lifetime cancer risk from the respective radiation exposure.

Several studies have been published recently using this approach to determine the risks from radical radiotherapy and to compare different treatment plans in radiotherapy. The risk estimates derived using this method yield very high values which may be up to two orders of magnitude higher than the risk derived directly from the epidemiological studies described below. The reasons for this discrepancy are the extraordinary dose inhomogeneities within individual organs and between organs. Epidemiological and experimental evidence actually shows that the probability of cancer induction decreases dramatically as the dose inhomogeneity in an irradiated organ increases. It is mainly for this reason that the ICRP strongly advises not to use the effective dose method to estimate the risks of radiation-induced cancer in situations of very large dose inhomogeneities with peak doses well above doses that would cause acute or chronic radiation effects (i.e. doses >5 Gy); see ICRP 60 (1991) and ICRP 103 (2007). The ICRP also recommends that data derived directly from epidemiological investigations on radiotherapy patients are better suited to estimate the risk of induction of second cancers by the radiation treatment of the first cancer.

Such data can best be collected by the comparison of the rate of second cancers in large patient cohorts who have been cured from the first cancer either by radiotherapy or by surgery. Conditions of suitability are:

- the first cancer has to be common
- the first cancer must have a good chance of cure (≥50 per cent)
- the chance of cure has to be similar from surgery and radical radiotherapy and the decision of treating by radiotherapy or surgery should be largely independent of factors affecting cancer risks
- the life expectancy of a large proportion of the cured patients must be >10 years.

Two types of cancer fulfil these conditions particularly well: they are cancer of the cervix and cancer of the prostate. For both these cancers, large epidemiological studies have been conducted which provide the main source of data on second cancer risks after radiotherapy in patients of advanced age.

In addition, important information can also be derived from studies on the topographical relationship of primary cancer and second cancer in symmetrical organs, in particular in patients with a primary breast cancer and a secondary lung cancer. Moreover, studies on second cancers after radiotherapy of young people and their comparison with age-matched healthy populations also provide important information since they permit very long follow-up, yet their interpretation is difficult and may be misleading because of strong genetic susceptibility factors influencing risks and because other carcinogenic treatment modalities such as chemotherapy may also be given, which makes any identification of radiation risks difficult. However, in some cancers, in particular Hodgkin's lymphoma, testicular cancer and paediatric malignancies, it has been possible to separate out the contributions of radiotherapy and chemotherapy and their interaction.

Suit *et al.* (2007) have made the most comprehensive analysis of the problem, putting the question of second cancers after radical radiotherapy into the context of radiobiological studies on cell transformation *in vitro*, radiation-induced cancers in experimental animals from mice to monkeys, the Japanese atomic bomb survivors, radiation workers, patients treated for benign diseases and those treated with radiotherapy for cancer. Estimating RR values in comparison with the general population and with patients treated with non-radiation modalities, they demonstrated that some (but not all) cured cancer patients have a higher risk of developing cancer than the general population. They concluded that 'radiation can induce malignant transformation of mammalian tissue.... The relationship between radiation dose and risk of cancer is clearly complex and is not amenable to a simple definition applicable to all mammalian species, all members of a species, or even all organs in one inbred strain of a species.... Due to quite large and undefined heterogeneity in the patient populations studied, no precise quantification of the risk of radiation-induced secondary cancer is available at present. However, the clear implication of this review . . . is that the basic concept for planning radiation treatment should be that the risk of radiation-induced secondary cancer would be reduced by any dose decrement to uninvolved normal tissues, at least down to around 0.05 Gy. The factorial decrease in risk would be greatest for reduction in dose levels below 2 Gy.'

By pooling data from 14 published radiotherapy series and by concentrating on RR, inevitably some details of the presented information which might be important for the assessment of the clinical relevance of the data was lost in the Suit *et al.* review. This is particularly so if one considers the dose response of individual organs at risk for second cancer induction since the spectrum of critical organs differed between the various studies. In the following, we have adopted a different approach in which the largest and most detailed studies of second cancers after radical radiotherapy have been selected to derive information that could be used not so much for risk estimation, but in the critical evaluation of treatment decisions and of dose–volume histograms in radiotherapy treatment planning.

Carcinoma of the cervix

The first analysis on the risk of second cancers after radical radiotherapy of primary cancers was a multi-institutional study on long-term survivors of cancer of the cervix. The study of Kleinerman *et al.* (1995) was a cohort study of the incidence of second cancers in 66 541 patients with cervical cancer reported to 13 population-based cancer registries in five countries. Out of this patient group, 49 828 (75 per cent) were treated with radiotherapy and 16 713 (25 per cent) were treated surgically. The average follow-up was 10.4 years. More than 2000 second cancers were recorded and analysed. The results are tabulated in Table 25.2 and are consistent with the results of a case–control study on the same patient population by the same investigators (Boice *et al.*, 1988).

The results of this study are remarkable in several aspects. In contrast to all studies which form

Table 25.2 Results of the cohort study on second cancers after radiotherapy of cervical cancer

Site of second cancer	Radiation dose (Gy)	Number of second cancers after radiotherapy/surgery	Relative risk after <10 years
Rectum	30–60	274/33	2 after 10 years; 4 after 30 years
Colon	24	296/56	No increase
Bladder	30–60	265/23	>2 after 10 years; 6 after 30 years
Stomach	2	143/19	1.2
Lung	0.3	276/91	No increase
Breast	0.3	366/114	Decrease 20–40% after 10 years and 30 years
Leukaemia	4.5	82/15	2

Data from Kleinerman *et al.* (1995).

the basis of radiation protection regulations such as the atomic bomb survivor studies or the ankylosing spondylitis studies (United Nations Scientific Committee on the Effects of Atomic Radiation: UNSCEAR, 2000, 2006), the greatest risk occurs in the bladder (which, although significantly related to radiation exposure in the atomic bomb survivors, has a small organ weighting factor) and in the rectum (which has not been shown to be sensitive to the induction of cancer by radiation). The colon, which also receives considerable doses in radiotherapy of cervical cancer, did not show increased second cancer rates. In addition to the bladder and rectum located in the high-dose volume, only two organs found in the low-dose volumes show significantly increased cancer rates. These are the stomach, receiving a mean dose of 2 Gy, and the bone marrow, receiving a mean dose of 4.5 Gy. The leukaemia risk per Gy derived from these data is less than 10 per cent of the risk per Gy estimated from the atomic bomb survivor study, demonstrating the overriding importance of dose inhomogeneity on second malignancy risks.

Carcinoma of the prostate

Several small studies on the risks of second cancers after radical radiotherapy of prostate cancer have yielded inconclusive results. Yet the results of the very large cohort study on more than 120 000 prostate cancer patients (Brenner *et al.*, 2000)

Table 25.3 Results of the study of second cancers after radiotherapy of prostate cancer

	Surgery only	Radiotherapy
Number of patients	70 539	51 584
Person-years at risk	312 499	218 341
Mean survival time (years)	4.4	4.2
Mean age at therapy (years)	71.4	70.3
Mean age at second cancer (years)	77	75.3
Percentage of persons at risk after:		
5–10 years	35.8	33.5
>10 years	10.8	9.8
Number of second malignancies:		
At all times after treatment	5055	3549
After >5 years	1646	1185
After >10 years	393	305

Data from Brenner *et al.* (2000).

clearly demonstrate the extent of the problem for clinical radiotherapy. The study was a cohort study on 122 123 patients with prostate cancer registered in the SEER (the National Cancer Institute's Surveillance, Epidemiology and End Results) programme who had either surgery or radiotherapy. The results of this study are summarized in Table 25.3.

Table 25.4 Risk of radiation-induced second cancer after radiotherapy of prostate cancer

	Relative risk	
	After >5 years	After >10 years
All second cancers	1.11 ($p < 0.007$)	1.27 ($p < 0.002$)
Bladder	1.55 ($p < 0.0001$)	1.77 ($p < 0.01$)
Rectum	1.35 ($p < 0.06$)	2.05 ($p < 0.03$)
Lung	1.22 ($p < 0.01$)	1.42 ($p < 0.02$)
Leukaemia in first 10 years:		
Surgery patients	Irradiated patients	Relative risk in 10 years
39 in 343 690 person-years	25 in 112 422 person-years	2 ($p < 0.05$)

Data from Brenner *et al.* (2000).

Comparing second cancer rates of patients treated with either radiotherapy or surgery at different follow-up times, the risk of radiation-induced second cancer and its dependence on follow-up can be calculated. Results are shown in Table 25.4. Out of the approximately 17 000 prostate cancer patients who survived more than 5 years after radical radiotherapy, 1185 (7 per cent) developed a second cancer. More than 1000 of those second cancers (>85 per cent) result from the increased lifespan after cure from the first cancer. Just about 120–150 of those second cancers among 51 584 prostate cancer patients (0.3 per cent) are related to radiotherapy:

- approximately 50 cases of bladder cancer
- approximately 15 cases of cancer of the rectum
- approximately 50 cases of lung cancer
- approximately 12 cases of leukaemia.

As was observed in the cervix studies, bladder and rectum cancers found in the high-dose volume are most frequent. The unexpected large number of radiotherapy-associated lung cancers is probably related to the older treatment techniques using large fields delivered mostly with ^{60}Co and a mean lung dose of 0.5 Gy has been estimated that is related to scattered radiation. This is in agreement with the risk of radiation-induced lung cancer from the atomic bomb survivor studies. Modern conformal treatment protocols lead to much lower lung exposure of about 10 per cent of the doses estimated in the Brenner *et al.* (2000) study. However, lung doses from some techniques such as intensity-modulated radiotherapy (IMRT) of prostate cancer may be close to those doses and may possibly be associated with similar risks of second lung cancer. This is due to the use of more treatment fields and higher monitor units greatly increasing both collimator and phantom scatter, as well as leakage from the linear accelerator head.

The most important result of the prostate cancer study is that half of all radiation-induced second cancers occur in the high-dose volumes and the other half in the volumes exposed to those radiation doses commonly associated with radiation carcinogenesis. It is very likely that two entirely different mechanisms are involved in the high- and low-dose volumes. In the low-dose volumes, we may assume the same molecular and cellular mechanisms as in other situations of low-dose radiation carcinogenesis which have been extensively explored in radiation protection research (UNSCEAR, 2006). However, radiation doses given to the bladder and the rectum very often lead to chronic radiation injury, which is characterized by progressive microvascular damage, parenchymal atrophy and chronic inflammation. This condition has been recognized for more than 100 years as a precancerous lesion. Therefore, one may classify the radiation-induced second cancers in the high-dose organs as secondary to chronic radiation injury. This attribution would have pronounced impact on the dose–risk relationship and on the optimization of treatment plans, as discussed in the concluding paragraph.

Breast cancer

Patients treated with postoperative radiotherapy for breast cancer receive significant radiation doses of more than 5 per cent of the target dose to

Table 25.5 Ipsilateral and contralateral second lung cancers in patients treated with postoperative radiotherapy of breast cancer

Duration of follow-up (years)	Number of second cancers		Lung cancer mortality ratio
	Ipsilateral	Contralateral	
<10	161	134	1.2
10–15	65	44	1.5
>15	57	21	2.7

Data from Darby *et al.* (2005).

the contralateral breast. New trial protocols are addressing this problem and studies such as the IMPORT High trial, using partial breast irradiation for high-risk patients, are suggesting a mean dose of 1 Gy as a dose constraint to the contralateral breast. Since second cancers in the contralateral breast occur more frequently than expected and constitute nearly half of all second cancers in women with breast cancer, a causal relationship with the radiation exposure from the treatment of the first cancer has been suggested. However, a nested case–control study by Storm *et al.* (1992) on 529 patients who developed contralateral breast cancer 8 or more years after diagnosis of the first cancer (being part of a cohort of more than 50 000 breast cancer patients in Denmark) provided evidence that there is little, if any, risk of radiation-induced breast cancer associated with exposure of the contralateral breast in postoperative radiotherapy. However, most patients in this study were over 45 years old and therefore at an age when the radiosensitivity of the breast with regard to cancer induction has been shown to be very low. In contrast, in a study on women under the age of 45 years, Boice *et al.* (1992) estimated that one in 10 of second breast cancers could be attributed to prior radiotherapy. Modern treatment planning permits a much lower dose to the contralateral breast than was the case in both these studies and their findings indicate that it is particularly in young breast cancer patients that the dose to the contralateral breast should be carefully controlled.

Patients treated with postoperative radiotherapy for breast cancer receive very different doses to the ipsilateral compared with the contralateral lungs. Darby *et al.* (2005) have reported a cohort

study on 308 861 women, included in the SEER programme, who were treated for breast cancer between 1973 and 2001 and of whom 115 165 (37 per cent) received radiotherapy as part of their primary treatment. Of these treated women, 482 (0.4 per cent) later died from lung cancer for which the affected side was clearly defined in the records. The main endpoint was which side of the lung developed a second cancer in relation to which breast was originally treated. More than 1000 cases of lung cancer (0.5 per cent) occurred in women who did not receive radiotherapy, and there was no difference between the rates of ipsilateral and contralateral lung cancers. Conversely, of the 482 cases of lung cancer that occurred in women who received radiotherapy, 283 cases (59 per cent) were ipsilateral and 199 (41 per cent) were contralateral. From these findings the risk of radiation-induced lung cancer can be estimated. The proportion of ipsilateral second lung cancers in women who had received radiotherapy increased with increasing follow-up time from a ratio of 1.2 less than 10 years after treatment to 2.7 more than 15 years after treatment (Table 25.5). Among women diagnosed with breast cancer during 1973–1982 and receiving postoperative radiotherapy, there were 112 deaths from ipsilateral lung cancer and 51 from contralateral lung cancer, indicating a mortality ratio of about 2. Taking into account also that the contralateral lung received considerable radiation doses from scatter, the RR of second cancer in the lung from postoperative radiotherapy of breast cancer would increase even further. The estimated RR is about 3, which would translate into an absolute risk of lung cancer from postoperative radiotherapy of <0.6 per cent. There is a non-significant suggestion that, in recent years, using more advanced radiotherapy techniques, the risk of second lung cancer after postoperative radiotherapy of breast cancer after >10 years is reduced compared with the older cohort.

25.3 RADIATION-INDUCED SECOND CANCERS AFTER COMBINED RADIOCHEMOTHERAPY TREATMENT OF MALIGNANCIES IN YOUNG ADULTS

Hodgkin's lymphoma

The treatment results of Hodgkin's lymphoma have improved significantly since the introduction of intensive radiotherapy, which was mainly based on the work of Kaplan at Stanford and of Musshoff in Freiburg in the 1950s. As a result, there are now thousands of long-term survivors of Hodgkin's lymphoma who are at risk for late effects of therapy including second cancers. Wolden et al. (1998) described the incidence of second cancers in 697 patients who were less than 21 years old at the time of treatment in Stanford – some were followed up for more than 35 years. Eighty patients (11 per cent) developed 85 new malignant tumours. Twenty-five (31 per cent) were non-melanoma skin cancers. The second most frequent second cancer was breast cancer (16 patients), followed by sarcomas (13 patients). Eight second leukaemias occurred, all but one within 10 years and all eight patients had received chemotherapy with alkylating agents. The actuarial risk of second cancer at 20 years after treatment for Hodgkin's lymphoma, at a mean attained age of 36 years, was 9.7 per cent for males and 16.8 per cent for females with more than half of their risk being breast cancer (9.2 per cent). The incidence of breast cancer was similar for patients who received both radiotherapy and chemotherapy versus radiation only as initial therapy. The most remarkable finding of this important single-institution study was that, among the 48 solid second cancers, 43 (90 per cent) occurred within the radiotherapy treatment field or in the penumbra region, and 40 (83 per cent) developed in volumes that had received at least 35 Gy. The authors stress

that treatment policies for Hodgkin's lymphoma have changed dramatically over the past 30 years, putting more emphasis on multiagent chemotherapy and reduced radiation doses and treatment volumes to involved sites. Thus, the second malignancy rates seen after long follow-up in this study may not represent the risk for patients treated in the modern era. It should be noted that patients were more than twice as likely to die from their primary Hodgkin's lymphoma than from a second cancer (11 per cent versus 4 per cent).

Dores et al. (2002) reported results of a large international study on 32 591 Hodgkin's lymphoma patients with 2861 patients followed up for more than 20 years and 1111 patients for more than 25 years; mean age at treatment was 37 years. Second malignancies developed in 2153 patients (7 per cent) which, compared with the age- and sex-adjusted general population, was an increase of more than a factor of 2. The risk of late-developing solid cancers was particularly increased after radiotherapy while second leukaemias were mostly related to chemotherapy. After more than 25 years' follow-up, there was evidence of a decrease in RR for all second cancers from a RR of 4.4 in the 20- to 24-year period to a RR of 2.4. The highest absolute excess second cancer risk was for cancers of the lung and breast. Whereas the RR of all second cancers decreased with increasing age at diagnosis of Hodgkin's lymphoma, the absolute excess risk of second cancers increased with increasing age from 30 cases per 100 000 person-years for under 21-year-old patients to 107 cases per 100 000 person-years in the 51- to 60-year-old patients. This was not seen for second breast cancer, where the risk was highest in patients treated when they were under 30 years old. The authors calculated a 25-year cumulative risk of treatment-induced second cancers of 11.7 per cent, most of which was related to radiotherapy.

In a case–control study of British patients, Swerdlow et al. (2000) demonstrated that MOPP chemotherapy also leads to a dose-dependent elevated risk of lung cancer and that this risk was not further increased if radiotherapy was given together with MOPP.

In their review of late effects after treatment for Hodgkin's lymphoma, Swerdlow and van Leeuwen (2005) concluded that the substantial increase in solid tumour risk with time since diagnosis necessitated careful, lifelong medical surveillance of all patients. Since the absolute excess risk of lung cancer was much greater among smokers than non-smokers, physicians should make a special effort to dissuade Hodgkin's disease patients from smoking. Women treated with mantle field irradiation before the age of 30 years are at greatly increased risk of breast cancer. In many centres, from 8 years after irradiation onwards, the follow-up programme of these women includes yearly breast palpation and mammography; however, the efficacy of these measures in this specific population has not yet been demonstrated.

Testicular cancer

In a large international study on nearly 29 000 patients with testicular cancer who survived more than 1 year, Travis *et al.* (1997) analysed the dependence of 1406 observed second cancers (which was an overall excess of 43 per cent) on time since treatment and on treatment modality with special emphasis on the histology of first and of second tumour. The 25-year cumulative risk after treatment of seminoma was 18 per cent compared with that of an age-matched normal population and greater than that of non-seminomatous testicular cancer which was 11 per cent compared with 6 per cent in an age-matched normal population. Compared with the general population, the excess cancer risk increased steadily for at least 30 years. The most pronounced significantly increased second cancer rates among the 3306 patients surviving more than 20 years were related to cancer of the bladder, which receives the highest radiation dose of all organs at risk. Seventy bladder cancers were diagnosed among the total of 276 cancer cases in this group, mostly related to radiotherapy with a RR of >3. In a later study, Travis *et al.* (2000) related the risk of treatment-induced leukaemia to the type of treatment. Both radiotherapy and chemotherapy with cisplatin increased leukaemia risk in a dose-dependent way. After cisplatin chemotherapy, leukaemia risk was nearly twice that of radiotherapy; however, the absolute risk was small after both treatment modalities (15 years

cumulative risk about 0.1 per cent) compared with the risk of treatment-induced solid second cancers, most of which resulted from radiotherapy.

25.4 RADIATION-INDUCED SECOND CANCERS AFTER TREATMENT OF PAEDIATRIC MALIGNANCIES

The chances of children with cancer being cured and having a near-normal life expectancy have reached a level unimaginable 30 years ago. But the price for this progress is high. Several large studies have demonstrated that both radiotherapy and chemotherapy, and in particular the combination of both, cause a significant risk of developing a second malignancy. Leukaemia predominates in the first 10 years whereas various solid cancers develop later in life. The latter risk increases steadily with increasing survival; therefore, a major effort is needed to identify those factors that determine the size of this risk. For chemotherapy it is mainly the type of drug; for radiotherapy it is, in the first instance, the dose and the dose distribution as well as the volume irradiated.

Neglia *et al.* (2001) investigated a cohort of 13 581 children from the Childhood Cancer Survivor Study register in the USA who survived at least 5 years with a median follow-up of 15 years. A total of 298 second malignancies were observed after a mean latency of 12 years. Whereas the risk of secondary leukaemia (24 cases) increased to a peak after 5–9 years, the risk of solid second cancers, in particular breast (60 cases), thyroid (43 cases) and central nervous system (CNS; 36 cases), was significantly elevated during the entire follow-up period of up to 30 years. The authors concluded that second malignant neoplasms are infrequent but extremely serious events following therapy for primary cancers. In particular, female survivors of childhood cancer are at a significantly increased high risk of developing secondary breast cancer. Yet the authors also warned not to compromise the effectiveness of treatment of the first cancer as <2 excess malignancies were recorded per 1000 years of patient follow-up (0.2 per cent).

The study of de Vathaire *et al.* (1999) is the only one which has looked at the impact of radiotherapy for childhood solid malignancies on the risk of second cancers. They analysed the second cancer risk in 4400 3-year survivors treated in eight centres in France and the UK, 3109 (71 per cent) of whom received radiotherapy. For 2831 (91 per cent) of these children, individual radiation doses at 151 points of the body were determined, based on the individual treatment plans using a computer phantom. A total of 113 patients (4 per cent) developed a solid second malignant tumour (non-melanoma skin cancers excluded). The cumulative incidence of treatment-associated second solid tumours increased dramatically as the patients progressed into their thirties. Twenty-five years after treatment of the primary malignancy, the cumulative risk was about 5 per cent, 5 years later it approached 8 per cent. In 543 patients who had already attained an age >30 years, 16 second cancers were diagnosed while only 3.3 were expected – a five-fold increase. The most critical organs for radiation-induced second cancers in paediatric radiotherapy are breast, brain, bone, soft tissues and thyroid. More than 80 per cent of all second solid tumours occurred in those organs and tissues, yet there were great differences in sensitivity with age and in dose dependence: while sarcomas and brain tumours tended to develop in the high-dose volumes, carcinomas tended to occur in the intermediate to low-dose volumes.

Neglia *et al.* (2006) reported a case–control study in 40 children from the Childhood Cancer Survivor Study who developed a secondary glioma after a mean interval of 9 years from primary radiotherapy and in 66 meningiomas diagnosed after a mean interval of 17 years. Local radiation dose at the site of the second brain tumour was the most important risk factor. No cases were observed at <10 Gy, and the maximal risk (RR >10) was related to a mean brain dose of >30 Gy. The risk of secondary glioma was particularly high in children given radiotherapy at age <5 years, which may be attributed to greater susceptibility of the developing brain to radiation. In a cohort study on 14 372 participants in the Childhood Cancer Survivor Study, 108 children were diagnosed with second sarcoma at a median of 11 years after the diagnosis of childhood cancer. In a multivariate model, increased risk of secondary sarcoma was significantly associated with radiotherapy (RR = 3.1) but also with treatment with higher doses of anthracyclines (RR = 2.3) or alkylating agents (RR = 2.2).

The evolving progress of treatment in paediatric oncology is associated with rapidly changing treatment schedules, regarding both chemotherapy (drugs, their combination and dosage) and radiotherapy (with a tendency to decrease target volumes and doses). The epidemiological data on the risk of second cancers are therefore, inevitably, those resulting from outdated treatment techniques. Whether the methods used today are associated with a lower or possibly even higher risk cannot be directly answered and any conclusions appear premature and speculative. The short latency of leukaemias may permit the investigation of this problem for relatively recent chemotherapy schedules since chemotherapy is mainly associated with secondary leukaemia arising within <10 years. Identifying the criteria determining risk in radiotherapy may be more difficult because of the long latency periods of solid cancers. Location of these solid cancers, matched to the patient's planned dose–volume distributions, may be used in the future.

As a caveat it should be mentioned that all studies on treatment-induced second cancers after radiotherapy of paediatric malignancies, so far, show only the tip of the iceberg. The vast majority of study members are still under the age of 50 years; yet from the atomic bomb survivor studies we may conclude that, even though RR may decrease with time, most radiation-induced cancers will occur only when the cured patients reach an age >60 years. For this reason, it is of utmost importance for paediatric radiation oncology that these studies be continued for at least another 20 years.

25.5 CONCLUSIONS

Considering the evidence presented in this chapter, there can be no doubt that radical radiotherapy of malignant diseases may cause second cancers many years later. The risk of radiotherapy-induced second cancers varies considerably with the type of primary cancers (paediatric malignancies posing the highest risk), and between different treatment techniques. However, by necessity, all data on second cancer risks after radiotherapy of first cancers relate to techniques which are more than 20 years old, and most are outdated. This poses two important questions:

1. Is the risk of radiotherapy-induced second cancers too high a price to be acceptable in the decision-making process for treating the first cancer?
2. Can the risk of radiotherapy-induced second cancer be reduced by optimizing the treatment techniques and the dose–volume distributions?

In answer to the first question, the risk of radiotherapy-induced second cancers is well below 1 per cent after radical radiotherapy of most adult cancers, such as cancers of the cervix and prostate. The risk of dying from uncontrolled local recurrences within a few years after radiotherapy is much higher than the risk of developing a second cancer 10 or 20 years later. This conclusion also applies to postoperative radiotherapy of breast cancer. For cases of juvenile and childhood malignancies, the answer has to be more guarded. Certainly, radiotherapy has made a great impact on long-term survival in these patients. After a 20-year follow-up, the risk of recurrence of the primary cancer is higher than the risk of developing a radiotherapy-induced second cancer. However, if this RR persisted throughout the remaining lifespan that those patients have been granted by the success of the radiation treatment in the first place, the risk of radiotherapy-induced second cancers would rise to levels that would cause serious concern. These considerations are based entirely on speculations on what the results of ongoing epidemiological studies may show 10 or 20 years from now and the true picture remains to be uncovered.

In answer to the second question, it is very likely, and it can be deduced from the evidence presented, that different treatment techniques are associated with different risks of radiation-induced second cancers. These variations in risk would be primarily caused by differences in dose–volume relationships. Many studies have been published in recent years which have determined the radiation doses within and outside the target volume as part of the treatment planning optimization process. The findings of the epidemiological studies in patients treated for cervix and prostate cancers suggest that two different

mechanisms, leading to radiation-induced second cancers, may exist which show very different relationships with radiation dose. One mechanism is related to chronic radiation damage in organs, such as rectum, bladder and skin, that develop acute, chronic and consequential radiation damage after high and very high radiation doses. Atrophy as a hyperproliferative disorder is known to be a precancerous lesion, in particular if associated with chronic inflammation. In the epidemiological studies on second cancers after radiotherapy for cervix and prostate cancer, about half of all radiation-induced second cancers are probably caused by this mechanism. Therefore, treatment optimization which aims at reducing the risk of severe chronic radiation damage might also reduce or minimize the risk of radiation-induced second cancer effected by this mechanism.

The epidemiological studies on second malignancies after radiotherapy of children and adolescents demonstrate that the vast majority of second, radiotherapy-induced cancers occur in tissues and organs not commonly associated in radiation protection with a great risk of radiation carcinogenesis such as brain and connective tissue. Moreover, nearly all radiotherapy-induced second cancers developed after high doses of just over 30 Gy and these doses are not sufficiently high to cause atrophy and chronic inflammation, which appears to be the mechanism of second cancer after high radiation doses in adults. In contrast, radiation exposure of organs outside the target volume is usually more homogeneous, giving mean organ doses of only a few Gy. It is in these organs that the characteristic mechanisms of radiation carcinogenesis at low radiation doses may become critical.

We conclude that there are at least three different mechanisms of radiation carcinogenesis after radiotherapy, each of which is critical at different dose levels, in different organs and in different age groups. It seems inconceivable that a single dose–volume risk relationship would be suitable to describe the treatment-related cancer risk in all clinical situations.

Owing to the relatively short latency and its distribution across the whole body, the mean radiation dose to the bone marrow appears to be the most critical factor in the majority of radiotherapy treatment plans; however, the results of the clinical studies suggest that the data from the atomic bomb survivors should not be used unchecked. The inhomogeneous dose distribution of bone marrow doses in most radiotherapy treatment plans leads to a reduction of risk by approximately a factor of 10 compared with atomic bomb survivor data.

The most critical organs in the low-dose volume with regard to radiation-induced second cancers are the lung and the stomach. In contrast to the organ-weighting factors proposed in the ICRP model, the organs shown in the post-radiotherapy studies to be at highest risk are very different: in none of the studies has the colon been found to be critical, and in many studies the breast was by far the most critical organ. The results of the various epidemiological studies of second cancers after curative radiotherapy demonstrate clearly that any optimization process has to be based on these results rather than on the mathematical models designed for radiation protection purposes for the general population or radiation workers.

Mean organ doses, or, even worse, effective doses, are not a valid predictor of second cancer risk. Individual dose–volume distributions in the different organs, both in the target volume and in the low-dose volumes, have to be critically assessed, taking into account age, sex, the specific anatomy and biology of the organ and any other factor such as chronic inflammation, all of which will potentially influence second cancer risk. So far, no criteria for optimization of dose–volume distributions have been published which would permit an evidence-based application in modern treatment planning of cancer. It is obvious that the most critical step in this process is the evaluation of the heterogeneity of doses in the various critical organs such as bone marrow, lung, bowel, breast and, particularly in children, brain and soft tissues. The assumptions made in many published evaluations of second cancer risks from different treatment plans, such as the comparison of conformal versus intensity-modulated radiotherapy, have to be regarded with caution as they are not consistent with the results of the clinical data presented above.

The development of evidence-based criteria for the optimization of treatment plans that include the risk of induction of second cancers in long-term survivors must await the results of comprehensive case–control studies on the relationship between second cancer risks in specific organs and treatment parameters, in particular dose–volume distributions in the respective critical organs. Few such studies have been performed to date, yet such studies are most likely to yield clinically useful information, particularly if they are embedded in large, single-institution cohort studies or in suitable randomized clinical studies with life-long follow-up of those cancer patients who have been cured by radiotherapy.

Key points

1. In radical radiotherapy, the radiation exposure to non-involved organs and tissues may cause second cancers several decades later.
2. In adult cancer patients, the risk of radiation-induced second cancers is much smaller than the risk of recurrent primary cancer.
3. In adult cancer patients, more than 90 per cent of second cancers occurring after radiotherapy are the consequence of increased life expectancy because of cure from the first cancer.
4. The risk of radiation-induced second cancers is much greater in young and very young cancer patients. Increased cancer rates may persist life-long.
5. Most radiation-induced second cancers occur in organs and tissues in the high-dose volume but some may also appear in the low dose ($<2\,Gy$) volume. There are pronounced differences in the types of radiation-induced second cancers between children, young adults and elderly patients treated with radiotherapy. Moreover, the types of second cancers after radiotherapy are different from those induced by low-dose total body irradiation (e.g. in Japanese atomic bomb survivors).
6. There are at least three different biological mechanisms leading to second cancers after radiotherapy, depending on dose distribution and age of the irradiated patient. The

dose–risk relationship, therefore, is unlikely to follow a simple mathematical function.

7. The risk of radiation-induced second cancers from radiotherapy should not be estimated using the effective dose method proposed by the ICRP for radiation protection purposes.

■ BIBLIOGRAPHY

Boice JD, Engholm G, Kleinerman RA *et al.* (1988). Radiation dose and second cancer risk in patients treated for cancer of the cervix. *Radiat Res* **116**: 3–55.

Boice JD, Harvey EB, Blettner M, Stovall M, Flannery JT (1992). Cancer in the contralateral breast after radiotherapy for breast cancer. *N Engl J Med* **326**: 781–5.

Brenner DJ, Curtis RE, Hall EJ, Ron E (2000). Second malignancies in prostate carcinoma patients after radiotherapy compared with surgery. *Cancer* **88**: 398–406.

Darby SC, McGale P, Taylor CW, Peto R (2005). Long-term mortality from heart disease and lung cancer after radiotherapy for early breast cancer: prospective cohort study of about 300,000 women in US SEER cancer registries. *Lancet Oncol* **6**: 557–65.

de Vathaire F, Hawkins M, Campbell S *et al.* (1999). Second malignant neoplasms after a first cancer in childhood: temporal pattern of risk according to type of treatment. *Br J Cancer* **79**: 1884–93.

Doll R, Peto R (1981). The causes of cancer: quantitative estimates of avoidable risks of cancer in the United States today. *J Natl Cancer Inst* **66**: 1191–308.

Dores GM, Metayer C, Curtis RE *et al.* (2002). Second malignant neoplasms among long-term survivors of Hodgkin's disease: a population-based evaluation over 25 years. *J Clin Oncol* **20**: 3484–94.

ICRP (1991). 1990 Recommendations of the International Commission on Radiological Protection. ICRP publication 60. *Ann ICRP* **21**: 1–201.

ICRP (2007). The 2007 Recommendations of the International Commission on Radiological Protection. ICRP publication 103. *Ann ICRP* **37**: 1–332.

Kleinerman RA, Boice JD Jr, Storm HH *et al.* (1995). Second primary cancer after treatment for cervical cancer. An international cancer registries study. *Cancer* **76**: 442–52.

Neglia JP, Friedman DL, Yasui Y *et al.* (2001). Second malignant neoplasms in five-year survivors of childhood cancer: childhood cancer survivor study. *J Natl Cancer Inst* **93**: 618–29.

Neglia JP, Robison LL, Stovall M *et al.* (2006). New primary neoplasms of the central nervous system in survivors of childhood cancer: a report from the Childhood Cancer Survivor Study. *J Natl Cancer Inst* **98**: 1528–37.

Storm HH, Andersson M, Boice JD Jr *et al.* (1992). Adjuvant radiotherapy and risk of contralateral breast cancer. *J Natl Cancer Inst* **84**: 1245–50.

Suit H, Goldberg S, Niemierko A *et al.* (2007). Secondary carcinogenesis in patients treated with radiation: a review of data on radiation-induced cancers in human, non-human primate, canine and rodent subjects. *Radiat Res* **167**: 12–42.

Swerdlow AJ, Barber JA, Hudson GV *et al.* (2000). Risk of second malignancy after Hodgkin's disease in a collaborative British cohort: the relation to age at treatment. *J Clin Oncol* **18**: 498–509.

Swerdlow AJ, van Leeuwen FE (2005). Late effects after treatment for Hodgkin's lymphoma. In: Dembo AJ, Linch DC, Lowenberg B (eds) *Textbook of malignant hematology*. Abingdon: Taylor & Francis, 758–68.

Travis LB, Curtis RE, Storm H *et al.* (1997). Risk of second malignant neoplasms among long-term survivors of testicular cancer. *J Natl Cancer Inst* **89**: 1429–39.

Travis LB, Andersson M, Gospodarowicz M *et al.* (2000). Treatment-associated leukemia following testicular cancer. *J Natl Cancer Inst* **92**: 1165–71.

UNSCEAR (2000). Annex I: Epidemiological evaluation of radiation-induced cancer. *Sources and Effects of Ionizing Radiation* **2**: 297–450.

UNSCEAR (2006). Annex A: Epidemiological studies of radiation and cancer. *Effects of Ionizing Radiation* **2**: (in press).

van Leeuwen FE, Travis LB (2005). Second cancers. In: DeVita VT, Hellman S, Rosenberg SA (eds) *Cancer: principles and practice of oncology*, 7th edn. Philadelphia: Lippincott Williams & Wilkins, 2575–602.

Wolden SL, Lamborn KR, Cleary SF, Tate DJ, Donaldson SS (1998). Second cancers following pediatric Hodgkin's disease. *J Clin Oncol* **16**: 536–44.

■ FURTHER READING

Henderson TO, Whitton J, Stovall M *et al.* (2007). Secondary sarcomas in childhood cancer survivors: a report from the Childhood Cancer Survivor Study. *J Natl Cancer Inst* **99**: 300–8.

Mody R, Li S, Dover DC *et al.* (2008). Twenty-five year follow-up among survivors of childhood acute lymphoblastic leukemia: a report from the Childhood Cancer Survivor Study. *Blood* **111**: 5515–23.

Mudie NY, Swerdlow AJ, Higgins CD *et al.* (2006). Risk of second malignancy after non-Hodgkin's lymphoma: a British Cohort Study. *J Clin Oncol* **24**: 1568–74.

Parkin DM, Whelan SL, Ferlay J, Teppo L, Thomas DB (eds) (2002). Cancer incidence in five continents. Volume VIII. *IARC Sci Publ* **155**: 1–781.

Glossary of terms in radiation biology

α/β **ratio** The ratio of the parameters α and β in the linear-quadratic model; often used to quantify the fractionation sensitivity of tissues.

Abortive cell division The limited number of divisions of cells that are radiation damaged (so-called doomed cells). The residual proliferative capacity of these cells contributes significantly to overall cell production during radiation-induced repopulation in normal tissues.

Accelerated fractionation Intensification of radiation therapy by increasing the average rate of dose delivery, typically by increasing the dose per fraction, by delivering multiple fractions per day, or by increasing the number of treatment days per week; a schedule in which the average rate of dose delivery exceeds the equivalent of 10 Gy per week in 2-Gy fractions.

Accelerated proliferation Increase in the stem cell (clonogen) proliferation rate after radiation or cytotoxic chemotherapy relative to its pretreatment value.

Acute hypoxia Low oxygen concentrations associated with changes in blood flow through vessels (e.g. by transient closing of blood vessels). Also called *transient* or *perfusion limited* hypoxia.

Analogue A chemical compound structurally similar to another but differing by a single functional group.

Angiogenesis The process of formation of new blood vessels.

Anoxia The absence of oxygen.

Apoptosis A mode of rapid cell death after irradiation characterized by chromatin condensation, fragmentation and compartmentalization, often visualized by densely-staining nuclear globules. Sometimes postulated to be 'programmed' and therefore a potentially controllable process.

ARCON therapy The use of *A*ccelerated *R*adiotherapy with *C*arb*O*gen and *N*icotinamide.

Asymmetrical divisions Divisions of stem cells into, on average, one new stem cell and one transit or differentiating cell. These divisions are called asymmetrical, as two 'different' cells are generated.

Asymmetry loss Switch of stem cell divisions from an asymmetrical to a symmetrical pattern during radiation-induced repopulation in normal tissues.

Autophagy A process in which cellular components are self-digested through the lysosome pathway. This process can extend cell survival during starvation conditions and remove damaged organelles, but can also lead to cell death.

Autoradiography Use of a photographic emulsion to detect the distribution of a radioactive label in a tissue specimen.

BER Base excision repair – DNA repair pathway for repairing damage to DNA bases.

Biologically effective dose (BED) In fractionated radiotherapy, the total dose that would be required in very small dose fractions to produce a particular effect, as indicated by the linear-quadratic equation. Otherwise known as *extrapolated total dose* (ETD). BED values calculated for different α/β ratios are not directly comparable. For time–dose calculations, EQD_2 is preferred.

BNCT Boron neutron capture therapy.

Brachytherapy Radiotherapy using sealed radioactive sources placed next to the skin, or inserted into a body cavity or through needles into tissues.

Bragg peak Region of maximum dose deposition near the end of the tracks of protons, α-particles and heavier ions. This phenomenon enables very precise spatial definition of dose in radiotherapy using ion beams.

Cancer stem cell A cell within a tumour that possesses the capacity to self-renew and to generate the heterogeneous lineages of cancer cells that comprise the tumour. In the context of cancer therapy, this definition translates into a cell which can cause a tumour recurrence.

CDK Cyclin-dependent kinase. These proteins are responsible for movement through the cell cycle and are inactivated by various mechanisms during the DNA damage response, to cause cell-cycle checkpoints.

Cell-cycle checkpoint Cellular control mechanism to verify whether each phase of the cell cycle has been accurately completed before progression to the next phase. An important function is to continually assess DNA damage detected by *sensors*.

Cell-cycle time The time between one mitosis and the next.

Cell death In the context of radiobiology, cell death is generally equated with any process that leads to the permanent loss of clonogenic capacity.

Cell loss factor The rate of cell loss from a tumour, as a proportion of the rate at which cells are being added to the tumour by mitosis. Sometimes designated by the symbol ϕ. Cell loss factor $= 1 - T_{pot}/T_d$, where T_{pot} is potential doubling time and T_d is the cell population doubling time.

CGH Comparative genomic hybridization – a large-scale method to detect amplifications and deletions in different regions of the genome by comparison with a reference cell or tissue using microarray technology (arrayCGH).

CHART Continuous hyperfractionated accelerated radiation therapy; a schedule delivering 54 Gy in 36 fractions, with three fractions per day on 12 consecutive days (i.e. including a weekend).

Chromatin The complex of DNA and proteins comprising the chromosomes.

Chromosomal instability An effect of irradiation in which new stable and unstable chromosomal aberrations continue to appear through many cell generations.

Chronic hypoxia Persistent low oxygen concentrations such as those existing in viable tumour cells close to regions of necrosis. Also called diffusion limited hypoxia since it arises at distances greater than approximately $150 < \mu$m from blood vessels.

Clonogenic cells Cells that have the capacity to produce an expanding family of descendents (usually at least 50). Also called 'colony-forming cells' or 'clonogens'.

Clonogenic survival Defined as the fraction of cells that survive following exposure to, or treatment with an agent that causes cell death. Only cells that are able to form colonies (clonogenic cells) are considered to have survived the treatment (*see* Cell death).

Colony The family of cells derived from a single clonogenic cell.

Complementation Identification of whether a (radiosensitive) phenotype in different mutants is caused by the same gene. Studied by means of cell fusion.

Consequential late effects Late normal-tissue complications which are influenced by the extent (i.e. severity and/or duration) of the early response in the same tissue or organ.

DDR The DNA damage response. A network of biological responses to DNA damage.

Direct action Ionization or excitation of atoms within DNA leading to free radicals, as distinct from the reaction with DNA of free radicals formed in nearby water molecules.

D_0 A parameter in the multitarget equation: the radiation dose that reduces survival to e^{-1} (i.e. 0.37) of its previous value on the exponential portion of the survival curve.

Dose-modifying factor (DMF) When a chemical or other agent acts as if to change the dose of radiation, the DMF indicates the ratio of dose without to dose with the agent for the same level of effect.

Dose-rate effect Increase in isoeffective radiation dose with decreasing radiation dose rate.

Dose-reduction factor (DRF) Term which has been used with different meanings, depending on context. For example, in low dose-rate exposures, has been used to indicate the percentage or fraction reduction in dose to achieve the same effect, if the dose rate is raised (gives

DRF values <1). Alternatively, has been used in studies of radioprotection as the ratio of dose with to dose without the protecting agent for the same level of effect (gives DRF values >1).

Double trouble   A hot-spot within a treated volume receives not only a higher dose but also a higher dose per fraction, which means that the biological effectiveness of the dose is also greater.

Doubling time   Time for a cell population or tumour volume to double its size.

Early endpoint   Clinical manifestation of an early normal-tissue response to radiation therapy.

Early normal-tissue responses   Radiation-induced normal-tissue damage that is expressed in weeks to a few months after exposure (per definition within 90 days after onset of radiotherapy). α/β ratio tends to be large (>6 Gy).

ED$_{50}$ Radiation dose that is estimated to produce a specified (normal tissue) effect in 50 per cent of subjects irradiated ('effect-dose–50 per cent').

Effectors   Proteins with the specific task of effecting (carrying out) the response to damage, e.g. apoptosis, cell-cycle arrest, or DNA repair.

Elkind repair   Recovery of the 'shoulder' on a radiation dose cell-survival curve when irradiation follows several hours after a priming dose.

EQD$_2$ Equivalent total dose in 2-Gy fractions. Note that the EQD$_2$ depends on the endpoint considered.

EQD$_{2,T}$ Equivalent dose in 2-Gy fractions but adjusted for a possible difference in overall treatment time by using a reference overall time, T.

EUD   Equivalent uniform dose. Conversion of a non-uniform dose distribution within a organ to a uniform dose, which would result in the same biological effect. This is a model-dependent quantity.

Exponential growth   Growth according to an exponential equation: $V = V_0 \exp(kt)$. The volume or population doubling time is constant and equal to $(\log_e 2)/k$.

Extrapolated total dose (ETD)   Calculated isoeffective dose, at an infinitely low dose rate or fraction size (*see* Biologically effective dose).

Extrapolation number   A parameter in the multitarget equation for cell survival versus dose: the point on the surviving fraction axis to which the straight part of the curve back-extrapolates.

Field-size effect   The dependence of normal-tissue damage on the size of the irradiated area (particularly in skin); in modern literature typically referred to as the 'volume effect'.

FISH   Fluorescence *in situ* hybridization. Fluorescent dyes are attached to specific regions of the genome, thus aiding the identification of chromosomal damage.

Flow cytometry   Analysis of cell suspensions in which a dilute stream of cells is passed through a laser beam. DNA content and other properties are measured by light scattering and fluorescence following staining with dyes or labelled antibodies.

Fractionation sensitivity   The dependence of the isoeffective radiation dose on the dose per fraction. Usually quantified by the α/β ratio – a high fractionation sensitivity is characterized by a low α/β ratio (*see* α/β ratio).

Free radical   A fragment of a molecule containing an unpaired electron, therefore very reactive.

Functional imaging   Imaging methods aimed at detecting physiological changes, for example metabolism or blood flow, in a tissue (in contrast to structural or anatomical imaging). Examples are glucose metabolism (detected by ^{18}F-labelled FDG-PET) or oxygen consumption [blood oxygen level dependency (BOLD) MRI], or vascular function detected by dynamic contrast enhanced (DCE) CT (*see* Molecular imaging).

Functional subunits (FSUs)   A concept of a (minimal) functional tissue structure (such as the alveolus in the lung). Their radiation-induced inactivation results in the reduced tissue function responses that can be seen after radiotherapy. Alternatively called tissue rescuing units (TRUs).

Genomic or genetic instability   The failure to pass an accurate copy of the whole genome from a cell to its daughter cells, for example seen after irradiation.

Genomics   Study of selected genes or the entire genome of the cell (DNA level).

Gray (Gy)   1 Gy is the SI unit equivalent to 1 J of energy per 1 kg of mass. The gray is most commonly used to refer to absorbed radiation dose and has replaced the previous unit, the rad (1 Gy = 100 rad).

Gray equivalents (GyE) or cobalt gray equivalents (CGE): GyE or CGE for densely ionizing radiation is equal to the measured physical dose in gray multiplied by the RBE factor.

Growth delay   Extra time required for an irradiated versus an unirradiated tumour to reach a given size.

Growth fraction   The proportion of cells in a population that are cycling.

Hierarchical tissues   Tissues comprising a lineage of stem cells, transit cells, and postmitotic (differentiating or mature) cells.

HR   Homologous recombination – DNA repair pathway for double-strand DNA breaks by using an undamaged homologous (identical) DNA sequence, usually from the sister chromatid.

Hyperbaric oxygen (HBO)   The use of high oxygen pressures (2–3 atm) to enhance oxygen availability in radiotherapy.

Hyperfractionation   Reduction in dose per fraction below a conventional level of 1.8–2.0 Gy.

Hyperthermia   The heating of tumours above normal physiological temperatures, to treat cancer.

Hypofractionation   The use of dose fractions larger than the conventional 2 Gy per fraction.

Hypoplasia   Reduction in cell numbers in a tissue (e.g. owing to radiation-induced impairment of proliferation in early-responding tissues).

Hypoxia   Low oxygen tension; usually refers to the very low levels that are required to make cells maximally radioresistant.

Hypoxic cell cytotoxins   Any agents, typically bioreductive drugs, that preferentially kill hypoxic cells.

Hypoxic fraction   The fraction of hypoxic cells within a tumour. This term is used in different contexts. Historically, it refers to the fraction of viable radioresistant hypoxic cells in a tumour. More recently it has been used to represent the frequency of oxygen measurements below some arbitrary threshold of oxygen tension (e.g. 5 mmHg).

Image segmentation   The process of separating out mutually exclusive (i.e. non-overlapping) regions of interest in an image, for example outlining the lungs on a computed tomography (CT) scan.

IMRT   Intensity-modulated radiation therapy – irradiation technique using non-uniform radiation beam intensities for delivering radiation therapy. This allows high conformality treatment plans often with considerable sparing of critical organs at risk. Sometimes a distinction is made between IMXT (intensity-modulated X-ray therapy) and IMPT (intensity-modulated proton therapy).

Incomplete repair   Increased damage from fractionated radiotherapy when the time interval between doses is too short to allow complete recovery.

Indirect action   Damage to DNA by free radicals formed through the ionization of nearby water molecules.

Initial slope   The steepness of the initial part of the cell survival curve, usually indicated by the value of α in the linear-quadratic model.

Interphase death   The death of irradiated cells before they reach mitosis. Sometimes used as a synonym for apoptosis.

Ionization   The process of removing electrons from (or adding electrons to) atoms or molecules, thereby creating ions.

IRIF   Ionizing radiation-induced foci. Used to describe the accumulation of DNA damage-response proteins that localize to sites of DNA damage after irradiation.

Isoeffect plots   Graphs of the total dose for a given effect (e.g. ED_{50}) plotted, for example, against dose per fraction or dose rate.

Labelling index   Proportion or percentage of cells positive for a certain signal (e.g. fraction of cells within the S phase, labelled by ^{3}H-thymidine or other precursors such as bromodeoxyuridine).

Late endpoints   Clinical expression of late normal-tissue responses.

Late normal-tissue responses   Radiation-induced normal-tissue damage that in humans is expressed months to years after exposure (per definition later than 90 days after the onset of radiotherapy). The α/β ratio tends to be small (<5 Gy).

Latent time/period or latency interval   Time between (onset of) irradiation and clinical manifestation of radiation effects.

$LD_{50/30}$ Radiation dose to produce lethality in 50 per cent of a population of individuals within 30 days; similarly $LD_{50/7}$, etc.

Linear energy transfer (LET) The rate of energy loss along the track of an ionizing particle. Usually expressed in keV/μm.

Linear-quadratic (LQ) model Model in which the effect (E) is a linear-quadratic function of dose (d): $E = \alpha d + \beta d^2$. For cell survival: $S = \exp(-\alpha d - \beta d^2)$.

Local tumour control The complete regression of a tumour without later regrowth during follow-up; this requires that all cancer stem cells have been permanently inactivated.

Log-phase culture A cell culture growing exponentially.

Mean inactivation dose (D_{bar} or $\bar{D}$) An estimate of the average radiation dose to inactivate a cell. It is calculated as the area under the survival curve, plotted on linear coordinates.

Microarray An array of DNA spots of known sequence, usually on a glass slide, used to quantify amounts of genomic DNA or cDNA (made from mRNA) in cells or tissue. Can hold up to 50 000 spots, capable of monitoring expression of all known genes and their variants. Also, referred to as gene expression microarrays or 'chips'.

MiRNA MicroRNAs – small 19–22 nucleotide single-stranded non-coding RNAs expressed in cells which can regulate expression of genes by interacting with mRNAs.

Mitigation Interventions to reduce the severity or risk of radiation side-effects, applied during or shortly after exposure and before clinically manifest symptoms occur (i.e. during the latent time).

Mitotic catastrophe Improper completion of cell division because of unrepaired or misrepaired DNA damage. Mitotic catastrophe occurs frequently after irradiation and is a major cause of cell death.

Mitotic delay Delay of entry into mitosis, resulting in an accumulation of cells in G2, as a result of treatment.

Mitotic index Proportion or percentage of cells in mitosis at any given time.

MMR Mismatch repair – DNA repair pathway for repairing mismatched bases in DNA, usually occurring through misincorporation by DNA polymerases.

Molecular imaging (Medical) imaging visualizing the spatial distribution of molecular targets, signalling pathways or cellular phenotypes. This is in contrast to traditional structural or anatomical imaging. Examples could be PET or SPECT with an appropriately labelled tracer, MR spectroscopy or optical imaging (*see* Functional imaging).

Molecular-targeted drugs *See* Targeted agents.

Multitarget equation Model that assumes the presence of a number of critical targets in a cell, all of which require inactivation to kill the cell. Surviving fraction of a cell population is given by the formula $1 - [1 - \exp(D/D_0)]^n$.

Necrosis Cell death associated with loss of cellular membrane integrity. Occurs in anoxic areas of tumours and is also a cause of cell death after irradiation.

NER Nucleotide excision repair – DNA repair pathway for repairing bulky DNA lesions such as thymine dimers or cisplatin adducts.

NHEJ Non-homologous end-joining DNA repair pathway for repairing double-strand DNA breaks without using any homologous sequence as template.

Non-stochastic effect An effect where the severity increases with increasing dose, perhaps after a threshold region; also called a *deterministic effect*.

NTCP Normal-tissue complication probability – generally a term used in modelling normal-tissue radiation response.

Oxygen enhancement ratio (OER) The ratio of dose given under anoxic conditions to the dose resulting in the same effect when given under some defined level of oxygen tension. If oxygen tensions >21 per cent are used, the OER measured is usually termed the 'full OER'. An OER of about half the full OER is usually obtained when the oxygen tension is between 0.5 and 1 per cent.

PET Positron emission tomography.

Plateau-phase cultures Cell cultures grown to confluence so that proliferation is markedly reduced (also known as 'stationary phase').

Plating efficiency (PE) The proportion or percentage of *in vitro* plated cells that form colonies.

Potential doubling time (T_{pot}) The (theoretical) cell population doubling time in the assumed absence of cell loss.

Potentially lethal damage (PLD) repair Operational term to describe an increase in cell survival that may occur during an interval between treatment and assay, caused by post-irradiation modification of cellular physiology or environment (e.g. suboptimal growth conditions).

Prodromal phase Signs and symptoms in the first 48 hours following irradiation as a part of the response to partial or total-body irradiation ('radiation sickness').

Programmed cell death Cell death that occurs as the result of an active process carried out by molecules in the cell. Examples include apoptosis, autophagy, senescence, and in some cases even necrosis.

Proteomics Study of the proteins expressed in cells, including structure and function.

Quasi-threshold dose (D_q) Dose point of extrapolation of the exponential portion of a multitarget survival curve back to the level of unity. Surviving fraction: $D_q = D_0 \ln(n)$.

Radiation modifier A substance (e.g. drug or gas) which in itself does not evoke an effect on cells or tissues, but which changes the effect of radiation.

Radioresponsiveness The clinical responsiveness to a course of radiation therapy. This depends on multiple factors, one of them hypothesized to be cellular radiosensitivity.

Radiosensitizer In general, any agent that increases the sensitivity of cells to radiation. Commonly applied to electron-affinic chemicals that mimic oxygen in fixing free-radical damage, although these should more correctly be referred to as *hypoxic cell sensitizers*.

Radiosensitivity, cellular The sensitivity of cells to ionizing radiation *in vitro*. Usually indicated by the surviving fraction at 2 Gy (i.e. SF_2) or by the parameters of the linear-quadratic or multitarget equations.

Reassortment or Redistribution Return towards a more even cell-age distribution, following the selective killing of cells in certain phases of the cell cycle.

Recovery *At the cellular level* – an increase in cell survival as a function of time between dose fractions or during irradiation with low dose rates (*see* Repair). *At the tissue level* – an increase in tissue isoeffective total dose with a decrease in dose per fraction or for irradiation at low dose rates.

Regression rate The rate at which the tumour volume shrinks during or after treatment.

Relative biological effectiveness (RBE) Ratio of dose of a reference radiation quality (usually ^{60}Co γ-rays or 250 keV X-rays) and dose of a test radiation that produce equal effect.

Reoxygenation The processes by which surviving hypoxic clonogenic cells become better oxygenated during the period after irradiation of a tumour.

Repair Restoration of the integrity of damaged macromolecules (*see* Recovery).

Repair saturation A proposed explanation of the shoulder on cell survival curves on the basis of the reduced effectiveness of repair after high radiation doses.

Repopulation Describes the proliferation of surviving clonogenic tumour cells during fractionated radiotherapy. Rapid repopulation of clonogenic tumour cells during therapy is an important factor in treatment resistance. Also describes the regeneration response of early-reacting tissues to fractionated irradiation, which results in an increase in radiation tolerance with increasing overall treatment time.

Reproductive integrity Ability of cells to divide many times and thus be 'clonogenic'.

Senescence A permanent arrest of cell division associated with differentiation, aging, or cellular damage.

Sensitizer enhancement ratio (SER) The same as *dose-modifying factor* (DMF), but typically used to describe radiosensitizing agents so that SER >1.

Sensors Proteins with the specific task of sensing damage to DNA.

sievert (Sv) Dose-equivalent in radiation protection. Dose in grays multiplied by a radiation quality factor.

SF_2 Surviving fraction of cells following a dose of 2 Gy.

SNP Single nucleotide polymorphism – variations in DNA sequence between individuals at a single nucleotide that is the major source of genetic variation. Can affect protein function and expression, and thus response to damage.

Spatial cooperation The use of radiotherapy and chemotherapy to hit disease in different anatomical sites.

Spheroid Clump of cells grown together in tissue-culture suspension.

Split-dose recovery Decrease in radiation effect when a single radiation dose is split into two fractions separated by times up to a few hours (also termed *Elkind recovery*, or recovery from sublethal damage).

SSBR Single-strand break repair – DNA repair pathway for repairing a break occurring in only one of the two DNA strands.

Stathmokinetic method Study of cell proliferation using agents that block cells in mitosis.

Stem cells Cells with an unlimited proliferative capacity, capable of self-renewal and of differentiation to produce all the various types of cells in a lineage.

Stochastic (non-deterministic) effect An effect where the incidence, but not the severity, increases with increasing dose (e.g. mutagenesis, carcinogenesis, teratogenesis).

Sublethal damage (SLD) Non-lethal cellular injury that can be repaired. Interaction between SLD in a cell can result in cytolethality. This process is described in the linear-quadratic model by the quadratic β term.

Supra-additivity or synergism A biological effect caused by a combination that is greater than would be expected from the addition of the effects of the component agents.

Symmetrical division Division of each stem cell into two stem cell daughters, occurring during radiation-induced repopulation in normal tissues.

Target cell A cell whose response to radiation is responsible for the clinical manifestation of a radiation response (e.g. in a normal tissue or tumour).

Targeted agents Small molecules or antibodies that inhibit cellular pathways that are specific to cancer cells or substantially overexpressed in malignant cells compared with normal cells.

Targeted radiotherapy Treatment of cancer by means of drugs that localize in tumours and carry therapeutic amounts of radioactivity.

Target theory The idea that the shoulder on cell-survival curves results from the number of unrepaired lesions per cell.

TBI Total-body irradiation.

TCD$_{50}$ The radiation dose that gives a 50 per cent tumour control probability.

TCP Tumour control probability – generally a term used in modelling tumour radiation response.

Telangiectasia Pathologically dilated capillaries, observed in all irradiated tissues and organs in association with late radiation effects.

Theragnostics Use of molecular imaging to assist in prescribing the distribution of radiation dose in four dimensions (i.e. the three spatial dimensions plus time).

Therapeutic index or ratio Denotes the relationship between the probability for tumour cure and the likelihood for normal-tissue damage. An improved therapeutic ratio represents a more favourable ratio of efficacy to toxicity.

Time–dose relationships The dependence of isoeffective radiation dose on the overall treatment time and number of fractions (or fraction size) in radiotherapy.

Time factor Describes the change in isoeffective total dose for local tumour control or normal-tissue complications that follows a change in the overall treatment duration.

Tolerance dose The maximum radiation dose or intensity of fractionated radiotherapy that is associated with an acceptable complication probability (usually of 1–5 per cent). Actual values depend on treatment protocol, irradiated volume, concomitant therapies, etc., but also on the status of the organ/patient.

Transcriptomics Study of genes which are expressed in cells at the RNA level.

Transient hypoxia Low oxygen concentrations associated with the transient closing of blood vessels. Also called *acute* or *perfusion limited* hypoxia.

Tumour bed effect (TBE) Slower rate of tumour growth after irradiation owing to stromal injury in the irradiated 'vascular bed'.

Tumour cord Sleeve of viable tumour growing around a blood capillary.

Vascular targeted therapies Treatments designed to specifically target tumour vasculature; includes angiogenesis inhibitors and vascular disrupting agents.

Volume doubling time Time for a tumour to double in volume.

Volume effect Dependence of radiation damage on the volume of tissue irradiated and the anatomical distribution of radiation dose to an organ.

Xenografts Transplants between species; usually applied to the transplantation of human tumours into immune-deficient mice and rats.

Index

Abbreviations: RT, radiotherapy. Page numbers in **bold** refer to the glossary.